# THE CARTULARY OF
# ST LEONARD'S HOSPITAL, YORK

## RAWLINSON VOLUME

The officers of the Yorkshire Archaeological Society would like to thank
the Trustees of the Elisabeth Exwood Memorial Trust for
a grant towards this publication and
their continuing support for the Record Series

THE YORKSHIRE
ARCHAEOLOGICAL SOCIETY
*FOUNDED* 1863   *INCORPORATED* 1893

RECORD SERIES
VOLUME CLXIII
FOR THE YEARS 2014–15

THE BORTHWICK INSTITUTE FOR ARCHIVES
BORTHWICK TEXTS AND STUDIES 42

# THE CARTULARY OF
# ST LEONARD'S HOSPITAL, YORK

## RAWLINSON VOLUME

## II

EDITED BY

DAVID X CARPENTER

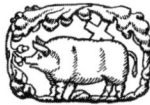

YORKSHIRE ARCHAEOLOGICAL SOCIETY
AND THE BORTHWICK INSTITUTE FOR ARCHIVES

THE BOYDELL PRESS

2015

First published 2015

A publication of the Yorkshire Archaeological Society
and The Borthwick Institute for Archives
in association with The Boydell Press
an imprint of Boydell & Brewer Ltd
PO Box 9, Woodbridge, Suffolk IP12 3DF, UK
and of Boydell & Brewer Inc.
668 Mt Hope Avenue, Rochester, NY 14620–2731, USA
website: www.boydellandbrewer.com

ISBN 978 1 903564 22 6

A CIP catalogue record for this book is available
from the British Library

The publisher has no responsibility for the continued existence or
accuracy of URLs for external or third-party internet websites referred to
in this book, and does not guarantee that any content on such websites is,
or will remain, accurate or appropriate.

This publication is printed on acid-free paper

Printed and bound in Great Britain by
TJ international ltd, padstow, Cornwall

MIX
Paper from
responsible sources
FSC
www.fsc.org    FSC® C013056

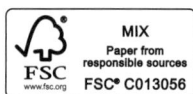

# Contents
## II

# East Riding

The East Riding division of the Rawlinson cartulary runs from f. 155 to f. 232 (R476 to R688). The heading is *Estriding'* throughout.

## *Brouneflete* [Broomfleet, par. South Cave]

## [Beningbrough, par. Newton-on-Ouse, NR]

**R476.** Confirmation [by Roger de Mowbray (and Nigel his son ?) to the hospital] of the land which William son of Warin [of Beningbrough] gave of the grantors' fee, being that between the close between *Fulsic* and the high wood, and the [river] Ouse, and a toft and common pasture just as William and his eldest son gave it, saving the grantors' service for 2 bv., should they wish it, according to the chirograph between them [1148 × 1156]

[*previous folio missing* . . .] [**f. 155ʳ**] de Ebor' deo deservientibus terram quam Willelmus filius Warini eis de nostro feudo dedit, videlicet que est inter clusa inter Fulsic et altum nemus et Usam in bosco et prato et terra arata et i. tophete infra villam et communem pasturam animalibus et pecoribus sicut ipse et filius suus primogenitus eis eam concesserunt salvo nostro servicio de ii. bovatis terre si illud habere voluerimus sicut est cirographum inter illos. Testibus istis existentibus Sampsone de Alb(ino) et Rogero de Flamvilla et Waltero de Rivera, apud Cavam.

The description of the brethren in the first words remaining indicates that they had not been named previously in the deed, and that only the salutation and a few additional words have been lost. The unnamed vill is Beningbrough (NR), rather than Broomfleet, to which place the deed was presumably assigned because of the grantor and the place-date. There can be little doubt that it was issued by Roger de Mowbray, who had interests in Beningbrough as well as North and South Cave. Each of the three witnesses attested Roger's deeds repeatedly in the mid-twelfth century (*Mowbray Charters*, passim), including an occasion in '1142 × 1157, probably 1154', when all three attested with Augustine prior of Newburgh and Robert master of the hospital (ibid., no. 240). There were several deeds relating to Beningbrough, including references to William son of Warin and his son Henry, in the Missing volume (M: Beningbrough [MS Dods. 120b, ff. 49ᵛ–51ᵛ]). Beningbrough was amongst the earliest possessions of the hospital. Meadow and land, with a *mansura* in Beningbrough was confirmed to the hospital by the pope in 1148. The bulls of January 1157 and 1173 confirm meadow and a *mansura*, with 2 bv. (C178–C180 [*EYC*, I, nos 179, 186, 197]).

The first witness, Samson d'Aubigny, was Roger de Mowbray's chaplain and his cousin. According to Greenway he first occurs before 1129; his last positively dated occurrence was in April 1153, and no deed in which he appears has a terminal date later than 1157, excepting only a notification issued by Samson d'Aubigny, canon of Newburgh, in 1161 × 1179, which shows he had retired to that monastery, 'probably . . . *c.*1154' (*Mowbray Charters*, pp. lxv–lxvi, 128–29). The date range given is that suggested by the papal confirmations, which is compatible with the men named in the deed.

Beningbrough was in the Arches fee, which by 1166 was a subtenancy of the Mowbray fee, and which was held for a time by the second witness, Roger de Flamville, by right of his wife JUETTA DE ARCHES.[1] The chronology of Juetta's life has until recently been obscure. Dugdale deduced erroneously that she married firstly Roger de Flamville, and secondly Adam de Brus I. In an unsuccessful attempt to remove the chronological difficulties which Dugdale's genealogy entailed, Farrer, followed by Clay, reversed the order of her husbands (*Baronage*, I, 448; *EYC*, II, 12; *EYF*, pp. 2, 29). Juetta was in fact married firstly to Roger de Flamville, and secondly to Adam de Brus II (Blakely, 'Bruses of Skelton', passim). The date of death of ROGER DE FLAMVILLE has also been the subject of confusion. Farrer based his assertion that Roger de Flamville died in 1168 or 1169 on the claim Alan de Flamville made in Yorkshire in the year to Michaelmas 1169 against Roger de Milliers for right in unidentified land, speculating that Roger de Milliers had married Flamville's widow Juetta (*EYC*, I, 415, 420; YAS, MS 869/7;[2] *PR*, 15 Hen. II, pp. 35–36). Clay stated that Roger de Flamville died not later than Easter 1169, but the evidence cited shows only that a different Roger de Flamville acquired his tenancy-in chief in [Whittingham in] Northumberland at about that time (*EYF*, pp. 30, 32; *PR*, 16 Hen. II, p. 49). The date of death of Roger de Flamville, Juetta's husband, cannot currently be ascertained more narrowly than 1166 × 1173. He was named in the carta of Roger de Mowbray in the former year (*Mowbray Charters*, no. 401), and was said to be of *bone memorie* in the latter (*EYC*, III, no. 1888).

Juetta must have been married to her second husband Adam de Brus II by 1176. Adam de Brus died between 1197, when an agreement was made in his court (*EYC*, II, 14; *Ctl. Gisborough*, no. 482), and Michaelmas 1198, when Peter de Brus I, his son and heir by Juetta, accounted for 500*m.* for his father's land, showing he was then of age (*PR*, 10 Ric. I, pp. 31, 43). The marriage may have come about as a result of the rebellion of 1173–74. Brus had remained loyal to Henry II, but Roger de Mowbray, to whom Juetta's marriage belonged, had joined in the rebellion, and as a result a portion at least of his lands were in the king's hands for a time. Henry II would certainly have gained from the marriage, which effectively transferred 7 k.f. from a rebel baron to a loyal one (*PR*, 20 Hen. II, p. 143; Blakely, *Brus Family*, pp. 42, 44; *Mowbray Charters*, pp. xxix–xxxi). Juetta died in 1209 × 1212. She paid 3½*m.* towards the debt of William de Mowbray in the former year (*PR*, 11 John, p. 131); the Arches interests had passed to her son Peter de Brus by the latter (*CRR*, 1210–1212, p. 345).

In view of the early date of the present deed, and the survival of Juetta de Arches until 1209 × 1212, it is open to question whether Roger de Flamville was holding the Arches fee at the time it was given.

[1]   Because *i* and *j*, and *u* and *v* are not differentiated in medieval scripts, it is often difficult to state with certainty whether *Iuetta* represents the name Juetta or Ivetta. F.M. Stenton favoured Ivetta (Stenton, *Facsimiles*, p. 45, citing Thorvald Forssner, *Continental Germanic personal names in England* (Uppsala, 1916), p. 168), but Charles Johnson, in his review of Stenton's book, said that Juetta was more likely, arguing that the name was the source of the surname Jewitt (*Antiquaries Journal*, XI (1931), 179–80; cf. *Dictionary of British surnames*, comp. P.H. Reaney (1958), s.n. Jowett). Juetta would appear to be correct for the Arches heiress, as she is called *Joeta* in a contemporary record (*CRR*, I, 349). But in other cases Ivetta may be preferred (see e.g. R589, where the form *Yveta* is used).
[2]   Farrer's unpublished notes for the Mowbray fee, intended for the *EYC* series.

# [Broomfleet resumes]

Broomfleet is not mentioned in Domesday, and Greenway suggested that it and other places south of Cave were reclaimed from the fens along the Humber (*Mowbray Charters*, p. li). Broomfleet is not mentioned in the hospital's confirmation of 1148, but in January 1157 Adrian IV confirmed 'Broomfleet, with meadow and fisheries and all appurtenances just as Roger de Mowbray confirmed by his deed' (C179 [*EYC*, I, no. 186]). Henry II's confirmation made in 1155 × 1158 includes 'by the gift of Roger de Mowbray all the land of Broomfleet' (C12 [*EYC*, I, no. 173]); the confirmation of Archbishop Theobald of 1154 'all the land of Broomfleet with all appurtenances just as Roger de Mowbray gave it, as witnessed by his deed [. . .] and whatever is between Broomfleet and that land which the Templars hold of Roger, just as Roger gave it to that house, with the consent of Alice his wife, as his deed witnesses [. . .]' (C194 [*EYC*, I, no. 185]). Mowbray's gift of Broomfleet can therefore be assigned to 1148 × 1154. In 1154 × 1157 Archbishop Roger confirmed the surrender by 'Robert of the hospital' of the tithes of the fisheries of Broomfleet to John, canon of York, to whose prebend the church of [South] Cave belonged (*EEA*, xx, no. 136). The 'grange of Broomfleet, with the pasture and other appurtenances', is included in the 1204 confirmation of Innocent III (C182 [*Letters Innoc. III*, no. 562]). In 1228 the master of the Templars in England impleaded the master of the hospital concerning a broken bridge in Broomfleet, which he said was damaging to his interests in Faxfleet. This or a similar case continued into the following year, when a fallen bridge in Wallingfen was the subject of dispute (*CloseR*, 1227–1231, pp. 94, 227). In 1280 the hospital had four ploughs, with pasture, meadow, and other appurtenances in Broomfleet, worth £60 annually (R901). The extent of 1287 gives Broomfleet's value as £50 11s. 1d., excluding fixed rents and the mill (R903). Walter of Langton, master of the hospital, and the brethren were granted free warren in their demesne lands in Broomfleet and other places in 1294 (*CalCh*, 1257–1300, p. 435). In 1431, at the inquisition following the death of Thomas Broomfleet, knight, he was stated to hold a capital messuage ('worth nothing yearly') and other property in Broomfleet of the hospital (*CalInqPM*, xxiii, no. 551). In 1535 Broomfleet was valued at £37 15s. annually (R905). In the post-Dissolution accounts of the hospital's lands the 'manor of Broomfleet with Goole' included the farm of the manor or grange of Broomfleet with demesne lands and rents there, rents in South Cave and North Cave, rents in Goole in Marshland, and the farm of a fishgarth in the Humber (*Dissolved Houses*, IV, 224). The tenure of the hospital's manor in Broomfleet after the Dissolution is discussed in *VCH Yorks ER*, IV, 45.

The inquisition which follows is the only Broomfleet deed remaining in the cartulary. In view of hospital's extensive possessions in the vill it is probable that several pages from the missing gathering contained Broomfleet deeds, including the two Mowbray deeds mentioned in Theobald's confirmation, but none have been recovered from other sources.

**R477.** Court held at Brouneflete before John Grenewode, bailiff and coroner of the liberty of St Leonard, York. Inquisition held by John Cras, Peter Watson, Robert Hobson, Peter Sandholme, John Flete, John Coll', Peter Doddyng, Thomas Robertson, Thomas Sandeholme, Robert Jakson, Peter Robertson and Robert Fote of Brouneflete, who say on their oath that William Doddyng the elder of Brouneflete died on Tuesday 30 July in the vill of Brouneflete, and the cause of death was the left wheel of his cart, and the axle of the cart, by which cart and axle William Doddyng was killed. The jurors valued the wheel

and axle at 2s. sterling. The parties individually affix their seals. 5 August 1409.
No rubric.

. . . apud Brounceflete quinto die august' anno regni regis Henrici iiii^ti decimo . . .

The value of an animate or inanimate thing which had caused death, known as the
deodand or bane, was to be handed over to the king for pious uses. The law survived
until the middle of the nineteenth century (*Hist. Engl. Law*, II, 473–74). This entry is
not separated from that preceding it by coloured capital or rubric, which gives the
impression that it is a continuation, but it is hard to see how this could be the case.

## *Buttyrwyc'* [Butterwick, par. Foxholes]

For Butterwick, where the count of Mortain had 12 ct. in 1086, which later passed to the Fossard fee, see *EYC*, II, 378 and *VCH Yorks ER*, II, 193–94. The hospital's property in Butterwick is absent from the regal and papal confirmations, the rental and extents of the later thirteenth century and the *Valor Ecclesiasticus*, but a rent in Butterwick was included in the account of 1542 (*Dissolved Houses*, IV, 226).[1] All that can be said of the gift of a toft in Butterwick [by Geoffrey of Butterwick] is that it was made some time in the mid-twelfth century. Durand of Butterwick confirmed his father's gift, and gave the hospital another toft and common pasture in *c.*1155 × *c.*1180 (R478). In 1568 the Crown granted land in Butterwick, once held by St Leonard's hospital, York, together with much other property elsewhere, to Percival Bowes and John Moyser (*CalPat*, 1566–1569, p. 281).

Farrer and Clay give brief accounts of the descendants of Durand of BUTTERWICK, who was a benefactor of Whitby and St Mary's, York, in *c.*1120 × *c.*1135 (*EYC*, II, 378–79, 381; *EYF*, pp. 11–13). Durand of Butterwick's gift to Whitby of 1 ct. in Butterwick [held of Fossard] and a mill and 2 bv. in Scampston [held of Eustace Fitz-John], was made with his heir Geoffrey, with the consent of his wife and all his sons. Walter and five other sons were named as witnesses. With Geoffrey and Walter his heirs, Durand offered the gift on the altar at Whitby Abbey (*EYC*, II, no. 1071). Geoffrey had succeeded his father by '1136 × 1150' when William Fossard [I] confirmed to Whitby 1 ct. given by Durand, in the grantor's fee in Butterwick, now held by Geoffrey son of Durand (*EYC*, II, no. 1047). By a deed dated by Farrer to *c.*1157 × 1166, but possibly somewhat later, Durand son of Geoffrey of Butterwick confirmed to Whitby the gift of 1 ct., a mill and 2 bv. made by his grandfather Durand (*EYC*, II, no. 1074).

Farrer, followed by Clay, assumed that the Durand son of William who held 2 k.f. of William Fossard in 1166 (*EYC*, II, no. 1003) was a member of this family, but this is not easy to reconcile with other evidence. William is not included in the long list of sons attesting Durand's deed to Whitby, and does not otherwise appear as a member of the Butterwick family.[2] The difficulties are removed if we accept Saltmarshe's identification of Durand son of William as the ancestor of the Hotham family, which held 2 k.f. of Fossard in 1242–43, rather than a member of the Butterwick family (FN: Hotham). This revision makes the Durand of Butterwick who attested a confirmation of William Ingram to Gisborough in 1180 × 1195[3] (*EYC*, II, no. 717) the son

[1] There is also a township called Butterwick in the parish of Barton-le-Street, in Rydale wapentake (NR), with which Butterwick, par. Foxholes, Dickering wapentake (ER), is occasionally confused or conflated (e.g. Faull and Stinson, *Domesday*, index of places). Kirkby's inquest shows that in 1284–85 Butterwick in Dickering wapentake was in the Mauley fee (previously held by Fossard), but Butterwick in Ryedale wapentake was not (*KI*, pp. 54, 118). Robert Fossard's confirmation of Durand of Butterwick's benefaction to Whitby (*EYC*, II, no. 1072) proves that Durand's interest was in Butterwick, par. Foxholes, as does Durand's grant to St Mary's Abbey which mentions a priest in the chapel of Butterwick, which belonged to the church of Foxholes (ibid., no. 1073).

[2] The William of Butterwick who gave 100 a. and other property in Butterwick to William of Howden in *c.*1180 × October 1184 was of Butterwick, co. Durham (*EEA*, XXIV, no. 72). William son of Durand, who attested a deed of William of Octon of '1170 × *c.*1185' with Richard of Seamer the rural dean of Dickering (*EYC*, II, no. 1065), is too late.

[3] Also attested by Geoffrey, abbot of Newminster (indicating 1180 × 1195), and Geoffrey, abbot of Sallay (1172 × 1198), dated by Farrer 1184 × 1188, presumably in the belief that Durand had been succeeded by his son Robert in 1189, as indicated by his suggested dates for *EYC*, II, no. 1076.

of Geoffrey of Butterwick, and grandson of the Durand of Butterwick who held in the reign of Henry I. It is unclear why no representative of the Butterwick family is named in the Fossard carta. Perhaps their holding was too small to notice, or a subtenancy, or not held by military service.

In 1202 × 1220[4] Robert son of Durand of Butterwick confirmed to the monks of St Mary's, York, the grant of the advowson of Butterwick made by his father (*EYC*, II, no. 1076). Robert of Butterwick, knight, was one of those asked to verify an essoin of *malo lecti* in Flamborough in 1218–19, and Durand of Butterwick appears as a pledge for Robert of Boythorpe in a Flotmanby case in the same period (*Yorkshire Eyre Rolls*, nos 22, 227).

**R478.** Confirmation to the hospital by Durand of Butterwick of a toft in Butterwick, which his father gave before, and gift of another toft which was Aileword's, between the first-mentioned toft and the grantor's culture, and common pasture for sixty sheep, three head of cattle, a horse, and six pigs [*c.*1155 × *c.*1180]

PRINTED: *EYC*, II, no 1075, where dated 1160 × *c.*1175.

[**f. 157ʳ**] *Carta de Buttirwica de ii. toftis et communi pastura.*
Sciant et intelligant universi filii sancte matris ecclesie quod ego[5] Durandus de Butterwyc' concedo et dono deo et pauperibus beati Petri hospitalis Ebor' unum toftum in Butterwyc, quod pater meus eis prius in elemosinam dederat, et aliud toftum quod fuit Ailewordi inter prenominatum toftum et culturam meam, et cum hiis toftis communem pasturam predicte ville lx. ovibus et iii. animalibus et uno equo et sex porcis. Hanc elemosinam dedi deo et predictis pauperibus liberam et quietam et immunem ab omni seculari et humano servicio preter orationes in cristo imperpetuum. Hoc feci pro animabus patris et matris mee et propria salute mea in vita et in morte et uxore mea et heredum meorum et omnium parentum meorum et amicorum, ut simus participes omnium orationum predictorum pauperum. Hii sunt testes, Nicholaus et Henricus sacerdotes, Thomas Ageilun, Willelmus filius Thome, Warinus, Robertus de Buttirwyc, Willelmus frater eius, Ailericus de Wivertorp' et plures alii.

The witnesses to the present deed are difficult to place, so a rather wide range of date has been assigned.

**R479.** Agreement between the master and brethren of the hospital of St Leonard, York, and William de Helmiswell of Butterwyke, whereby the master and brethren granted to William and his legitimate heirs that land in Butterwyc lying between the land of Sir Ralph son of William on the south side, the land of Thomas le Ferrour on the north side, the land of William Chaupenays on the east side, and the highway on the west side, paying the master and brethren 3*s.* yearly, half at St Martin in winter and half at Pentecost, for all service. Right of re-entry if rent in arrears. Warranty. Copies alternately sealed

---

4    The first witness was Thomas of Wilton, doubtless attesting in his capacity as steward of St Mary's. His predecessor was Walter of Boynton, who occurs as steward in 1202–03 (St Mary A2, f. 28ʳ) and his successor was Robert of Skegness, who occurs as steward in 1220 (FN).
5    MS: *ego* repeated.

by Adam de Midilton, then warden (*custos*) of the hospital, and by the cellarer of the hospital, and by William. No witnesses or dating clause [1305 × 1307]

*Magister et fratres hospitalis sancti Leonardi Ebor' de terram in B(utterwyke).*

Adam Middelton, who was of the Stockeld family, was appointed attorney to Walter Langton, bishop of Coventry and Lichfield, and master of St Leonard's, in 1305 and is recorded as warden in 1306 and in summer 1307 or later. Langton was removed from the mastership in August 1307 and doubtless Sir Adam was removed at the same time. He was referred to as 'formerly warden of the hospital' before the end of 1307 (*CalPat*, 1301–1307, p. 385; Beardwood, *Trial of Langeton*, pp. 1, 132, 244, 294).

**R480.** Release and quitclaim to the hospital by Richard son of William Sotheby of Butterwick of a toft with croft in Butterwick which he once held by the hospital's deed [later thirteenth century]

*Resignatio terre in Butterwyc ad hospitale.*
Universis cristi fidelibus presentes litteras inspecturis vel audituris Ricardus filius Willelmi Swthiby de Butterwyk' salutem in domino sempiternam. Noverit universitas vestra me reddidisse et omnino quiet'clamasse de me et de heredibus meis imperpetuum unum toftum cum crofto in Butterwyk' cum omnibus pertinenciis suis infra villam et extra magistro et fratribus hospitalis sancti Leonardi Ebor' et eorum successoribus imperpetuum, illud scilicet toftum cum crofto quod quondam de eis tenui per cartam eorundem, ita quod nec ego nec heredes mei nec aliquis nomine meo vel heredum meorum aliquod ius vel clam(eum) in dicto tofto cum crofto aliquo tempore poterimus exigere vel vendicare. In cuius rei testimonium presenti scripto sigillum meum apposui. Hiis testibus, Willelmo Barde, Iohanne de Hettona manente in Butterwyk', Willelmo Swan de eadem, Ricardo filio Ranulf', Winfray Keste Staike[6] et multis aliis.

The grantor and the witnesses are somewhat obscure, so the deed is difficult to date. William Barde of Butterwick was a juror in 1285, and a pledge for Simon of Pattishall in 1295 (*YI*, II, 36; ibid., III, 11n). William Bard and Richard Randolf were listed in Butterwick, wap. Dickering, in the lay subsidy of 1297 (*Lay Subsidy 1297*, p. 135).

---

[6] Apparently sic.

EAST RIDING

## *Brunneby'* [Burnby, near Pocklington]

There were several tenancies in Burnby in 1086. The archbishop had 4 ct., which was held of him by Geoffrey; the king had 1½ ct. as soke of his manor of Pocklington; Robert Malet had 2 ct., the jurisdiction being in Pocklington; William de Percy had 2 ct. 7 bv., with another 2½ ct. in Hayton belonging to Burnby. In 1284–85 it was said that Edmund de Aincourt held 1 k.f. there of the archbishop, and the church was endowed with 2 bv. There was also a Mowbray tenancy, apparently of 1 ct. 6 bv., held by four subtenants. In 1302–03 the archbishop held 3 ct. 4 bv., where 20 ct. made a fee, held by nine separate tenants; Mowbray had 1 ct. 1 bv., held by four separate tenants (*KI*, pp. 78, 81, 255). The archiepiscopal feodary of *c.*1225 × *c.*1245¹ has Gerard de Fancourt holding 1 k.f. in Burnby, doubtless as a subtenancy of Aincourt. Members of the Aincourt family paid homage to the archbishop for their tenancy in Burnby on several occasions in the fourteenth century (ibid., pp. 390, 404, 409, 416), and it was doubtless Burnby which Walter de Aincourt held as 2 k.f. of the archbishop in 1166 (*EYC*, I, no. 38). Apart from the three deeds which follow, no trace has been found of the hospital's tenancy in Burnby.

The FANCOURT family, which has been investigated by Foulds (*Ctl. Thurgarton*, pp. cxxviii–cxxxiv) took its name from Fallencourt, in Seine-Inf., arr. Neufchâtel, cant. Blangy (*ANF*, p. 41). Ellis de Fancourt held 1½ k.f. of Walter de Aincourt in 1166 (*Red Bk*, pp. 380–81); and the family held Burnby for 1 k.f. as undertenant of Aincourt. Ellis de Fancourt occurs as a knight in Yorkshire in 1203 (*CRR*, 1203–1205, p. 2), but was dead in 1212, when Gerard [II] de Fancourt held ½ k.f. in Scopwick (Lincs.) of Aincourt (*Bk of Fees*, p. 178). Gerard [II] de Fancourt last occurs in 1243. Foulds was unable to establish his relationship to Gerard [III] de Fancourt, who first appears in 1261.

**R481.** Gift to the hospital by Gerard de Fancourt of the toft in Burnby which Osbert son of Esa held [1203 × *c.*1220]

[f. 158ʳ] *Girardus de Fanncurt' de uno tofto in Brunnby.*

Sciant omnes presentes et futuri quod ego Girardus de Fannkurt pro salute anime mee et uxoris mee et antecessorum et heredum nostrorum dedi concessi et hac presenti carta mea confirmavi deo et pauperibus hospitalis sancti Petri Ebor' illud toftum cum pertinenciis in Brunneby quod Osbertus filius Ese tenuit, scilicet tenendum sibi imperpetuum in puram et perpetuam elemosinam libere et quiete ab omni servicio et ab omni exactione sicut elemosina ulla liberius et melius potest dari. Et ego predictus Girardus et heredes mei debemus warantizare et adquietare predictis pauperibus totum predictum toftum cum omnibus pertinenciis eius infra villam et extra imperpetuum contra omnes homines ut nos simus participes omnium bonorum que fiunt vel facienda sunt in prefata domo dei. Hiis testibus, magistro W. Dekerdun, Stephano celerario, Herberto, Anketino, Godefrido, Waltero et aliis fratribus ipsius domus, Thoma, Alexandro et aliis capellanis suis, T[homa] de Langwat,² Willelmo, Iohanne et multis aliis.

---

¹ For the date, see p. 521 n. 15.
² MS: *C. de Langwat.*

This deed was probably given after the succession of Gerard de Fancourt in 1203 × 1212 (FN). Thomas de Langwath attested *c.*1190 × *c.*1230, usually as master after *c.*1220. Godfrey attested *c.*1200 × *c.*1230; Stephen occurs as cellarer during the rectorships of Paulinus and Ralph, and in 1214 × 1217.

**R482.** Gift to the hospital by Peter son of Thomas of [Nun]burnholme of ½ a. in Burnby, being the land which lies next to the court of Benedict the clerk towards the west, between the road and the stream [1204 × 1212]

*Petrus filius Thome de dimidia acra terre in Bruneby.*
Sciant omnes presentes et futuri quod ego Petrus filius Thome de Brunnun pro salute anime [mee][3] et antecessorum et successorum meorum dedi concessi et hac carta mea confirmavi deo et pauperibus hospitalis sancti Petri Ebor' dimidiam acram terre in Brunneby, scilicet illam terram que iacet iuxta curiam Benedicti clerici versus occidentem inter stratam et rivulum, scilicet tenendam et habendam cum omnibus liberis pertinenciis suis predictis pauperibus in puram et perpetuam elemosinam libere integre honorifice et quiete ab omni servicio et exactione sicut ulla elemosina liberius potest dari, ita quod ego et heredes mei warantizabimus et adquietabimus predictis pauperibus predictam elemosinam cum liberis omnibus pertinenciis suis sine omni impedimento et retenemento contra omnes homines imperpetuum, ut nos et antecessores et successores sive heredes nostri simus participes omnium bonorum que fiunt vel facienda sunt in predicta domo dei. Hiis testibus, Roberto de Everingham, Elia de Fanec', Waltero de Ruddest', Thoma de Thanest', Willelmo capellano, Rogero capellano, Hugone capellano, Thoma de Langwat, Rogero nepote magistri Radulfi,[4] Roberto filio Elie de Fanecurt, Petro filio Cecil' Laurenc' et Adam clerico de Brunneby et multis aliis.

It seems from the witness Roger nephew of master Ralph, who appears only in this deed and the confirmation which follows, that Ralph of Nottingham was then rector of the hospital. Ellis de Fancourt was dead in 1212 (FN).

**R483.** Confirmation to the hospital by Richer of [Nun]burnholme of the gift of his brother Peter (R482) [1204 × 1212]

*Confirmatio Richeri de Brunnhum de dimidia acra terre quam pater eius dedit hospitali in Brunneby.*
Universis cristi fidelibus cartam istam visuris et audituris, Richerus de Brunnehum salutem. Noveritis me ratam et gratam habere donationem quam Petrus frater meus dedit pauperibus hospitalis sancti Petri Ebor' de dimidia acra terre in Brunnebi iuxta curiam Benedicti clerici, quare volo et firmiter concedo quod pauperes terram illam cum omnibus liberis pertinenciis suis teneant et habeant in bene et in pace in puram et perpetuam elemosinam sicut ulla elemosina liberius potest concedi. Et ut hoc eis imperpetuum ratum habeatur hanc donationem predictis pauperibus pro me et pro heredibus meis presenti sigillo meo confirmavi, ut nos et antecessores et successores nostri simus participes omnium bonorum que fiunt vel facienda sunt in predicta domo dei. Hiis testibus, Roberto de Everigham, Elia de Fanecurt, Waltero

---

3  *mee* supplied.
4  MS: *Rad'o.*

de Ruddest', Thoma de Thanest', Willelmo capellano, Rogero capellano, Hugone capellano, Thoma de Langwt, Rogero nepote magistri Rad(ulfi), Roberto filio Elie de Fanec', Petro Cecil filio Laurenc' et Ada clerico de Brunnebi et multis aliis.

The same occasion, and witnesses, as R482.

## *Buggethorp'* [Bugthorpe]

There were 4½ ct. in Bugthorpe in 1086, in the fee of Odo the crossbowman. The fee was held by the Chauncy family in the mid-twelfth century. Geoffrey of Bugthorpe held 1 k.f. of Chauncy in 1166 (*EYC*, II, no. 833). A later Geoffrey of Bugthorpe, also known as Geoffrey of Rufforth, who issued the following deed, was a substantial benefactor of the hospital in Rufforth (FN), but no further details of the hospital's property in Bugthorpe are available.

**R484.** Gift to the hospital by Geoffrey of Bugthorpe of a messuage in Bugthorpe, 210 ft in length and 86 ft in width, on the south side of the road which goes to Kirby Underdale, near the messuage which Walter Licement held [1211 × *c.*1220]

**[f. 158ᵛ]** *Galfridus de Buggethorp' de uno mesuagio in eadem.*
Omnibus presentes litteras visuris vel audituris Gaufridus de Buggethorp' salutem. Noveritis me caritatis et pietatis intuitu concessisse dedisse et presenti carta mea confirmasse deo et pauperibus hospitalis sancti Petri Ebor' unum mesuagium in villa de Buggethorp' ex aquilonali parte vie que protenditur usque ad Kirkeby in Hundolfdale prox(imum) mesuagio quod Walterus Licement tenuit, continens decies viginti pedes decem in longitudine et quater viginti pedes et sex in latitudine cum omnibus pertinenciis suis infra villam et extra in puram et perpetuam elemosinam liberam quietam et solutam ab omni seculari servicio et exactione sicut aliqua elemosina liberius et melius dari potest. Ego autem et heredes mei predictum tenementum predictis pauperibus in omnibus et contra omnes homines imperpetuum warantizabimus. In huius autem rei robur et testimonium huic scripto sigillum meum apposui. Testibus, Roberto de Colingham, Rogero, Iohanne, capellanis et fratribus, Radulfo de Fontibus, magistro Nicholao, Radulfo, capellanis secularibus, Thoma de Langwath', Roberto de Stowe, Waltero de Hundolfdale, Ricardo Fossard', Rogero de Hunton', Waltero de Beningburg', Alano coco et multis aliis.

Collingham and Stowe attest from *c.*1210; Langwath until *c.*1230, usually as master after *c.*1220. It is probable that Geoffrey of Bugthorpe succeeded his father Jordan in 1211 (FN).

## Brentingham [Brantingham]

In 1284–85 there were said to be 14 bv. in the Stuteville fee in Brantingham (*KI*, p. 88). Apart from the following deed there is no trace of the 2 bv. in Brantingham given to the hospital by Roger of Kent. The donor was presumably an ancestor of John of Kent, who held a twelfth part of 1 k.f. in Brantingham of the manor of Cottingham in 1282 (*YI*, I, 241; *EYC*, IX, 79).

**R485.** Gift to the hospital by Roger of Kent of 2 bv. which Herman held in Brant-ingham, and a toft of 1 a. in *Scortebuttes* which lies between [the tofts of] Hugh son of Geoffrey and Robert Pinel, excepting from the 2 bv. the land Daniel de Burgh holds of the donor [*c.*1200 × *c.*1220]

PRINTED: *EYC*, III, no. 1829, where dated 1190 × 1220.

**[f. 159ʳ]** *Rogerus de Kent' de ii. bovatis cum uno tofto in Brentingham.*
Sciant omnes presentes et futuri quod ego Rogerus de Kent' dedi et concessi et presenti carta mea confirmavi pro salute anime mee et patris mei et matris mee et parentum et antecessorum meorum deo et hospitali beati Petri Ebor' et pauperibus infirmatorii eiusdem loci ibidem deo servientibus, in puram et perpetuam elemosinam, liberam quietam et solutam ab omnibus geldis et consuetudinibus et exactionibus secularibus sicut ulla elemosina liberius dari potest, duas bovatas terre quas Hermannus tenuit in territorio de Brentingham et unum toftum unius acre terre in Scortebuttes quod iacet inter Hugonem filium Galfridi et Robertum Pinel, cum omnibus commoditatibus et pertinentibus ad predictam terram in pratis et pasturis et piscariis et lapifodinis et omnibus aisiamentis excepta terra Danielis de Burg' quam tenet de me que est de predictis duabus bovatis. Et ego et heredes mei warantizabimus et defendemus totam predictam terram predictis pauperibus cum omnibus pertinenciis suis imper-petuum contra omnes homines. Hiis testibus, Ada de Brentingh', Iordano, Dionisio de Elreb', Rogero clerico, Radulfus de Vals, Petro de Sanct', Ricardo clerico, Silvario, fratre Roberto capellano, Girardo, Godefrido fratribus dicti hospitalis, Willelmo, Petro, Lamberto capellanis, Thoma de Langwad', Willelmo de Notingh' cleric(is), Waltero, Ricardo, servientibus hospitalis et multis aliis.

Thomas de Langwath attests before *c.*1230, usually as master after *c.*1220; Girard had ceased to attest when Langwath became master. William of Nottingham witnessed between *c.*1195 and *c.*1220, once with Langwath as master. Godfrey indicates *c.*1200 × *c.*1230.

*Catton'*
# [Catton, near Stamford Bridge]

For High and Low Catton, south of Stamford Bridge, see *VCH Yorks ER*, III, 147–58. It is not always easy to distinguish references to Catton in Topcliffe (NR) from those to Catton near Stamford Bridge (ER), as both places were held by Percy. In 1086 there were four manors in Catton (Topcliffe), comprising altogether 6 ct., held by William de Percy. Catton (Stamford Bridge) was in 1086 the head of an extensive manor in the fee of Earl Hugh, which [with its soke] comprised 40 ct. In 1284–85 there were said to be 2 k.f. in Catton (Stamford Bridge), where 23 ct. made 1 k.f., held by Percy of the honour of Chester (*KI*, p. 86). It was a residence of the Percy family, and the birthplace in the mid-twelfth century of Maud de Percy, daughter and coheir of William de Percy II (*EYC*, XI, 5). In the division of the Percy barony made in 1175, Catton, like Stamford Bridge, was shared between the two coheirs (*EYC*, XI, no. 89). Deeds were dated at Catton by Henry Percy in 1331 and 1359 (*Ctl. Percy*, nos 517, 637). The manor house was apparently moated in 1258–59 (*VCH Yorks ER*, III, 151). The hospital had minor holdings in Catton (Topcliffe) and Catton (Stamford Bridge), but the only evidence for them is contained in the two deeds which follow.

Farrer gives many references to men described as 'OF CATTON' (Stamford Bridge), but there is no obvious line of descent, and it is probable that more than one family which had lands in the manor of Catton took that name (*EYC*, II, 251–52). Several men of the neighbourhood had the given name Ilger, and it is difficult to distinguish between them. The consistency of spelling in Osbert son of Ulger's deeds to the hospital (R680–R683), and the occurrence of his son as Ilger of Wilberfoss, son of Osbert son of Ulger, make Farrer's tentative identification of Ulger with the priest Ilger of Catton somewhat unlikely (*EYC*, II, 251, and nos 913–14; cf. FN: Wilberfoss). Ilger, parson of Catton, was amongst the witnesses to a confirmation of Jocelin de Louvain and his son Henry to Fountains made in 1175 × 1180 (*EYC*, XI, no. 71). Ilger of Catton owed 30*m.* in 1176 for a breach of an assize. In 1181, when he was described as a priest, Ilger was dead, with nothing paid against the debt (*PR*, 22 Hen. II, p. 109; ibid., 27 Hen. II, p. 37). Jeremy and Isaiah, sons of Ilger of Catton, witnessed Ilger son of Ascur's gift of land in Stamford Bridge to the hospital in *c.*1175 × 1192 (R645). Isaiah son of Ilger of Catton gave 2 bv. in Catton to Agnes daughter of Reginald of Catton in 1175 × 1184[1] (*Ctl. Percy*, no. 308).

Reginald son of Osbert of Catton, who with his sons Thomas and Ilger gave land in Catton to the hospital in *c.*1164 × *c.*1185 (R486), may have been the same man as Reinald of Catton, who attested a confirmation of Amfrey de Chauncy to Byland in or before 1181[2] (*EYC*, II, no. 838). Reginald of Catton owed ½*m.* for a disseisin in 1193 (*PR*, 5 Ric. I, p. 71). He appears to have been succeeded by his son Ilger. In 1199 Ilger of Catton impleaded the abbot of Byland for 1 bv. in Catton, which he claimed Reginald his father had pledged to the abbot for a term which had expired; and 1 bv. to which Ilger said the abbot had entry only by Pain of Catton, who had sold it to him, but Pain only held the land from year to year by lease of the same Reginald (*RCuria*, II, 37). The matter was settled by a fine made in January 1200, whereby the abbot acknowledged the 2 bv. belonged to Ilger of Catton, who then granted the land to the abbot for ½*m.*, at a rent of 2*s.* annually, retaining only a toft

---

[1] After the division of the Percy lands, and before the death of William earl of Warwick (*EYC*, XI, 4–5).
[2] Addressed to the archbishop and chapter, whilst Robert was dean.

and 2 a. which Reginald of Catton had held (*PF John*, p. 2).³ Richard de Percy was attached by Ilger of Catton and Ralph his brother in 1223, and by Ilger of Catton and Ralph of Catton in 1229 (*CRR*, 1223–1224, no. 1303; ibid., 1227–1230, no. 2120).

It can be suggested, because of their attestations to deeds issued by members of the Percy family, and the assize of mort d'ancestor mentioned below, that Raven of Catton, who witnessed deeds of Alan de Percy and his son William de Percy concerning Stamford Bridge in *c.*1130 × 1136 (R642–R643), was an ancestor, perhaps the father, of Pain of Catton. Pain of Catton attested Wilberfoss deeds in *c.*1160 × *c.*1171 and *c.*1170 × *c.*1190 (R681–R683), a Catton deed in *c.*1164 × *c.*1185 (R486), a deed of Jocelin of Louvain and Henry his son in 1175 × 1180 (*EYC*, XI, no. 71) and a deed of Adeliza de Percy in 1167 × '*c.*1175' (M: Collingham [*EYC*, XI, no. 297]). Pain of Catton, with Walter of Catton, attested a deed of Maud, countess of Warwick, in 1175 × 1194 (*EYC*, XI, no. 62). Pain of Catton and Walter his son attested a deed of Adam son of Copsi in 1175 × 1184 (ibid., no. 240). In 1185 Pain's son Walter held the ½ ct. in Catton which Pain had given to the Templars (*MA*, VI, 830b; Lees, *Templars*, p. 125). Pain was dead by Easter 1192,⁴ the latest date for a deed issued by Amfrey de Chauncy witnessed by Walter son of Pain of Catton (*EYC*, II, no. 836). The land of Walter of Catton is named in an abutment in a fine of 1208 (*PF John*, p. 152). In 1218–19, there was an assize of mort d'ancestor to determine if Hagen son of Raven [of Catton ?], was seised in demesne as of fee of 2 bv. in Stamford Bridge on the day he died, and if he died before or after the death of Henry II. Maud, daughter of Hagen and wife of Robert of Wheldrake was claiming the land against Walter of Catton, who held it. Walter claimed the assize should not be held without Maud's two surviving sisters Alice and Greta, but Robert and Maud replied that they were both dead. The outcome does not appear (*Yorkshire Eyre Rolls*, no. 220). There was another Walter of Catton, who as Walter son of Erneis of Catton, with the consent of his lord Richard de Percy, gave the nuns of Wilberfoss 1 bv. in Catton in 1239 × 1244⁵ (MS Dods. 7, f. 352ᵛ).

**R486.** Gift to the hospital by Reginald son of Osbert of Catton, and his sons Thomas and Ilger, of 6 perches in Nab in the fields of Catton, from the marsh to the [river] Derwent [*c.*1164 × *c.*1185]

PRINTED: *EYC*, II, no. 915, where dated 1180 × 1200.

**[f. 160ᵛ]** *Reginaldus filius Osberti de vi. perticatis in Catton'.*
Universis filiis sancte matris ecclesie Reginaldus filius Osberti de Catton' salutem. Notum sit vobis me et Thomam et Ilgerum filios meos concessisse et dedisse deo et pauperibus hospitalis sancti Petri Ebor' sex perticatas terre in Nab in campis de Cattona a marisco usque ad Derwente in puram et perpetuam elemosinam liberam et quietam ab omni seculari servicio preter orationes pauperum. Has autem sex perticatas terre eis contra omnes homines warentizabimus. Hiis testibus, Radulfo presbitero de Burnus, Normanno de Bocala, Thoma clerico de Bernaburg', Stephano de

³ It was doubtless in connection with these case that Ilger of Catton owed 1*m.* in 1199 for a writ of summons at Westminster, described, apparently incorrectly, as concerning *j bovata terre in Catton' versus Reginaldum de Catton'* (*PR*, 1 John, p. 53).
⁴ The approximate date of death of Amfrey de Chauncy (FN).
⁵ Before the death of Richard de Percy in or before 1244 (*CP*, X, 452), and during the tenure of Robert de Chauncy in 1239–46 (*EYC*, II, 177).

Bulemer, Thurstino clerico, Pagano de Cattona, Thoma filio Warini, Petro de Walbegata, Osberto filio Hugonis.

The witnesses Ralph priest of Burnus and Thurstan the clerk attested a Lead deed in 1166 × c.1175 (R255); Ralph chaplain of Burnus and Thurstan the clerk attested a Saxton deed in 1166 × 1177 (R392); Ralph the priest and Thurstan the clerk attested c.1175 × 1194 (R630). Pain of Catton first occurs before c.1171, and was probably dead in 1192 (FN). By a deed of c.1170 × 1181 attested by Thurstan the monk of Byland, William the clerk of Dalton, Erneis of Catton and others, the witness Thomas son of Warin confirmed to Pontefract Priory land in Catton which he had sold to Alice wife of Hugh son of Fulk, his *domina*, and she had subsequently given to the priory (*EYC*, XI, no. 227).[6] Thomas son of Warin can probably be identified with the man of that name who confirmed his brother Jordan's gift of a toft in Tadcaster to Sallay after Jordan's death (*Ctl. Sallay*, no. 622). Jordan had been granted the land by William de Percy in 1164 × 1175 (*EYC*, XI, no. 29).

## [Catton, par. Topcliffe, NR]

**R487.** Confirmation by William de Argentom to the hospital of 2 bv. in Catton with croft and toft, which David his kinsman previously gave to the hospital [c.1160 × 1185]

COPY: *b* Rawl., f. 160ᵛ. ABSTRACT: *c* Torre's catalogue, B18 N3, p. 66 [old], p. 475 [Burton], f. 239ᵛ.[7] *c* has a rough drawing of seal, round, a knight on horseback brandishing a sword, labelled SIGILLUM WILL. DE ARGENTON. PRINTED: *EYC*, II, no. 904, where dated 1170 × 1185, from *b*. NOTED: Drake, *Eboracum*, p. 335, via Torre's collections.

*Carta Willelmi de Argent' de Cattona de ii. bovatis in Catton' cum tofto et crofto.*
Sciant omnes videntes et audientes has litteras quod ego Willelmus de Argentom' concessi et dedi et hac presenti carta mea confirmavi deo et pauperibus hospitalis beati Petri Ebor' duas bovatas terre in Cattuna cum crofto et tofto et omnibus pertinenciis suis in villa et extra, in puram et perpetuam elemosinam liberam et quietam et ab omni seculari servicio et consuetudine solutam et immunem preter orationes pauperum quas videlicet bovatas David propinquus meus et heredes sui prius in liberam hospitali concesserant elemosinam. Hanc concessionem feci ego predictis pauperibus ut in vita et in morte et heredes mei simus participes omnium bonorum in illa domo. Hiis testibus, Radulfo presbitero, Nicholao presbitero, Ricardo Mala

---

6   Clay identified the 3½ ct. in Catton held by Hugh son of Fulk, which was assigned to the share of Jocelin de Louvain in the division of the barony in 1175, as lying in Catton, Topcliffe, and so assigned Thomas' grant to that place. This conclusion appears to rest on the proximity of Catton to Asenby in Topcliffe, where Hugh son of Fulk had land (*EYC*, XI, 264, 298). But an exchange made between Richard de Percy and the monks of Byland of lands in Catton, including gifts to the monks of 3 r. by Thomas son of Warin and 3 r. by Rainald of Catton; and 2 a. Richard de Percy held of the monks of Sallay, and 8 a. in his demesne tillage towards Burton (*Ctl. Percy*, no. 236) must belong to Catton (Stamford Bridge). Burton, later Hundburton, lay to the east of Stamford Bridge (*VCH Yorks ER*, III, 148, 151). Both Sallay and Byland Abbeys held land in Catton (Stamford Bridge), or Stamford Bridge itself (*Ctl. Percy*, p. 474; *KI*, p. 86; *Ctl. Byland*, p. 47; *Ctl. Sallay*, II, 138), and do not appear to have held in Catton (Topcliffe). The witnesses to the exchange, which do not appear in *Ctl. Percy* but are given by Farrer from MS Dods. 91, f. 25 (*EYC*, II, no. 911n), are associated with Catton (Stamford Bridge).
7   The deed does not appear in Burton's transcripts.

Herba, Martino fratre eius, Willelmo de Askelb', Alexandro filio Thurstan(i) de Aceles, Iohanne filio Rogerii, Ingelero de Torp', Hugone de Trecss' pistore, Alexandro de Rievill'.

Farrer originally assigned this deed to Catton (Stamford Bridge), but later revised his opinion to Catton (Topcliffe).[8] Clay regarded it as certain that the Argentom interest was in the latter place. The evidence he cites is not entirely satisfactory but there is other circumstantial evidence (*EYC*, XI, 223 and n).[9] Farrer's account of the Argentom family shows that William de Argentom, the grantor of this deed, was holding 1 k.f. of Percy in 1166, and was living in 1179. He was dead in 1185, leaving two daughters (*EYC*, II, 244–46). For another gift to the hospital by William de Argentom, see M: Upleatham [MS Dods. 120b, f. 103$^r$]. David of Catton, possibly the kinsman of William de Argentom named in the present deed, or a relation, attested deeds pertaining to Catton (Topcliffe) and Dalton (Topcliffe) in the late twelfth or early thirteenth century (*EYC*, XI, 298, 303).

# [Cayton, NR]

The following deed belongs to Cayton, about 3 m. south of Scarborough. Cayton was divided between several fees: the hospital's land was probably part of the Percy holdings in the vill. There is no evidence for a Cayton section in the Missing volume, and no further notice of the hospital's Cayton property until 1542, when a rent there was included in the account of lands formerly belonging to the hospital (*Dissolved Houses*, IV, 226).

**R488.** Gift to the hospital by William son of Angot of a toft in Cayton, with common pasture [*c.*1160 × *c.*1190]

*Willelmus filius Angot de uno tofto in Catton'*[10] *cum communi pastura eiusdem ville.*
Notum sit omnibus sancte matris ecclesie filiis tam presentibus quam futuris quod ego Willelmus filius Angot et heredes mei concessimus et dedimus et hac presenti carta nostra confirmavimus deo et pauperibus hospitalis beati Petri Ebor' toftam unam in Cattuna[10] in puram et perpetuam elemosinam liberam et quietam et immunem et solutam ab omnibus geldis et consuetudinibus et exactionibus et ab omni seculari servicio preter orationes pauperum. Concedimus vero eis communem pasturam eiusdem ville cum omnibus aisiamentis in bosco et plano in aquis et in viis in turbariis et in omnibus libertatibus ad eandem villam pertinentibus, et contra omnes homines warantizabimus, ut simus participes omnium bonorum et orationum que fiunt in illa

---

[8]  It was presumably Farrer's initial identification which led Allison to claim that the hospital had 2 bv. in Catton (Stamford Bridge) (*VCH Yorks ER*, III, 152, citing erroneously *Ctl. Percy*, p. 463).

[9]  Clay cites a plea by which Emma, widow of Geoffrey of Otterington, sought against Gregory de Argentom 3 bv. in Catton (*Yorkshire Eyre Rolls*, no. 104). South Otterington is within 7 m. of Catton (Topcliffe). Gregory de Argentom attested deeds concerning Dishforth and Catton (Topcliffe) (*Ctl. Fountains*, pp. 168, 230). Gregory *de Argentel*, who is shown as holding 6 bv. in Catton (Topcliffe) in a Percy feodary of the mid-thirteenth century was possibly a relation (*Ctl. Percy*, p. 472; cf. *KI*, p. 95). Roger de Argentom held in Sandhutton, near Thirsk, in the early thirteenth century (*Ctl. Fountains*, pp. 624–27; the nuns of Arden (near Thirsk) held in the same place). Against the weight of this evidence stands only the attestation of Robert de Argent' to Osbert son of Ulger's gift to the hospital of property in Wilberfoss (R683).

[10]  sic, probably for *Caitona*.

sancta domo dei tam in vita quam in morte. Hiis testibus, Adam de Gartuna, Petro de Hugat, Odone sacerdote, Gollano filio eius.

Richard son of Angot [OF OSGODBY] occurs as a juror in a deed of 1157–58 (*EYC*, I, no. 402). He held 1 k.f. of Percy jointly with Durand of Cayton, Geoffrey son of Robert, Theobald son of Pain, and Gilbert de Arches in 1166. The fee included lands in Deepdale, Killerby, and Osgodby, par. Cayton, as well as Cayton (*EYC*, XI, 233). The present deed was given by Richard's brother William. By a deed of the 'late twelfth century' Richard son of Angot confirmed his brother William's gift to Whitby, which Beatrix, William's widow, offered when William's body was brought for burial at Whitby (*EYC*, XI, no. 185). Richard son of Angot of Osgodby notified the archbishop of his gift to Byland of ½ bv. land in Osgodby by a deed witnessed by Odo the priest, which Clay dated to *c.*1160 × 1181 (*EYC*, XI, no. 195).

## *Crauncewyk* [Cranswick, in Hutton Cranswick]

For Hutton Cranswick, in the Fossard fee, see *EYC*, II, 403. The identity of the donor of the hospital's messuage in Cranswick is not known. In 1504 × 1515[1] the hospital complained that William Whiting entered into the hospital's lands in Hutton Cranswick, comprising a capital messuage and 200 a. land, meadow and pasture, which the hospital had held 'time out of mind', pretending it to be his inheritance (Purvis, *Monastic Proceedings*, pp. 166–67). In view of its substantial size, it is curious that no further reference to the hospital's tenement in Cranswick has been found.

**R489.** Chirograph by which Thomas, rector, and the brethren of the hospital conveyed to Thomas of Applegarth a messuage in Cranswick, between the highway and the land of St John [of Beverley], for 2s. 6d. annually and a portion of chattels as an obituary payment [1263 × 1276]

[**f. 161ʳ**] *Copia carte de quodam mesuagio dimisso ad firmam in Crauncewik'.*
Omnibus cristi fidelibus presens scriptum visuris vel audituris Thomas rector et fratres hospitalis sancti Leonardi Ebor' salutem in domino. Noveritis nos concessisse Thome de Apelgarthe unum mesuagium in Crauncewyk', illud scilicet quod iacet inter stratam regiam ex una parte et terram sancti Iohannis ex altera, habendum et tenendum dicto Thome et heredibus suis de nobis et successoribus nostris libere quiete integre bene et in pace cum pertinenciis et aisiamentis suis infra villam de Crauncewyk' et extra, reddendo inde annuatim nobis et successoribus nostris duos solidos et vi. denarios argenti, medietatem ad festum sancti Martini in yeme et aliam medietatem ad Pent' pro omni servicio ad nos pertinente. Et nos et successores nostri dicto Thome et heredibus suis dictum mesuagium cum pertinenciis suis contra omnes gentes warantizabimus quamdiu carta donatoris nostri nobis warantizare poterit. Idem autem Thomas et heredes sui vel quicumque dictam terram tenuerint portionem catallorum suorum ipsos in obitu suo contingentem pauperibus domus nostre fideliter relinquent. Et hoc tactis sacrosanctis iuravit idem Thomas pro se et suis et affidavit. In cuius rei testimonium duo scripta unius tenoris ad modum cirograffi sunt confecta quorum unum residet penes nos sigillo dicti Thome signatum et aliud penes dictum Thomam communi sigillo nostro munitum. Hiis testibus, Iohanne filio Iohannis de Crauncewyk', Iohanne Cokes de eadem, Ada Fraunkeleyn' de eadem, Thoma Vicar' de eadem, Iohanne Hopel de Hoton', Hugone Lapostoyle de Baynton', Willelmo de Wynetop de eadem et aliis.

The limits of date are set by the rectorship of Thomas of Geddington. A bovate in Cranswick was said to have been given to St John of Beverley during the provostship of Alan, i.e. in 1202 × 1212 (*Beverley Act Bk*, II, pp. xix, 336).

---

[1]   During the mastership of John Constable, and whilst William [Warham] was chancellor and archbishop of Canterbury.

# *Driffeld* [Driffield]

For Driffield, held by the king in 1086 and usually by royal grantees thereafter, see the *VCH* draft on the manor.[1] There is no trace of the hospital's holding in Driffield in the papal confirmations, the extents of the later thirteenth century, the *Valor Ecclesiasticus*, or the account of 1542. The hospital acquired two tofts and 5 a. in Driffield by the gift of Adam of Driffield, in *c.*1209 × 1218 (R490). This property, with another toft, was subsequently in the hands of Adam's son Hamo, who issued a bond for payment of an annual rent of 3*s.* to the hospital in *c.*1235 × *c.*1260 (R491). Stephen son of Hamo of Driffield conveyed part of the property to William Merchant of Driffield in or before 1271, when he issued a quitclaim to the hospital in the 3*s.* rent (R492). The hospital confirmed the land to William in 1276 × 1280 (R493).

**R490.** Gift to the hospital by Adam of Driffield of two tofts in Driffield, one held by Fulk, the other adjacent on the south side, and 5 a. which belong to 12 bv. which the donor holds in Driffield [*c.*1209 × 1218, probably 1209 × 1213]

[**f. 161ᵛ**] *Ada de Driffelde de ii. toftis et v. acris terre in Driffeld'.*
Omnibus presentes litteras visuris vel audituris Adam de Driffeld' salutem. Noveritis me dedisse concessisse et presenti carta mea confirmasse deo et pauperibus hospitalis beati Petri Ebor' pro salute anime mee et animarum antecessorum et successorum meorum duo tofta in villa de Driffelde quorum unum tenuit Fulco et aliud illi proximo ex parte aquilonali et v. acras terre cum omnibus pertinenciis suis infra villam et extra, que quidem acre pertinent ad duodecim bovatas quas teneo in territorio de Driffeld', tenenda et habenda imperpetuum in puram et perpetuam elemosinam liberam solutam et quietam ab omnibus serviciis et exactionibus sicut aliqua elemosina liberius et melius dari potest. Ego vero predictus Adam et heredes mei totum predictum tenementum cum omnibus suis pertinenciis warantizabimus aquietabimus [et][2] defendemus contra omnes homines predictis pauperibus imperpetuum. Testibus, Hamone thesaurario Ebor', Henrico de Redeman, Hugone de Magneby, magistro Waltero de Driffeld', Philippo de Capella, Galfrido de Leseth', Ingeram filio suo, Stephano de Langetoft', fratre Roberto capellano, fratre Bernardo capellano, Thoma celler(ario), Girardo, Godefrido, Waltero, Ricardo, Willelmo Ruffo fratribus hospitalis, magistro Willelmo de Gerondon', Petro, Lamberto capellanis hospitalis et multis aliis.

Hamo was treasurer of York until 1217 or 1218. Thomas the cellarer, Godfrey, William of Garendon, Peter and Lambert all attested only after *c.*1200; Bernard attested after *c.*1210. The presence of Henry de Redman suggests the period 1209–1213, when he was undersheriff of Yorkshire.

**R491.** Bond to the hospital by Hamo son of Adam of Driffield to pay 3*s.* yearly for three tofts and 5 a. in Driffield [*c.*1235 × *c.*1260]

*Hamo filius Ade de Driffeld' de solutione iii.s. magistro et fratribus ut infra.*
Omnibus cristi fidelibus ad quos presens scriptum pervenerit Hamo filius Ade de Driffelde salutem. Noverit universitas vestra me et heredes meos teneri magistro et

---

[1]  Formerly available at the 'England's past for everyone' website.
[2]  *et* supplied.

fratribus hospitalis sancti Petri Ebor' ad solvendum eisdem annuatim pro tribus toftis et quinque acris terre cum pertinenciis suis in Driffeld' tres solidos, medietatem ad Pent' et medietatem ad festum sancti Martini in yeme. Ad omnia prescripta fideliter et sine dolo facienda pro me et heredibus meis tactis sacrosanctis iuravi et affidavi. In cuius rei testimonium huic scripto sigillum meum apposui. Hiis testibus, magistro I[ohanne] de Esingwalde, Petro de Thornhou', Michaele capellano Raulin', Simone de Alta Ripa et aliis

Master John of Easingwold occurs in 1238 and after 1247 (FN).

**R492.** Gift and quitclaim to the hospital by Stephen son of Hamo of Driffield of all right which he had in 3*s.* rent from the messuage in Driffield nearest his own messuage, which William Merchant formerly held of him. 1 May 1271.

*Stephanus filius Hamonis de Driffeld' de redditu trium solidorum annui redditus.*
Sciant presentes et futuri quod ego Stephanus filius Hamonis de Driffeud' dedi et concessi et omnino quiet'clamavi pro me et heredibus meis imperpetuum magistro et fratribus hospitalis sancti Leonardi Ebor' et eorum successoribus in puram et perpetuam elemosinam totum ius et clam(cum) quod habui vel aliquando habere potui in reddidu trium solidorum annui redditus de illo mesuagio quod iacet propinquius mesuagio meo quod Willelmus le Marshaunt aliquando de me tenuit in villa de Driffeud' cum omnibus aliis serviciis et pertinenciis ad me vel ad predecessores meos aliquo modo pertinentibus, ita libere et quiete quod nec ego nec heredes mei vel assignati mei de predicto mesuagio vel predicto annuo redditu nec aliquis nomine nostro aliquod ius vel clam(eum) in predictis mesuagio et redditu exigere vel vendicare poterimus imperpetuum. Et ego predictus Stephanus et heredes mei vel assignati mei predictum annuum redditum de predicto mesuagio predict(o) magistro et fratribus et eorum successoribus in puram et perpetuam elemosinam warentizabimus acquietabimus ac imperpetuum defendemus. In huius rei robur et testimonium presenti scripto sigillum meum apposui. Hiis testibus, Waltero le Ioeuene, Iohanne tunc temporis eiusdem ville ballivo, Roberto de Lehull', Roberto Spileman, Simone preposito, Willelmo le Tollare et aliis. Dat' apud Driffeud' die apostolorum Philippi et Iacobi anno domini millesimo CC^{mo} lxx° primo.

**R493.** Grant at fee-farm by Roger, rector, and the brethren of the hospital, to William Merchant of Driffield of a toft in Driffield which lies next to the toft of Stephen son of Hamo on the north side, paying 3*s.* annually, and ½*m.* for a portion of chattels as an obituary payment [1276 × 1280]

*De quodam tofto in Driffelde.*
Omnibus cristi fidelibus ad quos presens scriptum pervenerit, Rogerus rector hospitalis beati Petri Ebor' et fratres eiusdem loci salutem. Noveritis nos dedisse concessisse et hac presenti carta nostra confirmasse Willelmo le Marchaund' de Driffelde et heredibus suis vel eius assignatis quoddam toftum in Driffelde quod iacet iuxta toftum Stephani filio Hamonis ex parte boriali, tenendum et habendum eidem Willelmo et heredibus suis vel cui assignare voluerit exceptis iudeis et viris religiosis aliis a nobis cum omnibus pertinenciis libertatibus et aisiamentis suis libere quiete integre et pacifice, reddendo inde annuatim nobis et successoribus nostris tres solidos, videlicet medietatem ad Pent' et aliam medietatem ad festum sancti Martini in yeme pro omni servicio seculari et demanda. Predictus vero Willelmus et heredes sui vel eius assignati vel quicumque dictum toftum tenuerint seu manserint in eodem pro portione

catallorum ipsos in obitu suo contingente dimidiam marcam pauperibus domus nostre nomine testamenti fideliter persolvent. Nos vero et successores nostri dictum toftum cum pertinenciis suis prefato W(illelmus) et heredibus vel assignatis suis ut supradictum est contra omnes homines warantizabimus aquietabimus et defendemus quamdiu carta donatoris nostri quam inde habemus nobis illud toftum poterit warantizare defendere et aquietare. In cuius rei testimonium sigillum commune domus nostre et sigillum dicti Willelmi huic scripto cirographato apponi fecimus alternatim. Hiis testibus, Roberto Spileman', Willelmo Toller', magistro Roberto de Driffeld', Willelmo le Iouen', Stephano filio Hamonis, Nicholao de Crosseby de Kyllom' et aliis.

The date range is the period for Roger as master.

## *Ellerton'* [Ellerton on Derwent]

In 1284–85 there was said to be 1 ct. in Ellerton, held by Roger de Lascelles and Thomas of Greystoke of William, baron Greystoke, who held of Gant in chief (*KI*, p. 89). Ellerton does not occur in the hospital's papal confirmations, the extents of the later thirteenth century, nor in the *Valor Ecclesiasticus*, but Ellerton is mentioned twice in the account of 1542 (*Dissolved Houses*, IV, 224–25). These entries, however, appear to belong to Ellerton-on-Swale (NR), where the hospital also had an interest (C346, C347 [*EYC*, v, nos 129–30]). It is unclear which of the two places was referred to in 1558, when a free rent of 2*s*. from the lands of Henry Hall in Ellerton, and a messuage there in the tenure of Richard Nateby, late in the possession of St Leonard's hospital, York, were granted with other property to Thomas Reve of London, gentleman, and Christopher Bullit, yeoman (*CalPat*, 1557–1558, p. 41).

**R494.** Gift to the hospital by William son of Botilda of a toft with ½ a. land adjacent in Ellerton on Derwent, and common pasture, and a place in the [river] Derwent to make a fish garth [*c.*1160 × *c.*1180]

COPIES: *b* Rawl., f. 162ᵛ, *ι* (in two parts) Burton transcripts 2, ff. 143ᵛ, 170ʳ, pp. 251, 304, B25 N18, drawing of seal, round, 'on yellow wax an eagle about to flie, looking backwards'. PRINTED: *EYC*, II, no. 1173, from *b*, where dated 1180 × 1200. NOTED: Drake, *Eboracum*, p. 335, via Torre's collections.

**[f. 162ᵛ]** *Willelmus filius Botilde de i. tofto et dimidia acra et communi pastura in Ellerton' super Derwent et loco in eadem aqua ad piscariam faciendam.*
Notum sit omnibus videntibus et audientibus litteras has quod ego Willelmus filius Botilde et heredes mei concessimus et dedimus et hac carta nostra confirmavimus deo et pauperibus hospitalis beati Petri Ebor' toftum unum et dimidiam acram terre continuam predicto tofto in Elretuna super Derwentam et communem pasturam cum omnibus aisiamentis que ad eandem villam pertinent et unum locum¹ in Derwenta ad sepem piscatoriam faciendam, in puram et perpetuam elemosinam liberam et quietam ab omnibus geldis et consuetudinibus humanis preter orationes pauperum. Hanc autem elemosinam dedimus eis et contra omnes homines warentizabimus² ut simus participes omnium beneficiorum que fiunt in illa sancta domo dei tam in vita quam in morte. Hiis testibus, Radulfo presbitero de Burn',³ Iohanne presbitero, Thoma filio Ra(m)kil, Hugone filio Ranulfi presbiteri, Roberto genero suo,⁴ Willelmo cognato Adam de Rid', Tedbaldo Lorimer, Iohanne de Leitop et multis aliis.

Ralph chaplain of *Burnus* attested with John, chaplain, and Thurstan, clerk, in 1166 × 1177 (R392). Hugh son of Ranulf *sacerdotis* attested two deeds of *c.*1165 × 1181 (R447, R454).

---

¹  *c: locum unum.*
²  *b: guarantizabimus.*
³  *c: Burnam.*
⁴  *c: generoso eius.*

## *Frisemarise* [lost, near Patrington]

Frismarsh, which lay in or near Patrington in Holderness, a member of the arch-bishop's fee, was abandoned because of the frequent inundations of the Humber (*PN YorksER*, pp. 24–25). Apart from the following deeds, there is no notice of the place in the hospital's muniments.

**R495.** Gift to the hospital by Osbert of Frismarsh of a close of 3 a. in Frismarsh, being the close called Kirkcroft which Richard son of Saxe held of the donor, next to the land of Hugh de Fauconberg towards the west [*c.*1187 × 1207, possibly *c.*1195 × 1207]

PRINTED: *EYC*, I, no. 51, where dated 1187 × 1207.

**[f. 163r]** *Osbertus de Frisemaris de i. clos de tribus acris terre in F(risemaris).*
Notum sit omnibus visuris vel audituris litteras istas quod ego Osbertus de Frisemaris dedi et concessi et hac presenti carta mea confirmavi deo et hospitali sancti Leonardi Ebor' unum clos de tribus acris terre in Frisemaris, scilicet le clos quod Ricardus filius Saxe tenuit de me quod vocatur Kirkecroft' prox(imum) terre Hugonis de Facunberg' versus occidentem in puram et perpetuam elemosinam libere et quiete ab omnibus secularibus serviciis et exactionibus. Et ego Osbertus et heredes mei warantizabimus predictum clos prenominato hospitali contra omnes homines imper-petuum. Hiis testibus, Willelmo de Badlesmar', Waltero de Bouington, Thoma de Wilton', Laurencio clerico, Hugone filio Lewini, Simone de Muhaut et Roberto fratre eius, Hugone clerico, Iohanne Fulforde', Hugone clerico, Radulfo de Cawde et multis.

Farrer showed that Osbert of Frismarsh succeeded his father Walter in 1187 or before, and was apparently dead in 1207 (*EYC*, III, 112; *PR*, 33 Hen. II, p. 98). The first witness, who took his name from Badlesmere in Kent, attested the following deed as constable of York. His connection with Yorkshire, and whether he can be identified with the William de Badlesmere who was in rebellion against King John are matters of conjecture. For the Badlesmere family, see *Baronage*, II, 57; *CP*, I, 371–74. The overlap of witnesses suggests the same occasion as the following deed.

**R496.** Gift to the hospital by Osbert son of Walter of Frismarsh of land in Frismarsh called Kirkcroft [*c.*1195 × 1207]

PRINTED: *EYC*, I, no. 50, where dated 1187 × 1207.

*Osbertus filius Walteri de Frismareis de quadam terra.*
Omnibus has litteras visuris vel audituris Osbertus filius Walteri de Frismareis salutem. Noveritis me dedisse et concessisse et hac presenti carta mea confirmasse deo et hospitali sancti Petri Ebor' quandam terram in Frismareis que vocatur Kirkecroft' in puram et perpetuam elemosinam liberam et quietam ab omni servicio et exactione seculari cum omnibus pertinenciis et libertatibus in pratis, in pascuis, in aquis, in viis, in semitis et omnibus aliis aisiamentis. Hanc autem donationem ego et heredes mei warantizabimus predicto hospitali imperpetuum ut predecessores mei et ego et succes-sores mei participes simus orationum et elemosinarum que fiunt et fient in predicto hospitali. Hiis testibus, Waltero de Bouinton', Hugone de Alna clerico, Willelmo de

Badlesmar' constabulario Ebor', Thoma de Wilton', Suano, Astino, Roberto milite, fratribus, Petro capellano et multis aliis.

Peter the chaplain attested within *c.*1195 and *c.*1220, Robert *miles* within a similar period.

## *Gauneton'* [Ganton]

For Ganton, a member of the Gant fee, see *EYC*, IX, 175 n. 7. Apart from the following deeds, and a rent in Ganton included in the account of 1542 (*Dissolved Houses*, IV, 226), no evidence for the hospital's holdings there has been found. Richard of GANTON held 1 k.f. of a Percy undertenancy of Gant in 1175, which was located in Ganton and Staxton, par. Willerby. Richard was succeeded by his son Henry, who confirmed the gift his father had made in Staxton to Bridlington Priory. Maud of Ganton, the hospital's benefactor, was Henry's daughter and heir. She was married to Richard of BOSSALL [I], who held ¾ k.f. of Stuteville and was living in 1206. Maud was a widow in 1232, when she gave land in Fordon (near Staxton) to Whitby Abbey. In November 1234 Maud of Ganton, in widowhood, gave two tofts in Staxton to Maud, daughter of Richard of Bossall and Mabel his wife, 'which Mabel was a daughter of Robert de Stuteville'. The gift was confirmed by Richard of Bossall [II, son and] heir of the donor.[1] Richard of Bossall II was dead in February 1238 (*EYC*, IX, 174–77; ibid., XI, 355–56). The following deeds show that Maud of Ganton married William Francigena as her second husband.

**R497.** Gift to the hospital by Maud of Ganton, in widowhood, and Richard of Bossall [II] her son and heir, of a toft and croft in Ganton, being that which Robert the smith formerly held with common of pasture [*c.*1214 × *c.*1230]

NOTED: *Ctl. Gisborough*, II, 302n, via MS Dods. 120b, f. 32ᵛ.

**[f. 164ʳ]** *Carta Matilde de Gauneton' et Ricardi heredis sui de i. tofto.*
Omnibus presentes litteras visuris vel audituris Matilda de Gauneton' in propria potestate et viduitate constituta et Ricardus de Bozhale filius et heres eiusdem salutem in domino. Noverit universitas vestra nos caritatis et pietatis intuitu concessisse dedisse et presenti carta nostra confirmasse deo et pauperibus hospitalis sancti Petri Ebor' unum toftum cum crofto in villa de Gauneton', scilicet illud quod Robertus faber quondam tenuit cum communi pastura et omnibus libertatibus ad dictum tenementum pertinentibus infra villam et extra, tenendum scilicet et habendum predictis pauperibus in puram et perpetuam elemosinam liberam quietam et solutam ab omni servicio et exactione seculari sicut aliqua elemosina liberius et melius dari potest, ita quod nos et heredes nostri predictum tenementum cum prenominatis iamdictis pauperibus in omnibus et contra omnes homines warentizabimus acquietabimus et defendemus imperpetuum. Hoc autem pro nobis et heredibus nostris tactis sacrosanctis iuravimus et affidavimus. In huius autem rei robur et testimonium huic scripto sigilla nostra apposuimus. Testibus, Willelmo, Bernardo, Roberto, Rogero, Iohanne fratribus et capellanis, Anketino, Stephano, Waltero, Iohanne, Godefrido, Willelmo, Henrico et aliis fratribus, Radulfo de Fontibus, Fulcone, Radulfo capellanis secularibus, magistro Thoma de Langwath', Roberto de Stowe, Ricardo Fossard', Roberto de Bowes, Radulfo de Arundel et multis aliis.

The date is determined by the attestation of Thomas de Langwath as master.

---

[1]   Clay assumed that Richard, husband of Mabel, was Richard of Bossall II, but this is not explicitly stated, and Mabel may perhaps have been first wife to Richard of Bossall I (*EYC*, IX, no. 97).

**R498.** Confirmation to the hospital by William Francigena of Ganton, of the gift made by Maud his wife, in her full power, being the toft which Robert the smith formerly held in Ganton [*c.*1214 × *c.*1240]

NOTED: *Ctl. Gisborough*, II, 302n, via MS Dods. 120b, f. 32ᵛ.

*Willelmus le Franceys de i. tofto in Galmeton.*
Omnibus has litteras visuris vel audituris Willelmus Francigena de Galmeton' salutem. Noverit universitas vestra me ratam et gratam habere donationem quam Matilda uxor mea in propria potestate sua constituta fecit deo et pauperibus hospitalis sancti Petri Ebor' in Galmeton', scilicet illud toftum quod Robertus faber aliquando tenuit cum communi pastura et omnibus pertinenciis suis infra villam et extra in puram et perpetuam elemosinam. Ego autem tactis sacrosanctis iuravi et affidavi quod numquam eis inde movebo questionem vel calumpniam. In huius autem rei robur et testimonium huic scripto sigillum meum apposui. Hiis testibus, Ricardo Passeboys, Reginaldo fratre suo, Henrico de Wilardeby, Henrico de Bru(m)pton', Ricardo Bret, Henrico de Binington' et multis aliis.

Many of the witnesses attested deeds of a similar period belonging to Willerby, which is 2 m. east of Ganton (*Ctl. Bridlington*, pp. 100–39). Richard Bret, Henry of Binnington, and Richard Passboys of Boynton were amongst the witnesses to a Willerby deed of 1236 (ibid., pp. 106–7).

# *Grymmeston'* [North Grimston]

In 1302–3 there were said to be 3 ct. in [North] Grimston in the Brus fee, and 1½ ct. in the Mowbray fee (*KI*, p. 275). Apart from the following two deeds, and another misplaced in the Grimston 'in Elmet' (WR) section of the Rawlinson volume (R710), the hospital's interests in North Grimston are undocumented until 1542, when a rent in [North] Grimston was included in the Crown's account of the revenues of the hospital (*Dissolved Houses*, IV, 226).

In 1194 × 1198[1] Walter of GRIMSTON[2] witnessed a deed of William [of Firby], son of Ralph son of Ralph, concerning land in Firby (*Frithebi*) (*EYC*, I, no. 636). It was apparently his son, Richard son of Walter of Grimston, who gave the hospital a toft with croft and messuage in Grimston in *c.*1209 × *c.*1231 (R499), and 1 bv. and a toft in 1214 × 1245 (R710). Richard son of Walter of Grimston made gifts in Grimston and Rillington nearby to the priory of Malton (Malton cartulary, ff. 173/169ᵛ, 179/175ʳ). Before 1241 he gave 2 bv. in Grimston to the Vicars Choral in York (*CVC*, II, nos 27, 28). Richard's heir was apparently Walter son of Robert of Grimston, who sued Thomas of Watton in the king's court for 1 bv. and a toft in Grimston in 1241 × 1251. This was presumably the property Richard had given to the hospital in 1214 × 1245. Thomas called the hospital to warrant, and Walter issued a quitclaim after payment of 2*m.* (R500). It was presumably the same Walter who as Walter 'Grimet' son of Robert of Grimston quitclaimed 2 bv. in Grimston to John de Brunne for 5*m*. This was the land which had been given by Richard son of Walter to the Vicars Choral, who sold it to Robert (of Grimston) son of Thomas of Watton, reserving a 2*s*. rent. Robert then sold it to John son of Stephen de Westbrunne, who can doubtless be identified with John de Brunne, both forms of the name indicating Kirkburn, some 13 m. south east of North Grimston (*CVC*, II, nos 27, 29–31; *PN YorksER*, p. 166).[3]

An undated quitclaim made by Walter son of Robert son of Walter of Grimston to Malton Priory indicates that the younger Walter was a nephew of Richard son of Walter (Malton cartulary, f. 240/236ᵛ). Joan widow of Walter Grimston of Grimston quitclaimed to Malton Priory all right in 2 bv. in Sutton *iuxta Norton* which William de Redburn, her father, had given to Walter in frank-marriage, and which Walter had given to the priory (ibid., f. 61/59ʳ). Joan former wife of Walter Grimston of Grimston occurs in 1257 (ibid., f. 179/175ʳ).

**R499.** Gift to the hospital by Richard of Grimston of a toft with croft and messuage in Grimston, which toft lies between the beck and Basil's toft [*c.*1209 × *c.*1231]

**[f. 164ᵛ]** *Ricardus de Grimeston' de uno tofto cum crofto et mesuagio in eadem villa.*
Omnibus cristi fidelibus Ricardus de Grymmeston' salutem. Sciatis me dedisse concessisse et hac presenti mea carta confirmasse deo et pauperibus hospitalis sancti Petri Ebor' unum toftum cum crofto et mesuagio cum omnibus pertinenciis suis infra villam et extra in villa de Grymestona pro salute anime mee et antecessorum meorum, scilicet illud toftum cum pertinenciis suis quod iacet inter bec et toftum

---

[1]  Roger de Bavent, sheriff of York, attested.
[2]  Perhaps to be identified with Walter son of Anketin of Grimston, who gave 2 bv. in Raisthorpe to Malton Priory (Malton cartulary, f. 201/197ʳ).
[3]  Walter Grimet gave 2 bv. in Raisthorpe to Malton by an undated deed (Malton cartulary, f. 201/197ʳ).

Basilii, tenendum scilicet deo et predictis pauperibus hospitalis sancti Petri Ebor' de me et heredibus meis imperpetuum libere solute et quiete ab omni seculari servicio et exactione sicut aliqua elemosina liberius et melius potest teneri et haberi. Ego vero dictus Ricardus de Grymmeston' et heredes mei illud toftum cum omnibus pertinenciis suis warantizabimus deo et sepedictis pauperibus hospitalis contra omnes homines imperpetuum. In huius autem rei robur et testimonium huic scripto sigillum meum apposui. Hiis testibus, Roberto de Colyngham, Bernardo, Iohanne fratribus et capellanis illius domus, I[ohanne] celerario, Waltero celerario, Anketino, Swayno, Godefrido, Ricardo, Petro fratribus secularibus illius domus, Radulfo de Fontibus, Fulcone capellanis, Roberto de Stowa et multis aliis.

All but one of the witnesses attested a deed of John Malebisse of 1209 × 1231 (R95).

**R500.** Release and quitclaim to the hospital by Walter son of Robert of Grimston of all right in 1 bv. land and a toft in Grimston, being the bovate which he demanded of Thomas of Watton by writ of right, whereof Thomas called the master of the hospital to warrant, before Roger of Thirkleby and his fellow justices itinerant at York. The master and brethren gave 2m. [1241 × 1251]

*Quieta clamatio Walteri Grimeston' de una bovata terre in Grymestona.*
Sciant omnes presentes et futuri quod ego Walterus filius Roberti de Grimmeston' remisi et quietum clamavi de me et heredibus meis imperpetuum deo et pauperibus hospitalis sancti Petri Ebor' totum ius et clam(eum) quod habui vel habere potui in una bovata terre et tofto cum pertinentiis suis in Grymmeston', illam scilicet bovatam terre cum pertinenciis quam exigebam versus Thomam de Watton' per breve de recto, unde idem Thomas traxit magistrum dicti hospitalis ad warentum coram domino Rogero de Thurkilleby et sociis suis, iusticariis itinerantibus apud Ebor', tenendam et habendam predictam bovatam terre cum tofto et cum omnibus pertinenciis suis aisiamentis et libertatibus suis infra villam et extra libere integre et quiete imperpetuum, ita quod neque ego neque heredes mei aliquod ius vel clam(eum) in predicta bovata terre vel tofto cum pertinenciis suis aliquo tempore habere poterimus. Pro hac autem remissione mea et quieta clamatione dederunt michi magister et fratres dicti hospitalis duas marcas argenti. In huius vero rei robur et testimonium huic scripto sigillum meum apposui. Hiis testibus, Waltero de Wildeker, Iohanne de Hamirton', Petro de la Hay, Waltero de Perchay, Rogero Hay, Roberto Mangevilayn', Ricardo Trussebut, Waltero de Grendal', Simone de Lilling', Godefrido de Melsa, Willelmo Haget', Roberto Chambard' et multis aliis.

Roger of Thirkleby occurs repeatedly as a justice in Yorkshire in the period 1241–1252 (*YF*, 1232–1246, passim; ibid., 1246–1272, passim; Foss, *Judges*, II, 483–84; *General Eyre*, passim). The 1st, 2nd, 3rd, 7th, 9th, 11th and 12th witnesses were jurors in York in September 1251, and the 8th was party to a fine in October 1252, on both of which occasions Roger of Thirkleby was a justice (*YF*, 1246–1272, pp. 26n, 28n, 33n, 88). The fifth witness was presumably Roger Hay of Aughton, who died in 1247 × October 1251 (ibid., p. 76n; FN: Hay).

## *Guthmundham* [Goodmanham]

Except for the following entry, there is no trace of the hospital's property in Aughton (ER) and Goodmanham, which are about 12 m. apart. The gathering containing the Aughton deeds had been lost by the time Dodsworth made his abstracts and the Contents List was compiled. Roger son of Roger son of Alured held land in both places. Emma Hay, his sister and heir, was a benefactor of the hospital, and it is likely that the hospital's possessions in Goodmanham and Aughton were given by her or a close relation (FN: Hay).

**[f. 165ʳ]** *Cartas de Guthmundham quer' supra in Aghton'*

## *Heselyngton'* [Heslington near York]

The main text of Domesday tells us that Hugh son of Baldric held 5 ct. in Heslington, Thorpe [Hill] and Buttercrambe. A clearer picture is given in the summary, where Heslington is assessed at 12 ct. Hugh son of Baldric had 3 ct., Count Alan 5 ct. and the archbishop 4 ct. In 1284–85 Heslington was again assessed at 12 ct., and the holdings of 1086 are apparent, though the archbishop's holding, now held by the dean and chapter, had increased by 1 ct. at the expense of Count Alan. The hospital then had 5 ct., comprising 3 ct. held of Henry Copsi (in other texts *Suply*, *Capsy*), who held of the heirs of Mowbray, who held of the king;[1] and 2 ct. of Henry son of Conan, who held of the earl of Richmond (successor to Count Alan), of the king. The chapter of St Peter in York held 5 ct. given by Ulf *in libertate*, and the remaining 2 ct. were held by three tenants of Henry son of Conan, who held of the earl, who held in chief (*KI*, p. 63).

In 1148 Eugenius III confirmed to the hospital 'a carucate in Heslington with woodland pasture, and three others in the same vill' (C178 [*EYC*, I, no. 179]).[2] In 1154 Archbishop Theobald confirmed 'by gift of the same [Roger de Mowbray] five carucates in Heslington' (C194 [*EYC*, I, no. 185]). Adrian IV confirmed in 1157 'two carucates in Heslington with woodland pasture, and three other carucates in the same vill' (C179 [*EYC*, I, no. 186]). The wording of the confirmation of 1173 is the same (C180 [*EYC*, I, no. 197]). The 3 ct. held by Hugh son of Baldric in 1086 passed to Mowbray, and thence to Eustace FitzJohn, who gave them to the hospital in *c.*1145 × 1148 (R507). Eustace's gift was confirmed by Robert Boscer, apparently his former tenant in the land, who mentions a confirmation by Roger de Mowbray, which is not in the cartulary (R508). Robert son of Copsi gave the hospital 1 ct. in *c.*1140 × 1148 in exchange for land in Walburn (R502), and another 1 ct., reserving an annual rent of 10s., in 1148 × 1154 (R501, R503). The Domesday summary, in conjunction with the survey of 1284–85, shows that Robert must have held this land of the honour of Richmond. The confirmation of Robert's gift by Roger de Mowbray, and the confirmation by Archbishop Theobald of 5 ct. given by Mowbray, indicate that Mowbray acquired a mesne tenancy between Count Alan and Robert son of Copsi, which was subsequently extinguished. It is noteworthy that Eustace FitzJohn's name does not appear in connection with the gift of 3 ct. in Heslington in the papal confirmations, nor in the confirmation of Archbishop Theobald. The hospital must have had some difficulty with its tenure in Heslington after Robert son of Copsi's death, resulting in Henry II's writ of 1155 × 1166 ordering Torfin son of Robert son of Copsi to allow the brethren to hold their land in peace (R505). Towards the end of the twelfth century Torfin's son Conan issued a confirmation to the hospital, reserving the 10s. rent (R506).

Some of the Heslington land was kept in hand. An agreement of 1252 concerning tithes due on a newly broken tillage called *Le Breke* shows the hospital was improving its lands in Heslington (R509). But a large part was granted out at fee-farm. Master Swain granted 2 bv. in *Estorp* [in Heslington] to Stephen son of Walter son of Fagenulf; master Paulinus granted 4 bv. and two tofts to Ralph Damisel of York; and

---

[1]   The Yorkshire lands listed as belonging to Hugh son of Baldric at the Domesday survey passed largely to the Mowbray fee (*EYC*, v, 64n; *VCH Yorks*, II, 179).

[2]   When Clay calculated that 5 ct. were confirmed in 1148 (*EYC*, v, 64) he was misled by the punctuation in Farrer's transcript, so included *unam carrucatam de abbatia pro iii. solidis et i. denario per annum que dicitur Monachalandis*. Comparison with subsequent confirmations shows that this land should not be included in the Heslington tally.

master Hugh granted 2 bv. to Reginald of Warthill (*Reg. Gray*, p. 90). Master Hugh granted 8 bv. to Nicholas of Warthill in 1238 × 1245 (R514). The hospital made other grants at fee-farm during the thirteenth century. The Heslington section also includes several fourteenth- and early fifteenth-century documents, which is unusual in the Rawlinson volume.[3]

An extent of 1280 stated that the hospital had three ploughs in Heslington, worth £6 13s. 4d. annually, and £4 rent from certain other lands leased out for eleven years (R901). The extent of 1287 shows the hospital had rents of £9 14s. 10d. from Heslington; elsewhere the manor is said to be worth £20 7s. 7d., excluding fixed rents (R903, R904). In 1292 William Burnel, canon of Ampleforth, York, claimed James de Ispania, master of the hospital, and others were making waste in a turbary in Heslington which they held conjointly, and where all had right to reasonable estovers, by digging and selling turf (Baildon, *Monastic Notes*, I, 247). In 1348, the master of the hospital, John Giffard, holding land in Heslington, was summoned, with others, to appear before the king on complaint by the men of the towns of Wheldrake, Escrick, Deighton, Moreby [Hall] and Stillingfleet, that the dykes intended to take water from Heslington through Tillmire, and through the said towns, were derelict and so the fields of the said towns were frequently flooded (*CalPat*, 1343–1345, p. 593; Flower, *Public Works*, II, 239).

In 1404 Henry son of Thomas FitzHenry of Kelfield, knight, granted the 10s. rent in Heslington, which had been reserved in his ancestor's gift of the mid-twelfth century, to four trustees presumably acting on behalf of the hospital (R553). By indenture of 26 April 1520 the master and brethren of the hospital leased to William Mennell of Gykeshall, co. York, gentleman, their manor of Heslington, with lands and a close called 'Pighill', reserving pasture for one horse for the hospital's miller in *Brikkes* in summer, and a cartload of hay for the maintenance of the horse in winter, for forty-seven years at £10 annually. A twenty-one year lease in reversion of this property was sold in 1557 to Thomas Eynns, gentleman, for £20 down and £10 annually (*CalPat*, 1557–1558, p. 303). In 1535 the hospital's land in Heslington was assessed at £26 1s. 3d. (R905). In 1545 Thomas Kyddall of St Lawrence parish in York had a grant from the Crown of lands in Heslington, formerly belonging to the hospital (*LPFD*, 1545, XX (1), 682), and in 1548 Ralph Aunger, son and heir of Ralph Aunger, esq., was granted livery of his father's possessions including land in Heslington held of the king as of St Leonard's, by service unknown, worth £3 yearly (*CalPat*, 1553, p. 325). For the subsequent history of the former holdings of the hospital in Heslington, see *VCH Yorks ER*, III, 69. An undated copy of the Heslington section of the cartulary, which has no indication of copyist, apparently drawn up in the later sixteenth century was probably made in connection with the sale of the Crown's interest in Heslington (Borthwick, formerly YMD/York/5, now YM/D/YOR/5).

Several generations of the family of Robert son of Copsi, which held 2 k.f. of the honour of Richmond, are apparent in the Heslington deeds. The family is discussed by Brown and by Clay, and further notes on its Westmorland holdings are given by Burton (*Ctl. Gisborough*, II, 183–84n; *EYC*, V, 53–58; *EYF*, pp. 57–58; Burton, 'Bleatarn', passim). Robert son of Copsi and his descendants are frequently described without surname of place, but also occur variously as 'OF MANFIELD', 'OF KELFIELD',

---

3   See Introduction, p. lxiv n. 166 above, for the possibility that the Heslington deeds once formed part of the York division of the hospital's archive.

## DESCENDANTS OF ROBERT SON OF COPSI

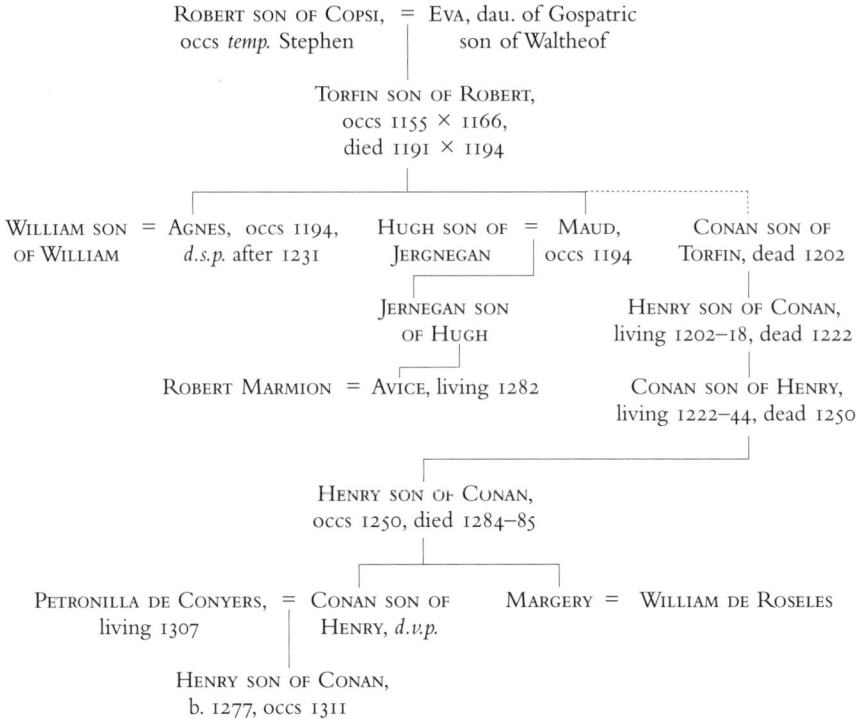

ROBERT SON OF COPSI,   =   EVA, dau. of Gospatric
occs *temp.* Stephen          son of Waltheof

TORFIN SON OF ROBERT,
occs 1155 × 1166,
died 1191 × 1194

WILLIAM SON  =  AGNES, occs 1194,      HUGH SON OF  =  MAUD,        CONAN SON OF
OF WILLIAM      *d.s.p.* after 1231        JERGNEGAN        occs 1194     TORFIN, dead 1202

JERNEGAN SON                        HENRY SON OF CONAN,
OF HUGH                            living 1202–18, dead 1222

ROBERT MARMION  =  AVICE, living 1282      CONAN SON OF HENRY,
living 1222–44, dead 1250

HENRY SON OF CONAN,
occs 1250, died 1284–85

PETRONILLA DE CONYERS,  =  CONAN SON OF      MARGERY  =  WILLIAM DE ROSELES
living 1307            HENRY, *d.v.p.*

HENRY SON OF CONAN,
b. 1277, occs 1311

'OF WARCOP', 'OF LIVERTON', and in the case of Torfin son of Robert son of Copsi,
'OF WAITBY' and 'OF BROUGH'.[4] The wife of Robert son of Copsi has not previously
been named. Describing herself as Eva daughter of Gospatric son of Waltheof, wife of
Robert son of Copsi, she gave her dower lands in Warcop (Westmorland) to Byland
Abbey, presumably after the death of her husband. The gift was made by the pledge
and witness of Torfin son of Robert, apparently her son, but not so described[5] (MS
Dods. 70, f. 65ᵛ, cited imperfectly *Ctl. Byland*, p. 24). Eva's grandfather was doubtless
Waltheof, lord of Allerdale, a son of Gospatric, earl of Northumbria under William I.[6]
Robert son of Copsi and Eva his wife made a gift to the hospital of land in Musgrave,
a mile or so from Warcop, in 1148 × 1157 (M: Musgrave [MS Dods. 124, f. 106ʳ]).
These transactions show that Robert's Westmorland interests were held by right of
his wife: his benefactions in the honour of Richmond do not mention her. His grant
of 1 ct. in Heslington to the hospital in exchange for land in Walburn was made in
*c.*1140 × 1148 (R502), and his subsequent gift of a further 1 ct., reserving a rent of
10s., in 1148 × 1154 (R501, R503).

4   *de Burgo*, probably for Brough in Catterick where the Marmion family later had an interest. Torfin son
    of Robert gave 1 bv. at Brough (*Burgum*) to the Templars, which Roger of Catterick was holding of
    them in 1185 for 2s. annually (Lees, *Templars*, pp. 127–28).
5   There must therefore be some doubt as to whether the pledge was actually her son. It is clear that
    there were two men named Torfin associated with Warcop in the second half of the twelfth century,
    both of whom had sons named Robert (*EYC*, v, 56n; Burton, 'Bleatarn', p. 30).
6   For Waltheof and Gospatric, see *Hist. Northumberland*, VII, 16–29, pedigree facing p. 104; *ODNB*, s.n.
    Gospatric, earl of Northumberland; *English Baronies*, p. 134.

In 1159 × 1171 Earl Conan restored the 2 k.f. in Manfield to Torfin son of Robert, as they had been held by Hermer his ancestor (*attavus*) or Gutherith, daughter of Hermer (*EYC*, IV, no. 55). The king's writ of 1155 × 1166 shows that the hospital faced some difficulty when Torfin succeeded to his father's land, but there are no details (R505). A feodary of the late twelfth century names Torfin as the tenant of 2 k.f. of the honour of Richmond (*EYC*, V, 13; *Red Bk*, p. 587). Torfin was living in 1191, when he accounted for 200m. to allow his daughter to marry as he wished, but he was dead in 1194, when William son of William and Hugh [son of] Jernegan owed 200m. for the land which belonged to Torfin son of Robert, whose daughters they had (*PR*, 3&4 Ric. I, p. 76; ibid., 6 Ric. I, p. 161). William and Hugh were husbands to Torfin's daughters and coheirs Agnes and Maud respectively. Agnes died without issue after 1231. Her sister Maud's granddaughter inherited not just the Manfield fee, but also the 2½ k.f. in Tanfield once held by Hugh son of Jernegan. In 1282, an inquiry into the knights' fees held of the honour of Richmond found that Lady Avice Marmion (daughter of Maud's son Jernegan, and widow of Robert Marmion) held 4½ k.f. in Tanfield and Manfield with the members, i.e. Hugh son of Jernegan's 2½ k.f. and Torfin's 2 k.f. (*EYC*, V, 40, 54, 56–58; *YI*, I, 234; *CP*, VIII, 507). Conan son of Torfin, who confirmed the land in Heslington held of him by the hospital (R506) was almost certainly illegitimate, but nevertheless acquired a substantial proportion of his father's holdings. An inquisition, probably of 1280, concerning castle guard at Richmond, states that Avice Marmion and Henry [Fitz] Conan [a descendant of Conan son of Torfin] held 2 k.f. in Manfield (*YI*, I, 228). Clay suggested that the descendants of Conan acquired the moiety belonging to Agnes, Conan's half-sister (*EYC*, V, 58). But Conan's gift of 2 bv. in Manfield to Marrick Priory almost certainly predates the death of his father Torfin (*EYC*, V, no. 168), and his confirmation to the hospital (R506) was made long before the death of his half-sister Agnes. It is more likely that Conan son of Torfin's holdings were acquired by subinfeudation, probably during his father's lifetime, and that his land was held originally of his half-sisters, who may have quitclaimed their interest to him or to the earl of Richmond.

Conan son of Torfin was dead in 1202, when the land of Henry son of Conan in Manfield was named in an abutment (*PF John*, p. 38). Henry son of Conan was a pledge, with other tenants of the honour of Richmond, for Roald son of Alan in 1207–08 (*RFine*, p. 444). He was a knight on a grand assize in Yorkshire in 1208 (*CRR*, 1207–1209, p. 295); and was a witness to William of Kilton's grant of the church of Kirkleatham (*Lyum*) to Gisborough, which was confirmed by King John in 1210 (*Ctl. Gisborough*, nos 745, 750). Henry had interests not far from Kirkleatham, in Liverton, which later evidence indicates he held as ½ k.f. of Brus. He served as steward to Peter de Brus I, and attested several of his deeds (Blakely, *Brus Family*, p. 118n). Henry son of Conan quitclaimed the advowson of the church of Liverton to Gisborough Priory in 1218. In an account of a dispute concerning the advowson of Liverton he is referred to as *miles*, and he appears as a knight in 1218–19 (*YF*, 1218–1231, pp. 5, 11n; *Ctl. Gisborough*, no. 923; *Yorkshire Eyre Rolls*, nos 19, 375, 505). Henry son of Conan was probably dead in 1214 × 1222,[7] when Conan son of Henry witnessed a deed of Peter son of Adam de Brus to Gisborough concerning Glaisdale (*Ctl. Gisborough*, no. 930). In 1223, 2 a. in Manfield were remised to Conan son of Henry, and in 1227 he was accused, with others, of a disseisin in Eppleby and Barforth, both of which

---

7 Peter de Mauley, who is named in an abutment, had lands in the locality through his marriage in 1214 to Isabel, daughter of Robert of Thornham, heiress of the Fossard fee (*ODNB*, s.n. Thornham; *VCH Yorks NR*, II, 345–47). Peter de Brus I was dead in February 1222 (*CalFine Hen. III*, 6/93).

are a few miles west of Manfield (*PatentR*, 1225–1232, p. 160). Conan of Kelfield was named as a recognitor in a case of 1244, but did not attend and so was amerced (*CRR*, 1243–1245, no. 1918).

Conan was dead in 1250, when Henry son of Conan had respite from distraint to become a knight for two years (*CloseR*, 1247–1251, p. 366). In 1257 Henry son of Conan was granted exemption for life from being put on assizes, juries, or recognitions, and being made sheriff (*CalPat*, 1247–1258, p. 582). Nevertheless he was a juror in 1268 (*YF*, 1246–1272, p. 158n). In 1271 Henry son of Conan had a grant of free warren in his demesne lands in Liverton, Kelfield, and [Kirkby] Fleetham (*CalCh*, 1257–1300, p. 166). The mill of Manfield was 'divided' between Henry, Avice Marmion, and the abbot of Easby in 1274–75 (*VCH Yorks NR*, I, 187, citing De Banco R., Mich. 3 Edw. I, m. 54). In 1279–81 Henry son of Conan was called upon to show by what warrant he had free warren in Kelfield, and cited the grant of 1271. He went on to explain the nature of his tenure in Liverton, [Kirkby] Fleetham, half of Manfield, and the manor of Kelfield (*YQW*, pp. 174–75). In 1281, in an adjustment to the division of the Brus barony, ½ k.f. in Liverton held by Henry son of Conan was allotted to the share of Marmaduke of Thwing and his wife Lucy (*CalCl*, 1279–1288, p. 106). The inquisition, probably of 1280, where with Avice Marmion, Henry [son of] Conan was said to hold 2 k.f. in Manfield of the earl of Richmond, has been noted above. The returns of 1284–87 show Henry son of Conan holding in Heslington, Kelfield, Stillingfleet, Liverton, Kirkby Fleetham, Eppleby and Great and Little Fencotes (*KI*, pp. 63, 65, 128, 150, 157, 169).

It seems that there was enfeoffment of a younger son in the middle of the thirteenth century, and there may be some confusion between individuals of similar names. Conan of Kelfield, a verderer of the hay of Langwath, was a juror in 1270 in an inquisition concerning that hay; and occurs again as a juror in another inquisition concerning the same in 1279–80 (*YI*, I, 111, 215). Sir Henry FitzConan, knight, William of Moreby, and Henry FitzConan of Kelfield were witnesses to a deed of 1283 (*KI*, p. 63, citing MS Dods. 9, f. 81r).[8]

Henry son of Conan was dead in August 1285, when the manor of Liverton, in the king's hand by his death, was ordered to be given to William Latimer (*CalFine*, 1272–1307, p. 219).[9] Henry's eldest son Conan had apparently predeceased him. In Michaelmas term 1285, the king's attorney, and Petronilla,[10] widow of Conan son of Henry, on behalf of her son, then under age and in the king's wardship, claimed the manor of Kelfield which had been seized by Margery, daughter of Henry son of Conan, and her husband William de Roseles. Petronilla stated that she had been married to Conan in the church of Sockburn, and that her son had been born in Sockburn and baptised in the same church (*YI*, II, 92, citing Coram Rege, no. 94, m. 29). In 1289 a writ was sent on the complaint of Petronilla, late wife of Conan son of Henry,[11] stating that Conan[12] had endowed her at the church door when he married her of all the lands of his father, that nevertheless the king had taken all the lands into his own hands, and committed them to William Latimer. The resulting

8    Dodsworth's source is St Mary JR, f. 348r.
9    The grave slab found at Liverton, bearing the arms of FitzConan, may have belonged to this Henry, or
      one of his thirteenth century predecessors (Anon., 'The Fitz Conan slab at Liverton', *YAJ*, XVIII (1905),
      417–19).
10   The usual Latin rendition of Parnel.
11   MS: Henry son of Conan.
12   MS: Henry.

inquisition, held in 1290, found that Henry father of Conan had empowered Conan to so endow his wife Petronilla, and he had received her and maintained her in his own house for three and a half years. At about the same time the earl of Richmond complained that the marriage of Henry, kinsman and heir of Henry son of Conan of Kelfield ought to belong to him, because the lands held of him were of more ancient acquisition that the lands he held of other lords. The jurors found that it was customary for the marriage of the heir to belong to the lord of the lands where he was found after the death of his ancestor. Henry son of Conan, on the death of the said Henry his grandfather, had been found at Liverton (*CalInqPM*, II, no. 743). Early in 1300 a proof of age was held for Henry, 'cousin' (elsewhere called grandson) and heir of Henry son of Conan, deceased, who claimed his lands which were in the custody of William Latimer senior. The younger Henry was said to have been twenty-two years old on 24 September 1299, which places his birth in 1277. The jurors agreed that he had been six years old at his grandfather's death, which was sixteen years previously. It was also said that his father Conan had been very young at the time of the pregnancy, which had caused much discussion (*YI*, III, 141–44). Petronilla of Kelfield occurs in 1297. Petronilla de Conyers and H[enry] her son together paid the lay subsidy in Kelfield in 1301. As the Conyers family had extensive interests in Sockburn, the place of Petronilla's marriage, it is apparent she was using her maiden name. In 1303 the lords of Kelfield were said to be the abbot of Selby, Henry son of Conan and Walter de Hamerton (*Lay Subsidy, 1301*, p. 105 and n; *VCH Yorks NR*, I, 450–51). In 1307, Archbishop Greenfield allowed Dame Petronilla, lady of Kelfield, an oratory in her manor there, as it was far from the parish church (*Reg. Greenfield*, III, 17). Henry son of Conan complained that game had been chased in his free warren in Kelfield in 1310. In 1311 he had licence to hold his woods of Liverton and Kelfield enclosed and emparked, as his ancestors had them, and in the same year had a grant of free warren in his demesne lands of Liverton, Kelfield, and [Kirkby] Fleetham (*CalPat*, 1307–1313, pp. 315, 356; *CalCh*, 1300–1326, p. 160). The *Nomina Villarum* of 1316 named John Marmion, the heirs of Henry son of Conan, and Amabel of Cleasby as the lords of Manfield; but the lord of Kelfield was said to be Henry son of Henry son of Conan, who also held Little Halton of the honour of Tickhill (*KI*, pp. 319, 336, 366). Conan son of Henry occurs in 1328, when he was granted protection for a year, as he was going on pilgrimage to the Holy Land (*CalPat*, 1327–1330, p. 229). In 1333 he received confirmation of the grant of free warren made in 1311, so far as it related to Kelfield and [Kirkby] Fleetham (*CalCh*, 1327–1341, p. 303). In 1343 the abbot of Selby claimed the custody of the manor of Kelfield, until Henry, son and heir of Conan of Kelfield, reached full age (Baildon, *Monastic Notes*, I, 200; *Ctl. Selby*, I, 342). A feodary of 1346 states that Henry son of Henry son of Conan, who was under age, and in the custody of the earl of Richmond, held half the fee in Manfield and Cloubeck (in Manfield), previously held by Roger Marmion and Conan son of Henry. Maud Marmion held the other half of the fee (*Feudal Aids*, VI, 240). For later references to the family, see *VCH Yorks ER*, III, 104; *VCH Yorks NR*, I, 187; *Ctl. Gisborough*, II, 183–85n.

**R501.** Gift to Robert warden of the hospital and the brethren by Robert son of Copsi and Torfin his son and heir, of 6 bv. land and 2 bv. which Aldred the priest holds in Heslington, with half the woodland pasture of the vill, for 10s. annually [1148 × 1154]

PRINTED: *EYC*, V, no. 156, where dated 'shortly before 1148'.

**[f. 167ʳ]** *Robertus filius Copsi de terra in Heselington'.*

Dominis et amicis suis et omnibus suis hominibus Robertus filius Copesi et Torfinus suus filius et heres salutem. Notum sit vobis omnibus tam futuris quam presentibus quod ego Robertus filius Copesi et Torfinus filius meus et heres et omnes post me mei heredes concedimus et damus Roberto custodi hospitalis sancti Petri Ebor' et fratribus ibidem deo servientibus vi. bovatas terre et duas bovatas quas Aldredus presbiter tenet plenar(ias) in Haslingtuna cum toftis omnibus ad eas pertinentibus et cum medietate virgulti eiusdem ville quietas et liberas et immunes ab omnibus geldis et consuetudinibus et auxiliis et ab omni servicio regis et com(itis) et omnium aliorum hominum, sic etiam quod ego et heredes mei omne servicium quod ad eandem terram pertinet semper faciemus et quod nos eam contra omnes homines eis semper guarentizabimus. Et eas habeant in elemosinam in feudum imperpetuum, singulis annis x. solidos pro eis reddendo michi et meis heredibus. Hiis testibus, Guillelmo presbitero de Ultra Usiam et Hugone presbitero et Roberto presbitero fratre Radulfi, militibus vero Thoma de Ultra Usiam, Gilleberto filio Nigelli, Iohanne de Walemure, Huctredo de Clivelande, bergensibus autem Hereberto nigro, Godefrido parmentario, Edwardo de Sancto Petro, Waldigo de Morbi, Gamello filio Bernulfi, Roberto filio Golle, Gudmundo et Stephano sacerdote eius filio.

As the witnesses to this deed, excepting the final five, attested Robert's gift of 14 bv. and 2 bv. held by the priest in Heslington (R503) it is evident that the two deeds were given on the same occasion. So both deeds refer to the second carucate in Heslington given by Robert son of Copsi, and must have been issued between the confirmation of 1148 and that of 1154. The similarity of phrasing suggests the present deed was written with reference to the earlier deed R502. Clay gives details for several of the witnesses.

**R502.** Gift in exchange to Robert warden of the hospital and the other brethren by Robert son of Copsi and Torfin his son, of 1 ct. land in Heslington, with half the woodland pasture of the vill, for 4 ct. 2 bv. in Walburn [par. Downholme, near Richmond, NR] which Robert and the brethren gave to Robert son of Copsi. If Robert son of Copsi could not warrant the land in Heslington, the brethren would have back the land in Walburn [*c.*1140 × *c.*1148]

PRINTED: *EYC*, v, no. 157, where dated 'shortly before 1148'.

*R[obertus] filius Copesi de i. carucata in Heselyngton'.*

Dominis et amicis suis et omnibus suis hominibus Rodbertus filius Copesi salutem. Notum sit vobis omnibus tam futuris quam presentibus quod ego Rodbertus filius Copesi et Torfinus meus filius et omnes mei heredes post me cambivimus et dedimus Rodberto custodi hospitalis sancti Petri Ebor' et ceteris fratribus eiusdem loci unam carucatam terre plenariam in Haslentona cum omnibus toftis ad eam pertinentibus et cum medietate virgulti eiusdem ville quietam et liberam et immunem ab omnibus geldis et consuetudinibus et auxiliis et ab omni servicio regis et com(itis) et omnium aliorum hominum, sic eciam quod ego et heredes mei omne servicium quod ad eandem terram pertinent semper faciemus et quod nos eam contra omnes homines eis semper guarantizabimus; scilicet pro iiii. carucatis terre et ii. bovatis in Walebrunna quas Rodbertus custos hospitalis et fratres eiusdem loci michi et heredibus meis concesserunt. Tali tamen pacto quod si ita evenerit quod nos predictam terram de Haslintona eis nullo modo quarantizare poterimus, fratres hospitalis ad suam prefatam terram de Walebrunna libere et quiete et sine omni contradictione redibunt et eam in pace possidebunt. Hiis inde existentibus testibus, Rualdo constab(ulario), Rodberto presbitero Caterici, Thiobaldo capellano, Alexandro Musard', Guihumero, Willelmo filio constab(ularii), Rodberto filio Rodberti, Harscoido filio constab(ularii), Eudone clerico, Gleio, Rualdo nepote constab(ularii), Dreuo filio Pinchun, Henrico clerico, Torfino filio Utthe,[13] Uhtredo, Guidone, Gaufrido, Hoilando, Philippo filio Thome de Burc'.

As the land in Walburn was not confirmed to the hospital in 1148, it is probable that it had already been exchanged for the land in Heslington. It is likely therefore that this deed refers to the carucate in Heslington given by Robert son of Copsi in that year or before. Torfin son of Robert died in 1191 × 1194, and so it is unlikely he would have been of an age to join with his father in this exchange much before 1140 (*EYC*, v, 55–56). There is no other trace of the hospital's estate in Walburn. Its substantial size suggests it was the gift of Count Alan, or his father Stephen whom he succeeded probably in 1135–36 (*EYC*, iv, 87–90; *CP*, x, 787–88), but it may perhaps have been given by the tenant of the 15 k.f. which originally made up the steward's fee. Walburn certainly formed part of this fee in later years, as it was held in 1286–87 by the heirs of Matthew of Thornton [Steward], to whom the steward's fee had passed (*EYC*, v, 17–26; *KI*, p. 157). In that year there were said to be 5 ct. in Walburn, of which 4 ct. were held by a number of tenants of the heirs of Thornton, of the earl of Richmond, of the king. The remaining carucate was held by three monasteries and the Knights Templar (*KI*, p. 157). A mill in Walburn was granted to the hospital by Robert son of William of Harmby in the first half of the thirteenth century (M: Walburn [MS Dods. 120b, f. 103ʳ]).

**R503.** Gift to Robert warden of the hospital and the poor of Christ there by Robert son of Copsi and Torfin his son and heir of 14 bv. land and 2 bv. which Aldred the priest holds in Heslington, with all tofts belonging and all the woodland pasture of the vill [1148 × 1154]

PRINTED: *EYC*, v, no. 158, where dated 'shortly before 1148'.

*Robertus filius Copsi de Heselington'.*
Dominis et amicis suis et omnibus fidelibus cristi Rotbertus filius Copesi et Torfinus filius suus et heres salutem. Notum sit vobis omnibus tam futuris quam presentibus quod ego et heredes mei concedimus et damus Rotberto custodi hospitalis sancti Petri Ebor' et pauperibus cristi in eodem degentibus xiiii. bovatas terre et ii. bovatas quas Aldredus presbiter tenet, plenarias in Hasaligtuna cum toftis omnibus ad eas pertinentibus et totum virgultum eiusdem ville, quietas et liberas et immunes ab omnibus geldis et consuetudinibus et auxiliis et ab omni servicio regis et comitis et omnium aliorum hominum, sic eciam quod ego et heredes mei omne servicium quod ad eandem terram pertinet semper faciemus, et eas habeant in feudum et elemosinam perpetuam, pro remissione omnium peccatorum nostrorum et pro animabus omnium antecessorum nostrorum et ut simus participes omnium beneficiorum que fiunt in supradicto hospitali, in missis in orationibus in elemosinis et hospitalitatibus imperpetuum. Testibus, Guillelmo presbitero de Ultra Usiam et Hugone presbitero et Rotberto presbitero fratre Radulfi et Thoma filio Ulluati et Gileberto filio Nigelli,

---

[13] Perhaps *Ucche*.

Huctredo de Clivalanda, Iohanne[14] de Walemure, Herberto nigro, Godefrido parmentario, Edwardo de Sancto Petro et multis aliis.

For the date, see R501.

**R504.** Confirmation to the hospital by Roger de Mowbray of the land with
woodland pasture which Robert son of Copsi gave them in Roger's fee in
Heslington, just as it holds other land in Roger's fee [*c.*1148 × 1154]

PRINTED: *EYC*, v, no. 160, where dated 'middle of 12th cent.'. CALENDAR: *Mowbray
Charters*, no. 303, where dated *c.*1154 × 1157.

*Confirmatio R(ogeri) de Mulbray de terra de H(esligtun).*
Rogerus de Mulbray omnibus hominibus suis et amicis universisque sancte matris
ecclesie filiis salutem. Sciatis me concessisse et confirmasse deo et fratribus et
pauperibus hospitalis sancti Petri terram illam cum virgulto quam Robertus filius
Copsi concessit eis de feudo meo in Hesligtun, sicut alias terras de meo feudo habent,
ita quod pro defectu servicii illius terre nullum namium capiam neque aliquo modo
eos distringam. Nam volo et firmiter precipio ut pauperes et infirmi illius sancte domus
omnes terras quas de meo feudo habent bene et libere et quiete et in pace teneant ut
pro me vivo et defuncto assidue deum exorent. Isti sunt testes, prior ecclesie sancte
Marie et Willelmus monachus et Daniel pater eius et Reginaldus Puher, Willelmus
de Wivilla, Rogerus de Condeio, Robertus capellanus, Radulfus Beler, Willelmus de
Crocheslei, Simon de Sancto Claro, Robertus[15] de Ripun, Radulfus[16] de Bellun,
Hamundus Beler. Valete.

It is likely that this deed precedes Archbishop Theobald's confirmation of 1154 which
included 5 ct. in Heslington 'by gift of Roger de Mowbray'. Greenway's dating is
based on the attestation of Ralph Beler, who was dead in 1157 (*EYC*, ix, 215), and
the high place in the witness list of William de Wyville, which may imply that he was
then Mowbray's steward, which position he was holding in 1154 (*Mowbray Charters*,
p. lxii). According to the Byland chronicle, Hugh Malebisse, Wyville's predecessor, was
holding the stewardship in 1147 (Burton, *Byland and Jervaulx*, p. 17).

**R505.** Writ of Henry II to Torfin son of Robert son of Copsi, ordering him to cause
the brethren of the hospital to hold peacefully the land which Torfin's father
Robert gave in Heslington and confirmed by his deed [1155 × 1166]

COPIES: *b1* Rawl., f. 167[r–v]; *b2* C14 [Cott., f. 4[r]]; differences as noted with further minor
variations of spelling. PRINTED: *EYC*, v, no. 159, from *b1*, *b2*, where dated 1155 × 1168.

*Henricus rex de terra de Heselington'.*
H.[17] rex Angl(orum) et dux Norm(annorum) et Aquit(anorum) et comes
And(egavorum) Turf(ino)[18] filio Roberti filii Copsi salutem. **[f. 167ᵛ]** Precipio quod

---

[14]  MS: *Iolianne*, but see R501.
[15]  MS: *Roberto*.
[16]  MS: *Radulfo*.
[17]  *b1*: *Henricus*.
[18]  *b2*: *Turstini*.

facias[19] fratres de hospitali sancti Petri Ebor' tenere in pace et iuste et libere terram totam de Heselingtona quam Robertus pater tuus eis concessit et dedit, et sic iuste ita libera et quieta sicut pater tuus eis concessit et carta sua confirmavit. Et habeant iuste illas consuetudines et libertates quas habuerunt tempore patris tui. Et prohibeo ne quis eis inde iniuriam vel contumeliam faciat. Quod nisi feceris Rogerus de Molbray faciat, et nisi fecerit comes Conanus faciat et nisi fecerit iusticia mea faciat fieri. T(este) R[oberto] episcopo Lincoln', apud Notingham.

The date range is given by the accession of Henry II, and the death of Robert Chesney, bishop of Lincoln, which is now believed to have occurred at the end of 1166 (*EEA*, I, p. xxxvi).

**R506.** Confirmation to the hospital by Conan son of Torfin of all land which the hospital held of him in Heslington, quit of all service beyond 10*s.* annually to Conan and his heirs [possibly *c*.1180 × *c*.1195]

PRINTED: *EYC*, v, no. 161, where dated '? post 1194'.

*Carta Conani de Heselingtun.*
Universis sancte matris ecclesie filiis Conanus filius Torfini salutem. Notum sit vobis me dedisse et concessisse et hac mea presenti carta confirmasse deo et pauperibus hospitalis sancti Petri Ebor' totam terram quam de me in Heseligtune tenuerunt, in liberam et puram et perpetuam elemosinam, solutam et quietam ab omni humano servicio preter x.s. annuatim michi et heredibus meis post me reddendos v.s. ad festum sancti Martini et v.s. ad Pent'. Hiis testibus, Eudone de Punchardun, Godefrido capellano, Richero fratre Henrici,[20] Roberto le Luue,[21] Petro filio Alani, Adam filio Laurencii, Iohanne de Manefeld', Petro filio Torfini, Alicia Burdun, Iueta uxore Conani.

Torfin died in 1191 × 1194, when the heirs to a large part of his holdings were his two daughters Maud and Agnes, but it is likely that Conan acquired his interests in Heslington during his father's lifetime. Conan had been been succeeded by his son Henry by 1202 (FN: FitzConan).

The first witness, Eudo de PUNCHARDON, held land in Grimston, adjacent to Heslington, and was apparently dead by the end of the twelfth century. Farrer gave a few references to some members of the Punchardon family in Yorkshire and Durham (*EYC*, I, 309). Whether they were related to others of that name who held in Devon, Hertfordshire, Hampshire, and Wiltshire in the late twelfth and thirteenth centuries is unclear, but the occurrence of the names Roger and Eudo in these places suggests a connection. Eudo de Punchardon is recorded in Hertfordshire in 1198 and 1214. Roger de Punchardon occurs in Devon in 1200; his widow Agnes entered a plea against William de Punchardon concerning Heanton in 1213 (*CRR*, I, 42, 356; ibid., 1213–1215, pp. 25, 233).[22] It is probable that the surname was derived from Pontchardon, Orne, arr. Argentan, in Basse-Normandie (*ANF*, p. 83). The occasional omission of *de* perhaps results from confusion with the patronymic Punchard.

---

[19] *b2: faciatis.*
[20] MS: *Henrico.*
[21] Possibly *Lune.*
[22] Some details of the Devon family are given in *ANF*, p. 83.

The descent of the Punchardon family, or families, of Yorkshire, Durham and Northumberland is elusive. It is probable, by the coincidence of names, that the Punchardons who served the bishop of Durham in the late twelfth and thirteenth centuries were tenants of the Bulmer (later Neville) fee in Yorkshire, but this has not been proved. Richard de Punchardon occurs in 1158, when he rendered account for £10 for a plea in Yorkshire (*PR*, 2–4 Hen. II, p. 148). The silence of the records between *c.*1140 and 1158, together with Richard de Punchardon's survival in Durham until at least March 1185[/86] (*Feod. Durham*, p. 142n), makes it unlikely that he is to be identified with Richard son of Eudo, who witnessed an act of Bishop G[eoffrey] of Durham in '1133 × 1141' (*Durham Charters*, no. 30). Matthew de Punchardon held a fifth part of a fee of Bertram of Bulmer in Yorkshire in 1166 (*Red Bk*, p. 429). The Bulmer fee included land in Sutton on the Forest, Whenby, and Grimston (*EYC*, II, 113–14).[23] Towthorpe on the Wold may probably be added to this list.[24] As Roger and Eudo de Punchardon appear to have held in each of those places in the first half of the thirteenth century, it is reasonable to suppose that Matthew was their predecessor.

There is no trace of a Punchardon tenancy in the return of fees made by the bishop of Durham in 1166 (*Red Bk*, pp. 415–18).[25] Richard, a knight, *a Pungente Carduo cognominatus*, was a judge in the bishopric who sentenced one Roger to be blinded and mutilated in 1174. Roger's subsequent recovery is listed amongst the miracles performed by Thomas Becket (Scammell, *Puiset*, p. 221; *Becket Materials*, I, 420–23). Eudo and Richard de Punchardon, who were contemporaries, appear frequently in the records of the bishopric of Durham, but the relationship between them is nowhere stated. Farrer's postulation that Eudo was son of Richard can be ruled out: they may perhaps have been brothers. Eudo, with his sons Roger, Robert and Walter; and Richard, with his sons Walter and William, attested several charters of the last quarter of the twelfth century, Eudo normally having a slight precedence over Richard. Richard de Punchardon and Walter his son witnessed acta of Hugh, bishop of Durham, in '*c.*1175 × *c.*1180' and '*c.*1180 × 1184' (*EEA*, XXIV, nos 72, 144). In *c.*1170 × *c.*1180[26] Eudo and Richard de Punchardon, with Walter and William, sons of Richard de Punchardon, witnessed together. Not long afterwards, Eudo de Punchardon, Roger, Robert and Walter his sons, Richard de Punchardon and Walter his son attested (*Feod. Durham*, pp. 124–25n). In '1183 × 1184' Eudo de Punchardon and Roger his son witnessed a further act of Bishop Hugh. Richard de Punchardon and Walter his son follow a little further down the witness list (*EEA*, XXIV, no. 151). Eudo de Punchardon and Roger his son attested again in 1189 (ibid., no. 91). Eudo Punchardon, [. . .] Conan of Manfield, Richard Punchardon, Hugh Punchardon, [. . .] Roger Punchardon, and William Punchardon witnessed a deed of Philip son of Hamund sheriff of Durham in *c.*1180 × 1195[27] (*Feod. Durham*, p. 126n). Walter

[23] Farrer also postulates that Bulmer held land in Kepwick (*EYC*, II, 114). This may be so, but it seems that the Punchardon interest there was gained by marriage to Joan, widow of Eustace de Laval, in the second half of the thirteenth century (see below, p. 608).

[24] See below, n. 34.

[25] The Punchardon tenancy of Bulmer suggests they may have been subtenants in the 5 k.f. held of the bishop of Durham by the son of Bertram of Bulmer. Sir Eudo (*Evayne*) de Punchardon of Thickley [Punchardon] occurs in a list of knights of the bishopric of Durham from the later thirteenth century, and was a witness to deeds (Holford, 'Knights of Durham', p. 212). Thickley Punchardon, now East Thickley, is close to Shildon in co. Durham.

[26] The deed is attested by Ralph Haget, sheriff [of Durham], to whom Snape assigns these dates (*EEA*, XXIV, p. xliv).

[27] The period assigned by Snape for the shrievalty of Philip son of Hamund is from before November 1180, possibly until the death of Bishop Hugh (*EEA*, XXIV, p. xliv).

Punchardon, with Roger, Robert, and Walter, sons of Eudo (*Ivonis*) de Punchardon witnessed a Stittenham (NR) deed of 1199[28] or soon afterwards (*Ctl. Rievaulx*, no. 303).[29] It is likely that both Eudo and Richard de Punchardon died towards the end of the episcopate of Hugh du Puiset (d. 1195). Several acts given towards the end of Puiset's life are attested by Roger, Robert or Walter de Punchardon (*EEA*, xxiv, nos 3, 43, 47, 66, 116); and a number of acts of Bishop Philip (1197–1208) are witnessed by Roger or Walter de Punchardon (*EEA*, xxv, nos 198, 211, 218, 228).

In 1208 × 1227[30] Henry de Neville, grandson of Bertram of Bulmer, whilst confirming his grandfather's gift of the site of Marton Priory, also confirmed the gift in his fee made by Roger de Punchardon son of Eudo de Punchardon of 10 bv. in *Sutton iuxta Tatecastra* (*MA*, vi, 199). This is somewhat difficult to understand. Sutton on the Forest, also called Sutton in Galtres, close to the priory, hardly fits the description 'by Tadcaster', but was part of the Bulmer fee. Stutton, 1 m. south of Tadcaster, may have been intended, but lay in the Percy and Arches fees, and no Bulmer interest there is known. Marton had £12 12s. 0d. rent in Sutton on the Forest, and £4 10s. 0d. rent in Stutton at the Dissolution (*MA*, vi, 199). Roger de Punchardon attested a Hewick deed in 1198 × 1200[31] (MS Dods. 92, f. 49ʳ). He witnessed the grant of Henry, prior of Marton, to Healaugh made in January 1203[/04] (*Ctl. Healaugh*, p. 11), and was a witness to a gift of land in Coney St., York, to the prior and monks of Durham in 1204 × 1209[32] (*EYC*, I, no. 246). Roger is named in the Yorkshire section of the pipe rolls of 1201 and 1212 (*PR*, 3 John, p. 155; ibid., 14 John, p. 38). Roger de Punchardon and Imania his wife gave 1½ bv. in Eppleby to Marrick Priory 'post *c.*1191' (*EYC*, v, no. 276). The gift to Marrick Priory by Roger de Punchardon and Imania his wife, of 2 bv. and two tofts and all the share which they had in wood and turbary in [Kirkby] Fleetham, is included in a general confirmation made in 1348 (*CalCh*, 1341–1417, p. 90).

In 1237 Eudo de Punchardon attorned John of Woodifield (*Wudingfeld*) and another concerning land in Whenby (*CloseR*, 1234–1237, p. 565). In 1240, fines were made between Eudo de Punchardon and William Haget, as to 1 ct. of land in Whenby, and between the same Eudo and the same William, whom Robert de Saunford, master of the Knights Templar in England, had called to warrant, also concerning 1 ct. in Whenby. William gave Eudo 11*m.* for a quitclaim (*YF*, 1232–1246, p. 63). Eudo de Punchardon, knight, gave 5 bv. in Towthorpe on the Wold to Simon le Grant, citizen of York, in 1247 × 1272[33] (MS Dods. 7, f. 327ᵛ).[34] Eudo (*Ivo*) de Punchardon was a juror on an inquisition in 1261, to determine who was the next heir to hold the serjeantry of the castle gate of York (*YI*, I, 87). In 1268 × 1270[35] Eudo de Punchardon, knight, son of Roger de Punchardon gave to St Peter's, York, for the souls of Sir James

---

[28] The deed mentions a deraignment before five justices, all of whom took part in the Yorkshire iter of that date (*General Eyre*, p. 59).

[29] Farrer is incorrect in stating that Eudo himself attested.

[30] The period when Henry de Neville was holding (*EYC*, II, 122, 128).

[31] When James Potern was sheriff of Yorkshire.

[32] With Robert Waleys, sheriff of Yorks.

[33] While John of Selby was mayor of York (ML).

[34] In 1283, ½ k.f. in Towthorpe [on the Wold], held by Simon le Grant of York and Ultarius of Wharram, was included amongst the possessions of the late Robert de Neville, who had succeeded to the Bulmer fee (*CalInqPM*, II, no. 483). In 1316 Ralph Neville and William Latimer were said to be lords of Towthorpe and Burdale nearby (*KI*, p. 315).

[35] This deed is best dated with reference to the witness John de Haulton, sheriff of Yorkshire in that period.

of Cawood, once canon of the same church, and others, all his manor of Grimston,[36] to be held of the nuns of Moxby (*Mollesby*) (*CVC*, II, no. 26). In the hundred rolls of 1274–75 it was said that St Peter's, York, had been enfeoffed with part of the vill of Newton-on-Ouse, and [illegible] which was Odo [recte Eudo] de Punchardon's in Grimston (*YQW*, p. 78). In 1284–85 two chaplains held 2 ct. in Grimston of the heirs of Punchardon, who held of Ranulf de Neville by military service (*KI*, p. 63).

There are no Punchardon attestations to surviving acts of Bishops Richard Marsh (1217–1226) and Richard Poor (1228–1237). Sir Eudo de Punchardon witnessed several acta of Bishop Walter Kirkham between 1249 and 1260, including examples of 1252, 1254 and 1259 (*EEA*, XXIX, passim). Not described as a knight, he witnessed a Coxhoe (near Kelloe, co. Durham) deed of 1260 (*Greenwell Deeds*, no. 38). He does not attest acts of Bishop Robert Stichill (1261–1274), but Sir Eudo de Punchardon, possibly a descendant rather than the same man, occurs again as a witness to acts of Bishop Robert of Holy Island, including examples of 1281 and 1283 (ibid., passim).

There does not seem to be anything to connect Sir Eudo de Punchardon to Sir Nicholas de Punchardon, who married Joan of Kepwick, and through her gained interests in Kepwick and elsewhere. Robert son of Meudre held 1 k.f. in Kepwick and elsewhere of Mowbray in 1224 × 1230 (*Bk of Fees*, p. 1460). His interest had passed to Joan of Kepwick by 1267–68 (*VCH Yorks NR*, II, 53, citing Assize R. 1051, m. 18d). Joan was married first to Eustace de Laval, who was dead by 1270, and was mother to Robert de Laval, who came of age in 1284 (*Hist. Northumberland*, IX, 167; ibid., XIV, 404–5). She had married Nicholas de Punchardon by 1276, when the couple sued John of Branton for custom and services in Branton in Northumberland (*Northumb. Pleas*, no. 425; *Hist. Northumberland*, XIV, 404–5). Nicholas de Punchardon, knight, was a juror in an inquisition quo warranto concerning the rights of the bishop of Durham in the manor of Howden and its outliers in 1279, and other inquisitions of approximately the same date concerning Easby (Langbargh wap.) and Whorlton (*YQW*, pp. 127, 130, 154; *Reg. Kellawe*, III, 54). He was witness to a Habton deed in 1279–80 (*YD*, V, no. 194), an Osmotherley deed in 1275 × 1280 (*CalCl*, 1279–1288, p. 62) and a deed pertaining to Newsham, 4 m. north-west of Thirsk, in 1281 (*YD*, II, no. 372). In 1283 Nicholas de Punchardon held ¼ k.f. in Kepwick, about 8 m. north of Thirsk, late of Robert de Neville (*CalInqPM*, II, no. 483). In the survey of 1284–85, there were said to be 3 ct. and 6 bv. in Kepwick held by Nicholas de Punchardon and Joan his wife, who held of Ranulf de Neville, of Roger de Mowbray, as ¼ k.f. (*KI*, p. 97). In 1285 Nicholas de Punchardon and Joan his wife granted the manor of Kepwick to Roger de Benson, to hold of the chief lords. Robert de Laval put in his claim (*YF*, 1272–1300, p. 73). Before 1310 the manor passed to the Knout family, who held it for most of the fourteenth century (*VCH Yorks NR*, II, 53).

**R507.** Gift to the hospital by Eustace FitzJohn of 3 ct. in Heslington [*c.*1145 × 1148]

*Eustachius filius Iohannis de Heselingtun.*
Eustachius filius Iohannis archiepiscopo et capitulo sancti Petri et omnibus hominibus et amiciis suis clericis et laicis presentibus et futuris francis et anglis salutem. Notum sit vobis me concessisse et in elemosinam imperpetuum dedisse hospitali sancti Petri Ebor' et pauperibus ibidem commorantibus iii. carrucatas terre in Haslintuna cum omnibus rebus eisdem pertinentibus quietas et immunes et liberas sicut elemosinam liberam ab omnibus consuetudinibus et geldis et auxiliis et omnibus aliis rebus terre

---

[36]  Described in the deed as 'between York and Stamford Bridge'.

pertinentibus, pro dei amore et sancti Petri et remissione peccatorum meorum et salute anime mee et uxoris mee et filiorum meorum et pro animabus patris et matris mee et omnium antecessorum meorum. Hiis testibus, Agustino priore de Novo Burgo et Reinero canonico suo et Hugone capellano suo et Willelmo de Traci capellano suo, Rogero de Condeio, Bernardo clerico, Willelmo de Vecci, Rogero de Flamvilla, Alitred(o) camerario, Willelmo de Traili, Amarma'duco de Arel, Henrico de Percy, Pagano de Cheuereci, Benedicto de Wimbeltun, Willelmo filio Turb(er)ti, Huctredo de Clivelande, David Hagghat, Ricardo de Essexia satrico[37] et multis aliis.

The 3 ct. given by this deed were those included in the confirmations of Eugenius III in 1148 and Adrian IV in 1157, and correspond to the 3 ct. held by the hospital in 1284–85 of Henry Copsi, who held of Mowbray, who held of the king (HN). Eustace FitzJohn acquired a substantial undertenancy of Roger de Mowbray during the reign of Stephen. After Ranulf earl of Chester captured Mowbray at the battle of Lincoln in 1141, he had been obliged to make a 'beneficial' grant of fourteen fees to Eustace FitzJohn. Greenway dates the feoffment to 'presumably . . . after [Eustace's] return from Scotland in 1143 or 1144, perhaps at about the time that he became constable of Earl Ranulf'. Much of this land was regained by Mowbray, and in 1166 William de Vescy, Eustace's son and heir, and probably the witness to the present deed, held only 2 k.f. of Mowbray (*Mowbray Charters*, pp. xxvii and n, 253–54).

An unspecified gift by Eustace FitzJohn is included in a purported charter of Henry I to the hospital (C23 [*EYC*, I, no. 168]); and in a doubtful charter of Stephen in similar terms, apparently made in 1136 × 1139 (C3 [*EYC*, I, no. 219]). It also appears in Henry II's probably genuine confirmation of 1155 × 1158 (C12 [*EYC*, I, no. 173]). The appearance of the gift in these charters suggests that the hospital was trying to improve an insecure tenancy by forgery (cf. R1n).

Several of the witnesses were closely linked to Roger de Mowbray. Roger de Cundy, Roger de Flamville, and probably Benedict of Wombleton were Mowbray tenants (*Mowbray Charters*, passim). Alfred was chamberlain to Nigel d'Aubigny, and continued in office after the succession of Roger de Mowbray, possibly until the early 1150s. He was succeeded by his son William before 1154 (*Mowbray Charters*, p. lxv). Newburgh Priory was a Mowbray foundation, and the description of the prior shows the deed was issued after c.1145, when the priory was moved from Hood to a site which came to be known as Newburgh, near Coxwold (*EYC*, IX, 206). It may have been made at the time of the gift in c.1145 × 1148, and certainly not later than 1157. In that year Eustace FitzJohn was killed (*ODNB*), and Richard was prior of Newburgh.

**R508.** Confirmation to the hospital by Robert Boscer of his 3 ct. in Heslington which Eustace FitzJohn had given and Roger de Mowbray had confirmed [c.1145 × 1148]

*Confirmatio Roberti Boscher de Heslinctun super tribus carrucatis terre in Hesel(ingtun).*
Dominis suis et amicis et omnibus sancte matris ecclesie filiis Robertus Boscer salutem. Sciatis me concessisse et in perpetuam elemosinam confirmasse pauperibus hospitalis sancti Petri meas tres carrucatas terre de Heslertuna quas Eustachius filius Iohannis eisdem pauperibus concesserat et in perpetuam elemosinam dederat et Rogerus de Molbrai carta sua confirmaverat. Et ego ipse idem concedo et confirmo et imperpetuum do. Huius concessionis testes sunt Geroldus canonicus, Walterus.

---

[37] sic, perhaps for *satyrico*.

Robert Boscer attested four deeds of Roger de Mowbray given in the 1140s (*Mowbray Charters*, p. 30n), and was presumably Mowbray's tenant in Heslington. The suggested date range is that of Eustace's deed.

**R509.** Settlement of a dispute between S[ewal de Boville], the dean, and the chapter of St Peter, York, and R[obert de Saham], master, and brethren of the hospital, touching the great tithes arising from the lands which the hospital was cultivating at the time of the agreement in a newly broken tillage called *le Breke*. The dean and chapter said the tithes belong to their church of St Laurence in Walmgate by parochial right. The master and brethren said they are not bound to pay them, because by papal privilege they are not bound to pay tithes from newly cultivated land, or small tithes. At length, out of respect for the dean and chapter, and to remove the cause of disputes, the master and brethren agreed to pay 10s. annually to the dean and chapter. The master and brethren would be immune from payment of small tithes in the parish of St Laurence, except for the tithes of orchard and garden which the dean and chapter held at the time of the agreement. Furthermore the master and brethren are not bound to pay the accustomed 4s. annually for small tithes. 21 June 1252.

*De x.s. pro []*[38]
Cum inter S[ewal'] decanum et capitulum beati Petri Ebor' ex parte[39] una et R[obertum] magistrum et fratres hospitalis sancti Leonardi ex altera, super decimis garbarum provenientium de terris quas dicti magister et fratres excolebant tempore compositionis istius in cultura quadam de novo exculta que dicitur le Breke, esset exorta materia quovis, quas quidem decimas decanus et capitulum dicebant ad ecclesiam suam sancti Laurenc' in Walmegath iur(e) parrochiali pertinere, dictis magistro et fratribus ex adverso dicentibus se ad earum prestationem non teneri, eo quod a sede apostolica eis est indultum ne ad prestationem decimarum novalium vel minutarum decimarum teneantur nec compellantur inviti. Tandem ob reverenciam decani et capituli, et pro bono pacis ut omnis tolleretur litis occasio, dicti magister et fratres constituerunt se solituros predictis decano et capitulo decem solidos annuos imperpetuum ad festum sancti Martini in yeme et ad Pent' per portiones equales. Et ipsi magister et fratres proventus decimarum illarum in suos versus convertent, et a prestatione minutarum decimarum in parrochia dicte ecclesie sancti Laurencii immunes existent, salvis sepedictis decano et capitulo decimis de virgultis et ortis quia in earum possessione fuerunt tempore compositionis istius. Nec ulterius tenebuntur magister et fratres ad solutionem quatuor solidos quos pro minutis decimis solvere consueverunt. In huius rei testimonium sigillum capituli Ebor' et sigillum magistri et fratrum hospitalis huic scripto in modum cirographi confecto alternatim sunt appensa. Dat' Ebor' xi. kal' iunii anno gracie millesimo CC^mo l^o secundo.

The hospital's land in Heslington was in the parish of St Laurence, Walmgate.[40]

See Reg. Mag. Album, f. 26^v, for similar instrument, concerning a different tillage, of the same date.

---

[38] Left incomplete.
[39] MS: *ex parte* repeated.
[40] The land in Heslington held by the archbishop in 1086 became a peculiar belonging to the Minster prebend of Ampleforth.

**R510.** Inspeximus by S[imon of Warwick], abbot of St Mary, York, of R509 [1258 × 1296]

*De x.s. solvendis pro decimis de nova cultura de Heselingt' que dicitur le Brec.*
Universis cristi fidelibus presentes litteras inspecturis S[imon] misericordia divina dictus abbas sancte Marie Ebor' salutem in domino sempiternam. Noveritis nos inspexisse quandam compositionem inter decanum et capitulum Ebor' et magistrum et fratres hospitalis sancti Leonardi Ebor' initam in hec verba: Cum inter S. decanum et capitulum et c. ut in proxima littera prescripta.[41] In cuius rei testimonium sigillum **[f. 168ʳ]** nostrum presentibus duximus apponendum.

The date range is the period for Simon of Warwick.

**R511.** Conveyance by Eva Roghes, formerly wife of John called 'lord of Walmgate', in widowhood, to Henry son of Roger the baker of Hambleton, of a toft in Heslington between the toft of Serlo of Staingate and [the toft of] Emma Roghes, the grantor's sister, and 5½ a. 1 r. of land and meadow, for a sum of money paid beforehand, and paying 1*d.* yearly to the grantor. If distraint be made in default of rent, the rent should be recovered from Serlo of Staingate and Nicholas of Warthill, because they ought to pay the rent for Eva and Henry at the exchequer of the hospital [*c.*1250 × *c.*1276]

*De terris in Heselyngton'.*
Sciant presentes et futuri quod ego Eva Roghes quondam uxor Iohannis dicti domini de Walmegate in mea libera viduitate concessi dimisi et hac presenti carta mea confirmavi Henrico filio Rogeri pistoris de Hamelton' unum toftum in villa de Heselingtona quod iacet inter toftum Serlonis de Staynegate ex una parte et Emme Roghes sororis mee ex altera[42] et quinque acras et dimidiam et rodam terre et pratum, duas scilicet in campo occident' de Heselington' quarum una pars iacet iuxta casulam Nicholai de Warthill' inter terram Serlonis de Staynegate ex una parte et terram Petri prepositi ex altera, et alia pars iacet iuxta Huarithsich' inter terras prenominatorum virorum, et alia acra iacet iuxta australem partem ville que se extendit usque ad Bounecroftsty et alius finis usque ad Watergote in Langhelandsich inter terras prenominatorum virorum, et duas acras in novo campo quarum una iacet in loco qui vocatur Thoneswayt[43] inter terras Serlonis de Staynegate et Helene filie mee et altera iacet in loco qui vocatur Besingholme inter terras predictorum Serlonis et Helene, et selionem ad Balc ad portam pincerne, et selionem ad finem pontis sicut iacet inter terras Serlonis prenominati et Petri prepositi, et dimidiam acram in australi campo apud Wandayles inter terras Petri prepositi et Iohannis famuli, et totum pratum quod pertinet bovate terre mee in occident' prato, unam dailam iuxta pontem sicut itur ad Ebor' inter Serlonem de Staynegate et Robertum de Cliftun', et iiiiᵒʳ daylas integras in occidentali campo inter prenominatos viros, pro quadam summa pecunie quam michi prorogavit, tenend(a) et habend(a) dicto Henrico et heredibus sive assignatis suis de me et heredibus meis libere et quiete pacifice et integre cum omnibus aisiamentis et libertatibus sine retinemento, reddendo inde annuatim michi et heredibus meis unum denarium scilicet obulum ad Pent' et obulum ad festum

---

[41] *ut . . . prescripta* in the red rubricating ink.
[42] MS: *ex altera* repeated.
[43] Possibly *Thoueswayt*.

sancti Martini in hieme pro omni servicio seculari exactione et demanda. Et si ita contingat, quod absit, quod in prenominatis quinque acris et dimidia et roda terre et prato pro defectu firme solutionis fiat districtio, de Serlone de Staynegate et heredibus suis et Nicholao de Warthill' et heredibus suis firma recipietur, q(ui)a predicti S(erlo) et N(icholaus) et heredes eorum Eve predicte et heredibus suis persolvent et Henrico prenominato et heredibus sive suis assignatis, prebebitur ut de firma ad saccarium sancti Leonardi valeant respondere. Ego vero Eva et heredes mei predictum toftum et predictas quinque acras et dimidiam et rodam terre et pratum prenominato Henrico et heredibus sive suis assignatis ut prescriptum est contra omnes homines et ubique warantizabimus defendemus et acquietabimus imperpetuum. In cuius rei testimonium presenti scripto sigillum meum apposui. Hiis testibus, Roberto filio Iohannis de Cawod', Willelmo de Thorp' de Heselington', Iohanne famulo in Heselington', Petro preposito de eadem, Henrico Waldman, Thoma de Galewayt, Nicholao clerico et aliis.

The grantee gave the land to the hospital in c.1263 × c.1276 (R512).

**R512.** Gift to the hospital by Henry, son of Roger the baker of Hambleton, of the land with a toft in Heslington, which he had by the grant of Eva Roges [c.1263 × c.1276]

*De terra in Heselington'.*
Sciant presentes et futuri quod ego Henricus filius Rogeri pistor(is) de Hameldone concessi dedi et hac presenti carta mea confirmavi deo et pauperibus ac magistro et fratribus hospitalis sancti Leonardi Ebor' pro salute anime mee et animarum antecessorum et successorum meorum totam illam terram cum topst'[44] et omnimodis pertinenciis suis in villa et in territorio de Heselington' quam habui ex concessione et dimissione Eve Roges in eadem, habenda et tenenda eisdem magistro et fratribus ac pauperibus et eorum successoribus omnia prescripta in liberam puram et perpetuam elemosinam cum omnibus pertinenciis suis infra villam de Heselington' et extra imperpetuum. Ego autem Henricus et heredes mei vel assignati mei omnia prescripta predictis magistro et fratribus ac pauperibus et eorum successoribus contra omnes gentes warantizabimus acquietabimus et in omnibus ubique defendemus imperpetuum. In cuius rei testimonium presenti scripto sigillum meum apposui. Hiis testibus, Serlone de Staynegate, Nicholao de Wardhill' civibus Ebor', Willelmo de Thorp', Roberto de Kawode, Roberto de Clyfton', domino Michaele capellano magistri, Willelmo de Beumes senescallo suo, Radulfo de Buhtton' presentium scriptore et aliis multis.

Ralph de Buhtton wrote many deeds for the hospital in the period c.1260 × c.1280. The four leading witnesses attested a quitclaim to the hospital in 1263 × 1276 (R543), and five of the witnesses attested a deed of Thomas, master of the hospital, with the same limits of date (R532).

**R513.** Release and quitclaim to the hospital by Eva Rokes, once wife of John Lauert[45] in Walmegate, of all right and claim in 6 a. in the west field of Heslington [c.1263 × c.1276]

[44] sic, probably for *tophto*, cf. R157.
[45] Possibly *Lanert'*.

*Quieta clamancia de Heselyngton'.*

Universis presens scriptum visuris vel audituris Eva Rokes quondam uxor Iohannis Lauert' in Walmegate salutem in domino sempiternam. Noveritis me concessisse reddidisse et omnino quiet'clamasse de me et heredibus meis imperpetuum magistro et pauperibus hospitalis sancti Leonardi Ebor' totum ius et clameum quod habui vel habere potui in sex acris terre iacentibus in occidentali campo de Heselington', quarum una acra iacet apud le Mar inter terram Serlonis de Staynegate et terram Petri prepositi de Heselington', et dimidia acra apud le Grethil inter terras prenominarorum Serlonis et Petri, et duo seliones, continentes in se tres rodas terre, iacent super Brakenhil inter terras prenominatorum Serlonis et Petri, et una roda super Uttretathe inter terras prenominatorum S(erlonis) et P(etri), et una dimidia roda apud Heselhouhd inter terras predictorum S(erlonis) et P(etri), et una acra apud Heselhouhd et Heykehoud' inter terras prenominatorum S(erlonis) et P(etri), et una roda in Yebeyeme inter terram dicti Serlonis et terram Roberti de Clifton', et una roda super Wytecroft iacens iuxta terram dicti Serlonis ex parte australi, et unus selio continens in se unam rodam et dimidiam inter terram dicti Serlonis et topstu'[46] Ade de Brunne, **[f. 168ᵛ]** et una acra et dimidia ex orientali parte campi iuxta terram dicti Serlonis ex parte orientali, tenend(as) et habend(as) dictis magistro et pauperibus et eorum successoribus integre et pacifice cum omnibus libertatibus aisiamentis et omnibus aliis pertinenciis suis infra villam de Heselington' et extra in liberam puram et perpetuam elemosinam sicut aliqua elemosina melius et liberius dari potest vel teneri. Ita videlicet quod nec ego Eva vel heredes mei seu aliquis ex parte nostra in dictis sex acris terre quas de eis tenui cum omnibus pertinenciis suis aliquod ius clam(eum) vel calumpniam decetero ponere poterimus aut exigere. In cuius rei testimonium presenti scripto sigillum meum apposui. Hiis testibus, Willelmo de Seleby, Serlone de Staynegate, Nicholao de Warthil, civibus Ebor', Willelmo de Thorp', Roberto de Kawod', Radulfo clerico presentium scriptore et aliis.

For the date, see R512, which has similar witnesses. The land does not appear to be that given by Eva to Henry son of Roger the baker by R511.

**R514.** Acknowledgement of receipt, with abbreviated recital, by Nicholas son of John of Warthill, of the deed of master Hugh, rector, and the brethren of the hospital, confirming to him 8 bv. in Heslington, of which 2 bv. lie in the field of *Estorp*, which once belonged to Thomas Roges, and 6 bv. lie in the field of *Westorp*, to be held according to the deeds of the hospital and of the other lords [1238 × 1245]

*Transcrip(tio) confirmationis date Nicholao de Warthill' de viii. bovatis terre in Heselington' etc.*

Sciant omnes presentes et futuri quod ego Nicholaus filius Iohannis de Warthill' recepi cartam hospitalis in hec verba: Omnibus cristi fidelibus ad quos presens scriptum pervenerit magister Hugo rector et fratres hospitalis sancti Petri Ebor' salutem. Noverit universitas vestra nos confirmasse Nicholao filio Iohannis de Warthyl' octo bovatas terre in Heselington', videlicet duas bovatas terre iacentes in campo de Estorp' que aliquando fuerunt Thome Roges et sex bovatas terre in eadem villa iacentes in campo de Westorp', tenend(as) et habend(as) sibi et heredibus suis cum omnibus pertinenciis suis libere et quiete secundum tenorem cartarum domus nostre et aliorum dominorum suorum quas inde habent. In cuius rei testimonium huic

---

[46] sic, for *tophtum*; cf. R157.

scripto sigillum nostrum apposuimus. Testibus, magistro Nicholao de Seleby, Radulfo persona de Neuton' etc. In cuius rei testimonium ego Nicholaus filius Iohannis de Warthill' huic scripto sigillum meum apposui.

The limits of date depend on the appointment of Ralph of Geddington as rector of Newton-on-Ouse in 1238, and the death of master Hugh in 1245. Master Nicholas of Selby, a canon of York, occurs in '1240 × 1244', 1246 and 1249 (*YMF*, II, 95). He was an executor of Hugh of Selby, formerly mayor of York, who died in 1245 × 1246 (ML). The abbreviation of the recital is perplexing. The obligations of the grantee are omitted, so the deed seems to serve no purpose.

**R515.** Gift to the hospital by Thomas de Galeway of Heslington of a toft, a croft, 6 a. land, and 3 r. meadow in Heslington [*c*.1285 × *c*.1300]

*De uno tofto cum uno crofto, vi. acris terre et iii. rodis prati cum pertinenciis.*
Sciant presentes et futuri quod ego Thomas de Galeway de Heselington' dedi concessi et hac presenti carta mea confirmavi magistro et fratribus ac pauperibus hospitalis sancti Leonardi Ebor' unum toftum, unum croftum, sex acras terre et tres rodas prati cum pertinenciis in villa et territorio de Heselington', illud videlicet toftum cum crofto quod iacet iuxta venellam que vocatur Hutgang' que ducit versus Ebor', videlicet ex parte occident(ali) eiusdem venelle, et illas sex acras terre et tres rodas prati que iacent in le Westfeld' et super le Windmylnehill', ubique in campo infra terras dicti hospitalis eiusdem ville, tenendum et habendum dictum toftum cum crofto et vi. acris terre et tribus rodis prati predictis cum omnibus pertinenciis suis prefat(is) magistro et fratribus ac pauperibus hospitalis predicti et eorum successoribus in liberam puram et perpetuam elemosinam imperpetuum. Ego vero Thomas et heredes mei predicta toftum, croftum, sex acras terre et tres rodas prati cum omnibus pertinenciis suis predictis magistro et fratribus ac pauperibus et eorum successoribus contra omnes homines warentizabimus acquietabimus et defendemus imperpetuum. In cuius rei testimonium sigillum meum presentibus apposui. Hiis testibus, Ada Werdenell', Nicholao de Langton', Willelmo le Forest', Iohanne de Warthil, Iohanne Waldeman', magistro Willelmo Coco, Henrico filio Willelmi de Thorp' et aliis.

The land of Thomas de Galeway in Heslington was mentioned in an abutment in a deed of *c*.1270 × *c*.1290 (R529). Galeway attested a Heslington deed in *c*.1250 × *c*.1276 (R511). Nicholas of Warthill and John his son attested on several occasions between 1278 and 1285. John of Warthill may have succeeded by March 1292[/93], when he attested without his father. If so, it was a different Nicholas of Warthill who attested in 1298. John of Warthill attested several York deeds of the 1290s and later, and on occasion described himself as John son of Nicholas of Warthill (Smith, *Merchant Adventurers*, pp. 108–11, 113). He was a bailiff of York in 1290–91 (ML), and in 1301 gave the tenement in Ousegate, York, formerly belonging to his father Nicholas, to the hospital (C838 [Cott., f. 167ᵛ]).

**R516.** Gift and quitclaim to the hospital by Henry, son and heir of Gilbert de Briggesic, of the toft and croft in Heslington which Robert of Fitling formerly held [*c*.1250 × *c*.1265]

*Henricus Brigesike in Hesel'.*
Sciant omnes presentes et futuri quod ego Henricus filius et heres Gilberti de Briggesic caritatis intuitu concessi dedi et hac carta mea confirmavi ac quietum clamavi

deo et pauperibus hospitalis sancti Leonardi Ebor' totum toftum cum crofto in Heselington' quod Robertus de Fitling' aliquando tenuit in eadem, habendum et tenendum eisdem pauperibus predictum toftum cum crofto et cum omnibus pertinenciis suis aisiamentis et libertatibus suis infra villam et extra in liberam elemosinam. Ita quod neque ego neque heredes mei vel aliquis alius per nos aliquod ius vel clam(eum) in predicto tofto cum crofto habere vel exigere poterimus imperpetuum. In huius autem rei robur et testimonium huic scripto sigillum meum apposui. Hiis testibus, Iohanne de Cawude, Willelmo de Thorp', Simone de Holebec, Benedicto de Hewrthe, Roberto dispensatore et multis aliis.

The four leading witnesses were the leading witnesses to a Heslington deed of 1250 × 1265 (R540).

**R517.** Quitclaim to the hospital by Peter of Heslington, called 'the reeve', of all right in the house in Heslington with the buildings, in which he used to live, and in 2 bv. of land which he used to hold of the hospital [*c*.1263 × *c*.1276]

*Quieta clamatio Petri de Heselynton' de ii. bovatis terre et una domo in eadem.*
Omnibus hoc scriptum visuris vel audituris Petrus de Heselington' vocatus prepositus salutem in domino sempiternam. Noveritis me concessisse et omnino quietum clamasse de me et heredibus meis[47] imperpetuum deo et pauperibus hospitalis sancti Leonardi Ebor' totum ius et clam(eum) quod habui vel habere potui in illa domo in Heselingtona cum edificiis et omnibus aliis pertinenciis suis in qua quondam mansi et in illis duabus bovatis terre cum suis pertinenciis quas de eodem hospitali quondam tenui in eadem villa, tenend(a) et habend(a) dictis deo et pauperibus et eorum successoribus libere quiete pacifice et integre, ita scilicet quod nec ego Petrus nec heredes mei nec aliquis pro me seu ex parte mea vel heredum meorum in predicta domo vel in predictis duabus bovatis terre cum pertinenciis aliquod ius clameum seu calumpniam decetero ponere poterimus vel exigere. In cuius rei robur et testimonium presens scriptum sigilli mei impressione munivi. Hiis testibus, domino Serlone de Staynegate, Nicholao de Warthil civibus Ebor', Willelmo de Thorp' in Heselington', Roberto de Cawode in eadem, Roberto de Greshop', Marmeduco de Disceford', armigeris magistri, Willelmo de Stokes tunc senescallo magistri, Radulfo de Buhtton' clerico presentium scriptore et aliis.

The four leading witnesses attested a Heslington deed of 1263 × 1276 (R543). Ralph de Buhtton indicates *c*.1260 × *c*.1280.

**R518.** Conveyance by Thomas, son of Henry Dibbel of Heslington, to John de Holt, parson of Althorp church, and Ralph de Hunkelby chaplain, of the grantor's messuage, lands and tenements in the vill and field of Heslington, which are held of the hospital of St Leonard, York, to hold of the chief lords of the fee by the customary services. Warranty and sealing clauses. 8 June 1349.

**[f. 169ʳ]** *Carta Thome filii Henrici Dibbel de terra in Heselyngton'.*

Hiis testibus, Iohanne de Warthil, Adam Verdinel, Roberto Bennesson', Ricardo de Heselington', Roberto de Lepington', Ricardo de Barneby, Petro Galewey et aliis.

---

47 MS: *meis* repeated.

Dat' apud Heselington' viii. die iunii anno regni regis Edwardi tertii post conquestum vicesimo tertio.

Holt and Uncleby were presumably acting on behalf of the hospital. Holt granted this land to the hospital in 1355 (R519–R520). Ralph of Uncleby acted in a similar capacity for the hospital in 1344 (C518 [Cott., f. 99ᵛ]). Holt, who may have taken his name from Holt, par. Bringhurst, Leics. (*VCH Leics*, v, 54), was closely associated with John Giffard, canon of York and master of the hospital from 1326 until 1349. Holt continued his association with the hospital after the death of Giffard, until his own death in 1356 (C693–C696 [Cott., ff. 135ᵛ–136ʳ]). As John Ward of Holt, clerk, he was presented by John Giffard to the church of Cotterstock in 1333, and as John Holt resigned it before December 1339 (*Reg. Burghersh*, nos 1464, 1618). In January 1339 Holt was instituted rector of Althorpe on Giffard's presentation as master of the hospital (*Reg. Burghersh*, no. 806).[48] John Giffard had interests in Cotterstock, in which place the Holt family had a manor (*VCH Northants*, II, 166, 555–56). In 1344–45 Sir Roger Neufmarché assigned the advowson of Barnby-upon-Don to John Giffard, canon of York, and John Holt, rector of Althorpe. The advowson was subsequently transferred to the college at Cotterstock, which Giffard had founded in 1339 (*Fasti Parochiales*, I, 29).

The manor of Stockholt, in Akeley (Bucks.), a possession of the Giffard family, was conveyed to John Giffard, canon of York, and John Holt, rector of Althorpe (Lincs.), and the heirs of John Giffard in 1347. In 1352 Holt granted Stockholt to Adam Lorimer of Leominster and his wife (*VCH Bucks*, IV, 146). Holt made his will on 5 May 1356 and it was proved on 24 May following (C693–C694 [Cott., ff. 135ᵛ–136ʳ]). In July 1356 Robert Hale of York quitclaimed to Peter Holt of Cotterstock, brother and heir of Sir John Holt, late parson of Althorpe, a messuage in Hale (par. Apethorpe), co. Northants., and the advowson of the church of Hale, and several lands which Sir John Giffard, late canon of York, and Sir John Holt had in Hale and Woodnewton by the grantor's feoffment, which descended to Peter on the death of Sir John Holt (A2A: W(A)/box 2/parcel IV/no. 2/f9).[49] For the manors and possessions held by John son of John Holt, knight, in 1391 and 1419, which included the advowson of the provostship of the collegiate church of Cotterstock, see *CalPat, 1388–1392*, pp. 285–86, and *CalInqPM, 1418–1422*, nos 123–26.

**R519.**    Conveyance to the master and brethren of the hospital of St Leonard, York, by John de Holt, parson of Althorp church, of the messuage and all the lands and tenements in Heselington which he holds of the hospital, which Thomas son of Henry Dibbel gave him and his heirs by his deed, to hold to the master and brethren and their successors from St Martin in Winter 1355 for sixty years, doing the customary services for John to the other chief lords of the fee during the term. Warranty and sealing clauses. 4 October 1355.

*Terra quondam Thome Dibbel dimissa ad firmam hospitali.*

Hiis testibus, Iohanne Russel de Naburn', Adam Verdenell', Ricardo de Barneby, Roberto de Grimeston', Roberto de Brunne, Thoma de Lepyngton', Ricardo de

[48]  The Templars, and later their successors the Hospitallers shared the advowson of Althorpe with the hospital, making alternate presentations (C1046 [Cott., ff. 216ʳ–217ʳ]).

[49]  Northamptonshire Record Office, Earl of Westmorland papers.

Holdernes et aliis. Dat' apud Heselington' die dominica proxima post festum sancti Michaelis archangeli, anno regni regis Edwardi tertii post conquestum Angl' vicesimo nono.

**R520.** Quitclaim to the master and brethren of the hospital of St Leonard, York, by John de Holt, parson of Althorp church, of all right in the messuage and lands and tenements in Heselyngton, which he formerly granted them for a term of sixty years, and which Thomas son of Henry Dibbel gave him. Sealing clause. 6 December 1355.

*Quieta clamatio de terra Thome Dibbel.*

Hiis testibus, Iohanne Russel de Naburn', Adam Verdenel, Ricardo de Barneby, Roberto de Grymston', Roberto de Brunne, Thoma de Lepington' et aliis. Dat' apud Heselington' die dominica prox' post festum sancti Andree apostoli anno domini millesimo CCC^mo quinquagesimo quinto, et regni regis Edwardi tertii post conquestum Anglie vicesimo nono.

**R521.** Appointment by John de Holt, parson of Althorp church, and Ralph de Hunkelby chaplain, of Thomas del Denes as their attorney to receive seisin of a messuage and the lands and tenements in the vill and field of Heselington which they have by the feoffment of Thomas Dibbel, within the fee of the hospital of St Leonard, York, according to a certain deed Thomas Dibbel made to them. Sealing clause. No witnesses. 13 June 1349.

*Littera attorn(ati) Iohannis de Holt et Radulfi de Hunkelby facta Thome de Denes.*

Dat' apud Ebor xiii. die iunii anno regni **[f. 169ᵛ]** regis Edwardi tertii post conquestum vicesimo tertio.

**R522.** Grant in exchange to the hospital by Peter, son of Henry of Heslington, of 2 bv. land in Heslington, being the 2 bv. between the land of Ranulf the reeve and Christine the widow, in exchange for 2 bv. which the hospital has given him [1214 × 1245]

*Petrus de Heselingtona de duabus bovatis terre datis in escambium.*
Sciant omnes presentes et futuri quod ego Petrus filius Henrici de Heselingtona dedi concessi et hac presenti carta mea confirmavi deo et pauperibus hospitalis sancti Leonardi Ebor' duas bovatas⁵⁰ terre in territorio de Heselingtona, videlicet illas duas bovatas terre que iacent inter terram Ranulfi prepositi et terram Cristine vidue in escambium pro duabus bovatis terre quas michi concesserunt, tenendas hereditarie, tenendas et habendas predictis pauperibus predictas duas bovatas terre cum omnibus pertinenciis ad easdem pertinentibus, in puram et perpetuam elemosinam libere integre et quiete ab omni servicio et exactione seculari, sicut aliqua elemosina liberius et melius teneri potest et haberi. Ego autem predictus Petrus et heredes mei predictis pauperibus antedictas duas bovatas terre warantizabimus adquietabimus et defendemus in omnibus et contra omnes homines imperpetuum. In cuius rei robur et testimonium huic scripto sigillum meum apposui. Hiis testibus, Iohanne de Warthil',

---

⁵⁰ MS: *bovatas* repeated.

Henrico de Sezevals, Thoma filio Orm', Gilberto Tillemir', Ranulfo preposito, Petro
Franceys, Willelmo de Creik, Rogero marscallo et aliis.

The hospital's grant in exchange was made in the time of rector Hugh (R523).

**R523.** Acknowledgement of receipt, with recital, by Peter son of Henry of Heslington
of the deed of master Hugh, rector, and the brethren of the hospital, granting
him 2 bv. in Heslington which Ranulf the reeve previously held, between
the land of John of Warthill and the land of Thomas Roges. Also three tofts,
which Henry son of Geoffrey, father of the said Peter, formerly held, which
lie between the toft of Eda of Stockton and the toft of Christine the widow,
paying 4s. 6d. annually, and a portion of chattels on death [1214 × 1245]

*Transcriptum carte Petri filii Henrici de Heselington' de duabus bovatis terre in Heselington'*
*et tribus toftis.*
Sciant omnes presentes et futuri quod ego Petrus filius Henrici de Heselingtona
recepi cartam hospitalis sancti Leonardi Ebor' in hec verba: Omnibus cristi fidelibus
ad quos presens scriptum pervenerit magister Hugo rector et fratres hospitalis sancti
Leonardi Ebor' salutem. Noverit universitas vestra nos concessisse et presenti carta
nostra confirmasse Petro filio Henrici de Hesclingtona duas bovatas terre in Heselingtona quas Ranulfus prepositus aliquando tenuit et que iacent inter terram Iohannis de
Warthil' et terram Thome Roges. Preterea concessimus eidem tria tofta que Henricus
filius Galfridi pater eiusdem Petri aliquando tenuit et iacent inter toftum Ede de
Stoctona et toftum Cristine vidue, tenend(a) et habend(a) predicto Petro et heredibus
suis cum omnibus pertinenciis suis aisiamentis et libertatibus suis infra villam et extra
libere integre et quiete ab omni servicio et exactione seculari, reddendo inde nobis
annuatim pro omni servicio ad nos pertinente iiii.s. vi.d., medietatem ad Pent' et aliam
medietatem ad festum sancti Martini in yeme. Predictus vero Petrus et heredes sui vel
quicumque in predicta terra manserint vel quicumque predictam terram tenuerint
portionem catallorum eos contingentem in obitu pauperibus domus nostre nomine
testamenti fideliter persolvent. Nos autem totum predictum tenementum predicto
Petro et heredibus suis warantizabimus adquietabimus et defendemus in omnibus et
contra omnes homines imperpetuum. In huius autem rei robur et testimonium huic
scripto sigillum nostrum apposuimus. Hiis testibus, Iohanne de Warthil', Henrico
de Sexdecim Vallibus, Iohanne de Cawod', Thoma filio Orm', Gilberto Tillemir',
Stephano filio Godefridi et multis aliis. In cuius rei testimonium ego predictus Petrus
huic scripto sigillum meum apposui.

The date range is the period for Hugh as rector.

**R524.** Quitclaim by Reginald son of Henry of Heslington, to Peter his brother and
his heirs, of all right in the 2 bv. which belonged to Henry son of Geoffrey,
the grantor's father, according to the hospital's deed which Henry had [1212
× 1245]

*Regin(aldus) filius Henrici de H(eselingtona).*
Sciant presentes et futuri quod ego Regin(aldus) filius Henrici de Heselingtona
concessi et quiet'clamavi de me et heredibus meis imperpetuum Petro fratri meo
et heredibus suis totum ius et clameum quod habui vel habere potui in illis duabus
bovatis terre que fuerunt Henrici filii Gedefridi[51] patris mei, tenendas et habendas illas

---

[51]  sic.

duas bovatas terre cum pertinenciis suis de magistro et fratribus hospitalis beati Petri
Ebor', libere integre et quiete secundum tenorem carte magistri predicti hospitalis
quam Henricus pater meus inde habuit. In huius rei robur et testimonium huic scripto
sigillum meum apposui. Hiis testibus, Hugone maiore civitatis Ebor', Iohanne de
Warthil', Ranulfo preposito, Thoma filio Orm', Thoma filio fabri, Gilberto Tillemire,
Stephano filio Godefridi, Henrico le Butiler, Rogero filio Holdewin' et multis aliis.

The extreme dates for Hugh of Selby as mayor are 1212 × 1246 (ML). The quitclaim
presumably predates the associated transactions R523–R524.

**R525.** Abbreviated copy of a purported grant by master Paulinus, rector, and the
brethren of the hospital, to Reginald of Warthill, of 6 bv. in Heslington, in
*Westhorp*, for 11*s*. annually, with free pasture for all his cattle in his house in
Walmgate in the hospital's common pasture of Heslington, and turbary in
Tillmire, with free entry and exit to the said house in York [probably fabri-
cated *c*.1400]

PRINTED: *EYC*, I, no. 320, where dated *c*.1180 × 1200.

*Magister Paulinus rector et fratres de vi. bovatis terre in Heselington'.*
Omnibus cristi fidelibus etc. magister Paulinus rector et fratres hospitalis sancti Petri
Ebor' salutem in domino. Noveritis nos concessisse et presenti carta confirmasse
Reginaldo de Warthil sex bovatas terre in Heselington' in Westhorp' cum omnibus
pertinenciis suis libertatibus et aisiamentis sine aliquo retenemento infra villam et
extra, tenend(as) et habend(as) sibi et heredibus suis libere quiete imperpetuum,
reddendo inde annuatim ecclesie nostre undecim solidos, medietatem ad Pent' et
alteram medietatem ad festum sancti Martini pro omnibus serviciis, sectis curie et
demandis. Concedimus etiam omnia averia sua in domo sua in Walmegate agistata
quieta de herbagio in nostra communi pastura de Heselington', et turbas suas in
turbario de Tilmyr' cum libero introitu et exitu ad dictam domum in Ebor' sine
aliquo impedimento ad ducendum. Hiis testibus, domino Rogero decano, Iohanne
Romano et aliis.

Problems of chronology show this deed to be a forgery. Paulinus was rector until 1203
at the latest, and Roger de Lisle did not become dean of York until 1220. John le
Romeyn becomes prominent in witness lists about 1220, and does not occur before
*c*.1200. There are also problems of style. This is the only deed in which Paulinus
occurs as *magister . . . rector* rather than *magister*, or *humilis minister*. The expressions
*alteram medietatem*, and *reddendo . . . ecclesie nostre* are otherwise unknown in the hospital's deeds. The reference to suit of court, and grant of common of pasture and
turbary are also exceptional. A dispute over these common rights, such as those
evidenced by court records from the early fifteenth century in this section of the
cartulary (R554, R557), must have provided the motive for the fabrication. 6 bv. in
*Westorp* were granted by rector Hugh to Nicholas son of John of Warthill in 1238 ×
1245 (R514), and it was presumably one of Nicholas' successors who was responsible
for the forgery. There is a record of a case in 1404 × 1405[52] between the hospital

---

[52]  The plea is addressed to [blank] bishop of Winchester and chancellor of England, and mentions
Richard Norton 'one of the justices'. Richard Norton first occurs as a justice in 1399 and died in
1420 (*ODNB*), which means the addressee was Henry Beaufort, bishop of Winchester 1404–47, and
chancellor 1403–05 (*HBC*, p. 87).

and Nicholas Warthill and John Neusom, esquires, concerning turbary in Heslington
(Purvis, *Monastic Proceedings*, pp. 163–64). If it was this case which occasioned the
forgery, the copy must have been a recent addition to the hospital's archive when the
cartulary was compiled.

**R526.** Gift and quitclaim to the hospital by Agnes, widow, formerly wife of Natefin,
of all her land in the field of Heslington which she formerly held of the
hospital, comprising 5½ a. land and meadow [*c.*1250 × *c.*1265]

*Agnes vidua de tota terra sua.*
Sciant omnes presentes et futuri quod ego Agnes vidua quondam uxor Natefini,
in mea propria potestate constituta, dedi concessi et hac carta mea confirmavi ac
quietum clamavi deo et pauperibus hospitalis sancti Leonardi Ebor' totam illam
terram meam in campo de Heselingtona quam de predicto hospitali aliquando tenui,
videlicet unam acram terre in le Brende, unam acram in Langethweit, unam acram
terre et prati in Langelandes et Bradebutes, unam acram **[f. 170ʳ]** in Croslandes et
le Syde, unam acram in Stretefurlang' iuxta viam, et dimidiam acram in Hungirhil,
habendum et tenendum dictis pauperibus totum predictum tenementum cum
omnibus pertinenciis suis, aisiamentis et libertatibus suis, infra villam de Heselington'
et extra, ita quod neque ego neque heredes mei aliquod ius vel clameum in predicta
terra vel tenemento antedicto habere poterimus vel exigere imperpetuum. In huius
rei robur et testimonium huic scripto sigillum meum apposui. Hiis testibus, Benedicto
de Hewrth', Willelmo de Thorp', Simone de Holebec, Willelmo de Fulford' clerico,
Thoma Neubond', Waltero Bret, Willelmo Dunyby et aliis.

The three leading witnesses attested together in 1250 × 1265 (R540). Innocent son of
Natefin of Heslington, who was presumably of the same family, quitclaimed all right
in a toft and croft and 2 bv. in Heslington in *c.*1263 × *c.*1276 (R537).

**R527.** Abbreviated transcript of a grant at fee-farm by Thomas, rector, and the
brethren of the hospital to Henry le Woldeman of Heslington of a toft with
croft, between the toft of Geoffrey Dibble and the toft of Henry Bochescollog
in Heslington, and 1 bv. in the same vill, being that which lies next to the
land of Geoffrey Dibble on the west side, paying 16*d.* annually, and a portion
of chattels as an obituary payment [1263 × 1276]

*Transcript(um) Henr(ici) le Woldman' de una bovata terre et uno tofto in Heselington'.*
Omnibus cristi fidelibus presens scriptum visuris vel audituris Thomas rector et
fratres hospitalis sancti Leonardi Ebor' salutem in domino. Noveritis nos concessisse et hoc presenti scripto nostro confirmasse Henrico le Woldman de Heselington'
unum toftum cum crofto iacens inter toftum Galfridi Dybyl et toftum Henrici
Bochescollog' in predicta villa de Heselington', et preterea unam bovatam terre in
territorio eiusdem ville, illam scilicet bovatam que iacet iuxta terram Galfridi Dibil'
ex parte occident(ali), habend(a) et tenend(a) dicto Henrico et heredibus suis de nobis
libere quiete integre bene et in pace cum pertinenciis et omnibus aliis aisiamentis suis
infra villam de Heselington' et extra, reddendo inde annuatim nobis et successoribus
nostris sexdecim denarios argenti, medietatem ad festum sancti Martini in yeme et
medietatem ad Pent' pro omni servicio ad nos pertinente. Dictus autem Henricus
et heredes sui vel quicumque dictam terram tenuerint vel in eadem manserint
portionem catallorum suorum ipsos in obitu suo contingentem pauperibus domus

nostre fideliter relinquent. Et hoc tactis sacrosanctis iuravit idem Henricus pro se et
suis et affidavit.

The limits of date are set by the period for Thomas as rector. The grant is in identical
terms to R528, apart from the name of the beneficiary and the description of the
land, and is probably of the same date, and similarly in chirograph form.

**R528.** Grant at fee-farm by Thomas, rector, and the brethren of the hospital, to
Geoffrey Dibble of Heslington, of a toft with croft, lying between the toft
of Henry le Woldman and the toft of Richard de Hamelton in Heslington,
and 1 bv. in the same vill between the land of Henry le Woldeman and the
land of William of Thorpe, paying 2s. annually, and a portion of chattels as an
obituary payment [1263 × 1276]

*Transcriptum carte Galfridi Dybil de una bovata terre et uno tofto in Heselington'.*
Omnibus cristi fidelibus presens scriptum visuris vel audituris Thomas rector et
fratres hospitalis sancti Leonardi Ebor' salutem in domino. Noveritis nos concessisse et hoc presenti scripto nostro confirmasse Galfrido Dibil de Heselington' unum
toftum cum crofto iacens inter toftum Henrici le Woldman' et toftum Ricardi de
Hamelton' in predicta villa de Heselington', et preterea unam bovatam terre in territorio eiusdem ville iacentem inter terram Henrici le Woldeman' et terram Willelmi
de Thorp', habend(a) et tenend(a) dicto Galfrido et heredibus suis de nobis libere
quiete integre bene et in pace cum pertinenciis et omnibus aliis aisiamentis suis infra
villam de Heselington' et extra, reddendo inde annuatim nobis et successoribus nostris
duos solidos argenti, medietatem ad festum sancti Martini in yeme et medietatem
ad Pent' pro omni servicio ad nos pertinente. Dictus autem Galfridus et heredes sui
vel quicumque dictam terram tenuerint vel in eadem manserint portionem catallorum suorum ipsos in obitu suo contingentem pauperibus domus nostre fideliter
relinquent. Et hoc tactis sacrosanctis iuravit idem Galfridus pro se et suis et affidavit.
Nos autem et successores nostri totum predictum tenementum cum pertinenciis
dicto Galfrido et heredibus suis contra omnes homines warantizabimus quamdiu
carta donatoris nostri nobis poterit warantizare. In cuius rei testimonium duo scripta
unius tenoris ad modum cirograffi sunt confecta, quorum unum residet penes nos
sigillo dicti Galfridi signatum, et aliud penes dictum Galfridum communi sigillo
nostro munitum. Hiis testibus, Willelmo de Thorp', Roberto de Cawod', Nicholao
de Wardhil, Serlone de Staingate, Stephano filio Nicholai, Petro filio Henrici, Iohanne
serviente de Heselington', Radulfo clerico presentium scriptore et aliis.

The date range is the period for Thomas as rector.

**R529.** Grant at fee-farm by the master and brethren of the hospital to John of Hornington and Maud his wife, of a toft and croft in Heslington, which lie in width
between the land of Henry son of Peter on one side, and the land of Thomas
de Galuwayth on the other, and in length from the highway in front, to the
bounds of the meadow of *Waytecroft* behind, paying 4s. 6d. annually, and ½m.
as an obituary payment [c.1270 × c.1290]

*Dimissio terre de Heselington' <de iiii^{or} s. vi.d.>*[53]
Omnibus hoc scriptum cirograffatum visuris vel audituris magister hospitalis sancti

---

[53] A later addition in black ink, apparently in the main hand.

Leonardi Ebor' et eiusdem loci fratres eternam in domino salutem. Noveritis nos communi assensu nostro dedisse concessisse et hoc presenti scripto confirmasse Iohanni de Hornyngton' et Matild(e) uxori eius unum toftum et croftum in villa de Heselington' que iacent in latitudine inter terram Henrici filii Petri ex una parte et terram Thome de Galuwayth' ex altera et in longitudine a regia strata ante, usque ad divisas prati de Waytecroft' retro, tenend(a) et habend(a) predictis Iohanni et Matild(e) uxori eius et eorum heredibus de nobis et successoribus nostris libere quiete integre et pacifice imperpetuum cum omnibus pertinenciis libertatibus communiis pascuis pasturis et aisiamentis ad predicta toftum et croftum pertinentibus infra predictam villam de Heselington' et extra ubique, reddendo inde annuatim nobis et successoribus nostris quatuor solidos et sex denarios argenti ad duos anni terminos, videlicet ad festum sancti Martini in yeme duos solidos et tres denarios, et ad Pent' duos solidos et tres denarios pro omni servicio seculari exactione et demanda. In fine vero obitus dictorum Iohannis et Matild' et heredum suorum unusquisque eorum pauperibus hospitalis predicti dimidiam marcam argenti pro obitu suo [persolvet].[54] Nos vero predicti magister et fratres et successores nostri dictum toftum cum crofto cum omnibus pertinenciis suis ut supradictum est predictis Iohanni et Matild(a) et eorum heredibus pro predicto servicio contra omnes gentes warantizabimus acquietabimus et defendemus imperpetuum. In cuius rei testimonium uni parti istius scripti cirograffati remanenti penes dictos Iohannem et Matild(am) sigillum nostrum commune apposuimus, et sigillum predicti Iohannis alteri parti penes nos remanenti est **[f. 170ᵛ]** appensum. Hiis testibus, Nicholao de Warthill', Ada Verdenell', Radulfo de Thorp', David de Cawode, Iohanne Waldman' et aliis.

The chirograph for grants at fee-farm was introduced while Thomas of Geddington was rector. The omission of the master's name is unusual, as is the expression *communi assensu nostro*. Rector Thomas made a chirograph *de communi consilio et assensu nostro* (C817 [Cott., f. 163ᵛ]), but this form of words is not otherwise used. Ralph of Thorpe succeeded his father William during or after the rectorship of Thomas (FN). Adam Verdenell and Ralph of Thorpe attested deeds by and to Nicholas of Warthill at the end of 1283 (R547, R549). Warthill and Thorpe witnessed together in 1282 × 1283 (R548).

**R530.** Release and quitclaim to the master and brethren of the hospital of St Leonard, York, by Robert, son of Geoffrey de Kirkebi in Kendale, of all right in the tenement and land in Heselington which the grantor and Thomas and Ellis his sons held for their lives by gift of the hospital, and had surrendered. Sealing clause. 15 October 1303.

*Quieta clamatio Roberti filii Galfridi de Kirkebi in Kendale.*

Hiis testibus, Ricardo Derley, Roland' de Thorneburgh', Baldewyno de Schepeshoued', Willelmo de Thornburgh', Rogero de Coquina et aliis. Dat' Ebor' die martis prox' ante festum sancti Luce evang', anno domini millesimo CCCᵐᵒ tertio et anno regni regis E[dwardi] xxxi°.

**R531.** Release and quitclaim to the master and brethren of the hospital of St Leonard, York, by Thomas son of Robert son of Geoffrey de Kirkeby in Kendale, of

---

[54] *persolvent* supplied.

all right in the tenement and land in Heselington which he, his father, and Ellis the grantor's brother held for their lives by gift of the hospital, and had surrendered. Sealing clause. 15 October 1303.

*Quiet(a) clamancia de terra in Heselington' facta magistro et fratribus.*

Hiis testibus, Ricardo de Derley, Rolando Thornburgh', Baldewyno de Schepesheued, Willelmo de Thornburgh', Rogero de Coquina et aliis. Dat' Ebor' die martis prox' ante festum sancti Luce evang' anno domini millesimo CCC^mo tertio, et anno regni regis Edwardi tricesimo primo.

**R532.** Gift by Thomas, rector, and the brethren of the hospital to Roger Botheme of a toft and 8 a. land in *Neufeld* in Heslington, paying 10s. annually and a portion of chattels as an obituary payment [1263 × 1276]

*Dimissio terre in villa de Heselington'.*
Universis presens scriptum visuris vel audituris Thomas rector et fratres hospitalis sancti Leonardi Ebor' salutem in domino. Noveritis nos concessisse et hoc presenti scripto nostro confirmasse Rogero Botheme unum toftum et octo acras terre cum pertinenciis in villa et territorio de Heselington', illud scilicet toftum quod iacet inter toftum quod fuit quondam Galfridi Fyn et toftum quod fuit Roberti de Stoketon', et octo acras terre iacentes in Neufeld' in duobus locis quarum iiii^or acre iacent inter terram Nicholai de Warthill' et terram Roberti de Clifton' et alie iiii^or acre iacent inter terram dicti Nicholai et partem predicti campi occidentalem propinquiores fossato, tenend(a) et habend(a) dicto Rogero et heredibus suis de nobis libere quiete integre cum omnibus aisiamentis et pertinenciis tanto tenemento spectantibus infra villam de Heselington' et extra, reddendo inde annuatim nobis et successoribus nostris decem solidos argenti medietatem ad Pent' et aliam medietatem ad festum sancti Martini in yeme pro omni seculari servicio ad nos pertinente. Predictus vero Rogerus et heredes sui vel quicumque eandem terram tenuerint vel in eadem manserint portionem catallorum suorum ipsos in obitu suo contingentem pauperibus domus nostre nomine testamenti fideliter relinquent. Et hoc iuravit idem Rogerus pro se et suis tactis sacrosanctis et affidavit. Nos autem et successores nostri predictum toftum et predictas octo acras terre cum pertinenciis dicto Rogero et heredibus suis contra omnes gentes warantizabimus quamdiu carta donatoris nostri quam inde habemus nobis poterit warantizare. In huius autem rei robur et testimonium duo scripta unius tenoris ad modum cirograffi sunt confecta, quorum unum residet penes nos sigillo dicti Rogeri signatum, et aliud penes dictum Rogerum communi sigillo domus nostre munitum. Hiis testibus, Serlone de Staynegate, Nicholao Warthill', civibus Ebor', Willelmo de Thorp', Radulfo filio eius, Roberto^55 de Kawode, Iohanne serviente de Heselyngton, domino Ingramo tunc capellano magistri, magistro Willelmo de Fodringheye, Radulfo de Buhtton' presentium scriptore et aliis.

The date range is given by the period for Thomas as rector. The deed has similar witnesses to R512, but there the master's chaplain is Sir Michael, rather than Sir Ingram.

---

55 MS: *Roberto* repeated.

**R533.** Acknowledgement of receipt, with recital, by Henry of Thixendale, citizen of
York, of the deed of master Hugh, rector, and the brethren of the hospital,
confirming to him 1 bv. in Heslington, which Henry has by the gift of Hugh
son of Gospatric, who held of the hospital by hereditary right, with a toft
belonging to the said bovate, paying 2s. annually and 1m. as an obituary
payment [1214 × 1245]

*Transcriptum carte Henrici de Sexdecim Vallibus de una bovata terre de Heselingtona.*
Sciant presentes et futuri quod ego Henricus de Sezevaus recepi cartam hospitalis
beati Petri Ebor' in hec verba: Omnibus cristi fidelibus ad quos presens scriptum
pervenerit, magister Hugo rector et fratres hospitalis sancti Petri Ebor' salutem in
domino. Noverit universitas vestra nos concessisse et presenti carta nostra confirmasse
Henrico de Sezevaus civi Ebor' unam bovatam terre cum pertinenciis in Heselingtona quam habet ex dono Hugonis filii Conspatricii, quam etiam idem Hugo tenuit
hereditarie de **[f. 171ʳ]** nobis et que iacet inter terram que fuit Thome filii Lamberti et
terram que fuit Roberti de Stoctona cum tofto in villa de Heselington' ad predictam
bovatam terre pertinente, tenendam et habendam predicto Henrico et heredibus suis
vel assignatis suis preterquam iudeis et viris religiosis aliis a nobis libere integre et
quiete iure hereditario imperpetuum, reddendo inde nobis annuatim duos solidos,
medietatem ad Pent' et aliam medietatem ad festum sancti Martini in yeme. Predictus
autem Henricus et heredes vel assignati sui vel quicumque predictam bovatam terre
tenuerint pro portione catallorum eos contingentem in obitu eorum pauperibus
domus nostre unam marcam argenti nomine testamenti persolvent. Hoc autem
fideliter observandum pro se et suis tactis sacrosanctis iuravit predictus Henricus
et affidavit. In huius vero rei robur et testimonium huic scripto sigillum nostrum
apposuimus. Hiis testibus, I[ohanne] de Warthil et aliis. In cuius rei testimonium ego
predictus Henricus huic scripto sigillum meum apposui.

The date range is given by the period for Hugh as master.

**R534.** Release and quitclaim to the hospital by Gilbert called 'Tillmire' of Heslington,
of 1 bv. land with toft and croft in Heslington, which Robert his father held
by hereditary right of the hospital [c.1240 × c.1275]

*Gilbertus Tyllemire de H(eselington').*
Sciant omnes presentes et futuri quod ego Gilbertus dictus Tillemire de Heselington'
concessi dedi ac presenti carta mea reddidi ac resignavi et omnino quiet'clamavi
magistro et fratribus ac pauperibus hospitalis sancti Leonardi Ebor' unam bovatam
terre cum tofto et crofto et cum omnibus pertinenciis suis in Heselington', illam
videlicet bovatam terre cum pertinenciis quam Robertus pater meus tenuit in feodo
et hereditate de eisdem, habendam et tenendam predictam bovatam terre cum tofto
et crofto et cum omnibus pertinenciis suis eisdem magistro et fratribus ac pauperibus
antedictis libere integre et quiete imperpetuum, ita quod neque ego neque heredes
mei vel aliquis per nos aliquod ius vel clam(eum) in predicta bovata terre cum pertinenciis suis habere vel exigere poterimus imperpetuum. In huius autem rei robur et
testimonium huic scripto sigillum meum apposui. Hiis testibus, Nicholao de Rauthe-
cliv', Benedicto de Hewrth', Willelmo de Thorp', Iohanne de Cawude, Simone
Holebec, Nicholao de Warthill', Serlone de Staynegate, Waltero de Fulford', Simone
fabro et multis aliis.

Tillmire was the wet area in the south of Heslington township (*VCH Yorks ER,* III,

68, 71). Gilbert Tillmire attested when Hugh was rector (R522, R523). Three of the witnesses attested a deed of 1250 × 1265 (R540).

**R535.** Quitclaim to the hospital by Agnes, daughter of John of Ellingstring, in maidenhood, of all right in 2 bv. land, a toft and a croft, in Heslington, which
Robert of Stockton formerly held of the hospital [*c.*1263 × *c.*1276]

*Quieta clamancia de Heselyngton'.*
Omnibus cristi fidelibus ad quos presens scriptum pervenerit Agnes filia Iohannis
de Ellingstrang' salutem in domino. Noverit universitas vestra me in virginitate et
ligia potestate mea constitutam concessisse et omnino quiet'clamasse de me et heredibus meis imperpetuum magistro et fratribus hospitalis sancti Leonardi Ebor' totum
ius et clameum quod umquam habui vel aliquo modo habere potui in illis duabus
bovatis terre, tofto et crofto et omnibus aliis pertinenciis suis in villa et territorio de
Heselington' que Robertus de Stoketon' quondam tenuit de predicto hospitali in
eadem villa, tenend(a) et habend(a) predictis magistro et fratribus ac eorum successoribus libere quiete integre et pacifice imperpetuum, ita quod nec ego dicta Agnes
nec heredes mei nec aliquis per nos aut nomine nostro in predictis duabus bovatis
terre tofto et crofto aut pertinenciis suis aliquid iuris clamii seu calumpnie ponere
habere exigere vel vendicare poterimus imperpetuum. In cuius rei testimonium
presenti scripto sigillum meum apposui. Hiis testibus, Serlone de Staynegate, Nicholao Warthill', Roberto de Cawod', Ieremia de Brettegate, Ieremia de Luda, Willelmo
de Thorp', Radulfo filio eius, Radulfo de Tresck' clerico presentium scriptore et aliis.

Five of the witnesses attested together in 1263 × 1276 (R543). Ralph de Buhtton,
clerk, wrote many of the hospital's deeds in *c.*1260 × *c.*1280, including examples
concerning Heslington. Ralph of Thirsk, clerk, who attested in 1272 × 1274 (R546),
was perhaps the same man (R537n).

**R536.** Surrender and quitclaim to the hospital by Agnes, widow of Walter of Fulford,
of her third part of the land of her husband in Heslington, which she had by
right of dower [1272 × *c.*1290]

*Quieta clamatio Agnetis uxoris Walteri de Fulford' de dote sua in H(eselington').*
Omnibus presens scriptum visuris vel audituris Agnes uxor Walteri de Fulford'
defuncti salutem in domino. Noveritis me reddidisse et omnino quiet'clamasse
magistro et fratribus hospitalis sancti Leonardi Ebor' totam tertiam partem terre
Walteri de Fulford' viri mei defuncti in villa de Heselington' quam habui vel habere
potui nomine dotis cum omnibus suis pertinentiis infra villam et extra, tenend(am)
et habend(am) dictis magistro et fratribus et eorum successoribus libere quiete et
integre in puram et perpetuam elemosinam, ita quod nec ego nec aliquis per me nec
nomine meo in dicta tertia parte terre et suis pertinenciis aliquid iuris vel clam(ei)
nomine dotis aut aliquo alio modo exigere aut vendicare possimus imperpetuum.
Et ut hec mea remissio et quieta clamancia firmitatis robur optineat imperpetuum
presens scriptum sigilli mei impressione duxi roborandum. Hiis testibus, Roberto de
Cawode, Radulfo de Thorp', Roberto Long' manent(e) in Kelkefelde, Willelmo de
Beaumes, Nicholao de Warthil et aliis.

Walter of Fulford is named in an abutment in 1263 × 1276 (R539). Thomas son of
Stephen of York granted 2 bv. and a rent of 4s. in Heslington to Walter son of Geof-

frey of Fulford, citizen of York, in 1253 × 1272 (R545). Walter quitclaimed the 2 bv. to the hospital in 1272 × 1274 (R546).

**R537.** Release and quitclaim to the hospital by Innocent, son of Natefin of Heslington, of all claim in the toft and croft with 2 bv. which he held of it [*c.*1263 × *c.*1276]

*Quieta clamacio de Heselingt'.*
Universis presens scriptum visuris vel audituris Innocent(ius) filius Natefini de Heslington' salutem in domino sempiternam. Noverit universitas vestra me concessisse remisisse et omnino quiet'clamasse de me et heredibus meis imperpetuum deo et pauperibus ac magistro et fratribus hospitalis sancti Leonardi Ebor' totum ius et clameum quod habui vel habere potui in illo tofto et crofto cum duabus bovatis terre in villa et territorio de Heslington' que de eis tenui in eadem, tenend(a) et habend(a) dictis magistro et fratribus et eorum successoribus libere quiete integre bene et in pace, in liberam puram et perpetuam elemosinam sicut aliqua elemosina melius et liberius dari potest vel teneri, ita scilicet quod nec ego Innocent(ius) nec heredes mei seu aliquis ex parte nostra in dicto tofto et crofto cum dictis duabus bovatis terre cum pertinenciis suis aliquo ius, clam(eum) seu calumpniam aliquo modo decetero ponere poterimus aut exigere. In cuius rei testimonium presenti scripto sigillum meum apposui. Hiis testibus, domino Serlone de Staynegate, Nicholao de Warthil, Willelmo de Thorp' in Heslington', Roberto de Cawode in eadem, Henrico Woldman, Iohanne Seriaunt[56] de eadem, Radulfo clerico presentium scriptore et aliis.

All the witnesses, except Henry Woldman, attested a deed of 1263 × 1276 (R532). Five of the witnesses attested another deed of the same period, with Innocent of Heslington (R539), who can doubtless be identified with the grantor of the present deed; Staingate, Warthill, Thorpe and Cawood witnessed a further deed within the same limits of date (R543).

As the last witness does not trouble to identify himself with a surname (cf. R539, R541), it is likely that there was only one Ralph writing deeds for the hospital during the period, and that Ralph of Thirsk, clerk, who wrote R535 and doubtless R701, and Ralph de Buhtton, clerk, who wrote many deeds between *c.*1260 and *c.*1280, were the same person. We may also speculate that *Radulfo filio Warini presentium scriptore*, the last witness to a deed in favour of the hospital drawn up in 1263 × 1276, was another manifestation of the same individual (M: Arrathorne [MS Dods. 7, f. 144ᵛ]).

**R538.** Release and quitclaim by George de Shupton to the master and brethren of the hospital of St Leonard, York, of all right in those lands and tenements, together with three tofts in Heslington', which Sir Robert de Percy had by demise of the said master and brethren. Sealing clause. No witnesses. 4 October 1320.

**[f. 171ᵛ]** *Quieta clamancia de Heselington'.*

Dat' Ebor' die sabbati prox' post festum sancti Michaelis anno regni regis Edwardi filii regis Edwardi xiiiimo.

---

⁵⁶  sic.

**R539.** Grant at fee-farm by Thomas, rector, and the brethren of the hospital to Adam de Brunne of a toft with croft in Heslington, being that which lies between the toft of Innocent of Heslington and the toft of Walter of Fulford, for 5s. annually and a portion of chattels on death [1263 × 1276]

*Carta Ade Brunne de uno tofto cum crofto in Heselingt'.*

Universis presens scriptum visuris vel audituris Thomas rector hospitalis sancti Leonardi Ebor' et fratres eiusdem domus salutem in domino. Noveritis nos concessisse et hoc presenti scripto nostro confirmasse Ade de Brunne unum toftum cum crofto in Heselington', illud scilicet toftum cum crofto quod iacet inter toftum Innocentii de eadem et toftum Walteri de Fulford', habend(a) et tenend(a) dicto Ade et heredibus suis de nobis libere quiete integre cum omnibus pertinenciis suis aisiamentis et libertatibus suis infra villam de Heselington' et extra, reddendo inde annuatim nobis et successoribus nostris quinque solidos argenti, mediatatem ad festum sancti Martini in yeme et medietatem aliam ad Pent' pro omni servicio ad nos pertinente. Portio vero catallorum dicti Ade et heredum suorum vel eorum quicumque dictam terram tenuerint ipsos in obitu suo quoquo modo contingens pauperibus domus nostre integre remaneat, ita quod ipsi vel eorum aliquis testandi de eadem nequaquam habeant facultatem. Et hoc tactis sacrosanctis iuravit idem Adam pro se et suis et affidavit. Nos autem dictum toftum cum crofto dicto Ade et heredibus suis warantizabimus quamdiu feoffator noster nobis warantizaverit. In cuius rei testimonium duo scripta unius tenoris ad modum cirograffi sunt confecta quorum unum residet penes nos sigillo dicti Ade signatum et aliud penes dictum Adam communi sigillo domus nostre munitum. Hiis testibus, Nicholao de Warthil, Willelmo de Thorp', Petro preposito, Henrico le Woldman', Iohanne serviente, Galfrido Dybel, Innocentio de Heselington', Radulfo clerico presentium scriptore et aliis.

The date range is the period for Thomas as rector.

**R540.** Acknowledgement of receipt, with recital, by Adam de Brunne, of the deed of Robert rector and the brethren of the hospital granting him a toft with croft in Heslington, which belonged to Thomas le Lung, and lies between the land of Walter the carpenter and the land of John Larde, for 7s. annually, and a portion of chattels as an obituary payment [1250 × 1265]

*Dimissio terre in Heselington'.*

Sciant omnes presentes et futuri quod ego Adam de Brunne recepi cartam hospitalis Ebor' in hiis verbis: Omnibus cristi fidelibus ad quos presens scriptum pervenerit, Robertus rector et fratres hospitalis sancti Leonardi Ebor' salutem. Noverit vestra nos concessisse et hac carta nostra confirmasse Ade de Brunne unum toftum cum crofto in Heselington' quod fuit Thome le Lung' et iacet inter terram Walteri carpentarii et terram Iohannis Larde, habendum et tenendum eidem Ade et heredibus suis predictum toftum cum crofto et cum omnibus pertinenciis suis et cum omnibus aisiamentis et libertatibus eidem ville de Hesellington' pertinentibus libere integre et quiete infra villam et extra, reddendo inde nobis annuatim pro omni servicio ad nos pertinente septem solidos, medietatem ad Pent' et medietatem ad festum sancti Martini in yeme. Predictus autem Adam et heredes sui vel quicumque in predicta terra manserit vel dictam terram tenuerit portionem catallorum ipsos in obitu contingentem pauperibus domus nostre nomine testamenti fideliter persolvent. Nos autem predictum toftum cum crofto predicto Ade et heredibus suis warantizabimus quamdiu carta quam inde habemus nobis warantizaverit. In huius rei testimonium huic scripto

sigillum nostrum apposuimus. Hiis testibus, Iohanne de Cawude, Willelmo de Thorp',
Simone de Holebec, Benedicto de Hewrth', Thoma et aliis. In cuius rei testimonium
ego Adam huic scripto sigillum meum apposui.

The date range is the period for Robert as rector.

**R541.** Quitclaim to Thomas rector and the brethren of the hospital by Juliana,
formerly wife of Thomas the smith of Heslington, for a sum of money, of all
right in the toft in Heslington, which Thomas held of the hospital, and which
lies nearest the hospital's garden towards the west [1263 × 1276]

*Quieta clamatio Iuliane uxoris Thome fabri de Heselington' super quodam tofto in eadem.*
Omnibus cristi fidelibus hoc scriptum visuris vel audituris Iuliana quondam uxor
Thome fabri de Heselington' salutem in domino sempiternam. Noveritis me concessisse et omnino quietum clamasse de me et de heredibus meis imperpetuum Thome
magistro et pauperibus hospitalis sancti Leonardi Ebor', pro quadam summa pecunie
quam michi dederunt in mea magna necessitate, totum ius et clameum quod habui
vel aliquo modo habere potui in toto illo tofto cum pertinenciis suis in villa de
Heselington' quod Thomas aliquando vir meus tenuit de eodem hospitali. Et iacet
propinquior capitali gardino suo versus occidentem, tenend(um) et habend(um)
dictis magistro et pauperibus et eorum successoribus libere quiete integre pacifice et
honorifice, ita videlicet quod nec ego Iuliana nec heredes mei vel aliquis ex parte
nostra seu pro nobis in predicto tofto cum pertinenciis suis aliquod ius clam(eum)
vel calumpniam decetero ponere poterimus aut exigere. Et ut hec mea concessio et
quieta clamatio perpetuum robur obtineat presens scriptum sigilli mei impressione
corroboravi. Hiis testibus, Willelmo de Thorp', Serlone de Staynegate, Nicholao de
Warthill', Roberto de Gresshop', Radulfo clerico et aliis.

The date range is given by the extreme dates for Thomas' rectorship. The following
deed may have been given on the same occasion.

**R542.** Quitclaim to Thomas, rector, and the brethren of the hospital by Maud,
daughter of Thomas the smith of Heslington, in maidenhood, of all right in
the toft in Heslington in which Thomas her father formerly lived, being that
which is nearest to the hospital's garden [1263 × 1276]

*Quieta clamatio Matild(e) filie Thome fabri super quodam tofto in Heselington'.*
Universis cristi fidelibus presens scriptum visuris vel audituris Matild(a) filia Thome
fabri de Heselington' salutem in domino sempiternam. Noveritis me in virginitate
mea et ligea potestate concessisse et omnino quietum clamasse de me et de heredibus
meis imperpetuum Thome magistro et pauperibus **[f. 172ʳ]** hospitalis sancti Leonardi Ebor' totum ius et clameum quod habui vel aliquo modo habere potui in toto
illo tofto cum pertinenciis in villa de Heslington' in quo dictus Thomas pater meus
quondam mansit, illud scilicet quod iacet propinquius capitali gardino dicti hospitalis,
tenend(um) et habend(um) dictis magistro et pauperibus et eorum successoribus
libere quiete integre et pacifice, ita scilicet quod nec ego Matild(a) nec heredes mei
nec aliquis ex parte nostra seu pro nobis in predicto tofto cum pertinenciis aliquod
ius clam(eum) vel calumpniam de cetero ponere poterimus aut exigere. In cuius rei
robur et testimonium presens scriptum sigilli mei impressione munivi. Hiis testibus,
Willelmo de Torp, Serlone de Staynegate, Nicholao de Warthil, Iohanne de Suttona,
Roberto de Greshop, Willelmo de Baumees et aliis.

The date range is set by the rectorship of Thomas.

**R543.** Quitclaim to Thomas, master, and the brethren of the hospital by Juliana, widow of Thomas the smith of Heslington, in widowhood, of all right in the toft with croft in Heslington, which is between the land of Henry son of Stephen and the land of Henry the carpenter [1263 × 1276]

*Quieta clamatio cuiusdam tofti in villa de Heselingtona.*
Omnibus cristi fidelibus presens scriptum visuris vel audituris Iuliana relicta Thome fabri de Heslington' salutem in domino sempiternam. Noverit universitas vestra me in libera potestate mea et viduitate constitutam concessisse et omnino quiet'clamasse de me et de heredibus meis imperpetuum Thome magistro et fratribus hospitalis sancti Leonardi Ebor' totum ius et clameum quod habui vel habere potui in toto illo tofto cum crofto et pertinenciis suis in villa de Heslington' quod iacet inter terram Henrici filii Stephani et terram Henrici carpentarii in longitudine et latitudine sine aliquo retenemento, tenend(um) et habend(um) dictis magistro et fratribus et illorum successoribus libere quiete bene et in pace, ita scilicet quod nec ego Iuliana neque heredes mei seu aliquis pro nobis aut ex parte nostra in predicto tofto cum crofto et suis pertinenciis aliquod ius clam(eum) vel calumpniam decetero ponere poterimus aut exigere. Et ut hec mea concessio et quieta clamatio perpetuum robur obtineat presens scriptum sigilli mei impressione corroboravi. Hiis testibus, Serlone de Staynegate, Nicholao Warthill', civibus Ebor', Willelmo de Thorp' in Heselington', Radulfo filio eius, Roberto de Kawode, et multis aliis.

The date range is the period for Thomas' rectorship.

**R544.** Quitclaim to Thomas, master, and the brethren of the hospital by Maud daughter of Thomas the smith of Heslington, in maidenhood, of all right in the toft with croft in Heslington which is between the land of Henry son of Stephen and the land of Henry the carpenter [1263 × 1276]

*Quieta clamancia de Heselington'.*
Omnibus cristi fidelibus presens scriptum visuris vel audituris Matild(a) filia Thome fabri de Heselington' salutem in domino. Noverit universitas vestra me in virginitate et ligea potestate mea concessisse et omnino quietum clamasse de me et heredibus meis imperpetuum Thome magistro et fratribus hospitalis sancti Leonardi Ebor' totum ius et clameum quod unquam habui vel habere potui in toto illo tofto cum crofto et omnibus pertinenciis suis in Heselington' quod iacet inter terram Henrici filii Stephani et terram Henrici carpentarii in longitudine et latitudine sine aliquo retenemento, tenend(um) et habend(um) predictis magistro et fratribus et eorum successoribus libere quiete integre bene et in pace, ita scilicet quod nec ego Matild(a) nec heredes mei seu aliquis pro nobis vel ex parte nostra in predicto tofto cum crofto et suis pertineciis aliquod ius clam(eum) vel calumpniam decetero ponere poterimus aut exigere. Et ut hec mea concessio et quieta clamacio perpetuum robur obtineat presens scriptum sigilli mei impressione roboravi. Hiis testibus, Serlone de Stainegate, Nicholao de Warthill', civibus Ebor', Willelmo de Thorp' in Heselington', Radulfo filio eius, Roberto de Cawode, et multis aliis.

The date range is the period for Thomas' rectorship.

**R545.** Gift by Thomas son of Stephen of York, to Walter son of Geoffrey of Fulford, citizen of York, of 2 bv. and a rent of 4s. yearly from a toft in *Brigkesiche* in Heslington, which Stephen the donor's father held, and the donor claimed to hold, of Nicholas of Warthill and his heirs, to be held by Walter of the same Nicholas, paying him yearly 17s. and 1*lb.* pepper annually [1253 × 1272]

*De terris in Heselington'.*
Omnibus cristi fidelibus hoc scriptum visuris vel audituris Thomas filius Stephani de Ebor' salutem. Noveritis me dedisse concessisse et hac presenti carta mea confirmasse Waltero filio Galfridi de Fulford' civi de Ebor' illas duas bovatas terre et redditum iiii$^{or}$ solidorum singulis annis recipiendum de tofto in Brigkesiche cum pertinenciis suis in Heselingtona, que Stephanus pater meus tenuit et ego clamavi tenere de Nicholao de Warthil et heredibus suis, tenend(a) et habend(a) eidem Waltero et heredibus suis vel quibuscumque assignare voluerit quocumque tempore vite sue de predicto Nicholao et heredibus suis in feodo et hereditate libere integre et pacifice cum omnibus liber-tatibus commun(ibus) et aisiamentis infra villam de Heselington' et extra ad predictas duas bovatas terre et redditui quatuor solidorum pertinentibus sine retenemento, reddendo inde annuatim dicto Nicholao et heredibus suis pro me et heredibus meis septemdecim solidos et unam libram piperis, scilicet octo solidos et sex denarios et unam libram piperis ad Pent' et octo solidos et vi. denarios ad festum sancti Martini in yeme, pro omnibus serviciis consuetudinibus auxiliis et demandis que de dicto tenemento et redditu exiguntur vel exigi poterunt. Et ego vero Thomas predictus et heredes mei predictas duas bovatas terre cum redditu iiii$^{or}$ solidorum et cum omnibus pertinenciis suis warantizabimus defendemus et adquietabimus prenominato Waltero et heredibus suis et eorum assignatis et eorum heredibus contra capitales dominos et contra omnes gentes in omnibus et per omnia imperpetuum per predictum servicium t(antu)m pro me et heredibus meis annuatim ut predictum est faciendum. In cuius rei testimonium presens scriptum sigilli mei appositione roboravi. Hiis testibus, Roberto Blundo tunc ballivo de Ebor', Willelmo de Holteby, Roberto de Eltoft', Hugone Blundo, Willelmo de Wixstowe, Henrico filio Uhttring de Heselington', Willelmo fratre eius, Stephano filio Matild(e), Ricardo clerico et aliis.

Robert le Blund first occurs as a bailiff of York when Gaceus de Chaumont was mayor, in 1253 × 1257. He served several terms, the last ending in 1277 (ML). This deed precedes Walter's quitclaim, and must have been issued before the appointment of the bailiffs who attested that deed (R546).

**R546.** Quitclaim to the hospital by Walter son of Geoffrey of Fulford of all right in 2 bv., which he had by gift of Thomas son of Stephen of York, in Heslington, in the east field, and in the toft with croft which Juliana Elvina held of the hospital in the same vill, paying Nicholas of Warthill 17s. and 1*lb.* pepper annually [19 August 1272 × 11 May 1274, probably Michaelmas 1272 × Michaelmas 1273]

**[f. 172ᵛ]** *De terris in villa et territorio de Heselyngton'.*
Sciant omnes presentes et futuri quod ego Walterus filius Galfridi de Fulford' concessi dedi et hac presenti carta confirmavi ac imperpetuum de me et heredibus meis omnino quiet'clamavi magistro et fratribus hospitalis sancti Leonardi Ebor' totum ius et clameum quod unquam habui vel aliquo modo habere potui in illis duabus bovatis terre quas habui de dono et concessione Thome filii Stephani de Ebor' in territorio

de Heselington' in campo orientali et in illo tofto cum crofto que Iuliana Elvine[57] tenuit de predictis magistro et fratribus in eadem villa, tenend(a) et habend(a) predictas duas bovatas terre et toftum cum crofto et cum omnibus pertinenciis libertatibus et aisiamentis ubique infra predictam villam de Heselington' et extra predictis duabus bovatis terre tofto et crofto pertinentibus sepedictis magistro et fratribus et eorum successoribus libere quiete integre pacifice et honorifice in liberam et perpetuam elemosinam, reddendo inde annuatim Nicholao de Warthil et heredibus suis pro me et heredibus meis vii[tem] et decem solidos argenti et unam libram piperis, scilicet octo solidos et vi. denarios et unam libram piperis ad Pent' et octo solidos et vi.d. ad festum sancti Martini in yeme, pro omni servicio seculari exactione et demanda, ita scilicet quod nec ego dictus Walterus nec heredes mei nec aliquis ex parte nostra in dicta terra tofto et crofto cum suis pertinenciis aliquid iuris clam(ei) vel calumpnie exigere habere vel vendicare poterimus imperpetuum. Et ego dictus Walterus et heredes mei totam predictam terram et toftum cum crofto et omnibus aliis pertinenciis suis ut predictum est predictis magistro et fratribus et eorum successoribus contra omnes gentes warantizabimus adquietabimus et defendemus imperpetuum. In cuius rei testimonium presenti scripto sigillum meum apposui. Hiis testibus, Iohanne Speciar' tunc maiore Ebor', Nicholao de Seleby, Henrico de Holteby et Rogero Basy tunc ballivis Ebor', Serlone de Staynegate, Roberto Blundo, Roberto de Cawod', Radulfo de Tresk' clerico et aliis.

This mayor and bailiffs occur in December 1272, and January and April 1273. Walter de Stokes was still mayor on 19 August 1272, and different bailiffs are named on 11 May 1274. The narrower date limits rest on the presumed appointment of new bailiffs at Michaelmas (ML).

**R547.** Release and quitclaim to the hospital by Nicholas of Warthill of a rent of 4s. which he used to receive from the hospital for a tenement which they held of the grantor in Heslington, in the fee of Robert of Clifton. 14 December 1283.

*Quieta clamatio Nicholai de Warthill' de annuo redditu iiii.s. in Hesel'.*
Sciant presentes et futuri quod ego Nicholaus de Warthill' concessi remissi et omnino quietum clamavi de me et heredibus meis rectori et fratribus hospitalis sancti Leonardi Ebor' et eorum successoribus imperpetuum quatuor solidos annui redditus quas percipere consuevi de dictis magistro et fratribus de quodam tenemento quod de me tenent in Heselington' de feodo Roberti de Clifton', ita quod nec ego nec heredes mei nec aliquis per nos aliquid de cetero de predictis iiii[or] solidis cum pertinenciis exigere vendicare nec habere poterimus. In cuius rei testimonium presenti scripto sigillum meum apposui. Hiis testibus, Ada Verdinell', Nicholao de Seleby, Roberto de Cawude, Radulfo de Thorp', Roberto Ster et aliis. Dat' Ebor' in crastino sancte Lucie virginis anno domini millesimo CC[mo] lxxx° tertio.

See R549 for Robert of Clifton's confirmation and quitclaim.

**R548.** Surrender and quitclaim to the hospital by Robert called 'of Clifton', living in York, of a toft and a bovate in Heslington [April 1282 × October 1283]

---

[57] Perhaps *Elvive*. Elvina and Elviva both occur as given names.

*Quieta clamatio Roberti de Clifton' de uno tofto et i. bovata terre in Heselington'.*
Omnibus cristi fidelibus ad quos presens scriptum pervenerit Robertus dictus de Clifton' manens in Ebor' salutem in domino. Noverit universitas vestre me pro me et heredibus meis reddidisse et omnino quietum clamasse magistro et fratribus hospitalis sancti Leonardi Ebor' unum toftum et unam bovatam terre cum omnibus pertinenciis suis que habui de dictis magistro et fratribus hospitalis predicti in villa et territorio de Heselington', tenend(a) et habend(a) eisdem magistro et fratribus et eorum successoribus libere quiete integre et pacifice in puram et perpetuam elemosinam, ita quod nec ego nec aliquis heredum meorum nec aliquis nomine nostro in dictis tofto et bovata terre cum eorum pertinenciis aliquid iuris vel clamei decetero exigere poterimus aut vendicare. Ego vero dictus Robertus et heredes mei dictum toftum et bovatam terre cum pertinenciis suis predictis magistro et fratribus et eorum successoribus contra omnes homines warantizabimus acquietabimus et defendemus. Et ut hec mea remissio et quietaclamatio firmitatis robur optineat imperpetuum presens scriptum sigilli mei impressione duxi roborandum. Hiis testibus, Iohanne de Lethegreines tunc vice-comite Ebor', Nicholao de Warthil, Iohanne Sampson', Iohanne apotecario, civibus Ebor', Roberto de Cawode, Radulfo de Thorp', Ada de Brunne de Heselington' et multis aliis.

John de Lithegraines was sheriff of Yorkshire between 1280 and 1285, and became keeper of the city after 13 April 1282, during the suspension of the mayorality in 1280–83. In October 1283 John Samson was named as mayor (ML). It is unlikely that Lithegraines would have attested this deed except as keeper of the city. Gascoigne has written *8: Ed: 1* in the margin next to Lithegraines' name, using his distinctive 'i' form for '1'.

**R549.** Release and quitclaim by Robert of Clifton, to Nicholas of Warthill and the hospital, of 4s. annual rent which he used to receive from a tenement in Heslington by the hand of Nicholas, which tenement the hospital holds of the grantor's fee in Heslington. 14 December 1283.

*Quieta clamatio Roberti de Clifton' de iiii⁰ʳ s. in Heselington'.*
Sciant presentes et futuri quod ego Robertus de Clifton' concessi remisi et omnino quietum clamavi de me et heredibus meis imperpetuum Nicholao de Warthil et hospitali sancti Leonardi Ebor', rectori et fratribus ibidem deo servientibus et imper-petuum servituris, iiii⁰ʳ s. annui redditus quos percipere consuevi de quodam tene-mento cum pertinenciis in Heselington' per manus dicti Nicholai, quod tenementum iidem rector et fratres tenent de feodo meo in eadem villa, ita quod nec ego nec heredes mei aliquid de predictis iiii⁰ʳ solidos cum pertinenciis decetero exigere poterimus vendicare nec habere. In cuius rei testimonium presenti scripto sigillum meum apposui. Hiis testibus, Ada Verdinel, Nicholao de Seleby, Roberto de Cawode, Radulfo de Thorp', Roberto Ster et aliis. Dat' Ebor' in crastino sancte Lucie virgine anno domini millesimo CCᵐᵒ lxxx⁰ tertio.

**R550.** Quitclaim by Gilbert son of Robert of Clifton, to Robert his father, of all the land in the territory of Heslington in *Westorp* whether in turbary or pasture, to hold to Robert, doing the customary service to the hospital, and to the grantor and his heirs a rose in the season for roses. Warranty against Christians and Jews [*c.*1270 × *c.*1290]

*Quietaclam(acio) Gilberti filii Roberti de Clifton' de terra in Hesel'.*

Sciant presentes et futuri quod ego Gilbertus filius Roberti de Clifton' pro me et heredibus meis concessi ac de me et heredibus meis omnino quietum clamavi imperpetuum Roberto de Cliftona patri meo et heredibus suis et assignatis **[f. 173ʳ]** totam illam terram cum pertinenciis in territorio de Heselington' iacentem in Westorp' tam in turbariis quam pasturis et omnibus aliis aisiamentis, tenendam et habendam totam predictam terram predicto Roberto et heredibus suis et assignatis ab omni actione mei seu heredum meorum quietam libere pacifice et integre imperpetuum, ita quod nec ego dictus Gilbertus nec heredes mei nec aliquis pro nobis seu nomine nostro aliquod ius vel clam(eum) in tota predicta terra cum suis pertinenciis nec in aliqua sui parte decetero habere vel exigere seu vendicare poterimus in futur(um), reddendo inde annuatim servicia exinde debita et consueta magistro hospitalis sancti Leonardi et michi et heredibus meis unam rosam tempore rosarum pro waranto tantum modo. Et ego vero dictus Gilbertus et heredes mei totam predictam terram cum pertinenciis predicto Roberto et heredibus suis et assignatis pro predictis serviciis contra omnes cristianos et iudeos warantizabimus acquietabimus et defendemus imperpetuum. In huius rei testimonium presentem cartam sigillo meo roboravi. Hiis testibus, Ada de Werdenel, Roberto de Cawode, Nicholao de Warthill', Radulfo de Thorp', Rogero de Bothum, Iohanne Waldeman', Thoma de Gaylewaithe, Roberto Albo clerico et multis aliis.

The witness Ralph of Thorpe was the son of William of Thorpe. William of Thorpe, sometimes called 'William of Thorpe in Heslington', and so associated with the place which gave its name to the fields of *Estorp* and *Westorp* (R514), attested many of the Heslington deeds which have been ascribed to *c*.1250 × *c*.1265 and *c*.1263 × *c*.1276. His land is mentioned in an abutment in a deed of 1263 × 1276 (R528). In 1263 × 1276 he attested with Ralph his son (R532, R535, R543). Ralph of Thorpe attested, presumably after his father's death, in *c*.1270 × *c*.1290 (R529), 1272 × *c*.1290 (R536) and 1282 × 1283 (R548). Henry son of William of Thorpe attested in *c*.1285 × *c*.1300 (R515). Adam Verdinel, Robert de Cawood, and Ralph of Thorp attested in 1283 (R547, R549). A date before *c*.1290 is indicated by the warranty against Jews, which was rendered obsolete by the Edict of Expulsion of 1290.

**R551.** Grant by John de Warthill of York to William son of Robert Oustyby of Hyldirthorp, smith, of St Leonard and his heirs and assigns, of one toft and croft with appurtenances in the vill of Heslington, which was formerly held of the grantor by Cecilia widow of John de Huntyngton, to hold to William, his heirs and assigns, excluding men of religion, of the chief lords of the fee by the due and customary services, in fields, meadows, pastures, moors and turbaries, paying the grantor and his heirs 4s. annually at Pentecost and St Martin in winter by equal portions for all service. Warranty and sealing clauses. Reversion to the grantor if William, his heirs or assigns, are unable to maintain the houses or pay the rent. 24 August 1317.

*De terris in Heselington'.*

Hiis testibus, Radulfo de Sylkyston' de Heselyngton', Iohanne Waldeman' de eadem, Henrico Dybbyll' de eadem, Henrico de Berley de eadem, Roberto dicto celerer man de eadem, Iohanne de Hessey de eadem, Petro de Neuton' clerico et multis aliis. Dat' apud Heselington' die mercur' in festo sancti Barthol' apostoli anno regni regis Edwardi filii regis Edwardi undecimo.

**R552.** Release and quitclaim by William, son of Robert Oustiby of Hilderthorp, smith, to the master and brethren of the hospital of St Leonard, York, and their successors, of all right and claim in one toft and croft with appurtenances in Heselingtone which he had by the gift of John de Warthill of York and which Cecilia widow of John de Huntyngtone held, to be held by the due and customary services. Warranty and sealing clauses [*c*.1325 × *c*.1340]

*Quieta clamancia Willelmi de Hilderthorp' de tofto et crofto in Heselington'.*

Hiis testibus, Roberto de Dalby, Willelmo de Lithingtone, Ricardo de Burtone, Willelmo de Thorp', Iohanne de Naburne, Roberto de Lepington', Iohanne Waldeman' de Heselingtone et aliis.

William Annaisburton of York, ironmonger, gave to William Hilderthorpe of York, smith, a rent of 8*s*. in Marketshire in 1316, which Hilderthorpe later quitclaimed to the hospital by an undated deed given before the first four witnesses to the present deed and others (C796–C798 [Cott., ff. 158ᵛ–159ʳ]). The witness Robert Dalby occurs in 1327, 1328, 1330, 1334[/35] (Smith, *Merchant Adventurers*, pp. 64, 65, 84, 90), 1337, 1338, 1342, 1343, and 1344 (C513–C518 [Cott., ff. 98ᵛ–99ᵛ]). He was a bailiff in 1332 (*CVC*, I, nos 180, 556). It was probably another Robert Dalby who attested in 1360 (C861 [Cott., f. 174ʳ]). Lithington, Burton and Thorpe witnessed together in 1330 (C478 [Cott., f. 90ʳ]).

**R553.** Grant by Henry son of Thomas FitzHenry de Kelfeld knight (*militis*), to Sir Nicholas de Bubwith, master Richard de Holme, master Alan Newerk, and John de Popilton the elder, clerks, of an annual rent of 10*s*. arising from all the lands and tenements in Heslyngton which the master and brethren of the hospital of St Leonard, York, hold of him, and which descended to him after the death of his father, the said Thomas, to be held of the chief lords of the fee **[f. 173ᵛ]** by the due and customary services. Warranty and sealing clauses. 12 April 1404.

*Carta Henrici filii Thome filtz Henrici de redditu annuo decem solidorum etc. ut infra.*

Hiis testibus, Gerardo Salvayn', Thoma Colvyll', Willelmo Rither, militibus, Iohanne Mergrave, Francisco Palmes, Nicholao Northfolk', Henrico Akelom', Willelmo Helmeslay, Rogero Shalford' et aliis. Dat' apud Heslyngton' duodecimo die mensis aprilis anno domini millesimo CCCCᵐᵒ quarto, et regni regis Henrici quarti post conquestum Anglie quinto.

A change in the quality of both red and black ink indicate that this deed, and those following in the Heslington section, were appended somewhat after the main period of compilation, but the hand is that of the original cartularist. The grantor was a descendant of Robert son of Copsi, who gave 1 ct. to the hospital in 1148 × 1154, reserving the 10*s*. rent quitclaimed by this deed (R501; *EYC*, v, 53–58; *Ctl. Gisborough*, II, 183–84).

**R554.** Inspeximus, dated 12 July 1403, by Henry [IV], of the record and process of a plea in his court of king's bench, by his writ, between master William Waltham, master of the hospital of St Leonard, York [the plaintiff] and William Strensall, Thomas Bernard, John Hert, Thomas Haukyn, Thomas de Banke, Thomas

Bateson, Thomas Hert and John Hornchilde [the defendants], concerning a certain trespass made on the plaintiff by the defendants.

Plea at Westminster before William Thirnyng and his fellows, justices, in Michaelmas term, 3 Hen. IV [1401], roll 203, York. The defendants were attached to answer the plaintiff as to why they, together with John Knapton senior, Thomas Shepherd of Heselynton, John Knapton junior, Thomas de Thorpe and John Revell, by force and arms, broke a close and embankment (*fossatum*) of the plaintiff at Heselynton, and depastured his grass to the value of £10 with certain beasts, to the damage of the plaintiff and against the king's peace. The plaintiff, by John Wyther his attorney, complains that the defendants, on Wednesday next after the feast of Holy Trinity, 2 Hen. IV [24 May 1401], by force and arms, that is swords, bows, and arrows, broke an enclosure and embankment and depastured the grass with horses, bulls, cows, draft animals, sheep and pigs, to the value of £40. And the plaintiff produces suit thereof. William Strensall, Thomas Bernard, Thomas Haukyn and John Hornchilde come in person and John Hert, Thomas de Banke, Thomas Bateson and Thomas Hert by John Bekwith their attorney. William Strensall says he is not guilty of entering by force and arms and all the trespass except entering the close. He denies breaking the embankment and depasturing the grass, and puts himself on the country. He says the place where the trespasses were made is called Thrusshawe, and is part of the moor of the vill of Heselyngton. He says that Maud, who was wife of John Verdynall, was seised of ½ bv. land with appurtenances in Heselyngton, and other land and tenements in the same vill. The said Maud, and all those with legal right in that ½ bv. and land and tenements from time beyond memory, had common in the said moor of Heselyngton of which the place called Thrusshawe was part, for every kind of animal, whatever the time of year. He says that the same Maud granted him that ½ bv. for a term of three years, from the feast of St Michael 1 Hen. IV [29 September 1400]. And because the master enclosed that place with embankments, William Strensall [f. 174ʳ] broke one of the embankments, and entered the enclosure and depastured the grass there as was his right. And he intended no injury. The other seven defendants all say they are not guilty. They say that William del Wode, prebendary of the prebend of Ampilford, in the cathedral church of St Peter's, York, has six messuages, a croft, 13½ bv. land, and other messuages, land and tenements in Heselyngton, by right of his prebend, which tenement had common in the moor from time beyond memory. And they say they hold separately of William del Wode, some at will, some for a term of years, and they held at the time of the alleged transgression, Thomas Bernard a messuage and a croft at will, John Hert a messuage and a croft at will, Thomas Haukyn a messuage and ½ bv. land for a term of years, John Hornechilde a messuage and ½ bv. land at will, Thomas de Banke a messuage and croft at will, Thomas Bateson a messuage and 2 bv. land at will, Thomas Hert a messuage and 2 bv. at will, by which they had common at the time of the supposed offence. The master, protesting he did not know a place called Thrusshawe, but that the place of the transgression is called Thrispole, otherwise called *separale* of the hospital of St Leonard's, York. [f. 174ᵛ] They put themselves on the country. Therefore it is ordered that the sheriff should have at the octave of St Hilary twelve [jurors] etc. On which Thomas Bernard, Thomas Haukyn, John Hornechilde and Thomas Banke mainprised William Strensall. And William Strensall, Thomas Haukyn, John Hornechilde and Thomas Banke mainprised the said Thomas Bernard. And William Strensall,

Thomas Bernard, Thomas Banke and John Hornchilde mainprised the said Thomas Haukyn. And William Strensall, Thomas Bernard, Thomas Banke, and Thomas Haukyn mainprised John Hornechilde to have their bodies before them at the said term. At which day the parties came etc. And the sheriff did not send the writ. Therefore it was ordered to the sheriff to come a month from Easter with twelve [jurors] etc. And so until this day, three weeks from Easter, 4 Hen. IV, unless the justices of the king take assizes in Yorkshire on Monday in the second week in Lent next at York. Afterwards, on the day stated, before William Gascoigne and Thomas Tyldesley, king's justices of assize in county York, came William Waltham, master of the hospital of St Leonard, by his attorney; William Strensall, Thomas Bernard, Thomas Haukyn and John Hornechilde in their own persons, and John Hert, Thomas de Banke, Thomas Bateson and Thomas Hert by John Bekwith their attorney. And the jurors come and say on their oath that the place where the enclosure and embankment was broken, and the grass depastured, is called Thrispole, otherwise called *separale* of St Leonard's hospital, York. And Maud who was wife of John Verdynall, of whom William Strensall holds for a term of years, had common in that place, as William Strensall alleged, and also that William del Wode, prebendary of Ampilford, and his predecessors had common, within which Thomas Bernard, Thomas Haukyn, John Hornechilde, John Hert, Thomas de Banke, Thomas Bateson and Thomas Hert hold of William del Wode, just as they alleged. And they say **[f. 175ʳ]** the defendants are guilty of the remaining offences specified in the writ. And they assess the damage at 10*m*. Therefore it is adjudged that master William Waltham should receive the damages from the defendants assessed at 10*m*. And the defendants should be taken etc. The king has caused the record to be exemplified, and made patent.

*De separali de Heslyngton'.*

Teste me ipso apud Westmonaster(iu)m duodecimo die iulii anno regni nostri quarto.

William Wood held the prebend of Ampleforth from 1389 until 1410.

**R555.** York. Recognition by John Langton of his debt to the king of 500*m*. to be paid next Michaelmas. In default the money to be raised on his lands and chattels in Yorkshire and elsewhere. The condition of the recognition was that if John, on the quindene of Michaelmas next came before the king in chancery in person to respond to all matters concerning the master and hospital of St Leonard, York, or if on that date he could show letters of Thomas, bishop of Durham, or Ralph, earl of Westmorland, that he and the master had come to an agreement, then the recognition would be void. 18 November [1416]

CALENDAR: *CalCl*, 1413–1419, p. 372.

*Recognitio Iohannis Langton'.*

T(este) r(ege) apud Westm' xviii. die novembris.

**R556.** Cancellation of R555, as the said earl by letters patent under his seal, filed in chancery, 5 [Hen. V], on the said quindene, certified that the parties were agreed. 13 October 1417.

CALENDAR: *CalCl*, 1413–1419, p. 372.

*Cancellatio eiusdem.*

**R557.** Plea at Westminster before William Babyngton and his fellows, justices of the king's bench, Easter term, 2 Hen. VI [1424], roll 394.

York. John de Langton' of Hodeleston in Yorkshire, knight, and Eufemia his wife were summoned to answer the master of the hospital of St Leonard, York, as to by what right they claimed common of turbary in the field of the master in Heslyngton. The master says by Thomas Sutton his attorney that John and Eufemia unjustly claim common of turbary in the field of the said master in Heslyngton, namely digging turves in 200 a. of moor of the said master, called Severell, lying between the common pasture of the vill of Foulford towards Le Cause in the same vill on the west side, and Le Tilmyre on the east side, in width, and from the common moor of Heslyngton as far as the closes called Ameriddynges in the vill of Heslyngton, at whatever time of year. The master had no right of common in the field of John and Eufemia, nor did they perform any service whereby they ought to have common in the field of the master. And the master thereby had damages of £40. And he produces suit thereof.

And John and Eufemia, by Robert Ben, their attorney, came and defended etc. They say that they have common of turbary in the said 200 a. for their fire at whatever time of year, as appendant to a messuage and 16 bv. land in Heslyngton. They were seised of the said common as of fee, and by right, in time of peace in the reign of Henry, former king of England, father of the now king, **[f. 175ᵛ]** as were all others who had an estate in the said messuage and land from time beyond memory. And the master is prepared to defend his right by the body of his free man John son of John Berkeworth, who is in court. And John de Langton and Eufemia are prepared to defend their right by the body of their free man Thomas son of Nicholas Gregory, who is in court. And Thomas son of Nicholas and John son of John are prepared to conduct the duel. Therefore it is considered that the duel should take place. John and Eufemia found pledges John Coventre and Richard Bukland, and the master found pledges John Bluet and William Kirkeby. And **[f. 176ʳ]** Friday the feast of St Augustin, apostle of the English [26 May 1424], is given. On this day the master came by his attorney with John son of John the champion. And John de Langton and Eufemia did not come. Therefore it is adjudged that the master should hold the said 200 a. as private land (*in separalite*), quit of John and Eufemia. And John and Eufemia, and their pledges of duel, are amerced.

[Hand D. The heading is in black ink, and no provision is made for a larger capital.]

COPIES: *b* Rawl. ff. 175ʳ–176ʳ; *c* Borthwick Institute, Yarburgh Muniments, YM/D/ HES/MISC/1, exemplification at the request of Thomas Eynns, esq., 1 February 1574, not collated.

*Placita apud Westm' coram Willelmo Babyngton' et sociis suis iusticiariis domini regis de banco de termino pasch' anno regni regis Henrici sexti post conquestum Anglie secundo. Rotulo CCC. lxxxxiiii.*

# Hugate [Huggate]

In 1086, the king had 8½ ct. in Huggate, and Earnwine the priest 8 ct. In 1284–85 there were said to be 10 ct. in the Greystoke fee in Huggate, which the prior of Watton held in free alms, having entry by Geoffrey de Mandeville (*KI*, p. 89).[1] Farrer identified these 10 ct. as the 8 ct. held by Earnwine at the Survey, together with another 2 ct. in Hawold nearby. The king's land in Huggate became part of the Fossard fee (*EYC*, II, 396–97). Forne son of Sigulf, the ancestor of the Greystoke family, came to prominence during the reign of Henry I, and acquired his fee piecemeal in the period between *c.*1110 and 1130, in which year he was dead (*EYC*, II, 505). The Mandeville tenancy of Greystoke is apparent in 1166, when Ernulf de Mandeville held 1 k.f. of Ranulf son of Walter [of Greystoke]. Ernulf is the only tenant named in Ranulf's *carta* (*EYC*, II, no. 1244). The descent of the fee in Huggate through Forne's daughter Edith, wife to Robert de Oilly, and Edith's presumed daughter Alice, wife to Ernulf de Mandeville, first established by Farrer (*EYC*, II, 505–06, 509) is discussed below.

There is no reference to Huggate in the papal confirmation to the hospital of 1148, but the confirmations of 1157 and 1173 include a grant made by Robert de Oilly and his wife of 20s. annually from Huggate (C178 C180 [*EYC*, I, nos 179, 186, 197]). As Robert de Oilly switched his allegiance to the empress after King Stephen's capture at Lincoln in February 1141 (*Gesta Stephani*, p. 117), and was dead in 1142, it is probable that the rent was granted in *c.*1136 × 1140. During the reign of Stephen the hospital granted the rent to Ellis de Amundeville in exchange for 4 bv. he held in the vill. If Amundeville was then holding Oilly's Greystoke fee, this transaction can be viewed as extinguishing a rent charge in exchange for land (R563). As a bovate is generally reckoned to comprise about fifteen acres, it is possible that the gifts of Edith, widow of Robert de Oilly, and her son Henry, of 68½ a. in Huggate (R558, R559) were actually confirmations of the exchange with Amundeville. Ernulf de Mandeville and Alice his wife confirmed the gift of Edith daughter of Forne, and Henry her son, adding a further 10 a. of their own gift (R561). These gifts were confirmed by Ernulf's son Geoffrey not long after Ernulf's death in 1178 (R560). The hospital appears to have let its land in Huggate at fee-farm. In *c.*1200 × *c.*1220 William son of Sybil of Huggate resigned and quitclaimed the land his ancestors held of the hospital to Roger son of Girard and Denise his wife (R562, R565), and in *c.*1200 × *c.*1230 Robert son of Arnold and his wife Helewise gave all the land they held of the hospital to John son of Roger of Millington in marriage with their daughter Christiana (R566). In 1263 × 1276 Nicholas son of John Scork surrendered and quitclaimed a toft and 8½ a. in Huggate which he and his father had held, which the hospital promptly regranted to Simon of York, carpenter (R567, R568). In the extent of 1280, *Parva Wald', Burtun, Lokyngton', Brunne et Hugate* were worth 22m. annually (R901). The *Valor Ecclesiasticus* makes no mention of land or rent in Huggate (R905), but a rent there appears in the post-Dissolution accounts (*Dissolved Houses*, IV, 226).

The Oilly tenancy in Huggate apparent in the hospital's deeds arose from the marriage of Edith, daughter of Forne son of Sigulf, to Robert de OILLY II, the constable of Oxford Castle, lord of the barony of Hook Norton.[2] A memorandum in the cartulary of Osney Abbey (Oxon.) states that Henry I gave Edith, daughter of Forne, his *amisia*,

[1] For the confirmation, made in 1235 or shortly before, by Thomas son of William [of Greystoke], of Geoffrey de Mandeville's gift of ½ k.f. in Huggate to Watton, see Anon., 'Grant to Watton'.
[2] For Robert de Oilly II, see *ODNB*.

to Robert de Oilly II in marriage, with all of Claydon (Bucks.). At Edith's urging, Robert founded Osney Abbey (*Ctl. Oseney*, v, 206). Robert issued a confirmation to Osney with the consent of Edith his wife and Henry and Gilbert his sons, probably not long before 1142³ (*Ctl. Oseney*, IV, 11). According to the annals of Osney, Robert de Oilly II died in 1142 (*Oseney Annals*, p. 24).

Robert's successor was his son Henry de Oilly I.⁴ There seems to be no evidence to support Postles' claim that Henry de Oilly I was in wardship between 1142 and 1154 (Postles, *Oseney Studies*, p. 12), though whether he had control of his fee much before the end of Stephen's reign is another matter. Several of Robert de Oilly II's deeds were given with the consent of his sons Henry and Gilbert, suggesting they were of age, or nearly of age, during their father's lifetime (*Ctl. Oseney*, I, nos 1, 12; ibid., IV, no. 9; v, no. 589d; *Ctl. St Frideswide*, no. 951; *Ctl. Thame*, nos 2, 3). In 1143 × 1147,⁵ witnessed by the earls of Gloucester, Hereford, Cornwall, and Salisbury, Robert FitzRoy (illegitimate son of King Henry I and half-brother of Henry de Oilly I), and Humphrey de Bohun [II] (Henry de Oilly's father-in-law), all prominent supporters of the empress, Henry confirmed the gift to Eynsham made by his father, of land in Moulsford, Berks. (*Ctl. Eynsham*, I, 75). In 1142 × 1148, at her stronghold of Devizes in Wiltshire, the empress included Henry's grant to Osney in a general confirmation (*Regesta*, III, no. 632). Henry de Oilly attested two charters of Duke Henry in 1153–54 (ibid., nos 306, 1000). On the duke's accession in 1154, or very soon afterwards, Henry de Oilly was made 'constable of the king', as his father had been. In several of his deeds Henry is so described, and it may be, as suggested by Salter, that the absence of the title indicates a date before about autumn 1154. According to the Osney annals, Henry de Oilly I died in 1163 (*Oseney Annals*, p. 33).⁶ Supporting evidence for his death at about that time is found in the pipe roll of 1164–65, when the unnamed wife (i.e. widow) of Henry de Oilly accounted in Oxfordshire for £4. In the same account the sheriff of Oxford accounted for £13 5s. 4d. [scutage] for the knights of Henry de Oilly (*PR*, 11 Hen. II, p. 71). Henry de Oilly I's wife Maud appears as a witness to her husband's confirmation to the hospital (R559). After Henry's death Maud married Walter son of Robert, lord of the barony of Little Dunmow in Essex, as his second wife.⁷ Maud was still living in 1201, but died in that year or soon afterwards.⁸

---

3 See Salter's note regarding the omission of Watlington church, which was lost to the Oilly family not long before Robert de Oilly II's death.

4 In recent years there has been an attempt to revise the traditional view that Henry, the eldest son of Robert and Edith, was the father of Henry de Oilly who died in 1232, and to insert another Henry between the two. The annalists and cartularists of Osney had no doubt that there were just two Henrys, using *primus* and *secundus* to distinguish between them. Dugdale, writing in the 1670s, agreed (*Baronage*, I, 460–61), as did D'Oyly Bayley, who published his book on the family in 1845 (D'Oyly Bayley, *D'Oyly*, pp. 10–13), and Herbert Salter, who edited the cartularies of Osney and other Oxfordshire houses in the first half of the last century. Ian Sanders appears to have been the inventor of the additional generation, going so far as to give the new intervening Henry a date of death of 1196 (*English Baronies*, p. 54). Keats-Rohan follows Sanders (Keats-Rohan, *Domesday Descendants*, s.n. de Oilli). Rosie Bevan has recently reasserted the traditional line of descent (FMG, Corrections to *Domesday Descendants*, s.n. de Oilly, 2003). There can be little doubt that the traditional account is correct. To the convincing evidence provided by the Osney records may be added a plea of 1225, in which Henry de Oilly claimed an interest in Ipsden had passed from Robert de Oilly to Henry de Oilly, and from Henry to his son Henry de Oilly, the claimant (*CRR*, 1225–1226, no. 1527).

5 Roger, earl of Hereford became earl after his father's death on 24 December 1143 (*CP*, VI, 453–54); Robert earl of Gloucester died at the end of October 1147 (ibid., v, 686).

6 Eodem anno obiit Henricus primus de Oyli, advocatus noster.

7 For Walter FitzRobert and his descendants see *Baronage*, I, 218–23; Morant, *Essex*, I (2), 338–39; Foss, *Judges*, I, 366–69; Round, 'Fitz Walter Pedigree'; *English Baronies*, pp. 129–30; *ODNB*, s.n. Fitzwalter.

8 In 1194, Maud, wife of Walter son of Robert, entered a plea concerning her dower which Henry de

A list of Yorkshire scutage payments in the pipe roll for 1161–62 shows that Henry de Oilly [I] was excused payment of 1*m*., which Farrer deduced was in respect of 1 k.f. he was holding of Greystoke in Huggate and Millington (*PR*, 8 Hen. II, p. 51; *EYC*, II, 506). But by 1166, as noted above, the Oilly tenancy of Greystoke had passed to Ernulf de MANDEVILLE, the illegitimate son of Geoffrey de Mandeville, first earl of Essex,[9] whose name is given variously as Ernulf, Arnulf, Arnold, or Ernold. Ernulf and his wife Alice jointly confirmed the gifts of Edith daughter of Forne and Henry d'Oilly (R561). Alice's rights in Huggate are also apparent in her demise to Osney Abbey of a mark's worth of land in Huggate, which Ernulf confirmed (*EYC*, II, no. 1256). It was doubtless this interest which caused Farrer to speculate that Alice was a daughter of Robert de Oilly and his wife Edith.[10] But it is more probable that Alice was a previously unnoticed daughter of Henry I. Robert FitzRoy, Henry I's illegitimate son by Edith daughter of Forne, has been mentioned above. John of Hexham tells us that he was at the siege of Winchester in 1141, describing him as *Robertus filius Ede et Henrici regis nothus* (John of Hexham, *Historia regum*, II, 310). One of Robert de Oilly's grants to Eynsham is witnessed by *Adeliza filia Reg'*. Salter expanded this to *Adeliza filia Reginaldi*, but the correct expansion is more likely to be *Adeliza filia regis* (*Ctl. Eynsham*, I, 73). If Alice was indeed a daughter of Henry I, then we may perhaps add her marriage to Ernulf to the list of concessions made to his father Geoffrey de Mandeville by the Empress Matilda in her attempts to secure his loyalty.[11] Geoffrey de Mandeville and Robert de Oilly II had been together in the company of King Stephen in Westminster in 1136 and in Oxford in 1136 × 1140 (*Regesta*, III, nos 626, 945, 947–48). About twenty years later Ernulf de Mandeville, his wife Alice and son Geoffrey were present when Henry de Oilly, constable of King Henry, confirmed the gift of two hides in Claydon which his mother Edith had made to Osney (*Ctl. Oseney*, V, 209).

As the sheriff of Wiltshire accounted at Michaelmas 1178 for a half-year's farm of Bratton 'which belonged to Ernulf de Mandeville', and a half-year's farm for [High] worth, due from Ernulf de Mandeville, it is evident that Ernulf died at about Easter of that year (*PR*, 24 Hen. II, pp. 28, 31). Geoffrey de Mandeville (Ernulf's son) accounted for the farm of [High]worth for three parts of the year at Michaelmas 1179 (ibid., 25 Hen. II, p. 56). The date of death of Geoffrey de Mandeville is not known. He was succeeded by his son, another Geoffrey. Details of their descendants may be found at Round, *Mandeville*, 232–33; *EYC*, II, no. 1260n; *VCH Wilts*, VIII, 160.

**R558.** Gift to the hospital by Edith, wife of Robert de Oilly, of a toft in Huggate and 68½ a. in the field(s) of Huggate, being 53 a. towards Wetwang, and 15½ a. in two other places, with common pasture for their livestock [*c.*1154 × 1163]

Oilly, her husband, had given her the day she was married. The dispute was unresolved in 1201, after which nothing more is heard (*RCuria*, I, 20; ibid., II, 59, 132, 183; *RFine*, p. 21; *CRR*, I, 173, 176, 293, 376–77, 420, 429).

9   The evidence that Ernulf was illegitimate is more than adequate. It was laid out by Holt under four headings: Ernulf appears as son, but not heir, of Geoffrey de Mandeville; he accepted enfeoffment from his two legitimate half-brothers; he attested deeds of Geoffrey's son and heir, also called Geoffrey; neither Ernulf nor his descendants disputed the claim of the younger Geoffrey to the earldom (Holt, 'Winchester', p. 298).

10  Farrer says nothing in the text, but in his genealogical table of the Greystoke family places Alice as a daughter of Robert de Oilly and Edith by a dotted line (*EYC*, II, 508).

11  For the career of Geoffrey de Mandeville, and his changing allegiances during the reign of Stephen, see *ODNB*.

PRINTED: *EYC*, II, no. 1238, where dated *c.*1145 × 1156.

**[f. 179ʳ]** *Edit uxor R(oberti) de Hugate de uno tofto et lxviii. acris et dimid' cum communi pastura in H(ugat).*

Notum sit omnibus sancte matris ecclesie filiis tam futuris quam presentibus quod ego Edit uxor Roberti de Oyli et heredes mei concessimus et dedimus deo et pauperibus hospitalis sancti Petri Ebor' in perpetuam elemosinam unum toftum in Hugat et in camp(is) eiusdem ville lxviii. acras terre et dimidiam acram videlicet versus Wetewanghe liii. acras et in aliis duobus locis xv. acras et dimidiam acram et communem pasturam pecoribus suis, pro salute anime mee et pro animabus patris et matris mee et Roberti de Oyli domini mei et pro heredibus meis sicut liberam et quietam et puram et perpetuam elemosinam et ab omnibus geldis et auxiliis et consuetudinibus et omni humano servicio immunem ut simus participes omnium beneficiorum et orationem que fiunt in illa sancta domo dei in vita et in morte. Isti sunt testes, Robertus presbiter, Nicholaus clericus, Robertus filius Arnaldi et Gamellus frater eius, Walterus filius Herberti et Rogerus frater eius, Robertus clericus, Robertus filius Iuonis, Robertus filius Sigherige, Robertus filius Gamelli, Arnaldus filius Cneuti, Gaufridus frater Nicholai, Willelmus clericus et multi alii.

As all the witnesses witnessed R559, it is clear the two deeds were given on the same occasion.

**R559.** Grant to the hospital by Henry de Oilly and his heirs of property in Huggate as described in R558 [*c.*1154 × 1163]

PRINTED: *EYC*, II, no. 1239, where dated *c.*1145 × 1156.

*Henricus de Oylli de Hugata de i. tofto et lxviii. acris et dimidia et communi pastura certo numero animalium.*

Notum sit omnibus sancte matris ecclesie filiis tam futuris quam presentibus quod ego Henricus de Oyli et heredes mei concessimus et dedimus deo et pauperibus hospitalis sancti Petri Ebor' in perpetuam elemosinam unum toftum in Hugat, et in camp(is) eiusdem ville lxviii. acras terre et dimidiam acram, videlicet versus Wetewanghe liii. acras et in aliis duobus locis xv. acras et dimidiam, et communem pasturam pecoribus suis, pro anima patris mei et pro matre mea et pro me ipso et uxore mea et pro meis heredibus sicut liberam et quietam et puram et perpetuam elemosinam et ab omnibus geldis et auxiliis et consuetudinibus et omni humano servicio immunem, ut simus participes omnium beneficiorum que fiunt in illa sancta domo dei in vita et in morte. Isti sunt testes, R[obertus] presbiter, Nicholaus clericus, R[obertus] filius Arnaldi et Gamellus frater eius, Walterus filius Herberti et Rogerus frater eius, R[obertus] clericus, R[obertus] filius Iuonis, R[obertus] filius Sigheride, R[obertus] filius Gamelli, Arnaldus filius Cneut, Gaufridus frater Nicholai, Willelmus clericus, Matild(a) uxor H[enrici] de Oilli, Nicholaus capellanus, Bard' filius Rogeri, Alicia filia Gamelli, Henricus, Willelmus filius Gilleberti.

As the witness Maud, wife of Henry de Oilly [II], was living as late as 1201, a date before *c.*1150 is improbable. The close connection between the hospital and King Stephen renders a date before the rapprochement between Stephen and Duke Henry at the end of 1153 unlikely, as Henry de Oilly was firmly in the Angevin camp. Farrer identifies Walter son of Herbert and Roger his brother as members of a local family. This indicates that the deed was given in Yorkshire, which also suggests a date after

1153. Henry de Oilly died in 1163; as he does not describe himself as constable, a date before *c.* Autumn 1154 may be indicated (FN).

**R560.** Confirmation to the hospital by Geoffrey de Mandeville and his heirs of a toft and 68½ a. in Huggate which his father gave, described as in R558, with another toft near [the land of] Robert of Wetwang, of the grantors' demesne culture, between two roads, 4 *perticas* wide and in length from the highway to the other road, and 10 a. land, being 5 a. next to the land of St Mary of Osney [Oxford], and 5 a. next to the land of the nuns of Watton, with common pasture for 160 sheep with their lambs to the next feast of St Martin, when the lambs will be separated from the ewes, and the hospital will have other animals and livestock as the other men of the vill [1178 × *c.*1188]

PRINTED: *EYC*, II, no. 1255, where dated 1178 × 1190.

*Galfridus de Mundavill' confirmat i. toftum in Hugat et lxviii. acras terre cum pastura certo numero animalium que pater eius dedit [in] H(ugat).*
Notum sit omnibus sancte matris ecclesie filiis tam presentibus quam futuris quod ego Gaufridus de Mandavilla et heredes mei concessimus et dedimus et presenti carta nostra confirmavimus deo et beato Petro et pauperibus hospitalis sancti Petri Ebor', in perpetuam elemosinam, terras quas pater meus dedit predictis pauperibus, videlicet unum toftum in Hugat et in campis eiusdem ville sexaginta octo acras terre et dimidiam acram, versus Wetewaghe quinquaginta tres acras, et in aliis duobus locis quindecim acras terre et dimidiam acram, et aliud toftum iuxta Robertum de Wetewaghe de dominica cultura nostra inter duas vias, habens latitudinem quatuor perticarum et longitudinem a regia via usque ad aliam viam, et decem acras terre, videlicet quinque acras propinquiores terre sancte Marie de Osanaia et quinque acras terre iuxta terram sanctimonialium de Watuna, et communem pasturam ad octies viginti oves cum agnis earum usque ad proximum festum sancti Martini et tunc agni seperabuntur a matribus ne numerus augeatur, et predicti pauperes habebunt animalia et aliam pecuniam sicut ceteri homines eiusdem ville. Hec omnia predicta confirmavimus prenominatis pauperibus in liberam et puram et perpetuam elemosinam, solutam et immunem et quietam ab omni humano servicio preter orationes pauperum. Hanc elemosinam warantizabimus sepedictis pauperibus contra omnes homines, et si contigerit nos non posse istam elemosinam warantizare, dabimus eis escambium ad valitudinem[12] in eadem villa. Hec omnia fecimus ut simus participes omnium beneficiorum et orationum que fiunt in illa sancta domo dei tam in vita quam in morte. Hiis testibus, Nicholao persona de Hugat, Petro filio Roberti, Waltero filio Arnoldi, Roberto de Sancto Iacobo, Arnoldo filio Cnut, Arnoldo clerico, Waltero Walrauen, Waltero de Wic', Nicholao Aticupe, Unfrido de Pasci, Radulfo de Tig(re)villa.

It is probable that this deed was made not long after the death of Ernulf de Mandeville *c.* Easter 1178 (FN). The mention of Osney indicates a date before the gift of the abbey's holdings in Huggate to Newburgh Priory, made by Hugh, abbot of Osney, with the consent of Geoffrey de Mandeville. Salter dated Abbot Hugh's deed to 1185 × 1188: Hugh became abbot in 1184, and it was assumed that the witness Ralph de St-Martin was dead in 1188, as he was no longer rural dean of Oxford in that year (*Ctl. Oseney*, VI, 180; *Oxford Charters*, no. 77n).

---

[12]  MS: *valitudinez.*

**R561.** Confirmation to the hospital by Ernulf de Mandeville and Alice his wife of a toft and 68½ a. in Huggate, described as in R558, and common of pasture for their livestock, which Edith daughter of Forne and Henry de Oilly her son gave before. And they add of their own gift a toft and 10 a. near [the land of] Robert of Wetwang [*c.*1153 × 1178]

PRINTED: *EYC*, II, no. 1254, where dated 1164 × 1178.

*Arnulfus de Mandavila de pluribus terris in territorio de H[ugate].*
Notum sit omnibus sancte matris ecclesie filiis tam futuris quam presentibus quod ego Arnulfus de Mandavila et uxor mea Aeliz et heredes mei concessimus et dedimus deo et beato Petro et pauperibus hospitalis sancti Petri Ebor', in perpetuam elemosinam, unum toftum in Hugat et in campis eiusdem ville lxviii. acras terre et dimid(ium) acre, videlicet versus Wetewanghe liii. acras et in aliis duobus locis xv. acras et dimid(ium) acr(e), et communem pasturam pecoribus suis, quam elemosinam Edit filia Forne et Henricus de Oyli filius eius eisdem pauperibus prius dederant, pro salute animarum nostrarum et pro animabus patrum nostrorum et matrum, parentum et propinquorum et omnium antecessorum nostrorum, sicut liberam et quietam et puram et perpetuam elemosinam et ab omnibus geldis et auxiliis et consuetudinibus et omni humano servicio immunem, ut simus participes omnium beneficiorum et orationum que fiunt in illa sancta domo dei in vita et in morte. Hiis testibus, Waltero de Barevila, Roberto de Hugat, Arnaldo filio Cneuth. Et preter h(ec) addimus ex dono nostro unum toftum et x. acras terre iuxta Robertum de Wetewanghe. [Testibus,] Radulfo de Gloucestr' pastoral' capellano, Waltero Palm', Petro de Hugate, Ricardo Nafrez', Waleranno, Lewino filio Turewif', **[f. 179ᵛ]** Gamello de Blaikestreta, Radulfo capellano, Patricio capellano, Henrico capellano, Iohanne capellano, Wydone diacono, Martino clerico, Gaufrido, Rogerio clerico, Thoma clerico, Willelmo clerico et multis aliis.

Farrer's *terminus a quo* depends on Ernulf de Mandeville acquiring his interest in Huggate after the death of Henry de Oilly I. But as it is likely that Ernulf had his land in Huggate in marriage with a daughter of Edith daughter of Forne an earlier date is possible. Ernulf died *c.* Easter 1178. For a similar interruption to the witness list, see R150.

**R562.** Resignation and quitclaim to the hospital by William son of Sybil of Huggate of all right in the land of Huggate which his predecessors held of the hospital, according to the deeds which they had from the hospital, by gifts of Edith daughter of Forne, Geoffrey de Mandeville, and Walter son of Herbert [*c.*1200 × *c.*1220]

PRINTED: *EYC*, II, no. 1258, where dated 1185 × 1200.

*Carta Willelmi filii Sibille de quieta clamatione de terra de Hugate.*
Notum sit omnibus videntibus et audientibus litteras has quod ego Willelmus filius Sibille de Hugate resignavi et quietum clamavi pro me et pro heredibus meis deo et pauperibus hospitalis beati Petri Ebor' et fratribus ibi deo servientibus omne ius meum et clameum quem habui in tota terra de Hugate quam antecessores mei tenuerunt de predicto hospitali secundum cartas quas habuerunt de predicto hospitalis ex dono Edit filie Forni et ex dono Galfridi de Mandevile et ex dono Walteri filii Herberti. Et ut hec quieta clamatio firmior sit testimonio sigilli mei corroboravi.

Hiis testibus, Rogero, Adam, Roberto, Willelmo capellanis, Stephano, Suano, Willelmo Balchi, Godefrido fratribus, Iohanne persona de Lonesdale, Ricardo clerico.

For a similar quitclaim by the same grantor, see R565. Godfrey attested within *c.*1200 × *c.*1230. William Balki attested about ten deeds, most of which can be dated within *c.*1195 × *c.*1225. He does not occur with Thomas de Langwath as master.

**R563.** Confirmation to the hospital by Ellis de Amundeville of 4 bv. in Huggate, for 20s. which the brethren were accustomed to receive by the gift of Robert de Oilly, who had held the vill, and by confirmation of Ellis' lord King Stephen [1142 × 1154]

PRINTED: *EYC*, II, no. 1243, where dated *c.*1160 × 1171.

*Elyas de Amundavilla de iiii<sup>or</sup> bovatis in Hugate.*
Notum sit archiepiscopo Ebor' totique capitulo ecclesie sancti Petri et omnibus hominibus meis et amicis cunctisque sancte matris ecclesie filiis tam futuris quam presentibus, quod ego Elias de Amundavilla et heredes mei concedimus et in perpetuam elemosinam damus deo et pauperibus hospitalis sancti Petri iiii. bovatas terre in Hugate plenar(ie) in mansuris et in campis et in pasturis, liberas et quietas et immunes ab omnibus geldis et consuetudinibus et auxiliis et ab omni humano servicio quod ad terram pertinet, sicut liberam elemosinam, pro remissione peccatorum meorum et pro animabus patris et matris mee et omni antecessorum meorum, et pro viginti solidis quos pauperes prefate domus singulis annis habere solebant ex dono et elemosina Roberti de Olei in eadem villa, que tunc temporis eius fuit, et ex concessione et confirmatione carte domini mei regis Stephani. Isti sunt testes, Serlo canonicus, David Lardanarius, Gocelinus de Areci, Teobaldus clericus et Murdacus frater eius, Walterus filius Faghenolfi, Eadwardus, Siwardus de Stangata, Arnaldus Sote Vagine et Osmundus.

Clay identified Ellis de Amundeville as a member of the Lincolnshire family, but was unable to explain the origin of his interest in Huggate. Amundeville attested a charter of King Stephen with Geoffrey de Mandeville and others in 1139–40 (*Regesta*, III, no. 690), and a deed of William, earl of York, in 1138 × 1143 (R578). By 1166 he was holding a fee in Lincolnshire of Simon de St Liz, earl of Northampton (*Red Bk*, p. 382). He succeeded to the family estates on the death of his brother William in the year ending at Michaelmas 1168, and was dead in 1179 (Clay, 'Amundeville', pp. 114–19). It seems that Amundeville somehow acquired the Greystoke fee in Yorkshire after Oilly went over to the Angevins, and that it was restored to Edith daughter of Forne on the accession of Henry II. The mention of Stephen's confirmation, which is not in the cartulary, suggests a date before the accession of Henry II at the end of 1154, when such confirmations ceased to have much value. The phrase *ex dono . . . Roberti de Olei in eadem villa, que tunc temporis eius fuit* shows Robert was dead or at least dispossessed in Yorkshire when the deed was given, so a date before 1141 is improbable. Serlo the canon, David Lardiner, and Walter son of Fagenulf occur in the reign of Stephen and later (*EYC*, I, nos 152, 243, 323). It is possible that Arnold Sottewain, not here described as canon, was the same man as the Arnulf Sottewain who attested amongst York canons in 1154 × 1162[13] and 1154 × 1157 (*EYC*, II, no. 1095; ibid., IX, no. 153).

---

[13] After the consecration of Roger, archbishop of York, and before John, treasurer of York, was elected bishop of Poitiers.

The witness Jocelin de ARECY had lands in Acaster [Selby] (*EYC*, III, no. 1854), and can possibly be identified with the man of that name of Harmston, Lincs., who occurs in 1178 (*PR*, 24 Hen. II, p. 8). With Helewise de Clere his wife Jocelin quitclaimed certain rights to Rievaulx in '*c.*1170 × 1176' (*EYC*, I, no. 611). He attested a deed of Roger de Clere [II] in '*c.*1170 × 1185' (ibid., no. 594). Jocelin was living in 1182, and had been succeeded in Acaster by his son Robert in 1194 × 1198[14] (ibid., III, nos 1855, 1857). Helewise de Clere, possibly the widow of Roger de Clere I, appears to have been the founder of the priory of Little Mareis, or Yeddingham, in 1158 or before, and probably before her marriage to Jocelin (Burton, *Monastic Order*, pp. 134–35; Clay, *Clere*, p. 16).

**R564.** Gift to the hospital by John, treasurer [of York Minster], addressed to Robert, clerk, and the men of Huggate, of the toft in front of the hospital's house, from the toft of Pain the clerk to the embankment [?], the hospital to pay the donor 12*d.* annually [1153 × 1162]

*Iohannes thesaur(arius) de uno tofto pro xii.d.*
Iohannes thesaurarius, Roberto clerico et omnibus hominibus de Hugate salutem. Sciatis me concessisse et dedisse fratribus hospitalis sancti Petri illud toftum quod est ante domum hospitalis, de tofto Pagani clerici usque ad vallem, reddendo michi singulis annis xii.d., t(antu)m pro omni re, dimidium ad festum sancti Martini et dimidium ad Pent'. Cuius rei hii sunt testes, magister Osbertus Arundel, Picotus presbiter, Willelmus Thilem', Walterus de Hugate, Petrus clericus de hospitali.

The date range is the period for John as treasurer of York. The origin of the treasurer's interest in Huggate is not known, but may have been associated with the Minster's holdings in the adjoining vill of Wetwang (*YMF*, II, 84). Osbert Arundel, a canon of Beverley, and William Tillemir were frequent witnesses to Archbishop Roger's acts (*Beverley Fasti*, pp. xx, 14; *EEA*, xx, pp. xliii–xliv).

**R565.** Quitclaim by William son of Sybil of Huggate to Roger son of Girard and Denise his wife, of all claim in the land in Huggate which his predecessors held of the hospital, according to the deeds which the hospital had by the gift of Edith daughter of Forne, Geoffrey de Mandaville, and Walter son of Herbert [*c.*1200 × *c.*1220]

PRINTED: *EYC*, II, no. 1259, where dated 1185 × 1200.

*W(illelmus) filius Sibille de Hugate quiet'clam(at) Rogero filio Ger(ardi) totum ius quod habuit in terra quam antecessores sui etc.*
Notum sit omnibus audientibus et videntibus litteras has quod ego Willelmus filius Sibille de Hugate resignavi et quietum clamavi Rogero filio Girardi et Dionisie uxori sue et heredibus suis omne ius meum et clam(eum) quod habui in tota terra de Hugate quam antecessores mei tenuerunt de hospitali beati Petri Ebor' in Hugate, secundum cartas quas predicta domus habet ex dono Edit filie Forne et ex dono et concessione Galfridi de Mandevile et ex dono Walteri filii Herberti de terris omnibus et toftis que predicta domus habet cum omnibus pertinenciis in predicta villa de Hugate. Hiis testibus, magistro hospitalis Ebor' cum toto suo capitulo, Rogero, Adam,

---

14 Witnessed by Roger de Bavent, sheriff.

Roberto, Willelmo, capellanis, priore de Watre cum suo capitulo, Iohanne persona, Ricardo clerico, Willelmo filio Petri, Roberto et Nicholao de Hugate et multis aliis.

This deed has been assigned the same date range as R562, which is witnessed by the same four chaplains.

**R566.** Grant by Robert son of Arnold and his wife Helewise, to John son of Roger of Millington, in marriage with Christiana their daughter, of all the land with the toft which the grantors held of the hospital, paying the grantors 2s. 9d. annually for all service [c.1200 × c.1230]

*Robertus filius Arnaldi et Helewysa uxor sua de tota terra cum tofto etc.*
Sciant omnes tam presentes quam futuri quod ego Robertus filius Arnaldi et Helewisa uxor mea dedimus concessimus et hac carta nostra confirmavimus Iohanni filio Rogeri de Midlington' totam terram cum tofto quam tenuimus de hospitali sancti Leonardi Ebor' in maritagium cum Cristiana filia nostra, tenendam et habendam ipsi Iohanni et Cristiane et heredibus de illis nascituris de nobis et heredibus nostris in feodo et hereditate, libere et quiete et honorifice cum omnibus pertinenciis suis et aisiamentis tam infra villam quam extra, reddendo inde annuatim nobis et heredibus nostris duos solidos et novem denarios pro omni servicio et seculari exactione, scilicet sexdecim denarios et obulum ad Pent' et sexdecim denarios et obulum ad festum sancti Martini. Et ego Robertus et Helewisa uxor mea et heredes nostri predicto Iohanni et Cristiane et heredibus de illis nascituris predictam terram cum pertinenciis contra omnes homines warantizabimus. Hiis testibus, domino Rogero capellano, domino Willelmo de Hamerton' milit(e), Roberto filio Galfridi, Nicholao filio Arnaldi, Willelmo de Sancto Iacobo, Gregorio filio Arnaldi, Willelmo filio Rogeri, Ricardo filio Petri et multis aliis.

Although the place is not named in the deed or rubric, the witnesses indicate that the deed has been placed correctly in the cartulary. Nicholas son of Arnold and Gregory his brother attested a Huggate deed of 1211 or before[15] (*EYC*, II, no. 1265); Nicholas son of Arnold attested a gift of Walter son of Geoffrey, knight, of Huggate, to Ellerton Priory in 1199 × 1225[16] (Burton transcripts 2, ff. 119$^r$–120$^r$, pp. 202–04, B17 N55). Richard son of Peter, William son of Roger, and Robert son of Geoffrey the knight appear in a deed of William de St-Jacques of Huggate by which he gave property in Huggate to Ellerton Priory, probably in or before 1225[17] (*EYC*, II, no. 1263n). William de St-Jacques[18] attested a Huggate deed made in 1204 × 1214[19] (*EYC*, II, no. 1261). Robert son of Geoffrey and William de St-Jacques attested a Huggate deed probably of similar date (*EYC*, II, no. 1262). Millington, which adjoins Huggate, appears as *Midlington* in 1227 (*PN YorksER*, p. 178).

The second witness, SIR WILLIAM OF HAMMERTON, appears to have gained his interests in Huggate and elsewhere in the East Riding by his marriage to Avice, whose ancestry is not known. He may have been related to the Hammertons of [Kirk] Hammerton

---

[15]  Witnessed by Jordan of Bugthorpe, who was murdered at the end of that year (FN: Rufforth).
[16]  Between the foundation of Ellerton and the death of William son of Peter (FN: Hay).
[17]  Witnessed by William of Goodmanham, i.e. William son of Peter (FN: Hay).
[18]  MS: *de sancto Iohanne.*
[19]  Between Ralph's accession to the mastership of the hospital and Simon de Apulia's election as bishop of Exeter.

(FN). He witnessed deeds concerning Cattal, where that family held land. A grant to Bridlington Priory of property in Cattal is witnessed by Sir William of Hammerton, knight, John of Hammerton, Hugh his brother, Alan of Hammerton; another by Sir J. of Hammerton and Sir W. of Hammerton; and a third by J. of Hammerton, knight, and Hugh son of Avice of Hammerton (*Ctl. Bridlington*, pp. 240–41).[20] In 1225 William of Hammerton, Avice his wife, and the heirs of Avice owed forinsec service for the tenement they held in Aughton (*Acton*) and in Huggate 'which is a member of Aughton'. The following year William of Hammerton, Avice his wife, and Romund Tirel, with Christiana his wife, granted 2 bv. in Laytham to Adam of Linton and Agnes his wife, to hold of the grantors and the heirs of Avice and Christiana. William of Hammerton occurs as a knight in 1231 (*YF, 1218–1231*, pp. 62, 75, 149n).

**R567.** Release and quitclaim to the hospital by Nicholas son of John Schork of Huggate of all claim in a toft and 8½ a. land in Huggate, which John his father formerly held of the hospital [1263 × 1276]

*Quieta clamat(io) Nicholai filii Iohannis Schork' de Hugate etc.*
Omnibus cristi fidelibus presens scriptum visuris vel audituris Nicholaus filius Iohannis Schork' de Hugate salutem in domino sempiternam. Noveritis me concessisse reddidisse et omnino quiet'clamasse de me et de heredibus meis imperpetuum magistro et fratribus hospitalis sancti Leonardi Ebor' totum ius et clam(eum) quod habui vel habere potui in uno tofto et in octo acris terre et dimidia cum suis pertinenciis in villa et territorio de Hugate que Iohannes pater meus quondam tenuit de dictis magistro et fratribus, tenend(a) et habend(a) predictis magistro et fratribus et eorum successoribus vel eorum assignatis libere quiete pacifice et honorifice, ita scilicet quod nec **[f. 180ʳ]** ego Nicholaus nec heredes mei seu aliquis pro nobis vel ex parte nostra in predictis tofto et octo acris terre et dimidia cum pastura communi et aliis pertinenciis suis aliquod ius clameum vel calumpniam de cetero ponere poterimus aut exigere. Et ut hec mea concessio redditio et quieta clamatio perpetuum robur obtineat presens scriptum sigilli mei munimine corroboravi. Hiis testibus, magistro Nicholao de Hugate, Willelmo de la Gasche, Henrico filio Willelmi, Willelmo de Herlthorp', Elia filio Gerardi, Willelmo filio Galfridi et aliis.

All the witnesses attest R568, the hospital's subsequent grant of the same land, presumably made on the same occasion. Nicholas son of master Nicholas of Huggate, with Ellen his wife, entered a fine concerning ¾ bv. in Burnby in 1296 (*YF, 1272–1300*, p. 115). Nicholas of Huggate, king's clerk, and provost of Beverley from 1318 until his death in 1338, was doubtless of the same family (*Beverley Fasti*, pp. xxi, 8).

**R568.** Grant at fee-farm (chirograph) by Thomas, rector of the hospital, and the brethren, to Simon of York, carpenter, living in Huggate, of a toft and 8½ a. in Huggate, which Nicholas son of John Scork formerly held, and quitclaimed to the hospital, paying the hospital 32*d.* annually and a portion of chattels as an obituary payment [1263 × 1276]

*Copia carte de terra in villa et territorio de Hugate dimissa ad firmam.*
Universis presens scriptum visuris vel audituris Thomas rector hospitalis sancti

---

[20] J[ohn] of Hammerton, knight, was probably the tenant of Green Hammerton, and not closely related to the Hammertons of Kirk Hammerton. He appears to have died in 1251 × 1253 (*EYC*, II, 81–82).

Leonardi Ebor' et fratres eiusdem domus salutem in domino sempiternam. Noveritis nos concessisse et hac presenti carta nostra confirmasse Simoni de Ebor' carpent(ario) manenti in Hugate unum toftum et octo acras terre et dimidiam in villa et territorio de Hugate, illas videlicet octo acras terre et dimidiam cum tofto quas Nicholaus filius Iohannis Scork quondam tenuit in eadem, et nobis postea per cartam quiet'clamavit, tenend(a) et habend(a) dicto Simoni et heredibus suis de nobis libere quiete integre bene et in pace cum omnibus pertinenciis suis infra villam de Hugate et extra, reddendo inde annuatim nobis et successoribus nostris triginta duos denarios argenti ad duos anni terminos, medietatem ad Pent' et aliam medietatem ad festum sancti Martini in yeme pro omni seculari servicio ad nos pertinente. Dictus autem Simon et heredes sui vel quicumque dictam terram tenuerint vel in eadem manserint portionem catallorum suorum ipsos in obitu suo quoquo modo contingentem pauperibus domus nostre nomine testamenti fideliter relinquent. Et hoc iuravit dictus Simon pro se et heredibus suis tactis sacrosanctis et affidavit. Nos vero et successores nostri dictum tenementum cum pertinenciis suis contra omnes gentes warantizabimus quamdiu carta donatoris nostri quam inde habemus nobis poterit warantizare. In cuius rei testimonium duo scripta unius tenoris ad modum cirograffi sunt confecta, quorum unum residet penes nos sigillo dicti Simonis signatum et aliud penes dictum Simonem communi sigillo nostro munitum. Hiis testibus, magistro Nicholao de Hugate, Thoma de Holme, Rogero socio[21] dicti Thome, Willelmo de la Gasche, Henrico filio Willelmi, Willelmo de Herlthorp', Elia filio Gerardi, Willelmo filio Galfridi, Radulfo de Buhtton' clerico presentium scriptore et aliis.

The date range is the period for Thomas of Geddington as rector.

---

[21] MS: *socro.*

## *Hundemanby'* [Hunmanby]

In 1086 Gilbert de Gant held 24 ct. in Hunmanby, with another 8 ct. in its outliers of *Ricstorp* and [Wold] Newton. In 1284–85 it was said there were 20 ct. in Hunmanby, in the fee of Gant, held of the king as 2½ k.f. (*KI*, pp. 52–53). Gilbert, the Domesday tenant, was succeeded *c.*1095 by his son Walter de Gant, the founder of Bridlington Priory. Walter died in 1139, having retired to Bardney Abbey (Lincs.) not long previously. His son and heir Gilbert II was then underage, but was created earl of Lincoln by Stephen in *c.*1147–48. On Gilbert's death in 1156 his interest passed to Alice de Gant, his daughter and heir, wife of Simon de St Liz III, earl of Northampton. Simon was recognised as earl of Huntingdon in 1174, and died in June 1184 (*EYC*, II, 432–36; *CP*, VII, 672–73; ibid., VI, 645). On Alice's death in 1185 her heir was Robert de Gant, brother of Earl Gilbert. Robert de Gant died in 1191, leaving a son Gilbert III who came of age *c.*1201–02. Gilbert de Gant III died in 1242 and was succeeded by his son Gilbert IV, who died in 1274, leaving Gilbert V who died in 1298. The heirs of Gilbert V were the children of two of his sisters (Sanders, *English Baronies*, p. 46).

Gilbert de Gant granted a rent in his mill of Hunmanby to the hospital in 1143 × 1148 (R569). The tithes of the mill had previously been granted to Bardney Abbey by Walter de Gant (*MA*, I, 630). The mill itself was included in Henry II's confirmation to the hospital of 1155 × 1170[1] (C10 [*EYC*, I, no. 175]), but does not appear in the papal confirmations of the twelfth century. In 1156 × *c.*1174 Simon earl of Northampton exchanged 5 bv. in Hunmanby for the mill (R570), and in 1204 'the land you have in Hunmanby' was included in the confirmation of Innocent III (C182 [*Letters Innoc. III*, no. 562]). The land was let at fee-farm by the hospital (R571–R573). In 1309, when the lands late of Robert Tattershall[2] were divided between his coheirs, 'the fees that the master of St Leonard's York holds in Hunmanby' fell to the share of Thomas de Cailly (*CalCl*, 1307–1313, p. 101). No reference is made to Hunmanby in the extents and rentals of the late thirteenth century, nor in the *Valor Ecclesiasticus*. A messuage in Hunmanby, now or lately in the occupation of Robert Lepington, formerly belonging to the hospital of St Leonard in York, was amongst property assigned by the Crown in letters patent of 16 July 1563 to Thomas Wood and William Frankland (A2A: YM/FD/1;[3] *CalPat*, 1560–1563, p. 576).

**R569.** Grant to the hospital by G[ilbert] de Gant of 10s. rent in a mill at Hunmanby, with any improvement in the value of the mill [1143 × 1148]

COPIES: *b* Rawl., f. 181ʳ; *c* MS Dods. 7, f. 329ʳ, differences as noted, with further minor variations of spelling. PRINTED: *EYC*, II, no. 1181, from *b*, where dated 1142 × 1147.

**[f. 181ʳ]** *G[ilebertus] de Gant de x. solidis redditus de molendino de Hundemandby'.*[4]
G[ilebertus] de Gant omnibus fidelibus hominibus suis francis et anglis salutem. Notum vobis[5] sit omnibus me concessisse et dedisse hospitali sancti Petri de Ebor'[6] redditum quendam decem solidorum in quodam molendino meo ad vivarium meum de Hundemanneby in elemosinam pro anima patris mei et matris mee et pro anima

---

[1] Nicholas Vincent's dating.
[2] For the Tattershall acquisition of the Gant interest in Hunmanby see *VCH Yorks ER*, II, 231.
[3] Borthwick Institute, Yarburgh muniments.
[4] *c* has rubric *Carta Gilberti de Gaunt*.
[5] *c: vobis* omitted.
[6] *c: Eboraci.*

mea et omnium parentum meorum. Hanc elemosinam concessi et dedi hospitali eidem liberam et quietam a me et omnibus heredibus meis. Hiis testibus, Rodberto decano, Radulfo de Novilla,[7] Willelmo nepote episcopi, Ricardo Scrop', Waltero filio Ivonis et Willelmo fratre eius, Almerico de Rictun, Gaufrido filio Malgeri, Willelmo filio Morcheri.[8] Hunc redditum molendini si emendare et proficere possunt bene concedo eis et molendinum et totum proficuum quod inde poterunt perquirere, eisdem testibus prenominatis.

Earl Gilbert's uncle Robert de Gant, who attested as dean of York, was chancellor to King Stephen. He became dean after March 1143 and probably retained the dignity until 1157–58 (Clay, 'Deans', pp. 366–70; *Regesta*, III, p. x).

**R570.** Grant to the hospital by Simon earl of Northampton, of Walter son of Arnald of Hunmanby with his children and chattels and tenement of 5 bv. in Hunmanby, in exchange for the mill in Hunmanby which Earl Gilbert had given to the hospital, to be held of the hospital by hereditary right, paying 1 *lb.* pepper annually [1156 × *c.*1174]

COPIES: *b* Rawl., f. 181[r]; *c* MS Dods. 7, f. 332[r]; differences as noted, further minor variations of spelling. PRINTED: *EYC*, II, no. 1186, from *b*, where dated 1156 × 1174.

*Carta Simonis comitis Norhamptune de quiet' clam' Walteri filii Arnaldi de Hundemanby' cum eius tenemento per molendinum eiusdem ville.*[9]
Universis filiis sancte matris ecclesie Simon comes Norhamtune salutem. Notum sit vobis me et heredes meos[10] concessisse et dedisse deo et pauperibus hospitalis sancti Petri Ebor'[11] Walterum filium Arnaldi de Hundemanabi cum omnibus liberis et catallis et toto tenemento suo, scilicet quinque bovatis terre in Hundemaneby plenariis in terra arabili pratis et pascuis aquis et viis et semitis et communi pastura eiusdem ville et omnibus aisiamentis que ad eandem villam pertinent, in puram et perpetuam elemosinam liberam et quietam ab omni seculari servicio preter orationes pauperum. Hoc autem eis feci qu(onia)m ipsi concesserunt michi et heredibus meis molendinum suum de Hundemaneby quod comes Gilebertus eis in puram et perpetuam[12] elemosinam dederat, tenendum de eis iure hereditario, reddendo illis annuatim unam libram piperis ad Pent'[13] pro omni servicio quod ad eos pertinet, et ut ego et uxor mea et antecessores et heredes nostri simus participes omnium bonorum que fient[14] in illa domo nunc et imperpetuum. Hiis testibus, Simone fratre comitis, Iuliano capellano, Rogero constabulario, Hereberto filio Alardi, Andrea de Muscampo, Ernisio de Nova Villa, Willelmo[15] filio Walteri, Roberto filio eius de Wella, Hugone filio Radulfi, Gaufrido Baard', Adam de Bouuingtona, Roberto de Rosel, Thoma pincerna, Ricardo dispensario, Ricardo coquo et multis aliis.

7    *c: Novavilla.*
8    *b: Mororheri.*
9    *c* has rubric *Carta Simonis comitis Norhamtunie.*
10   *c: et heredes meos* omitted.
11   *c: Eboraci.*
12   *c: et perpetuam* omitted.
13   *c: Penthecosten.*
14   *c: fiunt.*
15   *c: Gilleberto,* but see note.

In giving his suggested dates Farrer made the assumption that Simon would not style himself earl of Northampton after he gained the earldom of Huntingdon, but this is unproven. The witnesses, however, indicate Farrer's date range is reasonably safe. William son of Walter and Herbert son of Alard [of Orby, Lincs.] attested a deed of Gilbert de Gant before he became earl of Lincoln, i.e. before c.1147–48 (*Rufford Charters*, no. 668). Herbert son of Alard attested in 1149. According to the Hagnaby annals he did not die until 1194 (*HKF*, II, 98).[16] Tenants of Earl Simon in 1166 included William son of Walter, Hugh de Muschamp, Hugh son of Ralph, and Herbert son of Alard (*Red Bk*, p. 383). Andrew de Muschamp, Ernis de Neville, and Julian the chaplain are amongst the witnesses to a deed of Hugh son of Ralph son of Reinger dated 1173 (*Rufford Charters*, no. 745).

**R571.** Agreement between master H[ugh], rector of the hospital, and John de Hil of Hunmanby. The hospital has demised at farm to the said John all the land which John son of William held of it in Hunmanby. To be held to John de Hil, and his heirs (if John dies whilst John, son and heir of John son of William, who at the start of the agreement was almost three years old, is under lawful age); saving the third part to Agnes, widow of John son of William. John or his heirs pay to the hospital 4*m*. annually for the land. John son of John son of William will be in the custody of the master and brethren until he is of full age. And John de Hil has sworn that he will not sell or mortgage the land, and will keep the building and mill in good repair. 8 September 1217.

*Cirograph' de terra de Hundemanby concessa Iohanni de Hil [usque] her(es) fuerit legitime etatis.*
Anno ab incarnatione domini millesimo ducentesimo septimo decimo ad nativitatem beate Marie virginis, facta est conventio inter magistrum H[ugonem] rectorem hospitalis sancti Petri Ebor' ex una parte et Iohannem de Hil de Hundemaneby ex altera parte, quod magister et fratres dimiserunt predicto Iohanni ad firmam totam terram quam Iohannes filius Willelmi tenuit de illis in Hundemanby cum omnibus pertinenciis suis infra villam et extra, tenendam et habendam predicto Iohanni et heredibus suis, si ipse obierit donec Iohannes, qui in initio huius conventionis fuit fere trium annorum, filius et heres memorati Iohannis filii Willelmi, fuerit legitime etatis, salva per omnia tertia parte Agneti uxori quondam Iohannis filii Willelmi. Reddet autem predictus Iohannes vel eius heres pro predicta terra singulis annis predicto hospitali pro omnibus serviciis ad illud pertinentibus iiii[or] marcas argenti scilicet duas marcas ad festum sancti Martini et duas ad Pent'. Predictus autem Iohannes heres Iohannis filii Willelmi predicti in custodia magistri et fratrum erit usque ad legitimam pervenerit etatem. Sepedicto autem Iohannes de Hil tactis sacrosanctis iuravit quod nullo modo alienabit nec obligabit predictam terram un(de) a predicto hospitali et a vero herede elongetur, et quod omnia predicta fideliter observabit. Edificia autem et molendinum usque ad predictum terminum in bono statu conservabit. In huius autem rei robur et testimonium huic scripto utraque pars sigillum suum apposuit.

This is the earliest dated occurrence for rector Hugh. It is likely that the hospital needed many similar arrangements for the management of land during the minority of an heir, but this is the only such deed which survives. The clumsy drafting does not suggest the writer had drawn up many documents of this type.

---

[16] Farrer gives details of his family. See also Statham, 'Domesday Descendants', *DAJ*, NS II (2) pt 49, 291–95.

**R572.** Gift by John son of John *Iuuenis* of Hunmanby, to Walter de Stretton, or his
assigns, of 1 bv. land in Hunmanby, from the 5 bv. the donor holds of the
hospital, York, being the bovate which John son of Herbert formerly held of
the donor, excepting the toft, paying 4*d.* annually [*c.*1225 × *c.*1255]

*Carta Iohannis filii Iohannis Iuuenis.*
Omnibus sancte matris ecclesie filiis hanc cartam visuris vel audituris Iohannes filius
Iohannis Iuenis de Hundemanby salutem in domino. Noverit universitas vestra me
dedisse concessisse et hac presenti carta mea confirmasse Waltero de Stretton' vel
quicumque assignare vel legare voluerit unam bovatam terre cum pertinenciis in
territorio de Hund' de meis quinque bovatis quas teneo de domo sancti Leonardi
Ebor', et videlicet illam bovatam quam Iohannes filius Hereberti aliquando de me
tenuit cum omnibus aisiamentis ad dictam bovatam spectantibus infra villam et extra,
excepto tofto, scilicet in pratis et pascuis viis et semitis cum liberis introitibus et
exitibus, tenend(as) et habend(as) illi et heredibus vel assignatis de me et heredibus
meis libere quiete et honorifice, reddendo inde annuatim michi et heredibus meis iiii^{or}
denarios pro omnibus serviciis consuetudinibus et secularibus exactionibus, scilicet
ii.d. ad Pent' et duos denarios ad festum sancti Martini in yeme. Et ego Iohannes
et heredes mei warantizabimus defendemus et adquictabimus totam prenominatam
bovatam terre cum pertinenciis dicto Waltero vel assignatis contra omnes homines
imperpetuum. Et notandum quod dictus Walterus vel assignati nunquam in curia
mea venient nec aliquam reversionem pro sepedicta bovata terre ibi facient nisi
prenominatum servicium. Et ut ista mea donatio rata et stabila permaneat huic
presenti carte sigillum meum apposui. Hiis testibus, domino Willelmo de Ergum,
Ernaldo de Buketon', Willelmo filio eius, Willelmo vicario tunc de Hund', Galfrido
pincerna, Iohanne filio Walteri, Gilberto de Cave, Willelmo de Cresacre, Francisco
tunc temporis servient' domini Gilberti de Gaunt, Simon' **[f. 181^v]** filio Thorald',
Henrico serviente, Willelmo Faucun' et aliis.

It is difficult to establish precise limits of date for this deed. The donor, John son of
John *Iuuenis*, may be the man of that name who was tenant of 20 a. and a toft in
Selby in 1231 (*YF*, 1218–1231, p. 161n). John *Iuuenis* was a tenant in Wigginton in 1241
(*YF*, 1232–1246, p. 95). Arnald of Buckton and William de Erghum were witnesses
to a deed belonging to Willerby (near Staxton) made before 1242[17] (*Ctl. Bridlington*,
p. 134). Geoffrey Butler was named as a tenant in Hunmanby in a deed of 1198 ×
1226[18] (*YD*, VIII, no. 217). Walter and Geoffrey, sons of Arnald of Buckton, and John
son of Walter of Hunmanby witnessed in 1270 (*Ctl. Bridlington*, p. 63).

The first witness, William de ERGHUM, took his name from Argam, in the parish
of Hunmanby.[19] Members of the family witnessed several deeds in the Bridlington
cartulary and elsewhere pertaining to land in Burton Fleming, Buckton, Marton,
Folkton, Hunmanby, Sewerby and Reighton, all within about 5 m. of Argam (*Ctl.
Bridlington*, passim; *YD*, VI, 123–26; ibid., IX, 136–39; X, 37–38). William de Erghum

---

[17]  The witness Walter of Folkton, dean of Dickering, was apparently dead in 1242 (*Fasti Parochiales*, III,
      24).
[18]  Witnessed by Ellis, prior of Bridlington.
[19]  Arram (wap. Harthill, ER), Arram (Holderness, ER), Airyholme (Rydale, NR), Airy Holme (Langbargh
      West, NR) and Eryholme (Gilling East, NR) also appear as *Ergum* or *Erghum* in deeds of the thirteenth
      century. Brief notes on the family's interests in Argam and Reighton are given in *VCH Yorks ER*, II,
      6–7, 305.

quitclaimed to Simon de Hal 2 ct. in Reighton in 1219 (*YF*, 1218–1231, p. 23). Herbert de Erghum acted as attorney in a fine concerning Sewerby in 1234 (*YF*, 1232–1246, p. 20). Sir Arnulf of Buckton, Sir William de Erghum and John son of Walter of Hunmanby were amongst the witnesses to a deed citing a recovery made in 1234 (*Ctl. Bridlington*, p. 71). Arnald of Buckton and William his son attested a deed of Walter son of Herbert of Hunmanby and Cecilia his wife, which was confirmed by Cecilia in widowhood in January 1251[/52]. Sir William de Erghum, with his brother Herbert, witnessed her confirmation (*Ctl. Bridlington*, p. 314). In 1284–85 William de Erghum held 3 ct. in Argam and Bartin Dale nearby of the Gant fee (*KI*, p. 54). This was probably the William (son of Mauger) de Erghum who appears with Arnald (son of Walter) of Buckton, in 1291 and 1296, neither amongst the *milites*, and apparently of a later generation (*Ctl. Bridlington*, pp. 56, 64, 89). William (son of Mauger) de Erghum and his wife Eustacia occur in 1308 and 1310 (*YF*, 1300–1314, nos 369, 401; MS Dods. 7, ff. 228ᵛ–229ʳ).

**R573.** Grant at fee-farm by James de Ispania, master of the hospital, and the brethren, to Alice, widow of Henry Pakot of Hunmanby, of the 4 bv. land in Hunmanby which John son of Isabel of Hunmanby formerly held of the hospital, paying 40s. annually and 1m. as an obituary payment [1288 × 1293]

*De iiiiᵒʳ bovatis terre cum tofto et crofto etc ut patet inferius.*
Universis cristi fidelibus presens scriptum visuris vel audituris, Iacobus de Ispania magister hospitalis sancti Leonardi Ebor' et fratres eiusdem loci salutem in domino. Noverit universitas vestra nos concessisse dedisse et presenti carta nostra confirmasse Alicie relicte Henrici Pakot de Hundmanby illas quatuor bovatas terre cum tofto et crofto in Hundmanby quas Iohannes filius Isabelle de Hundmanby aliquando tenuit de hospitali nostro predicto, tenend(as) et habend(as) predicte Alicie et heredibus suis salvo iure cuiuscumque de nobis et successoribus nostris libere quiete integre et in pace cum omnibus pertinenciis libertatibus et aisiamentis ad dictam terram infra villam et extra spectantibus quamdiu servicium nobis inde debitum fideliter fecerint et reddiderint, reddendo inde annuatim nobis et successoribus nostris quadraginta solidos argenti, medietatem scilicet ad Pent' et aliam medietatem ad festum sancti Martini in yeme, pro omni servicio seculari consuetudine et demanda. Dicta vero Alicia et heredes sui vel quicumque dictam terram tenuerint vel in eadem manserint pauperibus hospitalis nostri predicti unam marcam argenti pro portione bonorum ipsos in obitu suo contingent(em) fideliter relinquent. Nec licebit predict(e) Alic(ie) aut eius heredes dictam terram seu aliquam partem eiusdem alicui dare vendere vel assignare sine licencia nostra speciali. Nos vero magister et fratres dictam terram cum tofto et crofto quantum in nos est predicte Alicie et heredibus suis contra omnes homines salvo iure cuiuscumque ut supradictum est warentizabimus acquietabimus et defendemus. In cuius rei testimonium sigillum nostrum commune et sigillum dicte Alicie presenti carte cirograffate alternatim sunt appensa. Hiis testibus, Waltero de Louthorp', Arnaldo de Buketon', Roberto de Wyeryn', Iohanne filio Iohannis de Hundmanby, Willelmo le Faucuner de eadem, Willelmo filio Rogeri, Henrico clerico, Willelmo filio Iohannis, Stephano de Pratis et aliis.

The date range is the period for James de Ispania as rector.

# HESLERTON

SIR THOMAS HESLERTON

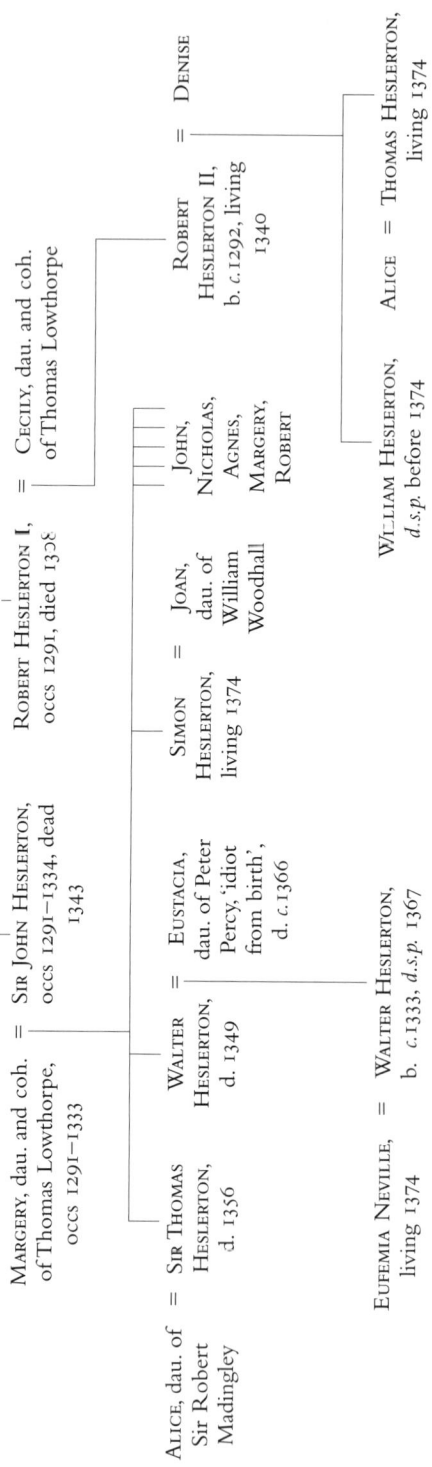

MARGERY, dau. and coh. of Thomas Lowthorpe, occs 1291–1333 = SIR JOHN HESLERTON, occs 1291–1334, dead 1343

ROBERT HESLERTON I, occs 1291, died 1338 = CECILY, dau. and coh. of Thomas Lowthorpe

ROBERT HESLERTON II, b. c.1292, living 1340 = DENISE

ALICE, dau. of Sir Robert Madingley = SIR THOMAS HESLERTON, d. 1356

WALTER HESLERTON, d. 1349 = EUSTACIA, dau. of Peter Percy, 'idiot from birth', d. c.1366

SIMON HESLERTON, living 1374 = JOAN, dau. of William Woodhall

JOHN, NICHOLAS, AGNES, MARGERY, ROBERT

WALTER HESLERTON, b. c.1333, d.s.p. 1367 = EUFEMIA NEVILLE, living 1374

WILLIAM HESLERTON, d.s.p. before 1374

ALICE = THOMAS HESLERTON, living 1374

## Harpham

For Harpham, a berewick of Burton Agnes in 1086, see *VCH Yorks ER*, II, 223–28. By 1265 Thomas of Lowthorpe held an estate in Harpham by service of a sixteenth part of a fee, of the manor of Burton Agnes, of Roger de Merlay, who held of Peter de Brus (*YI*, I, 101–2). The HESLERTON interest in Lowthorpe, Harpham and elsewhere arose from the marriage of John of Heslerton and Robert of Heslerton to the daughters and coheirs of Thomas of Lowthorpe, who was dead in 1279 (*VCH Yorks ER*, II, 273, citing PRO, Common Pleas, Plea Rolls CP 40/17 m. 41). John of Heslerton was the son of Sir Thomas of Heslerton, and a knight of the shire at the end of the thirteenth century;[1] Robert may have been his younger brother. There are several references to the moieties of the Lowthorpe inheritance, one held by Sir John of Heslerton, and afterwards by his son and heir Sir Thomas Heslerton (the senior line), the other by Robert of Heslerton and then by his son and heir, also called Robert (the junior line). Early in 1291 Robert of Heslerton and Cecily his wife claimed against John, son of Thomas of Heslerton, and Margery his wife, half of seven messuages, ninety-six tofts, five crofts, 122 bv. and 36 a., a watermill and a windmill in Lowthorpe, Harpham, Albourne, Foston, Muston, Thorpe and Carthorpe as the right of Cecily, which came to her by inheritance from Thomas of Lowthorpe, father of Cecily and Margery (Collier, 'Lowthorpe', p. 30, citing De Banco, Hilary 19 Edw. I). In the quo warranto inquiry of 1293–94, Richard Malebisse claimed to hold rights in Filey, which he shared with Margery wife of John of Heslerton, and Cecilia wife of Robert of Heslerton, from the inheritance of one Ralph,[2] his great-grandfather, and the great-great-grandfather of Margery and Cecilia (*YQW*, pp. 221–22). In 1299 Robert of Heslerton and John of Heslerton each held 2½ ct. in Lowthorpe (*YI*, III, 116). Robert Heslerton died on 3 March 1308. The resulting inquisition, taken in December 1308, found that he had, with other property, four tofts and 2 bv. in Harpham, held of Sir Roger Somervile by foreign service. His heir was his son, also named Robert, aged sixteen (*CalInqPM*, v, no. 121). On 15 February 1309 the king granted to William Clyff, to whom he had previously granted the marriage of the heir of Robert of Heslerton, deceased, any penalty incurred by the minor marrying without the king's licence (*CalPat*, 1307–1313, pp. 95, 99, 100). Clyff's relationship, if any, to Denise, to whom Robert of Heslerton was married before 1319 (R574), is unknown. Robert Heslerton presented master Robert Heslerton, son of Sir John Heslerton, knight, to Lowthorpe church in 1329 (*Fasti Parochiales*, III, 55).

The interest of the junior line in the advowson of Lowthorpe had been extinguished by 1333, when there was a fine between John Heslerton, knight, and Margery his wife, plaintiffs, and John Middelton, chaplain, defendant, regarding the church of Lowthorpe, whereby it was agreed that the advowson would remain to John and Margery for their lives, with remainders in succession to Thomas, Walter, John, Simon, Nicholas, Agnes, and Margery, sons and daughters of the said John Heslerton, and their heirs male (*YF*, 1327–1347, p. 60). Sir John Heslerton is last mentioned in 1334. His heir was his son, Sir Thomas Heslerton. Sir Thomas was married to Alice, daughter of the justice Sir Robert Madingley, through which marriage he acquired a manor in Barrington, co. Cambridge (*VCH Cambs*, v, 149). In 1343 there was a fine concerning the manor of Lowthorpe, 20 messuages, 18 a. land, rents and other

---

[1] For his career see Gooder, *Parliamentary Representation*, I, 29–32.
[2] Deduced by Farrer to be Ralph de Neville, but the surname is not in the record (*EYC*, II, 465; *PQW*, p. 217).

property, by which the manor was to be held to Thomas Heslerton, knight, and his wife Alice, with remainder to John, son of Gerard Salvayn, and John's wife Emma, and then to the right heirs of Thomas of Heslerton (*YF*, 1327–1347, p. 162). Thomas Heslerton died in February 1356 or shortly before (*CalFine*, 1356–1368, p. 14), when his heir was his nephew Walter Heslerton, son of Sir Walter Heslerton, son of Sir John Heslerton (*CalCl*, 1364–1368, p. 328).[3] For further details of the career of Sir Thomas Heslerton, see Gooder, *Parliamentary Representation*, I, 106–8.

Robert of Heslerton and Thomas of Heslerton were tenants in Burton Agnes in 1340–41 (*YF*, 1327–1347, pp. 140, 151). The second Robert of Heslerton of the junior line was apparently succeeded by a son William, who died childless. William's heir was his brother Thomas, who gave his land in Harpham to the hospital for an obit for himself, his wife Alice, and their parents (R575–R577). A licence was issued on 5 February 1374, for ½m. paid by Richard Ravenser, king's clerk and master of the hospital, for the alienation in mortmain by the trustees named in R575–R577 of three messuages and 2 bv. in Harpham to celebrate an anniversary for the souls of the father and mother of Thomas Heslerton in the hospital church (*CalPat*, 1370–1374, p. 409). The distribution of 13s. at the obit of Thomas Heslerton is noted in the *Valor Ecclesiasticus*, but Harpham is not mentioned (R905). A rent in Harpham was included in the account of 1542, and in May 1554, a messuage, garden, two crofts of pasture and 2 bv. of arable land in the tenure of Stephen Tovy in Harpham, formerly belonging to St Leonard's Hospital, York, were leased with other property to James Cokeson and others for twenty-one years (*Dissolved Houses*, IV, 224; *CalPat*, 1553–1554, p. 294).

**R574.** Surrender by William son of Thomas de Houton to Robert son of Robert of Heslerton, of Lowthorpe, and Denise his wife, and the heirs of their bodies, of all lands, tenements, rents, services of free tenants, with bondmen and their offspring and chattels, and all other lordships which he had before by gift of Robert, in the vill of Harpham, to hold of the chief lords by the service due. Reversion, in default of heirs of their bodies, to the right heirs of Robert [*c*.1313 × 1319]

**[f. 182ᵛ]** *Willelmus filius Thome de Houton' de terris et tenementis, redditibus et serviciis liberorum tenentium cum bondis et eorum sequelis catallis et omnibus aliis dominiciis.*
Sciant presentes et futuri hanc cartam indentatam visuri vel audituri quod ego Willelmus filius Thome de Houton' concessi et reddidi Roberto filio Roberti de Heslarton' de Louthorp' et Dionisie uxori eius omnia terras et tenementa redditus et

---

3 Walter Heslerton, Thomas's brother, married Eustacia, daughter and heir of Peter Percy, through whom he gained the lands of Percy of Carnaby (*CalInqPM*, VIII, no. 705; *EYC*, XI, 112). Walter died on 9 September 1349. He was survived by his wife and his son Walter, who was eighteen in 1351 (*CalInqPM*, IX, no. 639), and who was heir to his uncle Thomas Heslerton in 1356. The elder Walter was stated to have been the son of Sir John Heslerton, and to have died on 24 August 1349 'in the pestilence', at a further inquisition held in Lent 1367. His widow Eustacia was then said to have been 'an idiot from birth' and to have died 'about a year ago' (*CalInqPM*, XII, no. 147 (a), (b)). Walter Heslerton the son died in September 1367, leaving a widow Eufemia, who was living in 1374 (*YD*, IV, no. 541), but no heir of his body. Walter's heir was thus his uncle Simon Heslerton, knight, 'aged fifty years and more' (*CalInqPM*, XII, no. 202). Not all the Percy lands reverted to the chief lords of the fee. Simon Heslerton held the manor of Ilkley in 1373 (*YF*, 1347–1377, p. 180); Sutton on Derwent went to Ralph Neville, said in 1394 to be Eufemia's heir and of full age, and the son of John Neville her brother (*VCH Yorks ER*, III, 175; *CalCl*, 1392–1396, p. 192). Simon Heslerton was the husband of Joan, daughter and heir of William Woodhall, through whom he acquired the manor of *Woodhall* (lost, near Beverley) and 6 bv. in Aike, held of the archbishop, in 1343 (*KI*, p. 419). For his career, see Gooder, *Parliamentary Representation*, I, 112–13.

servicia liberorum tenentium cum bondis et eorum sequelis catallis suis et omnibus aliis dominiis cum suis pertinenciis que prius habui de dono predicti Roberti in villa de Harpham, tenenda et habenda omnia predicta terras et tenementa cum redditibus et serviciis liberorum tenentium cum bondis et eorum sequelis et catallis et omnibus aliis dominiciis Roberto et Dionisie et heredibus de corporibus eorundem Roberti et Dionisie exeuntibus de capitalibus dominis feodi per servicia inde debita libere imperpetuum. Et si predicti Robertus et Dionisia sine heredibus de corporibus eorundem Roberti et Dionisie exeuntibus obierint, tunc omnia predicta terras et tenementa redditus et servicia liberorum tenentium cum bondis et eorum sequelis et catallis suis et omnibus aliis dominiis cum suis pertinenciis, ut predictum est, rectis heredibus dicti Roberti remaneant imperpetuum, tenenda de capitalibus dominis feodi per servicia debita imperpetuum. In cuius rei testimonium huic carte indentate sigillum meum apposui. Hiis testibus, domino Willelmo Constabulario de Flanesburch', domino Roberto filio suo militibus, Iohanne de Hasthorp', Thoma de Munceus, Willelmo de Roston', Willelmo de Rudstane, Normanno de Kernarby et aliis.

Robert Constable of Flamborough died in 1272 × 1274 and was succeeded by his son, William Constable, the first witness, who occurs in 1274 and died in 1319. William's son Robert, the second witness, was living in 1338–39 (*EYC*, xii, 147–49). The grantor may have been of the family of Thomas de Houton, living in 1303, who was husband to Lettice, a sister of William Constable (*EYC*, xii, 149). Robert son of Robert of Heslerton came of age *c*.1313 (FN).

**R575.** Appointment by Walter de Nafferton, rector of the churches of St Margaret and St Mary in Walmegate, York, Thomas de Kirkeby, vicar choral of the cathedral church of St Peter, York, John de Braweby and John de Allerthorp chaplains, of Thomas Rose as their attorney to take seisin and possession of the lands and tenements with appurtenances which formerly belonged to Thomas de Heslarton, in the vill and territory of Harpham, according to the form and effect of the deed of feoffment which Thomas de Heslarton made to the grantors, as is there more fully set out. Sealing clause. 5 October 1373. No witnesses.

*Littera attorn' ad capiend(um) seisinam et possessionem.*

Dat' apud Ebor' quinto die Octobris anno domini M°CCC^mo septuagesimo tertio,[4] et regni regis Edwardi tertii post conquestum quadragesimo septimo.

**R576.** Enfeoffment by Thomas de Heslarton of Sirs Walter de Nafferton, rector of the churches of St Margaret and St Mary in Walmegate, York, Thomas de Kirkeby, vicar choral of the cathedral church of St Peter, York, John de Braweby and John de Allerthorp chaplains, with three messuages, 2 bv. land with appurtenances in the vill and territory of Harpham, which descended to the grantor by hereditary right after the death of William de Heslarton his brother, to be held to the beneficiaries, their heirs and assigns, of the chief lords by the due and customary service. Warranty and sealing clauses. 6 October 1373.

---

[4] There is apparently a brief erasure between *M* and *CCC*, probably caused by the removal of an additional and erroneous *C*.

*Carta Thome de Heslarton' de tribus mesuagiis et duabus bovatis terre.*

Hiis testibus, Marmaduco Conestable, Simone de Heslarton' militibus, Iohanne Mounseaux, Thoma de Carthorp', Willelmo de Cotum, Galfrido Randolf', Ricardo Randolf' et aliis. Dat' apud Harpham vi. die octobris anno domini millesimo CCC$^{mo}$ septuagesimo tertio, et regni regis Edwardi tertii post conquestum quadragesimo septimo.

**R577.** Grant by Walter de Nafferton rector of the churches of St Margaret and St Mary in Walmegate in York, Thomas de Kirkeby vicar choral of the cathedral church of St Peter, York, John de Braweby and John de Allerthorp chaplains, to the master and brethren of the hospital of St Leonard, York, and their successors, of a certain annual rent of 100s., for a term of thirty years from the date of the present deed, to be paid at St Martin in Winter and Pentecost by equal portions, from all their lands and tenements which they had by gift and feoffment of Thomas de Heslarton in the vill and territory of Harpham, on the following form and condition; that is that the brethren and their successors will perform two separate obits annually, one for the souls of Robert de Heslarton and Denise his wife, mother and father of the said Thomas de Heslarton, and all their benefactors (*beneficiorum*), and another for the souls of the father and mother of Alice, wife of the said Thomas de Heslarton, and all their benefactors, during the life of the said Alice and Thomas. And after their deaths the said obits will be made separately from year to year for the souls of Thomas and Alice and their mothers and fathers and all their **[f. 183ʳ]** benefactors, and all faithful deceased forever. And the chaplain brothers performing the obits shall have from the 100s. rent, for each obit 6s. 6d. shared equally between them, and the clerk who rings the bells at each obit 2d., and each bed of the cremetts (*lectus cremettorum*) in the infirmary-house (*domus infirmarie*) of the hospital ½d.; and whatever remains of the rent to be paid to the exchequer of the hospital towards the work and advancement (*proficuum*) of the hospital. Right of distraint if the rent is in arrears, in full or in part, at any term. Warranty. The grantors have handed over a silver penny of the said rent to the master and brethren in the name of seisin and possession. Alternate seals of grantors and master and brethren to the indentures. No witnesses. 10 October 1373.

*De quodam annuo redditu centum solidorum.*

Dat' apud Ebor' decimo die octobris anno domini millesimo CCC$^{mo}$ septuagesimo tertio, et regni regis Edwardi tertii post conquestum quadragesimo septimo.

## Hedon'

The origins of the town of Hedon are obscure. It does not appear in the survey of 1086, but in 1115 Stephen, count of Aumale, gave his churches and tithes in Holderness and elsewhere, together with his demesne tithes and other property, including a *hospitem*[1] on the river Hedon, with free transit on the Humber, to the abbey of Beauvais (dép. Oise, Picardie). This indicates that Hedon was already either the main port of Holderness or expected shortly to become so (*EYC*, III, no. 1304). About twenty years later the hospital similarly acquired property in Hedon in order to transport its tithes, or thraves, from Holderness. An acre of land in Hedon was given to the hospital, with 1m. from the toll of the town, by William earl of York, Count Stephen's son and successor, in 1138 × 1143 (R578, R579). Soon afterwards the hospital had two *mansuras* in the town, which were confirmed by Pope Eugenius III in 1148 (C178 [*EYC*, I, no. 179]). The confirmation of 1157 names the donor of this property as the earl of Aumale (C179 [*EYC*, I, no. 186]), but there is no trace of the second *mansura* in the earl's deeds. In 1204 the hospital's buildings in Hedon, with land and appurtenances, were confirmed by Innocent III (C182 [*Letters Innoc. III*, no. 562]). William de Forz [II], earl of Aumale, confirmed his grandfather's gifts to the hospital in 1214 × 1231 (R582), and in 1235 came to an agreement whereby he granted the hospital 1m. from Lob Wood, by the hand of the prior of Bolton, in exchange for the rent from the toll of Hedon (R595). William's son, William de Forz [III], confirmed the 1 a. plot to the hospital, and granted five of the hospital's tenants there freedom from toll and other exactions (R580). The confirmation by William de Forz [II] in 1214 × 1231 of ¼ a. in Hedon by gift of Alice daughter of William son of Hagen suggests this was a new benefaction, but Alice herself uses the verb *reddidi*, indicating it was a surrender of land previously held of the hospital (R581, R586). Other deeds in this section of the cartulary include three grants at fee-farm (R585, R587, R594), and several deeds illustrating the hospital's interest in controlling conveyances by its tenants (R588–R592). A plot of 1 a. 0 r. 27 p. in the south east of the town, on Woodmarket Lane, was called variously St Leonard's, Leonard Close, and Leonard Goit Close, 'the latter from its proximity to the drain which, on its north side, ran into the Fleet'. Boyle mistakenly believed there was a hospital on the site (Boyle, *Hedon*, p. 208 and n). The plot's size, and its proximity to the Fleet and Hedon Haven, make it likely that this was the acre given in 1138 × 1143 (R579). In 1389–90 the grassland on the bank of the Fleet 'as far as the houses of St Leonard' was being let at 5d. annually (Boyle, *Hedon*, p. xlix). In the time of Henry IV Leonard's Goit was found to be defective and was to be repaired by the master of St Leonard's Hospital and William Alnwick (ibid., p. 208n). A rent in Hedon is mentioned in the account of 1542 (*Dissolved Houses*, IV, 226), and 'Saint Leonard's rent' of 4s. annually, which may possibly be identified with the rent mentioned in R594, was still being paid in 1561–63 (Boyle, *Hedon*, pp. xl, xlii).

The career of WILLIAM OF AUMALE, and his role in Yorkshire during the reign of Stephen, is explored by Dalton.[2] Though his father Stephen of Aumale, who last occurs in 1127 and was apparently dead in 1130,[3] was sometimes styled *comes* of

---

[1]   Farrer gives the translation 'settler'. The context suggests 'warehouse' or 'lodging', cf. *DML*, s.v. *hospes, hospitatio*.

[2]   Dalton, 'William Earl of York', passim; Dalton, *Yorkshire*, esp. pp. 148–84; *ODNB*; cf. Crouch, *Stephen*, p. 160 and n.

[3]   Orderic lists Stephen of Aumale amongst those who gave succour to William Clito s.a. 1127 (Orderic,

Aumale in an English context (*CP*, I, 352), William of Aumale was not so described and was ranked far below the English earls in the witness clause of a royal charter issued at Easter 1136 (*Regesta*, III, no. 271).[4] According to Richard of Hexham, William of Aumale was granted the earldom of York by King Stephen after the battle of the Standard in August 1138 in recognition of his military services (Richard of Hexham, *Historia*, III, 165; cf. John of Hexham, *Historia regum*, II, 295).[5] It appears from a entry in a version of the Anglo-Saxon Chronicle that the king had entrusted York to William before the battle (*ASC*, II, 232). For a time it seems William held almost regal power in York. Following the death of Thurstan in 1140 he offered to procure the archbishopric of York for his kinsman Waldef of Kirkham, who had been rejected by Stephen. When Waldef refused, he informed the chapter that the king wished William FitzHerbert, treasurer of York and the king's nephew, to be elected, who was duly chosen (Knowles, 'St William', p. 165). Coins were apparently issued in William's name in the city.[6] The earl called himself 'a brother and the guardian' of the hospital when issuing his grant of thraves in Holderness (C297 [*EYC*, III, no. 1305]). William of Newburgh tells us that north of the Humber he was more of a king than Stephen himself, but on Henry II's command resigned the lands Stephen had granted him, including Scarborough, with the fortress he had built there (Will. Newburgh, *Historia*, I, 103–4). This resignation doubtless took place in 1155.[7]

Although he retained his rank as an English earl, William does not appear as earl of York after the accession of Henry II. Even in Stephen's time he was rarely so described. A writ, issued probably in 1140 × 1143, addressed to 'William earl of York and all his [the king's] men and burgesses of York', demanded that the hospital should have the king's peace and freedom from lawsuits until the consecration of a new archbishop at York (C2 [*Regesta*, III, no. 991]). It was probably *c.*1143, or not long afterwards, that Stephen ordered 'the earl of York and his ministers' to allow the prior of Bridlington to hold the port of Bridlington in peace, as he had held it previously (*Regesta*, III, no. 124). As earl of York, William attested royal charters of '1139–40' (ibid., no. 16), '1142' (ibid., no. 100; *EYC*, I, no. 100), '1138–39' (*Regesta*, III, no. 638), and '1138 × 1143' (ibid., no. 803), and a deed of Everard son of Peter de Ros of 1138 × early 1140 (*EYC*, III, no. 1330). But he attested a royal charter of 'Christmas 1141' as earl of Aumale (*Regesta*, III, 276). Even if we accept Round's proposition that an earl's description in a witness clause was no more than a matter of differentiation from others of the same Christian name (Round, *Mandeville*, pp. 145, 273), it seems unlikely that William himself gave deeds in which he described himself as *comes Ebor'* or *comes Albemarl'* entirely at random during the period 1138 to 1155. Farrer prints only four deeds given by William as earl of York. His grant of thraves to the hospital is probably of a similar date to the gift of the plot in Hedon (C297 [*EYC*,

---

VI, 368–69). William of Aumale rendered account of 154*m.* for an unspecified plea concerning his land in Holderness in 1130 (*PR*, 31 Hen. I, p. 29).

4   Clay discusses the title *comes*, with particular reference to Brittany and the lords of the honour of Richmond, in *EYC*, IV, 97–101.

5   Willelmum de Albamarla in Eboracensi et Robertum de Ferrers in Derbiensi scyra comites fecit.

6   A coin bearing the name 'William', belonging to a distinctive series struck at York during the reign of Stephen, was purchased *c.*2005 by the Fitzwilliam Museum in Cambridge.

7   English and Dalton follow Howlett's imprecise marginal summary, which is not supported by Newburgh's text, when they say that Henry 'received back Yorkshire' from the earl (English, *Holderness*, p. 22; *ODNB*, s.n. William le Gros). Farrer notes that the sheriff of York accounted for the issues of the county only from Henry's accession, but this was by no means unique to Yorkshire. Farrer also suggests that the £68 rent for Great Driffield, accounted for in 1155 and later, was Aumale's compensation for his resignation of Scarborough and Pickering (*EYC*, I, 285; *Red Bk*, pp. 648–58).

III, no. 1305]). Two deeds to Bridlington are more difficult to date but may have been issued *c.*1143 or shortly afterwards[8] (*EYC*, I, no. 362; ibid., III, no. 1306). In the deeds by which he founded Meaux Priory in 1149–50, William describes himself as earl of Aumale, and the chronicle of Meaux makes no mention of the earldom of York despite stating that William was *quasi dominus totius provincie Eboracensis* (*EYC*, III, nos 1379–1381; *Chron. Meaux*, I, 76). Amongst the chroniclers, apart from Richard of Hexham, whose account of William's ennoblement after the battle of the Standard is mentioned above, only John of Hexham describes William as earl of York, which he does when recounting events of *c.*1141–43 (John of Hexham, *Historia Regum*, II, 307–8, 312–13, 315).[9]

**R578.** Gift to the hospital by William earl of York, of a toft in Hedon and 1*m.* annually from his toll of Hedon [1138 × 1143]

COPIES: *b* Rawl., f. 184ʳ; *c* MS Dods. 7, f. 13ʳ; *d* PRO, C53/80, Charter R., 22 Edw. I, no. 18, m. 9; differences as noted, with further minor variations of spelling. PRINTED: *EYC*, III, no. 1313, where dated 1138 × 1142, from *b*. CALENDAR: *CalCh*, 1257–1300, p. 440, no. 11, from *d*. NOTED: Poulson, *Holderness*, II, 156, from *c*.

[f. 184ʳ] *Comes Albemarle de terra de Hedon', scilicet de uno tofto et una marca.*[10]
Guillelmus comes Ebor'[11] archiepiscopo Ebor'[12] et[13] decano et toti capitulo sancti Petri et dapifero et vic(ecomiti)[14] suo omnibusque baronibus suis francis et anglis et omnibus ministris et hominibus suis salutem. Sciatis me concessisse et dedisse in elemosinam imperpetuum fratribus hospitalis sancti Petri unum toftum[15] in Haduna[16] quietum et liberum ab omnibus geldis et auxiliis et omnibus consuetudinibus et serviciis cum omni libertate et consuetudine quas habet hospitale sancti Petri, et unam marcam argenti unoquoque[17] anno de theloneo meo reddendam in eadem villa pro remissione peccatorum meorum et pro animabus patris et matris mee et omnium antecessorum meorum, quare volo et firmiter precipio vic(ecomiti) meo quicumque vicecom(itatum)[18] teneat quod annuatim omni occasione postposita sicut me timet et diligit ad festum sancti Michaelis illam marcam reddat apud Ebor'.[19] T(estibus), Guillelmo decano[20] et Radulfo de Sancta Columba et Thoma Sothewaina, Varnero[21] capellano, Ricardo[22] de Curci, Helia de Mundevilla et Radulfo fratre suo, Ricardo de Otringeham, Stephano Pincerna, Girardo de Fana Curia, Alano de Muncels.

---

8 No. 1306 was made *pro restauratione dampni quod feci eis*, which may refer to William's occupation of the priory in 1143.
9 G.W. Watson drew a parallel with the count of Meulan, who was created earl of Worcester by Stephen, where 'again the English title was soon dropped' (*CP*, I, 353n).
10 *c* has rubric *Carta Guille(l)mi comitis Eboraci.*
11 *c: Eboraci.*
12 *c: Eboracensi.*
13 *c: et* omitted.
14 *b:* in full.
15 *c: thoftum.*
16 *c: Heduna.*
17 *b: unoque.*
18 *c: vicecomitum.*
19 *c: apud Ebor'* omitted.
20 *c: damori.*
21 *c, d: Garnero.*
22 *c: Rogero.*

The date is after William was created earl of York following the battle of the Standard, and before mid-March 1143, when William de Sainte-Barbe, dean of York, was elected bishop of Durham. He was consecrated three months later.

**R579.** Gift to the brethren of the hospital by William earl of Aumale, at the request of master Robert, of a toft of 1 a. in Hedon, for the gathering of corn and other alms for the use of the infirm of the hospital, and its men gathering their alms, with entry and exit for them and their boats, carts and wagons, with 1*m.* annually of his toll of Hedon [apparent date 1138 × 1143, possibly an amplification of 1155 or later]

COPIES: *b* Rawl., f. 184ʳ; *c* PRO, C53/80, Charter R., 22 Edw. I, no. 18, m. 9; minor variations of spelling. PRINTED: *EYC*, III, no. 1314, where dated 1138 × 1142, from *b*. CALENDAR: *CalCh*, 1257–1300, p. 440, no. 9, from *c*.

*Comes Albemarlie de tofto uno in Hedun et libertatibus multis et una marca annua.*
Guillemus comes Albemarl' archiepiscopo Ebor' et decano et toti capitulo sancti Petri et dapifero suo et vic(ecomiti) omnibusque baronibus suis francis et anglis et omnibus ministris suis et omnibus sancte matris ecclesie filiis salutem. Sciatis me dedisse et concessisse et hac presenti carta mea confirmasse in puram et perpetuam elemosinam imperpetuum amore dei et exoratu magistri Roberti, deo et fratribus hospitalis sancti Petri Ebor' unum toftum unius acre terre in Hedona ad colligendum ibi bladum suum et alias elemosinas ad opus infirmorum predicti hospitalis et hominibus suis ibi manentibus et elemosinam suam colligentibus, et ut ipsi et homines sui ibi manentes sint liberi quieti et immunes ab omnibus geldis et auxiliis et ab omnibus consuetudinibus et serviciis et exactionibus cum omni libertate et consuetudine quam habet hospitale sancti Petri, et liberum introitum et exitum sibi et omnibus suis et navibus et bigis et quadrigis suis, quare volo et firmiter precipio ut ipsi et homines sui in eadem terra manentes et conversantes habeant meam firmam pacem per totam terram meam. Et ne quis ministrorum meorum in terram illam invasionem faciat ad namium capiend(um) vel contumeliam faciendum neque aliquis illos iniuste calumpniet vel implacitet super forisfacturam meam. Preterea vero sciendum est me similiter dedisse et concessisse eidem hospitali unam marcam argenti redditus de meo theloneo de eadem villa, pro remissione peccatorum meorum et pro animabus patris mei et matris mee et omnium antecessorum et successorum meorum, quare volo et firmiter precipio vicecomiti meo quicumque vicecomitatum teneat quod annuatim omni occasione remota sicut me timet et diligit ad festum sancti Michaelis illam marcam reddat eis apud Ebor'. Testibus, Guillelmo decano et Radulfo de Sancta Columba et Thoma Sotwaina, Gwarnero capellano, Ricardo de Curci, Helia de Munda villa et Radulfo fratre suo, Ricardo de Otringham, Stephano Pincerna, Gerardo de Fana Curia, Alano de Muncell'.

The differences between the present deed and R578 are intriguing. It was granted by William as earl of Aumale rather than York; William does not describe the sheriff as 'his' in the address; we learn that the gift was made at the entreaty of master Robert; the size of the plot is stated; and a lot more is said about the use of the toft. This is distinctly odd, and is perhaps best explained if we consider the present deed as an amplification concocted after the death of King Stephen in 1154, at which time there is some evidence of tampering in an attempt to provide more secure title under the new regime. If so, the likely date is 1155 or soon afterwards, when Henry II was in the north commanding the surrender of royal demesne granted away by Stephen, and William of Aumale came under particular pressure (Will. Newburgh, *Historia*, I, 103–04). It may be that this deed, rather than R578, was that confirmed in 1157 by Pope Adrian, who names the donor as the earl of Aumale.

The deed, whether authentic or not, provides a rare insight into the hospital's collection of thraves. William had granted the plot in Hedon to allow the loading of corn from Holderness into boats for transportation down the river Hedon into the Humber and thence to York. His grant of thraves from Holderness was probably made at about the same date (C297 [*EYC*, III, no. 1305]).

**R580.** Confirmation to the hospital by William son of William de Forz, earl of Aumale, of a toft of 1 a. in the vill of Hedon, which it has by gift of Sir William le Gros, earl of Aumale, his ancestor, as the deed of that William shows. Also licence for five tenants living in the land, either themselves or their serjeants, to sell merchandise, or [practise] any craft within or without the said land, provided that their chattels are the property of the tenants, with freedom from toll or other exactions [1241 × June 1260, probably *c.*1255]

COPIES: *b* Rawl., f. 184ʳ; *c* PRO, C53/80, Charter R., 22 Edw. I, no. 18, m. 9; differences as noted with further minor variations of spelling. PRINTED: *MA1*, II, 394, abbreviated, with truncated witness list, from *c*; *MA*, VI, 612, no. 14, from *MA1*. CALENDAR: *CalCh*, 1257–1300, p. 440, no. 10, from *c*. NOTED: Poulson, *Holderness*, II, 156, from *b*.

*De uno tofto unius acre terre in villa de Hedon' etc. ut patet inferius.*
Universis cristi fidelibus hoc scriptum visuris vel audituris Willelmus filius Willelmi de Fort'²³ comes Albemarle salutem. Noveritis nos concessisse et caritative confirmasse deo et pauperibus hospitalis sancti Petri Ebor' unum toftum unius acre terre in villa de Hedona, quod habent ex donatione domini Willelmi le Gros comitis Albemarle antecessoris nostri in liberam puram et perpetuam elemosinam sicut carta eiusdem Willelmi quam inde habent testatur. Concessimus etiam ac confirmamus pro nobis et heredibus nostris eisdem pauperibus et hominibus suis ut²⁴ quinque tenentibus eorundem et eorum successoribus in illa acra terre manentibus, licet quinque fuerint mercator(es) mercatura(m), seu quodcumque opus artificiale, per se vel per servientes suos infra dictam acram terre vel extra exercentes, dummodo ipsa catalla sint propria dictorum quinque tenentium, ut liberi sint et quieti ac immunes ab omnibus et omnimodis geldis auxiliis teoloniis tallagiis stallagiis consuetudinibus exactionibus et de omnibus terrenis serviciis infra villam et extra de Hedona.²⁵ Et quod habeant omnes libertates communicates et liberas consuetudines ac omnimoda aisiamenta ad dictam villam de Hedona pertinencia. Et ne quis ministrorum nostrorum vel heredum nostrorum infra dictam acram terre invasionem faciat ad namia capienda vel contumelias faciendas neque aliquis illos iniuste calumpniet vel implacitet vel aliquod gravamen eis inferat super forisfacturam nostram. In huius autem rei robur et testimonium huic scripto sigillum nostrum apposuimus. Hiis testibus, domino Gileberto de Halteclo, domino Willelmo de Thorn', domino Adam de Sancto Martino, Yvone rectore ecclesie de Schipse, Henrico de Cesthunt tunc vicecomite Holderness', Nicholao Hog' rectore ecclesie de Bernestona, Iacobo de Wyhtona,²⁶ Roberto

---

²³  *c: Fortibus.*
²⁴  *b, c: ac.*
²⁵  *c: infra villam de Hedona et extra.*
²⁶  *c: Winton'.*

de Stivetona, Iohanne Dest, Stephano Passemer, Martino de Otringham, Ranulfo clerico et aliis.

The attestation of Henry de Cesthunt as sheriff shows that this deed was issued by William de Forz III, which provides the suggested range of date. Denholm-Young, who makes particular refererence to Holderness in his *Seignorial Administration*, provides a list of sheriffs from 1261 based on account rolls, but makes no attempt at a chronology before that date. His list gives Rémy of Pocklington (1261–63), William de la Twyere (1263–66), Richard Halstead (1266–67), Simon of Preston (1267–70), and Robert Hildyard (1270–89). After the wapentake was taken into the king's hands in 1268 these men were generally referred to as bailiffs rather than sheriffs (*op. cit.*, pp. 40, 47–48), but William de Walecote attested as sheriff in 1293 (MS Dods. 139, f. 54ᵛ).
      Amongst the earlier sheriffs of Holderness was Ranulf, who attested as sheriff in 1195 × 1212²⁷ (Poulson, *Holderness*, II, 204).²⁸ With others, Ralph, sheriff of Hedon, was accused of imprisonment and breach of the peace in 1214 (*CRR*, 1213–1215, pp. 74, 174). *Iohannes filius Randulfi tunc vicecom'* attested with Henry, dean of Holderness, who occurs with that title in 1241 (MS Dods. 139, ff. 48ᵛ, 61ᵛ). William English (*Anglicus*), sheriff of Holderness, attested a deed of William de Forz [III] with Sir Henry le Moigne, the steward, which can be dated to 1241 × 1251²⁹ (*CalCh*, 1257–1300, p. 381, no. 9). As Moigne attested as steward in 1241 × 1249 (*EYC*, VII, no. 40), it is clear that English was a predecessor of Henry de Cesthunt, who occurs as sheriff with a later steward, Sir Robert Daniel, in 1256 (*CalCh*, 1300–1326, p. 10, no. 3; Poulson, *Holderness*, II, 195).³⁰ Henry de Cesthunt also occurs as sheriff in 1251 (*BM Charters*, I, 373, citing BL, Harley Ch. 50 D. 38). To this list may perhaps be added Stephen Passemer, whom English calls sheriff when noting his possession of tenements in Hedon in 1235 × 1249 (English, *Holderness*, pp. 70, 76).³¹

The first witness, Gilbert de HALTECLO, held property in Caldbeck and Haltcliff in Cumberland, from where he took his name, including 31 a. in the king's forest of Haltcliff (*CalInqPM*, I, no. 495). It is clear from the earl's claim endorsed on a fine of 1255–56, to which Gilbert de Halteclo was a party, concerning property in Caldbeck and Haltcliff, that he had an interest in these places (Parker, 'Cumberland Fines', p. 225). This had been acquired after the death of Alice de Rumily in 1212 × 1215 and the subsequent division of her property between the heirs of her two sisters Amabel, wife of Reginald de Lucy, and Cecily, wife of William le Gros (*EYC*, VII, 14–19). Gilbert de Halteclo and his brother John occur in 1230 with the earl of Cornwall in the service of the king (*PatentR*, 1225–1232, p. 380). In October 1255 Robert de Brus was ordered to deliver the castle of Carlisle to the earl of Aumale or to Gilbert de Halteclo in his name (*CalPat*, 1247–1258, p. 445). Gilbert was dead in February 1261. His heir was his son William, aged twenty-one in May of that year (*CalInqPM*, I, no. 495; *RFine Excerpta*, II, 351). At an inquisition in 1305 Gilbert Halteclo was said

---

²⁷  The period for Baldwin de Béthune, who attests as earl of Aumale (*CP*, I, 354).
²⁸  Poulson's footnotes are incorrectly labelled. Burton cites the same deed, a grant by Nicholas de Chewincourt to Swine Priory, from 'Append. no. 10' (*Monasticon Eboracense*, p. 254). For the text, see Burton transcripts 3, f. 116ʳ, p. 205, B21 N43 or MS Dods. 7, f. 251ᵛ.
²⁹  From the accession of William de Forz III in 1241, and the dates here established for sheriff and steward; cf. A2A: SpSt/4/11/7/1, with similar witnesses, cited FN: Scures.
³⁰  For the careers of English and Cesthunt see *EYC*, VII, 289–90.
³¹  No reference is given. The source for the statement concerning property in Hedon is doubtless *Chron. Meaux*, II, 25, where Passemer is not called sheriff.

to hold 40*s*. of land in Haltcliff of Thomas Lucy, who was recently dead (*CalInqPM*, IV, no. 322).

**R581.** Confirmation to the hospital by William de Forz, earl of Aumale, of the toft containing ¼ a. in Hedon which it has by gift of Alice daughter of William son of Hagen [1214 × 1231]

NOTED: Poulson, *Holderness*, II, 156.

*Comes Albemarle de uno tofto in Hedon' continente unam acram terre.*
Universis sancte matris ecclesie filiis, hoc scriptum presens visuris et audituris Willelmus de Forc' comes Albemarl' **[f. 184ᵛ]** salutem. Noverit universitas vestra me concessisse et hac carta confirmasse deo et pauperibus hospitalis sancti Petri de Ebor' illud toftum in villa de Heddun quod habent ex dono Alicie filie Willelmi filii Hagne, pro salute anime mee et antecessorum et successorum meorum, quietum ab omni servicio et seculari demanda et re ad terram pertinente in liberam puram et quietam et perpetuam elemosinam. Et sciendum est quod predictum toftum continet quartam partem unius acre t(antu)m. Et ut hec mea confirmatio rata imperpetuum permaneat huic scripto sigillum meum apposui. Hiis testibus, Fulcone de Oyri, Petro de Faucunberg', Waltero de Scires,³² Willelmo Passem', Petro Grimb', Ioseph Grimb', Stephano Passem', Thoma de Holaim, He(n)r(ico) clerico, Petro clerico, Willelmo Truan clerico, Ricardo filio Siwarde, Stephano Guthemund'.

The grantor of R581 and R582 was William de Forz II, son of Hawise, the daughter and heir of William le Gros. The surrender by Alice daughter of William son of Hagen is R586. William de Forz II had seisin of his lands in 1214 and died in 1241 (*CP*, I, 355). The witness Fulk d'Oyry was dead in 1231 (Major, *D'Oyrys*, p. 23, from *MemR*, 14 Hen. III, p. 39).

**R582.** Confirmation to the hospital by William de Forz, earl of Aumale, of the gifts of his grandfather William earl of Aumale in Hedon according to his deeds [1214 × 1231]

COPIES: *b* Rawl. f. 184ᵛ; *c* MS Dods. 7, f. 15ʳ, with differences noted and further minor variations of spelling. *c* includes a drawing of the outline of a round seal on tag, separate drawing of seal (*secretum*), round, a shield bearing a cross clechée, legend not transcribed.³³

*Carta Willelmi comitis Albemarle et confirmatio eius.*³⁴
Universis sancte matris ecclesie filiis hoc presens scriptum visuris vel audituris Willelmus de Forc'³⁵ comes Albemar' salutem. Noveritis me ratas et gratas habere concessiones et donationes pauperibus hospitalis sancti Petri Ebor' caritative factas a predecessore meo Willelmo comite Albemarle avi mei, un(de) omnes eiusdem comitis concessiones et donationes et libertates secundum tenorem carte sue quam inde habent in omnibus caritative confirmavi, vicecomiti etiam meo et omnibus ballivis meis mandare dignum duxi ut ipsi fratres dicte domus et eorum homines res et

---

³² sic, for *Scures*.
³³ For this seal, see English, *Holderness*, pl. 10.
³⁴ *c* has rubric *Carta Willelmi de Forz comitis Albemarl'*.
³⁵ *c: Forz*.

possessiones et terras cum earum pertinenciis quas eis in villa de Hedun caritative dedi protegant manuteneant et defendant nec quicquam molestie contra libertates eis in carta memorata[36] concessas illis inferant vel inferri permittant, marcam autem annuam a predicto Willelmo comite de theloneo meo de Hedun pro salute animarum nostrarum et antecessorum et successorum nostrorum concessavi singulis annis ad festum sancti Michaelis secundum tenorem carte predicte sine contradictione predictis pauperibus solui volo et precipio. In huius autem rei robur et testimonium huic scripto sigillum meum apposui. Hiis testibus, Fulcone de[37] Oyri, Petri de[37] Faucunberg', Waltero de Scures, Willelmo Pasm(er'), Petro Grimb(ald'), Ioseph Grimb(ald'), Stephano Passem(er'), Thoma de Holam, Henrico clerico, Petro clerico, Willelmo Tran' clerico, Ricardo filio Siward', Stephano Guthemund' et multis aliis.

Identical witnesses to R581, and presumably the same occasion.

**R583.** Grant to the hospital by Roland de la Twyer of a rent of 4*d.* in Hedon, being the rent which Agnes daughter of William Hagen formerly paid to him [*c.*1214 × 1235]

NOTED: Poulson, *Holderness*, II, 156.

*Rollandus de la Tuier' de redditu iiii. denariorum in Hedon'.*
Sciant presentes et futuri quod ego Rollandus de la Tuire dedi et concessi et hac presenti carta mea confirmavi deo et pauperibus sancti Leonardi Ebor' in puram et perpetuam elemosinam redditum iiii[or] denariorum in villa de Hedon', pro salute anime mee et patris mei et matris mee, illud vero redditum quod Agnes[38] filia Willelmi Hagene michi quondam persoluit. Et ut hec donatio mea rata permaneat et firma, presens scriptum sigillo meo corroboravi. Hiis testibus, domino Willelmo de Redburne senescallo, Iohanne Pictavo, Petro Hog', Willelmo Hog', Thoma clerico, Amando Pasmer, Stephano Pulle, Henrico Hog', Stephano Lainde, Simone de Lavinton', Ricardo Siwarde et aliis.

Roland does not occur in Poulson's account of the Twyer family (Poulson, *Holderness*, II, 191–92). In 1226 he quitclaimed four messuages in Hedon to Peter de la Twyer (*YF*, 1218–1231, p. 87), and in 1256 attested an agreement between Sir William de la Twyer knight, and master Peter, rector of St Sepulchre's Hospital in Hedon (Poulson, *Holderness*, II, 195). Richard son of Siward was probably dead in 1235 (R588). English states that William Redburn occurs as steward of Holderness in 'about 1230', but gives no authority (English, *Holderness*, p. 66).

**R584.** Gift to the hospital by Hamo of Hollym of all his land in Hedon, which lies between the land of Ive le Mariner and that of Cecily Yokedog, with the buildings, paying Stephen Passemer 4*d.* annually [*c.*1214 × 1235]

COPIES: *b* Rawl., f. 184ᵛ; *c* Burton transcripts 1, f. 181ʳ, p. 309, B11 N42, trivial differences of spelling. NOTED: Drake, *Eboracum*, p. 335, via Torre's collections; Poulson, *Holderness*, II, 156, from *b*.

---

[36]   *c: memorata carta.*
[37]   *b: de* omitted.
[38]   sic, not Alice as in R581 and R586.

*Hamo de Holeyme de quadam terra in Hedona.*
Omnibus cristi fidelibus ad quos presens scriptum pervenerit, Hamo de Holeym salutem. Noverit universitas vestra me caritatis et pietatis intuitu et pro salute anime mee et animarum antecessorum et successorum meorum dedisse concessisse et presenti carta mea confirmasse deo et pauperibus hospitalis sancti Petri Ebor' totam terram meam in Hedona cum edificiis in ea contentis que iacet inter terram Ivonis le Mariner et terram Cicilie Yokedogge, tenendam et habendam predictis pauperibus cum omnibus pertinenciis suis aisiamentis et libertatibus suis infra burgum et extra, in liberam et perpetuam elemosinam libere integre et quiete ab omni servicio et exactione, reddendo inde annuatim Stephano Passemer iiii$^{or}$ denarios ad quatuor terminos, scilicet ad festum sancti Iohannis baptiste unum denarium et ad festum sancti Michaelis unum denarium et ad Natale unum denarium et ad Pascha unum denarium. Ego autem et heredes mei predictam terram cum pertinenciis predictis pauperibus warantizabimus in omnibus et contra omnes gentes imperpetuum. In huius autem rei robur et testimonium huic scripto sigillum meum apposui. Hiis testibus, Thoma de Holaym, Willelmo Hog', Henrico Hog', Petro homine vicecomitis, Stephano Pulle, Galfrido Passemer, Ougrim de Monte, Ricardo filio Siwardi, Stephano Pulcro, Roberto de Holaym, Stephano Lainde et multis aliis.

Richard son of Siward was probably dead in 1235 (R588). The witnesses suggest a similar date to R583 and R586.

**R585.** Acknowledgement of receipt with recital by Hamo of Hollym, of the deed of master H[ugh], rector, and the brethren of the hospital, granting him and Alice his wife, niece of Mabel Hog, the hospital's land in Hedon between the land of Stephen Laynde and the land of Ernis *ad Gote*, with the buildings, paying 12*d.* annually and a portion of chattels as an obituary payment. Reversion to the hospital on death of Hamo and Alice, quit of their successors [1214 × 1235]

*Hamo de Holeyme de terra de Hedona quam suscepit, habendam tota vita ipsius et uxoris sue.*
Omnibus sancte matris ecclesie filiis has litteras visuris vel audituris Hamo de Holeym salutem. Noverit universitas vestra me recepisse cartam hospitalis beati Petri Ebor' in hec verba: Omnibus cristi fidelibus ad quos presens scriptum pervenerit magister H[ugo] rector et fratres hospitalis sancti Petri Ebor' salutem. Noverit universitas vestra nos concessisse et presenti carta nostra confirmasse Hamoni de Holeym et Alicie nepti Mabille Hog' uxori sue terram nostram in Hedona cum edificiis in ea contentis que iacet inter terram Stephani Laynde et terram Ernisii ad Gote, tenendam et habendam dictis Hamoni et Alicie tota vita eorum de nobis libere integre et quiete ab omni servicio et exactione, reddendo inde nobis annuatim duodecim denarios, scilicet medietatem ad festum sancti Martini et medietatem ad Pent'. Predicti vero Hamo et Alicia vel quicumque in predicta terra manserint portionem catallorum eos contingentem in obitu suo domui nostro fideliter relinquent. Predictis autem Hamone et Alicie sublatis de medio redibit terra predicta domui nostre quieta et soluta de predictis **[f. 185ʳ]** Hamone et Alicia et de eorum successoribus imperpetuum. Et in huius rei testimonium huic scripto sigillum nostrum apposuimus. Hiis testibus, Batheman' de Hedona, Ernisio, Stephano Laynde, Thoma clerico, Ricardo filio Sywardi, Ricardo de Lavinton' et multis aliis.

Hugh became rector in 1214 or later. Richard son of Siward was probably dead in 1235 (R588).

**R586.** Surrender to the hospital by Alice daughter of William son of Hagen of Hedon, in her free power, of whatever right she had in the land which her father gave her in marriage next to the land of John Talun in Hedon. Confirmations by Walter brother of Alice, Peter Grimbald and William Hog [c.1214 × 1231]

NOTED: Poulson, *Holderness*, II, 156.

*Aliz filia Willelmi concedit hospitali totum ius quod habuit in maritagio suo in Hedon', et similiter alii tres super eodem.*
Sciant omnes presentes et futuri quod ego Aliz filia Willelmi filii Hahgen de Hedona in libera potestate mea reddidi et concessi et dedi et hac presenti carta mea confirmavi deo et hospitali beati Petri Ebor' quicquid iuris habui vel habere potui in terra quam pater meus michi dedit in maritagium in Hedona iuxta terram Iohannis Talun, scilicet tenend(am) et habend(am) predicto hospitali imperpetuum cum omni libertate et omnibus liberis pertinenciis, libere integre honorifice et quiete ab omni servicio et ab omni exactione, ut ego et antecessores et successores mei simus participes omnium orationum elemosinarum et aliorum beneficiorum que fiunt vel facienda sunt in prefata domo dei imperpetuum. Et ego Walterus frater predicte Aliz ratam et gratam habeo predictam donationem et eam sigillo confirmavi. Et ego Petrus Grimbald' similiter. Et ego Willelmus Hog' similiter. Hiis testibus, Willelmo Passemer tunc ballivo, Iosep Grimbalde, Petro Hog', Ricardo filio Siwarde, Waltero fratre eius, Ernisio filio Edmundi, Gilleberto de Holeim, Thoma de Holei(m), Willelmo clerico, Stephano Passem(er') et multis aliis.

This was doubtless the grant confirmed by William de Forz in 1214 × 1231 (R581).

**R587.** Agreement between Ralph, rector, and the brethren of the hospital and Stephen son of Robert of Hollym, by which the master and brethren grant to Stephen their toft in Hedon, which Stephen's sister Alice gave them. Stephen is to pay the hospital 5s. annually, and do all service due to the earl [of Aumale]. He would maintain the buildings in their current state, that is to the value of 40s., unless burnt by another's fire. If the buildings are burnt by their own fire, they and their heirs would replace them to the value of 40s. if they wished to remain, or pay 40s. if they wished to surrender the land [1204 × 1217]

NOTED: Poulson, *Holderness*, II, 156.

*Cyrograph' inter magistrum hospitalis et Stephanum filium Roberti de Hola(m) de uno tofto in Hedon' de quo redd(untur) annuatim hospitali v.s.*
Hec est conventio facta inter magistrum Radulfum rectorem et fratres hospitalis beati Petri Ebor' ex una parte et Stephanum filium Roberti de Holam ex alia parte, quod predicti magister et fratres dimiserunt predicto Stephano toftum suum in Hedun cum omnibus pertinenciis suis quod soror Alicia eis dedit, tenend(um) et habend(um) sibi et heredibus suis iure hereditario, libere et quiete de iam dicto hospitali, reddendo eidem hospitali pro omni servicio ad dictum hospitale pertinente quinque solidos, scilicet medietatem ad festum sancti Martini in yeme et medietatem ad Pent' singulis annis, et faciendo alia servicia pro hospitali ad ipsam terram pertinencia comiti et suis. Predictus etiam Stephanus et heredes sui sustinebunt edificia de suo in statu in quo ea invenerunt scilicet in precio quadraginta solidorum nisi combusta fuerint

igne alieno. Si autem combusta fuerint suo igne ipse et heredes sui propriis expensis ea reparabunt ad valenciam quadraginta solidorum si in terra predicta manere voluerint et firmam predictam solvent. Si autem terram illam relinquere voluerint, quadraginta solidos hospitali solvent. Totum vero predictum tenementum cum pertinenciis suis ut predictum est tenend(um) predicti magister et fratres predicto Stephano et heredibus suis concesserunt quamdiu firmam predictam ad terminos predictos bene persolverint, et legaliter eos se habuerint et conventionem predictam servaverint. Hoc autem tenend(um) pro se et pro heredibus suis predictus Stephanus tactis sacrosanctis iuravit. Et ut firmiter observetur imperpetuum utraque pars huic scripto sigillum suum apposuit. Hiis testibus, fratre Roberto capellano, Thoma celerario, Girardo, Godefrido, Waltero fratribus predicti hospitalis, Petro, Thoma, capellanis, Willelmo de Not(ingham), Henrico, Rogero cleric(is), Malgero, Ricardo, Waltero, Alano servientibus predicti hospitalis et multis aliis.

The date range is given by the period for Ralph as master. The detailed (and unique) clauses relating to fire suggest that it was a particular danger for this tenement, or that the premises had previously been damaged by fire.

**R588.** Acknowledgement of receipt, with recital, by Richard son of Walkelin of Hedon, of the deed of master Hugh, rector, and the brethren of the hospital, confirming the conveyance which Luke, son of Richard son of Siward of Hedon, made to him of all his land in Hedon with the buildings, paying the hospital 3s. yearly and a portion of chattels as an obituary payment. 1 August 1235.

NOTED: Poulson, *Holderness*, II, 156.

*Ricardus filius Walklini de illa terra in Hedon' quam habet de vendicione et dono Luce filii Ricardi filii Siwardi de predicta villa de Hedon'.*
Omnibus cristi fidelibus hoc scriptum visuris vel audituris Ricardus filius Walkelini de Hedon' salutem. Noveritis me cartam hospitalis beati Petri Ebor' in hec verba suscepisse: Omnibus cristi fidelibus ad quos presens scriptum pervenerit, magister Hugo rector et fratres hospitalis sancti Petri Ebor' salutem. Noverit universitas vestra nos ratam et gratam habere donationem et venditionem Luce filii Ricardi filii Siward' de Hedona quam idem Luc(as) fecit Ricardo filio Walkelini de tota terra sua in Hedona cum edificiis in ea contentis, sicut illa terra se extendit in longitudine et latitudine inter terram Germani ad Gota(m) et Stephani Minche, tenendam et habendam totam predictam terram cum omnibus pertinenciis suis dicto Ricardo et heredibus vel assignatis suis libere integre et quiete, reddendo inde annuatim nobis tres solidos, medietatem ad Pent' et medietatem ad festum sancti Martini in yeme, pro omni servicio et exactione ad nos pertinente. Predictus autem Ricardus vel quicumque in predicta terra manserint portionem catallorum eos contingentem in obitu suo pauperibus domus nostre fideliter persolvent. Et hec omnia fideliter observanda pro se et suis tactis sacrosanctis iuravit predictus Ricardus et affidavit. Et in huius rei robur et testimonium huic scripto sigillum nostrum apposuimus. Et sciendum quod ego predictus Ricardus omnia predicta a me et heredibus meis vel assignatis meis imperpetuum fideliter observanda tactis sanctis evangeliis iuravi et affidavi. Et in robur et testimonium istud scriptum sigillo meo roboravi. Testibus, Radulfo persona de Hemeleseya, magistro Iohanne de Tid, magistro Iohanne de Lada, fratre Iohanne de Notingha(m), fratre Simone, Germano ad Gota(m), Nicholao clerico et multis aliis. Actum apud Ebor' in festum sancti Petri ad vincula anno incarnationis dominice MCC. tricesimo quinto.

See R591 for an associated bond.

**R589.** Recital, noting the consent of the hospital, by Richard son of Walkelin of
Hedon, of a deed by which he gave to Thomas of Paull, in frank marriage
with his daughter Ivette, part of his land which he bought from Luke son of
Richard son of Siward in Hedon, being the part with buildings which begins
at the Goit and measures 83 ft eastwards on one side, 95 ft on the other, south,
side, and 124 ft in length, to hold to Thomas and Ivette and the heirs of their
bodies, paying the hospital 12*d*. annually, and ½*m*. for a portion of chattels
as an obituary payment. Richard agrees to make no further agreement with
Thomas without consent of the hospital [1238 × 1245]

*Trans(criptum) carte date Thome de Pagula de terra in Hedona et ne quid inter ipsum et
Ricardum sine assensu fratrum hospitalis.*
Sciant omnes presentes et futuri quod ego Ricardus filius Walkelini de Hedona dedi
Thome de Pagula cum filia mea Iueta quandam partem terre mee per voluntatem
et assensum magistri hospitalis et q(uod) idem **[f. 185ᵛ]** Thomas recepit cartam illius
terre in hec verba: Sciant omnes presentes et futuri quod ego Ricardus filius Walkelini
de Hedona dedi concessi et hac carta mea confirmavi Thome de Pagula in liberum
maritagium cum Yveta filia mea quandam partem terre mee quam emi a Luca filio
Ricardi filii Siwardi in Hedona, scilicet illam partem terre cum edificiis in ea contentis
que incipit a Gota et durat versus orientem quatuor viginti pedes et tres in uno latere
et in alio latere australi continet quatuor viginti pedes et quindecim et in longitudine
sexicies viginti pedes et quatuor, tenendam et habendam totam predictam terram
cum omnibus pertinenciis suis aisiamentis et libertatibus suis infra villam et extra
predicto Thome et heredibus de se et de Iueta filia mea procreatis libere integre et
quiete iure hereditario, reddendo inde annuatim magistro et fratribus hospitalis sancti
Petri Ebor' pro omni servicio et exactione ad eos pertinente duodecim denarios,
medietatem ad Pent' et medietatem ad festum sancti Martini in yeme. Predictus vero
Thomas et heredes sui vel quicumque in predicta terra manserint vel dictam terram
tenuerint pro portione catallorum eos contingente in obitu pauperibus dicti hospitalis
dimidiam marcam argenti nomine testamenti fideliter persolvent. Ego autem Ricardus
et heredes mei dictam terram antedicto Thome et heredibus predictis warantizabimus acquietabimus et defendemus in omnibus et contra omnes homines imperpetuum. In huius rei robur et testimonium huic scripto sigillum meum apposui. Hiis
testibus, etc. Et ne succedente tempore fiat alia conventio vel compositio inter me et
dictum Thomam sine voluntate et assensu magistri hospitalis predicti et fratrum. Hoc
scriptum sigillo meo et signo dicti Thome de Pagula roboratum magistro et fratribus
predicti hospitalis tradidimus ad habend(um).

The land conveyed appears to represent a quarter of the hospital's 1 a. plot on Woodmarket Lane. It is likely that the deed was given at the same time as R590.

**R590.** Acknowledgement of receipt with recital, by Thomas of Paull, of the deed
of master Hugh, rector, and the brethren of the hospital, confirming the
gift which Richard son of Walkelin of Hedon made to him, as in R589,
concerning the part of that land which Richard bought from Luke son of
Richard son of Siward, to hold to Thomas and the heirs of the bodies of
Thomas and Ivette, daughter of the said Richard, paying the hospital 12*d*.
annually, and ½*m*. as an obituary payment [1238 × 1245]

*Transcriptum Thome de Pagula de terra in Hedon'.*
Sciant omnes presentes et futuri quod ego Thomas de Pagula recepi cartam hospitalis sancti Petri in hec verba: Omnibus cristi fidelibus ad quos presens scriptum pervenerit magister Hugo rector et fratres hospitalis sancti Petri Ebor' salutem. Noverit universitas vestra nos ratam et gratam habere donationem quam Ricardus filius Walkelini de Hedona fecit Thome de Pagula de parte illius terre quam idem Ricardus emit a Luca filio Ricardi filii Siwardi continente in longitudine sexies viginti pedes et quatuor pedes, et in uno latere quatuor viginti pedes et tres et in latere australi quatuor viginti pedes et quindecim pedes, tenendam et habendam ipsam partem terre cum omnibus pertinenciis suis predicto Thome et heredibus suis de se et de Iueta filia predicti Ricardi exeuntibus, libere integre et quiete, reddendo inde nobis annuatim pro omni servicio ad nos pertinente duodecim denarios, medietatem ad Pent' et medietatem ad festum sancti Martini in yeme. Predictus vero Thomas et heredes sui vel quicumque in predicta terra manserint vel dictam terram tenuerint pro portione catallorum eos contingente in obitu pauperibus domus nostre dimidiam marcam argenti nomine testamenti fideliter persolvent. Hoc autem fideliter faciendum pro se et suis iuravit predictus Thomas et affidavit. In huius rei robur et testimonium huic scripto sigillum nostrum apposuimus. Hiis testibus, magistro Willelmo Passemer' canonico Ebor', domino Radulfo rectore ecclesie de Neutona, Nicholao de London', fratre I. de Notingham, fratre Roberto tunc celer(ario) et W. subceler(ario) et aliis. In cuius rei testimonium ego predictus Thomas huic scripto sigillum meum apposui.

The deed was issued between the institution of Ralph of Geddington as rector of Newton-on-Ouse in 1238 and the death of rector Hugh in 1245. William Passemer occurs as a canon in 1242 and 1243. For Nicholas of London, who occurs frequently as *magister*, see FN.

**R591.** Bond by Richard son of Walkelin of Hedon, promising to idemnify the hospital from all demands made by the earl of Aumale or his heirs on account of Richard or his heirs, and to submit to the jurisdiction of the dean and chapter of York. 1 August 1235.

*Obligatio Ricardi filii Walkini quod conservabit magistrum et fratres hospitalis indempnes erga comitem Albemarlie.*
Omnibus sancte matris ecclesie filiis hoc scriptum visuris vel audituris Ricardus filius Walkelini de Hedon' salutem. Noverit universitas vestra me promisisse concessisse et hac carta mea confirmasse pro me et heredibus meis magistro et fratribus hospitalis sancti Petri Ebor' quod ipsos conservabo indempnos super omnibus dampnis controversiis querelis questionibus motis vel movendis eisdem a comite Albemarlie seu heredibus suis occasione persone mee vel heredum meorum. Et si que expens(a) fuerint f(a)c(er)e vel faciende, seu si qua dampna sustinuerint pretextu memoratorum dampnorum questionum controversiarum querelarum eisdem, una cum heredibus meis satisfaciam, prout per eorum sacramentum prestitum dum habentes pre oculis velint iurare. Et ad predicta fideliter observanda obligavi ac subieci me et heredes meos iurisdictioni decani et capituli Ebor' omn(i) iuris beneficio tam civilis canonici appostollici cavillationi exceptioni dilationi et precipue regie prohibitioni renuncians, ita ut plenam habeant potestatem compellendi me et heredes meos per censuram ecclesiasticam ad antedicta in omnibus observanda. Et ut supradicta robur optineant firmitatis huic scripto sigillum meum apposui. Testibus, Radulfo persona de Hemeleseya, magistro Iohanne de Tid, magistro Iohanne de Leda, fratre Iohanne de Leda, fratre Iohanne de Notingham, Iohanne persona sancte Margarete, Germano de Hedon',

Nicholao clerico et multis aliis. Act' apud Ebor' in festo ad vincula sancti Petri, anno dominice incarnationis millesimo CC.xxxv. In super obligavi me et heredes vel attorn(atos) meos quod numquam terram quam teneo de hospitali predicto judeis vel viris religiosis assignabimus.

This bond was issued in association with R588.

**R592.** Will of Richard German of Hedon, made 26 January 1307[/08], and proved 26 March 1308. Amongst other provisions, he leaves his capital messuage to his wife Eda for life, and afterwards to his son John, paying the hospital 14*d*. annually; and leaves a house to his daughter Margaret, paying 2*s. 6d*.

NOTED: Poulson, *Holderness*, II, 156.

*Testamentum Ricardi German'.*
In nomine patris et filii amen. Ego Ricardus German' de Hedon' ordino et facio testamentum meum die veneris prox' post conversionem sancti Pauli anno domini millesimo CCC^mo septimo in hunc modum. In primis lego et commendo animam meam deo et beate Marie et omnibus sanctis eius et corpus meum ad sepeliendum in cimiterio sancti Augustini de Hed(on). Item **[f. 186ʳ]** pro mortuare meo meliorem supertunicam meam in salute anime mee. Item in pulsationibus vigillis oblationibus et aliis necessar(iis) circa corpus meum ii.s. vi.d. Item do lego Ede uxori mee et Iohanne filio meo cum predictam[39] Eda capitale mesuagium meum excepto furno cum terra appendente et aliis suis pertinenciis prout per bundas dividitur, habendum et tenendum dictum mesuagium cum pertinenciis et aisiamentis suis dicte Ede uxori mee in tota vita sua et post eius decessum predicto Iohanne filio meo et here-dibus suis vel suis assignatis quibuscumque, reddendo inde annuatim fratribus hospi-talis sancti Leonardi Ebor' quatuordecim denarios ad terminos consuetos. Item do lego Margarete filie mee illam domum que sita est iuxta venellam que vocabatur quondam venella Thome de Gardo cum furno et aliis suis pertinenciis et aisiamentis, habendam et tenendam predictam domum cum furno et aliis suis pertinenciis et aisiamentis predicte Margarete filie mee et heredibus suis vel suis assignatis, reddendo inde annuatim fratribus hospitalis sancti Leonardi Ebor' ii.s. vi.d. ad terminos debitos et consuetos. Ita do lego Ede uxori mee omnia utensilia ad domum meam pertinentia tam magna quam minuta possidenda in tota vita sua ita quod si necesse fuerit licite poterit ea vendere et commodum suum inde facere. Et si aliqua bona ad partem meam contingentia residua fuerint ea do lego integre predicte Ede uxori mee. Huius autem testamenti istos constituto executores meos, videlicet predictam Edam uxorem meam et predictum Iohannem filium meum quorum sigilla una cum sigillo meo in huius rei testimonium huic testamento sunt appensa.
*Probatio eiusdem testamenti.*[40]
In dei nomine amen. Admissis probationibus super confectione presentis testa-menti coram me W. clerico domini W. Wrayns[41] rector(is) ecclesie de Lounesburgh' sequestator(is) general(is) commissar(ii) testamentum ipsum rite probatum pronuncio exec(utoribus) in eodem nominat(is) liberam administrat(ionem) in forma statuti concedend'. Dat' apud Hedon' vii. kal' April' anno gracie millesimo CCC^mo octavo.

---

[39] MS: *cum predictam* repeated.
[40] These three words are in the red ink of the rubric, but there is no provision for a decorated capital.
[41] sic, for *Darrayns*.

William Darreyns, or Dareyns, rector of Londesborough, was appointed sequestrator in the archdeaconries of Cleveland and the East Riding in November 1306, and held the position until May 1308 (*Reg. Greenfield*, III, pp. xv, 124).

**R593.** Conveyance by John Frankys, burgher of the vill of Hedon, to Sir Richard de Ravens(er), archdeacon of Lincoln, master Walter de Syklagh', archdeacon of the East Riding, Sir John de Ravens(er), rector of the church of Algerkyrke [Lincs.], Sir Thomas de St-Martin (*sancto Martino*), rector of the church of Brandesburton, William de Holm' and John de Redenes, of one messuage with appurtenances in the vill of Hedon, which lies in length from the road called Marketgate towards the west, as far as Sutors road (*viam sutorum*) towards the east and in width from the lane called Destlane towards the north as far as the plot of John Shackyll' towards the south, to hold of the chief lords of the fee by the service due. Warranty and sealing clauses. 31 January or 7 February 1377[/78]

*Iohannes Frankys burgens de Hedon' de uno mesuagio in eadem villa.*

Hiis testibus, Stephano de Goldeman' tunc maiore, Iohanne de Burton', Roberto Chapman tunc ballivis, Thoma Iustisse et Thoma Mody et aliis. Dat' apud Hedon' in Holdernesse die dominica prox' []⁴² festum purificationis beate Marie anno domini millesimo CCC^mo septuagesimo septimo.

The leading grantee, Richard Ravenser, was then master of the hospital. Frankys was mayor of Hedon in 1376 and *c.*1390. His will, which included bequests to the church of St Augustine in Hedon, was dated 28 August 1391 and was proved on 5 January [1392 ?] (Boyle, *Hedon*, pp. 90n, l; *Test. Ebor.*, I, 161).

**R594.** Grant at fee-farm by Roger of Malton, rector of the hospital, and the brethren, to Roger Gayte of Hedon, of a toft in Westgate in Hedon, which toft Utting Fuller formerly held. Rent 4*s.* annually. Prohibition on alienation without the consent of the hospital [1276 × 1280]

*De uno tofto.*
Omnibus cristi fidelibus hoc scriptum visuris vel audituris Rogerus de Malton' rector hospitalis beati Petri Ebor' et fratres eiusdem hospitalis salutem in domino. Noverit universitas vestra nos unanimi consensu et assensu concessisse dedisse et hoc presenti scripto confirmasse Rogero dicto Gayte de Hedon' unum toftum in Westgate in Hedon' cum omnibus aisiamentis suis, quod quidem toftum Utting' Fullo quondam tenuit in eadem villa, tenendum et habendum predicto Rogero Gayte et heredibus suis libere hereditarie et pacifice imperpetuum, reddendo inde annuatim nobis et successoribus nostris iiii^or solidos, duos scilicet solidos ad Pent' et duos solidos ad festum sancti Martini in yeme pro omni servicio seculari. Et sciendum est quod licebit eidem predicto Rogero nec heredibus suis predictum toftum sine consensu et assensu nostri et successorum nostrorum alicui dare vendere aut alienare. Nos vero predicti Rogerus rector et fratres hospitalis antedicti et successores nostri predictum toftum cum aisiamentis suis prefato Rogero Gayte et heredibus suis warantizabimus acquietabimus et defendemus quamdiu carta nostri donator(is) quam inde habemus nobis illud warantizare acquietare et defendere poterit. In huius rei testimonium huic

---

⁴² *post* or *ante* omitted.

scripto ad modum cirographi confecto tam nos predicti Rogerus rector et fratres dicti hospitalis quam antedictus Rogerus Gaite sigilla nostra alternatim apposuimus. Hiis testibus, Nicholao de Crosseby, Willelmo de Beauuise,[43] Stephano de Frisemarays, Roberto de eadem, Ricardo German, Alano Salter', Iohanne de Garde et aliis.

The date is limited by the rectorship of Roger.

**R595.** Final concord between Hugh, master of the hospital, plaintiff, and William [de Forz II], earl of Aumale, defendant, by Stephen Passemer his attorney, concerning 1 *m.* rent in Hedon, whereof there had been a plea in the same court. The master released and quitclaimed that rent, and the earl gave the master 1 *m.* annual rent at Bolton, by the hand of the prior of Bolton, from 20*s.* rent which the prior was accustomed to pay the earl from Lob Wood [in Draughton]. 17 January 1235.

ORIGINAL: *a* PRO, CP 25/1/263/29, no. 136, not collated. COPY: *b* Rawl., f. 186[r–v]. CALENDAR: *YF*, 1232–1246, p. 34, from *a*.

*Cirographum de una marcata redditus percipiendo per manum prioris de B[oulton] pro comite Albemarl'.*[44]
Hec est finalis concordia facta in curia domini regis apud Ebor' die mercurii prox' post festum sancti Hillarii anno regni regis Henrici filii regis Iohannis decimo nono coram Rogero Bertram, Roberto de Ros, Ada de Novo Mercato, Willelmo de Ebor' et **[f. 186ᵛ]** Iollano de Nevill' iusticiariis itinerantibus et aliis domini regis fidelibus tunc ibi presentibus, inter Hugonem magistrum hospitalis sancti Leonardi Ebor' querentem et Willelmum comitem Alba Marl' deforcientem per Stephanum Pasem[er] positum loco suo ad lucrandum vel perdendum de una marcata redditus cum pertinenciis in Hedon', unde placitum fuit inter eos in eadem curia, scilicet quod predictus magister remisit et quiet'clamavit de se et successoribus suis et fratribus predicti hospitalis eidem comiti et heredibus suis totum ius et clam(eum) quod habuit in predicta marcata redditus cum pertinenciis imperpetuum. Et pro hac remissione quieta clamant(ione) fine et concordia idem comes dedit et concessit predicto magistro unam marcatam redditus singulis annis percipiend(am) apud Boulton' per manum prioris de Boulton' et successorum suorum ad duos terminos anni de viginti solidatis reddit(us) quos idem prior reddere consuevit predicto comite de bosco qui vocatur Libewych', scilicet medietatem ad Pent' et medietatem alteram ad festum sancti Martini. Et hec concordia facta fuit presente predicto priore et eam concedente et cognoscente se debere predictum redditum unius marce.

Lob Wood is about 1 m. south of Bolton Priory, on the west bank of the Wharfe. William de Forz II, earl of Aumale, inherited the honour of Skipton from his mother Hawise, who was daughter of Cecily de Rumilly and William le Gros, earl of Aumale (*EYC*, VII, pedigree facing p. 1). The rent from Lob Wood had presumably been reserved on some benefaction to the priory, it but is not apparent in the deeds of the lords of the honour of Skipton printed by Clay and by Legg (*EYC*, VII, passim; *Ctl. Bolton*, passim).

---

43 sic, doubtless for Beaumes. William de Beaumes was a regular witness to the hospital's deeds at this period, sometimes with Nicholas de Crosby; Beauvise does not otherwise occur.
44 In the margin: '*Evidenc' pro una marca in Bolton' in Craven Lobbwode*; also *de ann[u]o red' i. marce per annum pro bosco voc' Lobwyck*.

## *Howm'* [Holme on the Wolds]

In 1086, the fee of the bishop of Durham included 12 ct. in Holme on the Wolds, of which 6 ct. were held by Nigel. In '*c.*1125 × 1135' Alan de Percy [I] and William his son gave ½ ct. in Holme [on the Wolds] to Haslat of Leconfield for a rent of 3*s.* yearly, Haslat to do the forinsec service due to the bishop (*EYC*, II, no. 970; ibid., XI, no. 5). The gift of Alice de St-Quintin to Nun Appleton of the church of Holme indicates that land in Holme was included in the fee held of Percy by Robert son of Fulk (*EYC*, I, no. 543; ibid., XI, 91). An unidentified Walter de Percy gave 6 bv. and two tofts in Holme (*Howum*) to Bridlington Priory (*Ctl. Bridlington*, p. 201). By fine made in 1202, after an assize of mort d'ancestor, Robert de Vilers and Denise his wife quitclaimed to Henry de Percy, clerk, all right in 2 bv. in Holme (*Howum*) for 2*m.* (*PF John*, p. 38).

There is no further evidence for the hospital's holdings in Holme on the Wolds, but the hospital had interests in Lockington, Middleton-on-the-Wolds, Cranswick and North Dalton, all within a few miles of Holme.

**R596.** Gift to the hospital by Phip of Dalton of a fourth part of the toft belonging to his ½ ct. of land in Holme, being the eastern part [*c.*1200 × *c.*1215]

[f. 187$^v$] *Ph(ipp)us de Dalton' de iiii$^{ta}$ parte totius tofti pertinent(is) ad dimidiam caruc(atam) terre.*
Sciant omnes presentes et futuri quod ego Phippus[1] de Dalton' dedi et concessi et hac presenti carta mea confirmavi deo et pauperibus hospitalis sancti Petri Ebor' quartam partem totius tofti mei pertinentis ad dimidiam carrucatam terre mee in Howm', scilicet illam partem que est propinquior orient(i), tenendam et habendam predictis pauperibus in puram et perpetuam elemosinam, libere integre honorifice et quiete ab omni servicio et ab omni exactione sicut ulla elemosina liberius potest dari. Et ego predictus Ph(ipp)us et heredes mei warantizabimus et adquietabimus predicto hospitali totam predictam iiii$^{tam}$ partem tofti cum[2] commun(i) pastura et communa ipsius ville et cum omnibus aliis aisiamentis et liberis pertinenciis ad predictum tene-mentum pertinentibus infra villam et extra imperpetuum contra omnes homines, ut ego et antecessores et successores et heredes mei simus participes omnium orati-onum elemosinarum et aliorum beneficiorum que fiunt vel facienda sunt in prefata domo dei. Hiis testibus, Willelmo filio Petri, Marmaduc de Tueeng', Willelmo Salvein, Henrico de Perci persona de Giseburne in Craven, Waltero fratre eius, Hugone de Langethwett, Willelmo de Watton', Thurstino de Dalton', Rogero de Kava genero eius, Willelmo filio Thome, Gilleberto de Midelton' et multis aliis.

This deed is probably of approximately the same date as R597. The witness Henry de Percy, probably an illegitimate son of William de Percy II, became rector of Gisburn between 1190 and 1200 (*EYC*, XI, p. xi; M: Painley [MS Dods. 120b, f. 87$^r$]). His interest in 2 bv. in Holme is noted above. Henry was still rector in 1216, but Jordan of Bingley was collated in August 1228 (*Fasti Parochiales*, IV, 56). William son of Peter was living in 1220, but dead in 1225 (FN: Hay). For Marmaduke of Thwing [I], a justice itinerant in the 1220s, see *EYC*, XI, 205.

---

[1]   sic.
[2]   MS: *et.*

**R597.** Acknowledgement of receipt by Walter, son of Ingold of Holme, of the hospital's grant of the fourth part of the toft in Holme which Phip of Dalton gave it, paying 15*d*. annually. Walter will make the brethren a suitable building to receive and store their corn. A portion of chattels will be given as an obituary payment [*c.*1200 × *c.*1215]

*Walterus filius Ingold'*[3] *de xv. denariis annuatim reddend(is) hospitali de terra de Howm'.*
Sciant omnes presentes et futuri quod ego Walterus filius Ingolde de Howme recepi a magistro et fratribus hospitalis beati Petri Ebor' iiii^{tam} partem tofti in Howme quam Ph(ipp)us de Dauton' eis dedit in puram elemosinam, tenend(am) michi et heredibus meis, reddendo eis inde annuatim quindecim denarios, medietatem ad Pent' et medietatem ad festum sancti Martini, ita quod faciemus eis in ipsa terra competentem domum ad bladum suum recipiendum et deponendum. Et in obitu nostro reddemus ego Walterus et heredes mei predictis pauperibus integre nostram portionem catallorum nostrorum que habuerimus in predicta terra. Et hoc legitime tenendum pro me et pro heredibus meis iuravi affidavi et presenti carta mea confirmavi. Hiis testibus, Ph(ipp)o de Dauton', Roberto, Ada, Petro et aliis capellanis predicte domus, Alano, Roberto, Girardo, Willelmo, Waltero, Godefrido et alius fratribus ipsius hospitalis, Thoma de Languath', Willelmo, Eustac(io) et aliis clericis et multis aliis.

Thomas de Langwath normally attested as master after *c.*1220, and Girard had ceased to attest by the time Langwath gained the title. Godfrey cannot be shown to attest before 1200. Robert, Adam, Peter chaplains, Girard, William, Robert, brothers, and Thomas de Langwath, with others, attested a deed of *c.*1206 (R463). The present deed represents a preliminary stage in the development of the acknowledgement of receipt with recital which was first used during the rectorate of Hugh.

---

3   MS: *Sugold'*.

## *Northecave* [North Cave]

In 1086 Nigel [Fossard] held an estate of two manors comprising 6 ct. 2 bv. in [North] Cave of the count of Mortain. In 1284–85 the holding in North Cave of Peter de Mauley, who had succeeded to the Fossard fee, was assessed at 5 ct., of which the hospital held 2 bv. (*KI*, p. 85). In 1148 Pope Eugenius III confirmed 'a mill in North Cave of the Fossard fee' to the hospital (C178 [*EYC*, I, no. 179]). It may perhaps have been after this date that Roger Hay issued his grant of the mill (R598). Several mills were given to the hospital by tenants-in-chief during the reign of Stephen, and it is quite probable that the grant was instigated by Fossard rather than Hay.[1] The grant of the mill was twice confirmed by Roger's son Thomas (R599, R600). In *c.*1184 × *c.*1191 the hospital assigned half the mill of Cave to Osbert of Broomfleet for a rent of 4*s.* (R809). The 2 bv. in North Cave given by John Todhe in *c.*1210 × 1217, which were regranted to him by the hospital (R603–R606), appear to be distinct from the 2 bv. given by Lady Sybil Hay (R607–R609).[2] Smaller gifts were made in the first half of the thirteenth century by Simon Brabazon, David de Anford, Robert son of David of North Cave, Robert de Anford the younger, and Herbert son of Robert of North Cave (R610–R617). The hospital's possessions in North Cave are not mentioned in the extents of the late thirteenth century, or the *Valor Ecclesiasticus*, and were probably included in the manor of Broomfleet. In 1295 a commission of oyer and terminer was issued on complaint by Walter of Langton, master of the hospital, that Peter de Eyville, John of Cave and John de Eyville had carried away the crops and goods of the hospital at North Cave, and prevented the hospital's men from reaping and binding the corn there (*CalPat*, 1292–1301, p. 160). Sir Robert Babthorpe held a messuage, 10 bv. land, and a ruinous fulling mill in North Cave of the hospital at his death in 1436, which he had acquired by grant of Roger Airmyn (*CalInqPM*, XXIV, no. 705). In 1504 it was found by inquisition following the death of William Babthorpe that he had held six messuages, 90 a. land, meadow and pasture, and a fulling mill in North Cave, worth 10*m.*, of the hospital, by fealty, other service unknown (*CalInqPM Hen. VII*, II, no. 939). In 1602 Ralph Babthorpe and others sold an estate of two messuages, three cottages, and a watermill with lands in North Cave and Everthorpe, and 2*s.* rent issuing from a messuage in Kirkgate in North Cave (*YFTP*, IV, 188, 197).

The hospital's deeds show that there was difficulty in getting the local tenants to use the mill, which was presumably in an unattractive location. The statement in Roger Hay's deed of *c.*1135 × *c.*1154 that all those who had previously used the mill would do so henceforth (R598) suggests the tenants had an alternative. His son's confirmation of 1190 × 1212 notes the suit of mill from 4 ct. (R600), but the judgment of the chapter of York, probably made in 1204 × 1217, shows that the tenants continued to mill elsewhere (R602). In 1374 the hospital leased the millpond to John Tothe, and in its indenture detailed the obligation of suit. It is likely that the mill was then in considerable disrepair, as there is no mention of it, and the rent for the first eleven years was to be at a reduced rate (R601). In 1436, as noted above, it was described as a ruinous fulling mill.

---

[1]  It was not uncommon for a lord to reach an accommodation with a tenant to allow such a grant. Kirkstall Abbey was built on land belonging to William Peitevin, but his lord Henry de Lacy was the founder (FN: Peitevin of Headingley). William Fossard himself gave 3 ct. in Hawold to Watton Priory, making recompense to his tenant Roger son of Roger (*EYC*, II, no. 1095).

[2]  Although the hospital was said to hold 2 bv. in 1284–85, and 2 bv. land in North Cave were included in the Broomfleet rental of the late sixteenth century, it is clear from the inquisition of 1504 that the actual extent of the land was rather greater.

# Hay of Aughton

WILLIAM SON OF ANKETIN

CHRISTIANA = PETER SON OF WILLIAM

ROGER SON OF ALURED, dead 1162

THOMAS SON OF ROGER, benefactor of Thicket, dead 1190

EMMA HAY, occs 1176 × 1187, d. c.1200 = ROGER HAY, of Hunston and North Cave, occs c.1150, sheriff of Sussex 1163–1170, d. 1190 × 1196

ROGER SON OF ROGER, holding 2 k.f. of Fossard in 1166, founder of Thicket Priory, d.s.p. before 1190

ALICE or ALIVE = WILLIAM SON OF PETER, founder of Ellerton Priory, d.s.p. 1220 × 1225

THOMAS HAY, occs 1176 × 1187, d. 1226–27

ALICE = ROGER HAY, of Hunston, Sussex, occs 1196–1226, d.s.p. by 1230

AGNES, occs 1231, dead in 1246 = ADAM OF BURLAND or OF LINTON, died 1225 × 1231

THOMAS SON OF THOMAS SON OF ROGER, occs 1190, d.s.p. before 1196

OLIVIA, said to have married PETER DE LA HAYE, of Spaldington

ROGER OF LINTON

EMMA = SIR WILLIAM OF LINTON, occs 1252

MASTER JOHN OF HOWDEN, rector of Goodmanham, living 1268

ROGER HAY, d. 1247 × 1251 = CHRISTIANA

WILLIAM HAY, d.v.p.

JOHN HAY, succ. by 1251, d.s.p. 1252 × 1255

GERMAN HAY, succ. by 1255, living 1295 = MARGERY, occs 1273, 1286

NICHOLAS HAY, occs c.1261–1268

PETER, occs 1252

Unnamed daughters

A rental of the manor of Broomfleet (which belonged to the hospital before the Dissolution), probably made towards the end of the sixteenth century, lists appurtenances in North Cave including a water mill rented out for 8s. per annum, 2 bv. land, two messuages and other land (*YD*, II, no. 128).

The accounts of the family of HAY OF AUGHTON given by Farrer and Clay require revision (*EYC*, II, 423–24; *EYF*, pp. 40–42). Roger Hay first comes to notice in the mid-twelfth century, when he granted the mill in [North] Cave to the hospital, with a toft, for the health of himself, his wife, and his lord William Fossard (R598). Later evidence shows Roger had 4 ct. in North Cave, held as ¼ k.f., from which suit of the mill was due (R599; *KI*, p. 265). Roger son of Nigel confirmed to the hospital the land they held in North Cave, being a toft of his own gift, and another given by his man Walter Talun. It has been assumed that this was Roger Hay, or perhaps his father, but this remains unproven, and the authenticity of the deed is questionable (R622). It is curious that Roger Hay does not appear in the list of fees returned by William Fossard in 1166 (*EYC*, II, no. 1003).[3] If the quarter fee in North Cave had represented his entire holding it might not have been thought worthy of inclusion, as nothing less than ½ k.f. is listed. But later evidence suggests he held a further quarter fee of Fossard in Everthorpe. Possibly the land in North Cave was held as a subtenancy, perhaps through a grant in frank-marriage. Roger Hay's attestation to a deed of William Fossard [I] (*EYC*, II, no. 1047) seems to be his only other appearance in Yorkshire before 1190. His name follows that of Wimund *dapifer* amongst the witnesses. The deed cannot fall far outside Farrer's suggested dates of '1136 × 1150', as Wimund had been succeeded by his son Ralph by the end of Stephen's reign at the latest (FN: Wimund). Roger's absence from Yorkshire records is not difficult to explain: he was mainly resident in Sussex, and cannot have been a frequent visitor to the county.

There is no direct twelfth-century evidence to identify Roger Hay of North Cave with the man of the same name of Hunston, near Chichester, but thirteenth-century records leave no room for doubt. In both Yorkshire and Sussex contexts Roger Hay's wife is named as Emma, and his eldest son and heir as Thomas. In the 1230s the Yorkshire Hays inherited the remaining property of the Hays of Sussex, and soon exchanged it for more convenient holdings in Yorkshire.[4] Roger Hay held Hunston of William de St-Jean, lord of the honour of Halnaker, and was a benefactor of Boxgrove Priory, the remains of which still stand a few miles north-east of Chichester. Between 1176 and 1187[5] Roger Hay gave the mill of Hunston to the priory, for the health of his lord [William] de St-Jean and Emma the donor's wife and his children, by a deed attested by 'Emma and Thomas my son who themselves with me made that gift' (*Ctl. Boxgrove*, no. 26). Roger Hay attests many deeds in the Boxgrove cartulary dating from the 1170s and 1180s, and an act of Hilary, bishop of Chichester, made in 1147 × 1169 (*Chichester Acta*, no. 24). Roger was sheriff of Sussex from about Michaelmas 1163 until Easter 1170 (*PR*, passim), and so described attested a deed in favour of

3   As will be shown, Roger son of Roger, who held 2 k.f. of Fossard in 1166, was not the same man.
4   See below. Roger Hay, then holding the Yorkshire lands, exchanged the remaining Sussex interests for lands in South Kirkby and elsewhere in Yorkshire (*YF*, 1232–1246, p. 173). German Hay, a successor to the Yorkshire fee, was holding 100s. rent in South Kirkby in 1295 (*YI*, III, 18).
5   William de St-Jean confirmed Roger's grant by a deed which appears to precede another confirmation issued in 1187 (*Ctl. Boxgrove*, nos 5, 6). The mill does not appear in the general confirmation to Boxgrove issued by Bishop John Greenford in 1176 × 1180, but it is listed in the confirmation of Bishop Seffrid II of 1180 × 1190 (*Chichester Acta*, nos 58, 76). It is often difficult to discover the criteria for the date ranges suggested in *Ctl. Boxgrove*.

Lewes Priory between 1163 and 1166 (*Hatton's Bk of Seals*, no. 221). No satisfactory evidence is available from Sussex sources to confirm Roger's antecedents.[6] He reappears in Yorkshire in 1190, when Thomas son of Thomas son of Roger accounted for 100s. for having recognition of the death of his father, for land in Aughton and Goodmanham, of which land Roger 'de Hay' was deforcing him (*ei disforciat*) (*PR*, 2 Ric. I, p. 66).[7] Roger was dead in 1196, when Emma Hay accounted in Yorkshire for ½m. for a disseisin (*ChancR*, 8 Ric. I, p. 188).

Although Roger Hay made his gift to Boxgrove with his son Thomas, his successor in the Sussex holdings was another son, Roger. After his father's death, Roger Hay son of Roger Hay confirmed his father's gift of the mill to Boxgrove and made the additional gift of a virgate called *de quercu* in Hunston, which his father had wished to give with his body, by a deed which was confirmed by Bishop Seffrid II in 1187 × 1204 (*Ctl. Boxgrove*, no. 27; *Chichester Acta*, no. 78). By another deed to Boxgrove the younger Roger Hay gave the land called Woodcroft [in Hunston], for the health of his soul and that of Alice his wife (*Ctl. Boxgrove*, no. 140). It is noteworthy that despite frequent attestations by the elder and younger Roger in the Boxgrove cartulary there is no occasion on which father and son occur together. Nor does the younger Roger appear as Roger son of Roger Hay other than in his confirmation to Boxgrove. Roger did not inherit the Yorkshire lands, which passed to his brother Thomas. As Roger is not mentioned in the deed by which his father gave Hunston mill to Boxgrove we can be confident he was a younger son, and that a family arrangement was made whereby he inherited the Sussex lands, his older brother Thomas taking the more extensive Yorkshire interests.

Emma Hay's amercement for a disseisin in Yorkshire, for which she accounted in 1196 and 1197 (*ChancR*, 8 Ric. I, p. 188; *PR*, 9 Ric. I, p. 58), is not the only evidence that she, rather than her son Thomas, held much of the Yorkshire property after her husband's death. Between August 1197 and Michaelmas 1198 Emma Hay made a grant to the hospital, with the assent of Thomas Hay, her son and heir, for the health of their souls, and for the souls of Roger, her brother, whose heir she was, and Roger, her husband, of a rent of 6s. from ½ ct. in Oglethorpe, from the 2 ct. which Hugh son of William of Oglethorpe 'holds of us' (M: Oglethorpe [MS Dods. 95, f. 61ʳ]).[8] As Emma Hay she confirmed to the nuns of St Mary at Thicket 1 bv. in Cottingwith which Pigot had given (*EYC*, II, no. 1132). She made an agreement with William son of Peter concerning a gage, or mortgage, for land in Goodmanham and Aughton, which had been made by William's grandfather William son of Anketin to Emma's father Roger son of Alured, to which she appended her seal which Dodsworth described as 'an egle regardant to the dexter point wings partly [?] erected', 'SIGILL': EMME: DOMINE: DE: ACTONA+'. After her death an agreement made between Thomas Hay and William son of Peter speaks of the pledge 'redeemed in the time of Emma Hay, mother of Thomas' (*EYC*, II, nos 1129–30).[9] In 1251 John Hay claimed land in Aughton as Emma, his

---

[6]   It is unlikely that he was related to Robert de Haye, founder of Boxgrove and grandfather of William de St-Jean. Robert de Haye was given the honour of Halnaker by Henry I, and gave the church of Hunston with its lands and tithes to the abbey of Lessay in 1105 (*VCH Sussex*, IV, 156). Roger and his immediate descendants are almost never referred to as 'de Hay' or 'de la Hay', and probably derived their surname from an ancestor with personal name Hay, whereas Robert de Haye was of Haye-du-Puits in Normandy (*ANF*, p. 51).

[7]   The identity of Thomas son of Thomas son of Roger is discussed below.

[8]   An abbreviated copy is printed at *EYF*, no. 12.

[9]   From MS Dods. 7, f. 342ʳ⁻ᵛ. Farrer did not include Dodsworth's description of the seal when he printed the text of Emma's deed. A further copy of William son of Peter's agreement with Emma Hay, possibly from a different original, appears at MS Dods. 95, f. 57ʳ, together with a slightly different version of

ancestor, had been seised of it in the time of King Henry II (*YF*, 1246–1272, p. 76n).
If these lands had belonged to Roger Hay in his own right, they would have passed
directly to his son Thomas, Emma holding only a right in dower. That they did
not shows that they were the inheritance of Emma. Thus we must look to Emma's
ancestors, rather than those of her husband, to find the twelfth-century tenants of the
substantial Yorkshire lands later held by her descendants.

Emma's gift to the hospital, and the agreements with William son of Peter noted
above show that she was daughter of Roger son of Alured, and heir to her brother
Roger. Additional evidence is contained in King John's charter of 27 February 1204,
which confirmed the possessions of Thicket Priory. These included the place called
Thicket, and 4 bv. in Cottingwith given by Roger son of Roger; ½ ct. in the same
place given by Thomas son of Roger; 1 bv. in the same place given by Picot; 1 bv.
in Goodmanham given by Roger son of Roger; and 1 bv. in the same place given
by Emma[10] sister of Roger son of Roger. By a separate deed Emma Hay confirmed
to Thicket the gift of a bovate in Cottingwith and a toft in *Crossum* given by Picot
(*EYC*, II, no. 1131; *MA*, IV, 385–86, nos 1, 2). In William Fossard's return of fees made in
1166 we find Roger son of Roger holding 2 k.f. (*EYC*, II, no. 1003). From these details
it is clear that the tenant of 1166 and the founder of Thicket Priory was Roger son
of Roger son of Alured and not Roger Hay, to whom the foundation was ascribed
by Clay (*EYF*, p. 40).

Little can be ascertained of Roger son of Alured beyond the names of his children.
If he is to be identified with the man of that name who in 1166 was holding 3 k.f. of
Lacy and, with Roald, 1 k.f. of Vescy (*Red Bk*, pp. 422, 427) then the question arises
as to why he was not named as the tenant in the Fossard *carta*.[11] William Fossard's
deed of 1154 × 1162,[12] giving 3 k.f. in Hawold (in Huggate), held by Roger son of
Roger, to Watton Priory suggests that Roger son of Alured was dead by 1162 at the
latest (*EYC*, II, no. 1095).

It seems that Roger son of Roger's holdings did not pass directly to his sister
Emma Hay on his death. Thomas son of Roger's gift of ½ ct. in Cottingwith to
Thicket is noted above; the pipe roll entry of 1190, whereby Thomas son of Thomas
son of Roger paid 100s. into the exchequer for entry to his deceased father's lands in
Aughton and Goodmanham, of which Roger 'de Hay' was disseising him, indicates
he then held, or should have held, the fee (*PR*, 2 Ric. I, p. 66). But the tenures of
Thomas son of Roger and his son Thomas son of Thomas son of Roger must neces-
sarily have been brief, for Emma Hay calls herself heir to her brother Roger, not
Thomas, in her benefaction to the hospital noted above. If, as is likely, Roger 'de
Hay' was in fact Roger Hay, it is probable that he gained temporary possession of the

William's agreement with Thomas Hay, made in the court of Robert of Thornham, with a similar but
not identical list of witnesses.

[10]  In their notes of this deed, both Burton and Farrer called her Emma Hay, but the surname is not
included in the text of the deed (*Monasticon Eboracense*, p. 280; *EYC*, II, no. 1131). Burton is doubtless
the source for the account given in *Bulmer's History & Directory of East Yorkshire* (1892) where it is
stated that the site of Thicket was granted in 1542 to John Aske, esq., of Aughton, to whose family
the patronage of foundership had descended from the De La Hays, one of whom had married Emma,
sister of Roger Fitz Roger.

[11]  The difficulty is not insurmountable. Roger son of Alured could have resigned in favour of his son, or
enfeoffed him with Huggate and died at about the time of the returns of 1166, but further evidence
is required before the identification can be accepted. Farrer suggests that Roger son of Alured was
holding the Lacy fees as custodian of the lands of Humphrey de Veilli (*EYC*, III, no. 1583n). No
evidence has been found for Hay holdings of Lacy or Vescy in later years.

[12]  The deed is attested by Roger, archbishop, who was consecrated in 1154, and John, treasurer, who
became bishop of Poitiers in 1162.

fee during the minority of Thomas son of Thomas, under some arrangement with William Fossard II. Neither Thomas son of Thomas nor Roger Hay lived through the 1190s, for in 1196 it seems Emma Hay was holding the fee.

Thomas Hay confirmed his father Roger's gift of the mill in North Cave, with suit from the land of his fee there, namely 4 ct., by a deed dated by Farrer '*c.*1175 × 1188', but probably issued after 1190 when Roger Hay was still living (R599). Between *c.*1195 and 1204 Thomas issued a further confirmation of his father's grant, which was said to have been made 'in very remote times', mentioning the deed 'which I have seen' (R600). As there is no confirmation by his mother Emma Hay, and she does not join in Roger Hay's original gift, it is likely that the holding in North Cave had belonged to Roger Hay in his own right, and was not part of the fee of Roger son of Alured. The request in 1200 by Richard de Wyville[13] for record and judgment in his plea which had been in the court of Robert of Thornham[14] between him and Thomas Hay concerning 8 ct. in Everthorpe and *Hundecou'*,[15] which was placed in respite because Thomas was overseas on the king's service (*RFine*, p. 105; *PR*, 3 John, pp. 157–58), suggests that Roger Hay may have held ½ k.f. in those places in the mid-twelfth century.

Emma Hay last occurs in 1197 × 1198 when with her son Thomas she made the grant to the hospital mentioned above. There is no evidence that she survived into the thirteenth century. Over the years 1204–12 Thomas Hay paid off an amercement of 30*m. pro transgressione* (*PR*, passim). In 1197 × 1211[16] the agreement was made whereby Thomas released and quitclaimed Aughton and its members to William son of Peter [of Goodmanham] as his right and inheritance, which William son of Anketin, grand-father of William, had pledged to Roger son of Alured, Thomas's grandfather, which pledge had been redeemed in the time of Emma Hay, Thomas's mother. William son of Peter also gave his nephew William son of Adam of Burland (*Birland*) 6 bv. in Goodmanham in frank-marriage with Emma, Thomas's daughter, and gave his niece Christiana, daughter of Adam of Burland, to Roger, Thomas's eldest son, with 5 bv. of land and the capital messuage in Goodmanham which Emma Hay had held, in frank-marriage (*EYC*, II, no. 1130).[17]

There is other evidence, besides the pledge and the arrangement for marriages, of the close relationship between the families of William son of Peter and Thomas Hay. Both families appear to have had interests in Aughton, Goodmanham, Laytham, West Cottingwith, and Huggate. By an agreement made in 1225, Thomas Hay released to Adam of Linton and Agnes his wife (who can be shown by later evidence to be Adam of Burland and the sister and heir of William son of Peter respectively) a moiety of the land he had claimed against them, being 18 bv. in Aughton, 10 bv. in Good-manham, and 4 bv. in Laytham, which were to be held to Adam and Agnes and the heirs of Agnes, of Thomas, for the service of one knight (*YF*, 1218–1231, pp. 60–63).

---

[13]  For the Wyville family, see *EYF*, pp. 103–06. No evidence has been found to explain the Wyville interest in Everthorpe and North Cave. The family were Mowbray tenants, and do not appear in the Fossard *carta*.

[14]  Thornham held the Fossard fee by right of his wife Joan, daughter and heir of William Fossard. For Fossard and Thornham see *ODNB*.

[15]  Later evidence shows that the plea concerned Everthorpe and North Cave.

[16]  After the death of Emma Hay, and before 1211, when Robert of Thornham, whose steward Alan of Wilton attests, was dead (*ODNB*, s.n. Thornham).

[17]  Amongst the pedigrees added to the Norcliffe MS by Robert Glover is that of Hay, which states that Christiana, sister and heir of William of Linton married Roger Hay, son of Thomas Hay. The pedigree is not free from error, but this information was presumably based on a contemporary deed (*Flower's Visitation*, p. 365).

The 10 bv.[18] in Cottingwith given to Thicket by Roger son of Roger, Thomas son of Roger, and Picot, a tenant of Emma Hay, are of particular interest. In 1231 a fine was made between Eve, prioress of Thicket, and Agnes, daughter of Peter and sister and heir of William son of Peter, concerning 10 bv. in Cottingwith. These were said to have been given to the priory by William son of Peter, whose deed was produced by the prioress. Agnes had been called to warrant the property, in particular to render the services due at the county and wapentake courts. William's deed was almost certainly a confirmation of the 10 bv. previously given rather than a new gift, as in 1284–85 the prioress was holding no more than 10 bv. in Cottingwith, at that time of German Hay (*YF*, 1218–1231, pp. 135–36 and n; *KI*, p. 62). These details suggest that William son of Peter had inherited or acquired a moiety of the 2 k.f. held by Roger son of Roger in 1166. Whether there was a family connection between William son of Anketin and Roger son of Alured has not been determined.[19]

William son of Peter is chiefly remembered as the founder of the Gilbertine priory of Ellerton on Spalding Moor. His deed of 1199 × 1207,[20] made for the health of King John, Archbishop Geoffrey, Sir Robert of Thornham and Joan his wife, Geoffrey earl of Essex, Alan of Wilton and Mary his wife, and for the health of his own soul and that of his wife Alice and the souls of Peter his father and Christiana his mother, gave to the order of Sempringham, in order to set up a priory in Ellerton and to feed thirteen poor people there, all his land in Ellerton, a wood in Lathingholme, and 2 bv. in Laytham, with other property (*EYC*, II, no. 1133). At a later date William son of Peter gave to the convent of Ellerton reasonable estovers in his wood of Spaldington, and common pasture for their tofts which the priory had by the gift of four named donors (MS Dods. 7, fol. 333ᵛ). His deed was confirmed by Peter de la Hay of Spaldington[21] before 1228 (*EYC*, XII, no. 72). 4 bv. in Huggate, which had been given to Ellerton by William son of Peter, *advocatus noster*, were granted by the priory to Oliver of Gunby (MS Dods. 7, f. 334ʳ).[22] William also gave to the canons of Ellerton his mill in Goodmanham, and a piece of land next to the mill (MS Dods. 7, f. 336ʳ).[23] He made a grant of common pasture in Spaldington to another Gilbertine house, that of North Ormsby in Lincolnshire (*EYC*, XII, no. 67), and was connected with the Gilbertine priory of Watton, which granted him 6 bv. in Huggate, part of the 19 bv. which Walter son of Geoffrey had given to the priory (*EYC*, II, no. 1263). In 1189 × 1212[24] William son of Peter presented William Hay, clerk, to a third part[25] of the rectory of Goodmanham on a vacancy caused by the death of Roger of Lockington (*EYC*, II, no. 1122); and later presented John, clerk, who was inducted

---

[18]  Only 9 bv. can be accounted for, but perhaps 'the place called Thicket' comprised the additional bovate.

[19]  It might perhaps be suggested that Christiana, mother of William son of Peter, was a sister of Emma Hay. In this context the agreement between William son of Peter and Emma Hay could be seen not only as a redemption of the outstanding pledge made by William son of Anketin to Roger son of Alured, but also as part of a wider agreement about the division of the 2 k.f. For an alternative explanation of the agreement and the later settlement between Thomas Hay and William son of Peter as attempted resolutions of a long-running dispute, see P.R. Hyams, *Rancor and Reconciliation in Medieval England* (Ithaca, 2003), pp. 286–87. But placing Emma and Christiana as sisters opens questions about the legality of the marriages arranged between their respective descendants.

[20]  After the accession of King John, and before Archbishop Geoffrey, who attests, went into exile in 1207.

[21]  Said to have married Olivia, a daughter of Adam of Linton and Agnes, sister of William son of Peter (John Britton, et al., *The Beauties of England and Wales* (1812), XVI, 570).

[22]  Noted with witness list, *EYC*, II, no. 1263n.

[23]  Noted, *EYC*, II, 416.

[24]  During the time of Archbishop Geoffrey.

[25]  The other two thirds were held as part of the Percy fee (*EYC*, XII, 43).

by Simon, dean of York, in 1212 × 1214[26] (*EYC*, xii, no. 14). William son of Peter was living in 1220, when with the prior of Ellerton he accused Robert de Ros and his men of deforcing them of their common pasture in Laytham (*CRR*, 1219–1220, p. 198), but was either dead or retired by 1225, when Thomas Hay made the agreement with Adam of Linton and Agnes his wife (William's sister and heir).

During the period 1220 × 1225[27] Adam of Linton confirmed the gifts of William son of Peter to Ellerton, for the health of the souls of William son of Peter and Alive his wife (*MA*, vi, 976–77, no. 3). Adam was dead in 1231 when Agnes made the fine with Thicket Priory noted above. Dodsworth notes a damaged deed of Agnes, who describes herself as widow of Adam of Linton and sister and heir of William son of Peter, by which she gave property in Goodmanham to Ellerton Priory (MS Dods. 7, f. 339ʳ). Agnes was probably dead in 1246, when Sir Roger Hay and Sir William of Linton attested a deed to Ellerton (MS Dods. 7, f. 342ʳ) and was certainly dead in January 1252, when William of Linton and Peter his son made a fine with John Hay concerning lands in Laytham, Aughton, Goodmanham, Ellerton, Oglethorpe, Huggate, West Cottingwith, Sutton, and Spaldington (*YF*, 1246–1272, p. 76 and n).

We now return to the Hay family. Thomas Hay was living in November 1226, when he put in a claim concerning 2 bv. in Laytham (*YF*, 1218–1231, p. 75) but was dead in November 1227, when Roger Hay was in dispute with Ellerton Priory about a presentation to a vicarage of Aughton (*Reg. Gray*, p. 19). The dispute was resolved for a time by a fine of August 1230,[28] whereby Roger Hay agreed with John, prior of Ellerton, that the advowson of Aughton church was the right of Roger. Roger gave the priory ½ ct. in Goodmanham, and quitclaimed his right in the advowson of Ellerton church, formerly a chapel belonging to Aughton church, and granted a further 6 bv. and a yearly rent of 10s. in Goodmanham, for a term of ten years. The capital messuage in Goodmanham was excluded (*YF*, 1218–1231, p. 118). As Roger Hay was being impleaded by Nicholas de Yeland and Eustacia his wife[29] for 8 ct. in Everthorpe and [North] Cave by right of William de Wyville, ancestor of Eustacia, in Hilary and Michaelmas terms 1225 and Hilary term 1226, it is evident that Thomas had resigned his interest in those places to his son (*CRR*, 1225–1226, nos 14, 803, 1394, 2111).

We turn now to Roger Hay, the younger brother of Thomas, who inherited the Sussex interests. He occurs as a juror in Sussex in 1196, 1220, 1221 and 1226 (*CRR*, i, 30; ibid., 1219–1220, p. 287; 1220, pp. 6, 233; 1221–1222, p. 35; 1225–1226, no. 2230). Roger was dead in Trinity term, 1230, when an assize was held to determine if Roger Hay, uncle of Roger son of Thomas Hay, was seised in demesne of 7s. of rent, 4 virgates of land, and 8 a. of meadow and other property in Hunston. It was found that he was so seised, and that his nephew Roger son of Thomas Hay was his heir (*CRR*, 1230–1232, nos 148, 359).[30] The heir Roger Hay soon disposed of the Sussex property, making a fine with the prior of Boxgrove concerning 8 a. in Hunston in

---

[26] Clay dated this deed to 1197 × 1201, as it was attested by H[amo] the treasurer [of York] and A[dam de Thorner] archdeacon of York. Clay believed Adam had lost his archdeaconry for good in 1201. But as Simon the dean was acting *sede vacante*, it can only have been given after the death of Archbishop Geoffrey in 1212, and before Simon's consecration as bishop of Exeter in October 1214 (Carpenter, 'Paulinus', p. 17 and n).

[27] Attested by Roger de Lisle, dean of York, and Simon Hale then sheriff, amongst others.

[28] Assigned to 1228 by Parker, but the presiding justices show 1230 is the correct year (cf. *YF*, 1218–1231, p. 128; MS Dods. 7, f. 344ʳ).

[29] Eustacia was a daughter of Richard de Wyville, who was impleading Thomas Hay for the same land in 1200 (*EYF*, p. 104).

[30] In one of these hearings (no. 148) it is *Rogerus filius Thome Hay avunculus Rogeri*, rather than *Rogerus*

November 1235, in which his attorney was Ralph de Ralegh; and another in January 1237, by which he granted ½ k.f. in Hunston to Ralph de Ralegh and Mabel his wife, in exchange for 70m. and all their lands in South Kirkby and Barthorpe (par. Acklam), to be held of them and the heirs of Mabel by the service due (*Sussex Fines*, nos 288, 338; *YF*, 1232–1246, p. 173).[31] In 1242–43 Roger Hay was said to hold ½ k.f. in Aughton and ½ k.f. in Everthorpe and Cave of Peter de Mauley, who had succeeded to the Fossard fee (*Bk of Fees*, p. 1098). Roger occurs as a recognitor in April 1246 (*YF*, 1232–1246, p. 144n) and in 1246 and 1247 attested deeds to Ellerton Priory as *dominus* (MS Dods. 7, ff. 336ᵛ–337ʳ, 342ʳ). He was dead in October 1251, when John Hay claimed against the prior of Ellerton 12 a. land and 50 a. wood in Aughton as his right, claiming that Emma his ancestor had been seised in the time of Henry II. From her the right descended to Thomas her son and heir, and from Thomas to Roger as his son and heir, and from Roger to William as his son and heir, and from William, who died without heir of his body, to the same John as brother and heir (*YF*, 1246–1272, p. 76n). William had presumably predeceased his father, as he does not otherwise appear.

In January 1252 John Hay of Aughton was party to a fine by which he quitclaimed the fishery of *Alemare*[32] to the abbot of Fountains for 30m. (*YF*, 1246–1272, p. 65). In March 1252 he was granted free warren in his demesne lands of Aughton, Everthorpe and Laytham (*CalCh*, 1226–1257, p. 380) but he was dead in August 1255 when Peter de Mauley confirmed to Ellerton Priory property including 4 bv. in Goodmanham which German Hay ought to defend (*MA*, VI, 976, no. 2). German appears to have been brother to John Hay, as he calls himself German son of Roger Hay in a deed by which he quitclaimed two tofts and 2 bv. in North Cave to Watton Priory (MS Dods. 7, f. 335ᵛ). He was granted respite from becoming a knight for three years from Whitsunday 1256 and similarly in September 1268 was granted respite for one year, at the instance of John of Howden clerk[33] (*CalPat*, 1247–1258, p. 474; ibid., 1266–1272, p. 258). German Hay attested a deed, probably of 1261 or shortly before, with his brother Nicholas[34] (*CVC*, II, no. 9), and was named as patron of Thicket Priory in May 1264 (*MA*, IV, 386, no. 4). In 1275 he revoked his presentation of master William of Pickering to the church of North Cave, as he had no right (*Reg. Giffard*, p. 288); and in September 1280 he agreed with Joan, prioress of Thicket, that he would do

Hay, *avunculus Rogeri filii Thome Hay* (no. 359) who is said to have died, but the former is apparently an error.

[31] The lands in South Kirkby and Barthorpe are not apparent in the survey of 1284–85, but see the note below of the inquisition ad quod dampnum of 1295 concerning land in South Kirkby.

[32] In Wheldrake (*VCH Yorks ER*, III, 124). Hay's interest in the fishery presumably stemmed from his holdings in the adjoining townships.

[33] Master John of Howden was a member of the Linton family and uncle to German Hay. After 1254 (attested by John de la Hay of Spaldington, who succeeded in that year or later (*EYC*, XII, 88)) master John of Howden, rector of part of Goodmanham church, gave to Ellerton Priory, with his body, ½ ct. in Goodmanham, which lay between the land he had given to the daughters of Roger of Linton and the land of St Andrew's, York (MS Dods. 7, fol. 334ᵛ). The gift was confirmed and quitclaimed by German Hay, who describes master John of Howden as his uncle (MS Dods. 7, fol. 347ʳ). Master John of Howden and Roger of Linton his brother attested a deed made by William Franceys of Laytham to Ellerton (MS Dods. 7, fol. 345ᵛ); Sir William of Linton and master John his brother attested a deed of John son of Oliver of Gunby (MS Dods. 7, f. 341ᵛ). Master John of Howden also attested a deed of Peter de la Hay to Ellerton in the 'middle 13th cent.' (*EYC*, XII, no. 73), and a deed of Peter son of Peter de Mauley of 1255 (*MA*, VI, 976, no. 2); master John, parson of Goodmanham attested a deed of 1268 (MS Dods. 7, f. 343ᵛ). It is not impossible that he was same man as John, clerk, presented by William son of Peter in 1212 × 1214, but if so he must have held the rectory for more than half a century.

[34] Nicholas, son of Sir Roger Hay of Aughton, granted his windmill in Goodmanham to Ellerton Priory in November 1268 (MS Dods. 7, f. 343ᵛ, also at Burton transcripts I, f. 62ᵛ, p. 72, B20 N51).

the king's service arising from the messuage and 10 bv. she held of him in Thicket and Cottingwith (*YF*, 1272–1300, p. 45). He occurs several times in the period 1279 to 1293 as a juror (*YI*, I, II, passim) and at the inquisition after the death of Peter de Mauley in 1279 was found to hold 1½ k.f. in Aughton (ibid., I, 196). In the survey of 1284–85 he held lands in Cottingwith, Spaldington, Laytham, Aughton, Huggate, Everthorpe, and North Cave, all of Peter de Mauley (*KI*, pp. 62, 83–85). In 1295 there was an inquisition as to whether it would be to the king's damage if German Hay was to grant 100s. rent and land in South Kirkby to the prior and convent of St Oswald [of Nostell] (*YI*, III, 18). German's wife was Margery, with whom he gave 22 a. meadow in Seaton [Ross] to the priory of Warter, in exchange for 2 bv. with a toft and garden in North Cave. German Hay of Aughton and Margery his wife were disputing a tenement in Seaton [Ross] with the prior of Warter in 1273 (Warter cartulary, ff. 44ᵛ–45ʳ, 46ʳ, 83ʳ). Margery was compelled to live with her husband by archiepiscopal command in August 1286 (*Reg. Romeyn*, I, 191).

The descent after 1295 has not been ascertained, but there are many references to Hays at Aughton and Everthorpe during the fourteenth century. In 1386 German Hay, son of Godfrey Hay, quitclaimed the advowson of Aughton church to Ellerton and confirmed the possessions the priory held of his fee, called *Haysefee*, in Ellerton, Aughton, and Laytham (MS Dods. 95, f. 45ᵛ). German Hay was named as lord of Aughton in 1387–88 (*Year Book 11 Ric. II*, pp. 88–89). Plantagenet-Harrison gave a very detailed pedigree of the Askes of Aske in Richmondshire, the family of Owsthorpe, later of Aughton, being a cadet branch. He apparently saw the marriage settlement made by German son of Geoffrey Hay dated 1 October 1386, by which German entailed the manors of Aughton and Everthorpe on himself and Alice his wife, and the heirs of their bodies. In default of such heirs, Aughton was to remain to Alice's father John Aske and his heirs, and Everthorpe to German and the heirs of his body, with default to John Aske of Owsthorpe (Harrison, *Yorkshire*, I, 70, cited in Saltmarshe, 'Aske Family', p. 17). Ellis states that the Hay interests in Aughton and elsewhere passed on the death of Alice, daughter of John Aske (which John died in 1395) and widow of German Hay, to her nephew Richard, son of John Aske of Owsthorpe, who was aged ten at his father's death in 1429 (Ellis, 'Askes of Aughton', pp. 44, 46, citing 'Inq. at Durham').

Glover's pedigree of Hay also shows an earlier marriage between Richard Aske, father of John Aske of Owsthorpe and grandfather of Alice, and an unnamed daughter of Godfrey Hay (*Flower's Visitation*, p. 365). Richard Aske of Aughton occurs in 1444, when he was accused with others of slaying Thomas Dawson of Tadcaster (*CalPat*, 1441–1446, p. 297). In his will of 1497 Sir John Aske left his *dominium* in Everthorpe for the use of younger sons (*Test. Ebor.*, IV, 123–24). Lands formerly belonging to both Ellerton and Thicket priories were purchased by a later John Aske in 1542 (*VCH Yorks ER*, III, 115).

**R598.** Gift to the hospital by Roger Haid of a mill in Cave, worth 12s., with a toft. All those who went to the mill when it was in Roger's hands will go now. This for God, St Peter, and St Leonard, and William Fossard, Roger's lord. Entreaty to his lord, his friends, and his men to maintain the alms [*c.*1135 × *c.*1154]

PRINTED: *EYC*, II, no. 1123, where dated *c.*1135 × 1148.

**[f. 213ʳ]** *Rogerus Haide de molendino Cave.*
Notum sit omnibus tam futuris quam presentibus quod ego Roggerus Haid condo

et imperpetuum in elemosinam do[35] unum molendinum in Cava valentem xii^{cim} solid(os) cum uno tofto fratribus hospitalis sancti Petri. Et omnes qui iverunt ad eundem molendinum ad molendum quamdiu eum habui in manu mea ibunt modo. Et hoc pro amore dei et sancti Petri domini mei et sancti Leonardi et pro Wuillelmo Fossard domino meo et pro memetipso et pro sponsa mea et pro animabus antecessorum meorum. Qua propter precor dominum meum et amicos et homines meos ut h(ec) concedant et manuteneant quatinus huius elemosine participes sint. Hii sunt testes, Adam heremita, Ulfus presbiter de Actun, Walterus dapifer, Hugo de Hugcad, Tocca prepositus.

The deed may have been issued before 1148, when Pope Eugenius III confirmed 'a mill in North Cave of the Fossard fee' (C178 [*EYC*, I, no. 179]). The confirmations of 1157 and 1173 include 'a mill in North Cave and two *mansa*' (C179, C180 [*EYC*, I, nos 186, 197]). However the mention of St Leonard is suggestive of a date close to 1154, when the hospital's church of St Leonard was consecrated by Archbishop Theobald (C194 [*EYC*, I, no. 185]). This later date would also be more in keeping with the other early appearances of Roger Hay, who was apparently still living in 1190 (FN). It is suggested above that the gift of the mill may have been at the instigation of William Fossard I, the tenant in chief.

**R599.** Confirmation to the hospital by Thomas Hay of the mill in North Cave which his father Roger Hay gave to the hospital, with suit of the land of Thomas's fee in that vill, being 4 ct., to mill and give multure [1190 × 1212, possibly 1204 × 1212]

PRINTED: *EYC*, II, no. 1126, where dated *c*.1175 × 1188.

*Thomas Hai de molendino in Northcava cum eius sequela de tota terra sua scilicet de iiii. carucatis terre.*
Omnibus has litteras visuris vel audituris Thomas Hay salutem. Noverit universitas vestra me intuitu pietatis et caritatis concessisse et presenti carta mea confirmasse deo et pauperibus hospitalis beati Petri Ebor' in puram et perpetuam elemosinam illud molendinum in Northcave quod pater meus Rog(erus) Hay dedit predictis pauperibus in puram et perpetuam elemosinam cum sequ(e)la totius terre de feodo meo in predicta villa, scilicet iiii^{or} carucatarum que debent sequi et molere ad predictum molendinum et multuram dare. Ego vero Thomas et heredes mei debemus warantizare defendere et adquietare predictum molendinum cum sequela predicta et cum omnibus libertatibus et pertinenciis suis predictis pauperibus contra omnes homines imperpetuum ut simus nos participes omnium elemosinarum que fiunt et fient in prefata domo dei imperpetuum. Hiis testibus, Willelmo de Murers, Willelmo de Riplingham, Rogero Daniele, Iohanne de Dreuton', Willelmo de Santona, Simone f[ilio] Baudrai persona de Northcava, Osberto de Clif', Willelmo de Araines, Petro de Santona, Radulfo f[ilio] Syre, Reginaldo fratre suo, Thoma Brabazun, Willelmo f[ilio] Willelmi et multis aliis.

This deed was given after Thomas Hay succeeded his father in 1190 × 1196. John of Drewton died in 1208 × 1212; William de Araines in 1205 × 1214. It is probable that William of Sancton was the son of Alexander of Sancton who succeeded his

---

[35] MS: *deo*.

father in or before 1195 and was dead in 1218; Peter of Sancton may have been his brother, who occurs in 1198–1207, or the son of William son of Peter of Anlaby who succeeded in 1204–05 (FNs).

There are several references to the witness John of DREWTON early in the thirteenth century. John of Drewton and Robert his brother attested in 1191 or earlier[36] (*EYC*, x, no. 113). In '*c*.1180 × 1201'[37] John of Drewton attested a Kirby Grindalythe deed as the king's bailiff of Buckrose (*EYC*, II, no. 1081). John of Drewton was described as a knight in 1201 (Stenton, *Pleas*, III, nos 92, 512). In the year to Michaelmas 1205 he accounted for 40*s*. for an inquisition, and cleared the debt the following year (*PR*, 7 John, p. 52; ibid., 8 John, p. 200). He was a pledge in 1208 (*CRR*, 1207–1209, p. 261), and in the same year he was accused by Reiner of Garton and Philip de Beellum of wounding them, which he denied (Stenton, *Pleas*, IV, nos 3446, 3450). John was dead in Trinity term 1212, when Alice his widow claimed the third part of 13 bv., half a mill, and twelve messuages in Drewton against Eustace de Vescy, as her dower. In the same term a case against Hugh son of Andrew, for burning the houses of his lord John of Drewton, was abandoned (*CRR*, 1210–1212, pp. 350, 373).

Robert of Drewton,[38] probably the younger brother of John of Drewton, occurs as an attorney on Sancton business in 1201 and 1205 (*CRR*, I, 384; ibid., 1203–1205, p. 260), and as attorney for John le Gras in 1220 (ibid., 1219–1220, p. 302; 1220, p. 34).

**R600.** Confirmation to the hospital by Thomas Hay of the mill of [North] Cave with a toft and suit from all men and lands in his fee of [North] Cave, which mill with multure and suit Thomas's lord and father Roger Hay gave to the hospital in very remote times and confirmed with his deed, which deed Thomas has seen and confirmed [*c*.1195 × 1204]

ORIGINAL: *a* Northamptonshire Record Office, Fitzwilliam (Milton) Charters, F(M) Charter/2022, 17 cm. (wide) × 11 cm., stained, bottom turn-up, three slits for seal tag, seal gone. Medieval endorsements: (in the deed hand) *Thom' Hay de molendino de Kava; iij.; script'.* COPY: *b* Rawl., f. 213ʳ, no significant differences. PRINTED: *EYC*, II, no. 1127, where dated *c*.1175 × 1188, from *b*.

*Thomas Hay' de molendino de Cava.*
Universis cristi fidelibus cartam istam visuris vel audituris, Thom' Hay salutem. Noveritis me pro salute anime mee et omnium antecessorum et heredum meorum concessisse dedisse et hac presenti carta mea confirmasse deo et pauperibus hospitalis sancti Petri Eborac' in puram et perpetuam elemosinam molendinum de Kava cum tofto et cum tota sequela sua, scilicet omnium hominum et omnium terrarum existentium in feodo meo de Kava, quicumque terras ipsas coluerit vel tenuer(it), quod molendinum cum multura et sequela predicta dominus et pater meus Rogerus Hay predictis pauperibus mult(is) retroact(is) temporibus dedit in puram et perpetuam elemosinam, et carta sua confirmavit, quam cartam ego vidi et pia caritate concessi et presenti carta mea confirmavi pauperibus prefatis, libere integre et quiete sicut ulla elemosina liberius potest dari. Et ego predictus Thom' Hay et heredes mei warantizabimus et adquietabimus predictis pauperibus in perpetuum predictum molendinum

---

[36]  Clay gives sound reasons for this *terminus ad quem*. The difficulties concerning the age of John of Birkin have been resolved by a reassessment of the chronology of the Birkin family (FN).
[37]  Certainly issued before February 1204, when the grantor Ingram Aguillun was dead (FN).
[38]  Transcribed as *Drenton*, presumably for *Dreuton*, the normal form of the name.

cum tota sequela predicta in tofto et in omnibus aliis liberis pertinenciis suis contra omnes homines, ut ego et omnes antecessores et heredes mei simus participes omnium orationum elemosinarum et aliorum beneficiorum que fiunt vel facienda sunt in prefata domo dei. Hiis testibus, Stephano, Willelmo Balki, Roberto milite, Suano, Anketino, Willelmo, Gamello et aliis fratribus predicti hospitali, Willelmo, Roberto, Hugone et aliis capellanis ipsius domus, Rein(ero), Thoma de Languath et aliis clericis ipsius domus, Rogero de Dayvill', Petro filio Willelmi de Norcava,[39] Willelmo fratre eius,[40] Radulfo de Yuertorp, Reginaldo fratre eius et multis aliis.

The first lay witness Roger de Daiville was probably dead in 1204 (FN). Thomas de Langwath occurs from the time of master Paulinus: after *c*.1220 he is usually described as master. Most of William Balki's attestations can be dated within *c*.1195 × *c*.1225, and he does not occur with Thomas de Langwath as master. The attestations of brother Robert, knight, also fall within *c*.1195 × *c*.1225. A deed of Agnes, daughter of Reginald (*Rainaldi*) Syre of Everthorpe, made in 1226 × 1245 (R774), indicates that the witnesses Ralph and Reginald of Everthorpe were the sons of Syre who attested in 1190 × 1212, possibly 1204 × 1212 (R599). Reginald and William, sons of Syre, attested in *c*.1210 × 1217 (R603, R606).

**R601.** Indenture by which the master and brethren of the hospital of St Leonard, York, grant to John Tothe of Midelton and his heirs, the millpond with appurtenances in Northcave, as it lies on the Westbek, which millpond the hospital had by gift of Roger Hay, together with the suit of the land of his fee in the vill, that is 4 ct. of land, which owe suit and ought to mill there and give multure, paying for the first eleven years 4*s*. annually, by equal portions at Pentecost and St Martin in winter. After the first eleven years John and his heirs will pay 8*s*. at the same terms. Right of distraint if rent is in arrears for a fortnight, and right of re-entry if in arrears for half a year or more. **[f. 213ᵛ]** Alternate seals to alternate parts of the indenture. 11 September 1374.

*Indentura Iohannis Tothe de Midelton de molendino de Northecave.*

Hiis testibus, Iohanne Hay de Aghton', Roberto de Lychefeld' de Northcave, Ricardo de Clyf', Iohanne de Brantyngham de Northcave, Roberto de Danthorp' de eadem et aliis. Dat' apud Ebor' die lune proxima post festum nativitatis beate Marie virginis, anno domini millesimo trecentesimo septuagesimo iiiiᵗᵒ.

**R602.** Judgment of the chapter of St Peter, York, that whereas master R., rector, and the brethren of the hospital have complained that men living in the fee of Roger Hay in North Cave had deprived them of their suit of mill; so the parties were summoned before the chapter. Judgment in favour of the hospital, with taxed costs of 30*s*. [probably 1204 × 1217]

PRINTED: *EYC*, ii, no. 1125, where dated 1148 × *c*.1158.

*Summa de sequela molendini de Cava.*
Omnibus sancte matris ecclesie filiis presentes litteras visuris vel audituris capit-

---

39   *b*: *Nortkava.*
40   *b*: *suo* for *eius.*

ulum sancti Petri Ebor' salutem in domino. Ad universitatis vestre noticiam volumus
pervenire quod cum magister R. rector et fratres hospitalis sancti Petri coram nobis
conquesti fuissent quod homines manentes in feudo Rogeri Hay in Northcava eos
de sequela molendini sui de eadem villa iniuste spoliassent, iam dictos homines coram
nobis legitime citari fecimus. Tandem partibus coram nobis comparentibus et magistro
et fratribus mentionem suam fundantibus et asserentibus se per memoratos homines
manentes in feudo Rogeri Hay in Northcava de sequela molendini sui de eadem
villa iniuste spoliatos esse, procurator partis adverse huic eorum intentioni contradi-
cens directe litem contestatus est. Partibus igitur rite competentibus statutis diebus
ut debita gaudent testium productione, testes productos diligenter examinavimus, et
instrumenta coram nobis exhibita legi fecimus. Publicatis tandem attestationibus et
copia dicendi in testes et testificata concessa, diem statuimus ut sententialiter litem
terminaremus. Tandem diligentius inspectis attestationibus et instrumentis coram nobis
exhibitis et utriusque allegationibus attentius notatis et ponderatis cause meritis iuris
ordine per omnia observato communicato virorum prudentum consilio, sententialiter
adiudicavimus predictis magistro et fratribus possessionem sequele molendini predicti
ab omnibus hominibus manentibus in feudo Rogeri Hay in Northcava faciende,
condempnantes eosdem homines prenominatis magistro et fratribus nomine expensarum in lite factarum, moderata facta taxatione in summam triginta solidorum.

Farrer gave an early date to this act, assuming that master R. was Robert, the first
known master of the hospital. But the form *magister X. rector et fratres hospitalis* is
unknown before the time of rector Ralph of Nottingham.[41] The Cotton volume
contains other chapter acts which do not mention the dean, and have no witnesses.
Two of these date from *c*.1160 × *c*.1185, one from 1214 × 1220 and another possibly
from *c*.1210 × *c*.1235 (C69, C70, C96, C125 [*EYC*, I, nos 195–96, Cott., ff. 14ʳ, 18ᵛ]).
The present act is probably from Ralph of Nottingham's rectorship, but a date during
the rectorate of Robert de Saham (indicating 1250 × 1265) or Roger of Malton
(1276–1280) should not be entirely ruled out. The refererence to 'the fee of Roger
Hay' cannot be relied on to determine the date, as fees are not infrequently described
by the names of long-dead tenants.

**R603.** Confirmation by Reginald Todhe, that John his son and heir, in his presence,
had given to the hospital 2 bv. in North Cave, from the 6 bv. which Reginald
held there, being those nearest the south, with two tofts, one held by Ive and
the other by Ranulf. John's gift was made with the body of Reginald, who
has chosen to be buried in the hospital [*c*.1210 × 1217]

*Confirmatio Reginaldi Tothe de ii. bovatis et ii. toftis que Iohannes filius eius dedit hospitali*
*in Cava.*
Omnibus presentes litteras visuris vel audituris Reginaldus Todhe salutem. Noverit
universitas vestra Iohannem filium meum in presencia mea constitutum dedisse
concessisse et carta sua confirmasse deo et pauperibus hospitalis beati Petri Ebor'
duas bovatas terre in territorio de Northcave de vi. bovatis quas ego tenui in eadem
villa scilicet propinquiores soli cum omnibus pertinentibus ad illas duas bovatas et
duo tofta in predicta villa quorum unum tenuit Ivo et reliquum tenuit Ran(u)l(fus)
in puram et perpetuam elemosinam liberam quietam et solutam ab omni servicio et
exactione seculari sicut ulla elemosina liberius dari potest. Predictam autem dona-

---

[41]   The deed of Paulinus which uses this description is a forgery (R525).

tionem et concessionem fecit predictus Iohannes filius et heres meus pauperibus predicti hospitalis cum corpore[42] meo ubi elegi sepulturam. Hanc autem predictam donationem gratam et ratam habeo et habui et presenti carta mea confirmavi. Hiis testibus, Willelmo persona de Cava, Thoma Brabantione, Petro filio Petri, Reginaldo filio Syre, Willelmo filio Syre, Willelmo Talun, Radulfo Mot, Waltero de Alredale, Ricardo de Radeclive, Aluredo de Brung(er)flet et multis aliis.

See the note to R606, which has the same witnesses.

**R604.** Confirmation to the hospital by Thomas Hay of 2 bv. and two tofts in North Cave given by Reginald Tothe with his body [*c.*1210 × 1217]

*Thomas Hay de ii. bovatis et ii. toftis in Northcave.*
Omnibus has litteras visuris vel audituris Thomas Hay salutem. Noverit universitas vestra me concessisse et presenti carta mea confirmasse deo et pauperibus hospitalis beati Petri Ebor' duas bovatas terre et duo tofta in territorio de Northcave, tenend(a) predictis pauperibus cum omnibus pertinenciis suis infra villam et extra in puram et perpetuam elemosinam liberam solutam et quietam ab omni servicio et exactione et consuetudine sicut ulla elemosina liberior potest esse, scilicet quas duas bovatas et que duo tofta Reginaldus Tothe dedit predictis pauperibus in puram et perpetuam elemosinam cum corp(or)e suo. Hiis testibus, Willelmo de Daivilla, Petro de Santona, Ricardo clerico de Kave, Rogero f[ilio] Matill', Thoma Braibazun, Iohanne, Anketino, Ambrosio, Thoma Tuschet fratribus hospitalis et multis aliis.

The date range has been assigned by reference to other deeds in this series (R606n). The witness Roger son of Maud was also known as Roger of Cave. By a fine of November 1202 William of Sancton released all right in ½ ct. in Cave to Roger of Cave, and Roger quitclaimed 2 bv. in Cave to Peter, brother of William. Maud, mother of Roger, quitclaimed all right in dower to the same Peter (*PF John*, p. 66). According to Clay's translation of an assize roll of 1208, there was a case concerning the death of Roger son of Maud of Cave, but Stenton was unable to read the manuscript (*Three Yorks. Assize Rolls*, p. 30; Stenton, *Pleas*, IV, no. 3433).

**R605.** Confirmation by John Thodhe that he has received from Ralph, rector, and the brethren of the hospital 2 bv. in North Cave, from the 6 bv. which Reginald his father held, nearest the south, and two tofts in the same vill, of which Ive held one and Ranulf the other, paying 40*d.* annually, and ½*m.* as an obituary payment. John has done homage to master Ralph for the tenement [*c.*1210 × 1217]

*Iohannes Todde de xl. denariis annuatim reddendis hospitali pro ii. bovatis terre quas ten(et) de eis in North Cave. Et de dimidia marca pro catallis suis in fine.*
Omnibus presentes litteras visuris vel audituris Iohannes Thodhe salutem. Noverit universitas vestra me suscepisse a Radulfo rectore et fratribus hospitalis beati Petri Ebor' duas bovatas terre in territorio de Northcave de illis sex bovatis quas Reginaldus pater meus tenuit propinquiores soli et duo tofta in eadem villa quorum unum tenuit Ivo et reliquum Ranulfus, tenenda de illis cum omnibus suis pertinentiis, libere quiete honorifice iure hereditario, reddendo inde annuatim dicto hospitali

---

[42] MS: *opere.*

pro omni servicio et exactione quadraginta denarios, medietatem ad festum sancti Martini et medietatem ad Pent'. Ego autem et heredes mei in obitu nostro debemus reddere domui dicti hospitalis dimidiam marcam argenti pro portione catallorum nostrorum nos contingente. Fidelitatem autem servar(e) domui dicti hospitalis, et eidem firmam annuam predictam suis terminis fideliter solvere, et ut predictum est dimidiam marcam in obitu meo et heredum meorum domui hospitalis dicti reddere, tactis sacrosanctis pro me et pro heredibus meis iuravi et presenti carta mea confirmavi. De prenominato autem ten(emento) humagium feci magistro Radulfo. Hiis testibus, Roberto, Bernardo, fratribus et capellanis hospitalis, **[f. 214ʳ]** Girardo, Godefrido, Anketino, Waltero et aliis fratribus hospitalis, Petro, magistro Willelmo de Gerondon', magistro Willelmo de Aquila, capellanis, Thoma de Langwath', Roberto de Stowe, Ricardo de Flaxflet', Waltero de Alredale, Ricardo de Radeclive, Ricardo filio Roberti et multis aliis.

See R606 for John's gift of this land to the hospital. Ralph as rector indicates 1204 × 1217; Robert de Stowe c.1210 × c.1230.

**R606.**  Gift to the hospital by John Todhe, of 2 bv. in North Cave from the 6 bv. which his father held there, being nearest the south, and two tofts in the same vill, of which Ive held one and Ranulf the other [c.1210 × 1217]

*Iohannes Todde de ii. bovatis et de vi. bovatis in Northecave.*
Omnibus has litteras visuris vel audituris Iohannes Todhe salutem. Noverit universitas vestra me intuitu caritatis et pietatis dedisse et concessisse et presenti carta mea confirmasse deo et pauperibus hospitalis beati Petri Ebor' duas bovatas terre in territorio de Northecave de sex bovatis quas pater meus tenuit in eadem villa, scilicet propinquiores soli, cum omnibus pertinenciis ad illas duas bovatas et duo tofta in predicta villa, quorum unum tenuit Ivo et reliquum tenuit Ranulfus, in puram et perpetuam elemosinam liberam quietam et solutam ab omni servicio et exactione seculari sicut ulla elemosina liberius dari potest, ita quod ego et heredes mei totum predictum tenementum predictis pauperibus cum omnibus pertinenciis suis warantizabimus aquietabimus et defendemus contra omnes homines imperpetuum ut ego et successores mei et anime patris mei et aliorum antecessorum meorum simus participes omnium bonorum et elemosinarum que fient in prefato domo dei imperpetuum. Hiis testibus, Willelmo persona de Cava, Thoma Brabancione, Petro filio Petri, Reginaldo filio Syre, Willelmo filio Syre, Willelmo Talun, Radulfo Mot, Waltero de Alredale, Ricardo de Radeclive, Aluredo de Brug(er)fl(et) et multis aliis.

John's gift was confirmed by his father Reginald on the same occasion (R603), and later by Thomas Hay (R604). The hospital regranted the same property to John Tothe, probably immediately it had received it, by a deed of c.1210 × 1217 (R605). The second reissue of Magna Carta in 1217 prohibited an individual taking back as a tenant land he had granted previously to a religious house. The penalty was the voiding of the gift and the escheat of the land to the lord of the fee (Stubbs, *Select Charters*, p. 343, art. 43).

**R607.**  Release by Maud daughter of Sybil Hay, in her own power, to her mother, of 2 bv. land with a toft in North Cave, which Sybil gave her, being the 2 bv. which Roger the smith formerly held which lie next to the land of St Peter [of York], and the toft which William Cavun formerly held [c.1214 × 1232, possibly 1226 × 1232]

*Resignatio Matildis Hay de ii. bovatis terre in Northcava.*

Omnibus cristi fidelibus ad quos presens scriptum pervenerit Matildis filia Sibille Hay salutem. Noverit universitas vestra me in propria potestate constitutam resignasse Sibille matri mee illas duas bovatas terre cum uno tofto in Northcava quas predicta Sibilla michi dedit, scilicet illas bovatas quas Rogerus faber aliquando tenuit et que iacent iuxta terram sancti Petri, et illud toftum quod Willelmus Cavun aliquando tenuit, tenendas et habendas dicte Sibille et heredibus suis vel cuicumque assignare voluerit liberas quietas et solutas a me et heredibus meis imperpetuum, quod autem ego numquam predicte Sibille et heredibus suis vel assignatis suis inde movebo questionem vel calumpniam tactis sacrosanctis iuravi et affidavi. Et in huius rei robur et testimonium huic scripto sigillum meum apposui. Hiis testibus, Alano de Flamevill', Willelmo de Ayvill', Petro filio Petri, Iohanne de Thothe, Willelmo fratre suo, Simone Brabecun, Willelmo filio Willelmi, Petro filio suo, Simone filio Simonis, Petro Hasqui, Ricardo de Dreuton' et multis aliis.

See the note to R608, which has the same witnesses.

**R608.** Gift to the hospital by Lady Sybil Hay of 2 bv. and a toft in North Cave, comprising the 2 bv. which Roger the smith formerly held which lie next to the land of St Peter, and the toft which William Cavun formerly held [*c.*1214 × 1232, possibly 1226 × 1232]

COPIES: *b* Rawl., f. 214ʳ; *c* MS Dods. 95, f. 33ᵛ, no 38, first few lines only, from a slightly different original found in the rubble of St Mary's Tower, York.[43]

*Sibilla Hay de ii. bovatis terre in Northcava.*

Omnibus cristi fidelibus ad quos presens scriptum pervenerit, domina Sibilla Hay salutem. Noverit universitas vestra me caritatis et pietatis intuitu concessisse dedisse et presenti carta mea confirmasse deo et pauperibus hospitalis sancti Petri Ebor' duas bovatas terre et unum toftum in villa de Northcava, scilicet illas duas bovatas quas Rogerus faber aliquando tenuit et que iacent iuxta terram sancti Petri, et illud toftum quod Willelmus Cavun aliquando tenuit, tenendum et habendum predictum tenementum predictis pauperibus in puram et perpetuam elemosinam cum omnibus pertinenciis suis aisiamentis et libertatibus suis infra villam et extra libere integre et quiete ab omni servicio et exactione sicut aliqua elemosina liberius et melius teneri et haberi potest. Ego autem et heredes mei totum predictum tenementum cum omnibus prenominatis memoratis pauperibus warantizabimus adquietabimus et defendemus in omnibus et contra omnes gentes imperpetuum. In huius autem rei robur et testimonium huic scripto sigillum meum apposui. Hiis testibus, Alano de Flamevill', Willelmo de Ayvill', Petro filio Petri, Iohanne Tothe, Willelmo fratre suo, Simone Brabecum, Willelmo filio Willelmi, Petro filio suo, Simone filio Simonis, Petro Hasqui, Ricardo de Dreuton' et multis aliis.

Sybil's daughter Maud released the same 2 bv. to her mother, and issued a quitclaim to the hospital, on the same occasion (R607, R609). Alan de Flamville was dead in 1232 (*EYF*, p. 32). The first seven witnesses appear in a deed of *c.*1214 × 1232 (R612). An

---

[43] *c* reads: Omnibus cristi ad quos presens scriptum pervenerit, domina Sibilla Hay salutem. Noverint universi per presentes me pietatis intuitu concessisse dedisse et presenti [carta] mea confirm(asse) deo et pauperibus hospitalis sancti Petri Ebor' duas bovatas terre et unum toftum in villa de Northcava etc.

assize was held in 1227 to determine a case of novel disseisin brought by Sybil Hay against Richard de Murers concerning a tenement in Elvington (*PatentR*, 1225–1232, p. 160). Her description as *domina* in the present deed shows she was a person of some importance. The name of the wife of Thomas Hay (d. 1226 × 1227) is not known, so Sybil may perhaps have been his widow.

**R609.** Quitclaim to the hospital by Maud daughter of Sybil Hay, in her own power, of all right in 2 bv. with a toft in North Cave, which her mother gave [*c*.1214 × 1232, possibly 1226 × 1232]

*Quieta clamatio Matildis filie Sibille Hay de ii. bovatis in Northcava.*
Omnibus cristi fidelibus ad quos presens scriptum pervenerit Matildis filia Sibille Hay salutem. Noverit universitas vestra me in propria potestate constitutam caritatis intuitu concessisse et quietum clamasse deo et pauperibus hospitalis sancti Petri Ebor' totum ius et clam(eum) quod habui vel habere potui in duabus bovatis terre cum uno tofto in villa de Northcava, quas Sibilla Hay mater mea eis caritative contulit, tenend(a) et habend(a) in puram et perpetuam elemosinam. Quod autem ego numquam predictis pauperibus inde movebo questionem vel calumpniam tactis sacrosanctis iuravi et affidavi. Et in huius rei robur et testimonium huic scripto sigillum meum apposui. Hiis testibus, Alano de Flamevill', Willelmo de Ayvill', Petro filio Petri, Iohanne Tothe, Willelmo fratre suo, Simone Brabecun, Willelmo filio Willelmi, Petro filio suo et multis aliis.

The final three witnesses of R608 are omitted, but the deed was doubtless given on the same occasion.

**R610.** Gift to the hospital by Simon Brabazon of North Cave of a toft in North Cave, being the toft which stretches from the ditch of the grantor's garden as far as the high street towards the south, 12 perches long and 7 [ft][44] wide [*c*.1214 × 1232]

*Simon Brabacun de Northcava de uno tofto in eadem villa.*
Omnibus cristi fidelibus ad quos presens scriptum pervenerit, Simon Brabacun de Northcava salutem. Sciatis me dedisse et concessisse et hac mea presenti carta confirmasse deo et pauperibus hospitalis sancti Petri Ebor' unum toftum in Northcava, illud scilicet toftum **[f. 214ᵛ]** quod protenditur a fossato gardini mei usque ad publicam stratam versus austrum, continens duodecim perticatas in longitudine et septem [pedes][45] in latitudine, tenendum et habendum predictum toftum predictis pauperibus de me et heredibus meis, in puram et perpetuam elemosinam libere et quiete et honorifice sicut ulla elemosina liberius et melius dari potest cum omnibus libertatibus et aisiamentis ad predictam villam pertinentibus. Ego autem et heredes mei warantizabimus acquietabimus et defendemus predictum toftum prenominatis pauperibus contra omnes homines imperpetuum. In huius autem rei robur et testimonium huic scripto sigillum meum apposui. Hiis testibus, Alano de Flamivile de Northcava, Radulfo de Fontibus et Simone capellanis, Petro filio Petri de Northcava, Iohanne Thothe, Radulfo Mot de eadem, Willelmo filio Osberti de Brunkerfleth, Willelmo de [],[46] Rogero clerico et multis aliis.

---

[44] cf. R611.
[45] *pedes* supplied.
[46] MS: *Willelmo de Rogero clerico.*

The donor was the son of Thomas Brabazon (R612). Thomas Brabazon was party to a fine concerning North Cave in 1202 (*PF John*, p. 73), and with Peter son of Peter of Cave claimed he had been disseised in Cave in 1212 (*CRR*, 1210–1212, p. 333). Alan de Flamville was dead in 1232 (*EYF*, p. 32). The donor and first, fourth and fifth witnesses attested in *c*.1214 × 1232 (R609).

**R611.** Gift to the hospital, for the sustenance of the poor abiding there, by Simon Brabazon of North Cave, of a selion of arable land in the field of North Cave containing 3 *percatas*, stretching from the croft of William the carpenter of the same vill, as far as the headland towards the south, and a certain part of the donor's toft 12 perches long and 7 ft wide, nearest the house of Walter Ellus towards the east [*c*.1240 × *c*.1265]

*Carta de Northcave.*
Omnibus hoc scriptum visuris vel audituris Simon Brabazun de Northcave salutem. Noveritis me pro salute anime mee et antecessorum meorum dedisse et hac presenti carta mea confirmasse in puram et perpetuam elemosinam[47] deo et hospitali beati Petri Ebor', ad sustentationem pauperum ibidem commorantium, unam selionem terre arabilis in campo de Northcave continentem tres percatas, illam scilicet que protenditur a crofto Willelmi carpentarii eiusdem ville usque ad forarium versus austrum, et quandam partem tofti mei continentem xii^cim percatas in longitudine et septem pedes in latitudine, illam scilicet que iacet proxima domui Walteri Ellus versus orientem, tenendas et habendas dictas seliones et partem tofti cum omnibus libertatibus aisiamentis ad predictam villam pertinentibus, libere quiete et pacifice ab omni servicio seculari consuetudine exactione et demanda. Et ego Simon Brabazun et heredes mei dictas selionem et partem tofti ut prenominatum est contra omnes homines warantizabimus acquietabimus et defendemus. Et ut hec mea donatio et concessio rata et stabilis imperpetuum perseveret presens scriptum sigilli mei impressione corroboravi. Hiis testibus, Alexandro de Santona, Rogero fratre eius, Rogero Dayvile, Simone de Foro, Iohanne Tothe, Stephano Talun, magistro Petro de Kava, Radulfo Morte, Iohanne filio Walteri, Galfrido clerico et aliis.

The four leading witnesses occur in a South Cave deed of 1252 × 1255 (*YMF*, II, no. 56). Roger de Daiville succeeded his father in 1231 × 1251 and died in 1280 × 1290; Alexander of Sancton succeeded his father William in 1208 × 1218 (FNs).

**R612.** Gift to the hospital by Simon Brabazon, son of Thomas Brabazon of North Cave, of a toft and croft in North Cave, containing 1 a. and 14 perches, which lie between the donor's toft and croft and those of Martin Barn [*c*.1214 × 1232, possibly *c*.1226 × 1232]

*Simon Brabacun de Northcava de uno tofto in eadem villa.*
Sciant presentes et futuri quod ego Simon Brabecun filius Thome Brabecun de North-cave dedi concessi et presenti carta mea confirmavi deo et pauperibus hospitalis sancti Petri Ebor' unum toftum et unum croftum in villa de Northcava, que continent unam acram et quatuordecim perticatas terre et que iacent inter toftum et croftum meum et toftum et croftum Martini Barn, tenendum et habendum predictum tenementum cum omnibus pertinenciis suis et cum communi pastura eiusdem ville infra et extra

---

47 MS: *elemosinarum.*

dictis pauperibus in puram et perpetuam elemosinam liberam quietam et solutam ab
omni seculari servicio et exactione sicut aliqua elemosina liberius et melius teneri
potest. Ego autem Thomas et heredes mei warantizabimus predictum tenementum
cum omnibus prenominatis memoratis pauperibus in omnibus et contra omnes gentes.
Hoc autem fideliter observandum tactis sacrosanctis iuravi et affidavi. Et in huius rei
robur et testimonium huic scripto sigillum meum apposui. Hiis testibus, Roberto de
Colingham, Laurencio de Stowe, fratribus et capellanis, Radulfo de Fontibus, Radulfo
de Gaitington', Willelmo de Boghes capellanis secularibus, magistro Lamberto, Alano
de Flamengvill', Willelmo de Ayvill', Petro filio Petri, Petro de Santon', Iohanne
Thothe, Willelmo Tothe, Radulfo de Geveldal', Willelmo filio Willelmi, Willelmo filio
Hacun, Waltero de Alredal' et multis aliis.

The grantor's father was living in 1212 (FN); Alan de Flamville was dead in 1232 (EYF,
p. 32). Robert of Collingham indicates $c.1214 \times c.1245$; Ralph of Geddington attested
as chaplain from $c.1214$ until 1238, in which year he became rector of Newton-upon-
Ouse; William of Bowes attested from $c.1214$ until $c.1230$; Walter of Allerdale indicates
$c.1210 \times c.1235$. Six of the lay witnesses and the grantor attest a deed possibly given
in $1226 \times 1232$ (R608).

**R613.** Gift to the hospital, for the sustenance of the poor of the hospital, by David
de Anfordia, of a toft in North Cave which Alan Curbuil held, on the east
side of the land of Henry son of Alger in *Weltholm* [1197 × 1214]

*De terris in Northcave.*
Universis hanc cartam visuris vel audituris David de Anfordia salutem. Noverit
universitas vestra me concessisse et dedisse et hac presenti carta mea confirmasse deo
et hospitali sancti Leonardi Ebor' pro salute anime mee et antecessorum meorum ad
sustentationem pauperum eiusdem hospitalis, in liberam et perpetuam elemosinam,
quietam ab omni servicio et exactione, unum toftum in Nordcava quod Alanus
Curbuil tenuit iacens ex orientali parte terre Henrici filii Algeri in Weltholm. Et ego
et heredes mei deo et prefato hospitali sancti Leonardi Ebor' prefatum toftum contra
omnes homines warantizabimus. Hiis testibus, Simone decano sancti Petri Ebor',
Hamone thesaurario, magistro Erardo, Nicholao de Estutevill', Waltero de Barkeston',
Thoma Brebanzun, Petro filio Petri de Cava.

Simon de Apulia was dean between 1194 and 1214; the extreme dates for Hamo as
treasurer are 1197 to 1218.

**R614.** Gift to the hospital by David de Amford of a toft in North Cave, between
the toft which Peter son of William took with his wife, and the toft which
William son of Hacon held of the hospital [$c.1210 \times 1232$]

*David de Amford' de uno tofto in Northcava.*
Omnibus presentes litteras visuris vel audituris David de Amnford' salutem. Noverit
universitas vestra me caritatis et pietatis intuitu concessisse dedisse et presenti carta
mea confirmasse deo et pauperibus hospitalis sancti Petri Ebor' unum toftum in
Northcava, illud scilicet quod iacet inter toftum quod Petrus filius Willelmi cepit
cum uxore sua et toftum quod Willelmus filius Hacon' tenuit de predicto hospitali,
tenendum scilicet et habendum predictis pauperibus prenominatum toftum cum suis
pertinenciis libere integre et quiete in puram et perpetuam elemosinam [**f. 215ʳ**] sicut
aliqua elemosina liberius et melius dari potest. Ego autem et heredes mei predictum

toftum warantizabimus acquietabimus et defendemus predictis pauperibus in omnibus et per omnia contra omnes homines imperpetuum. Hoc autem pro me et pro here-dibus meis tactis sacrosanctis iuravi affidavi et sigillo meo confirmavi. Testibus, Alano de Flangvill', Petro de Saunton', Petro filio Petri, Thoma Brabaz', Gileberto filio Petri, Stephano, Ricardo, Radulfo, Iohanne cellerario, Galfrido, Thoma fratribus hospitalis, Ieronimo capellano, Roberto de Stowe, Waltero de Beningburg', Stephano et multis aliis.

Robert of Stowe indicates *c*.1210 × *c*.1230; Walter of Beningbrough *c*.1210 × *c*.1235; John the cellarer *c*.1210 × *c*.1230. Alan de Flamville was dead in 1232 (*EYF*, p. 32).

**R615.** Gift to the hospital by Robert son of David of North Cave of a toft in North Cave, between the tofts of William Bouer[48] and Henry the skinner, in length from the road called Eastholme Gate as far as Milnebeck [1250 × 1265]

*Carta de Northecave.*
Omnibus cristi fidelibus ad quos presens scriptum pervenerit Robertus filius David de Northcave salutem in domino. Noverit universitas vestra me dedisse concessisse et hac presenti carta mea confirmasse deo et pauperibus hospitalis sancti Petri Ebor', pro salute anime mee et animarum antecessorum et successorum meorum, unum toftum cum pertinenciis in villa de Northecave, illud scilicet quod iacet inter toftum Willelmi Bou(er) et toftum Henrici Pelliperii, sicut se extendit in longitudine a via que vocatur Estholmgate usque ad rivulum qui vocatur Milnebek', tenendum et habendum predictum toftum predictis pauperibus de me et heredibus meis, in puram et perpetuam elemosinam, cum omnibus pertinenciis aisiamentis et libertatibus suis ad predictam villam pertinentibus libere integre quiete pacifice et solute ab omni secu-lari servicio exactione et demanda, sicut aliqua elemosina melius et liberius teneri et haberi potest. Ego vero Robertus et heredes mei sive assignati predictum toftum cum omnibus pertinenciis aisiamentis et libertatibus predictis pauperibus warantizabimus adquietabimus et defendemus in omnibus et contra omnes homines imperpetuum. In cuius rei testimonium huic scripto sigillum meum apposui. Hiis testibus, Petro filio Petri, Radulfo Foliot', Rogero filio Willelmi Russel, Iohanne Toth', Willelmo Thothe, Petro clerico de Brung(er)flete, Henrico del Flet de eadem, Simone filio Roberti de Cave et aliis.

The witnesses, with the exception of William Tothe, attested the hospital's grants of the same land, made when Robert was rector (R619, R620).

**R616.** Gift to the hospital by Robert de Anford the younger of a toft with the build-ings on it in North Cave, in length from the road to the watercourse and in width from the well of St Helen to the toft which Alice Walker held [*c*.1230 × 1245]

*De uno tofto in Northecave.*
Omnibus cristi fidelibus ad quos presens scriptum pervenerit, Robertus de Anford' iunior salutem. Noverit universitas vestra me caritatis et pietatis intuitu et pro salute anime mee et animarum antecessorum et successorum meorum dedisse concessisse

---

[48] It is unclear whether the name is Bouer or Bon. In R615 and R620 it ends in a suspension mark frequently used for *er*. But in R619 it is *Bon* or *Bou*, without suspension mark.

et presenti carta mea confirmasse deo et pauperibus hospitalis sancti Petri Ebor'
unum toftum cum edificiis in eo contentis et cum omnibus pertinenciis suis in
Northcava iacens in longitudine a via usque ad cursum aque et in latitudine a fonte
sancte Helene usque ad toftum quod Alicia Walker tenuit, tenendum et habendum
predictis pauperibus in puram et perpetuam elemosinam cum omnibus pertinenciis
suis aisiamentis et libertatibus suis infra villam et extra libere integre et quiete ab
omni servicio et exactione seculari, sicut aliqua elemosina liberius et melius teneri
et haberi potest. Et ego et heredes mei predictum toftum cum omnibus pertinenciis
suis predictis pauperibus warantizabimus adquietabimus et defendemus in omnibus
et contra omnes homines imperpetuum. In huius autem rei robur et testimonium
huic scripto sigillum meum apposui. [Hiis testibus]⁴⁹ Radulfo Foliot, Willelmo Russel,
Iohanne Tothe, Willelmo Tothe, Willelmo filio Hacun, Roberto filio Thoraldi, Thoma
filio Iuliane et Hugone fratre eius, Waltero filio Iohannis et multis aliis.

The land was granted out at fee-farm by the hospital during the rectorate of Hugh
(R618). The first, third, and fourth witnesses, with Roger son of William Russell,
attested in 1250 × 1265 (R615).

**R617.** Gift to the hospital by Herbert son of Robert of North Cave of a certain land
called *Gaire* in Havercroft in the territory of North Cave [*c.*1210 × *c.*1217]

*Herbertus filius Roberti in Northecava de terra que vocatur Gaire in Havercroft'.*
Omnibus presentes litteras visuris et audituris Herbertus filius Roberti de Northecava
salutem. Noverit universitas vestra me caritatis et pietatis intuitu dedisse concessisse et
presenti carta mea confirmasse deo et pauperibus hospitalis beati Petri Ebor' in territorio de Northecave quandam terram que vocatur Gaire in Havercroft, habendam
scilicet et tenendam predictis pauperibus in puram et perpetuam elemosinam integre
libere quiete et solute ab omni servicio et exactione seculari, sicut ulla elemosina liberius et melius dari potest, ita quod ego et heredes mei totum predictum tenementum
predictis pauperibus warantizabimus aquietabimus et defendemus in omnibus et
contra omnes homines imperpetuum, ut ego et antecessores et successores mei simus
participes omnium bonorum que fiunt in prefata domo dei imperpetuum. Testibus,
Willelmo persona, Petro filio Petri, Willelmo Talon', Iohanne Todhe, Thoma Brabanc',
Simone Ruffo, Willelmo filio Willelmi, Petro Pugili, Willelmo filio Siri et multis aliis.

The five leading witnesses, and the last, occur in a deed of *c.*1210 × 1217 (R606).

**R618.** Acknowledgement of receipt, with recital, by Henry son of Ranulf of North
Cave, of the deed of master H[ugh], rector, and the brethren of the hospital,
granting him a toft in North Cave with the buildings on it, in length from
the road as far as the watercourse, and in width from the well of St Helen to
the toft which Alice Walker held, paying 12*d.* annually, and 6*s.* as an obituary
payment [*c.*1230 × 1245]

*Transcriptum Ranulfi Henrici⁵⁰ filii Ranulfi de uno tofto in Northecave.*
Sciant presentes et futuri quod ego Henricus filius Ranulfi de Northcava suscepi
cartam hospitalis beati Petri in hec verba: Omnibus cristi fidelibus ad quos presens

---

⁴⁹ Supplied.
⁵⁰ sic.

scriptum pervenerit, magister H[ugo] rector et fratres hospitalis beati Petri Ebor' salutem. Noverit universitas vestra nos concessisse et hac presenti carta nostra confirmasse Henrico filio Ranulfi de Northcava unum toftum cum edificiis in eo contentis et cum omnibus pertinentiis suis in Northcava, iacens in longitudine a via usque cursum aque et in latitudine a fonte sancte Helene usque ad toftum quod Alicia Walker tenuit, tenendum et habendum predicto Henrico et heredibus suis de nobis cum omnibus pertinenciis suis aisiamentis et libertatibus suis infra villam et extra libere integre et quiete, reddendo inde nobis annuatim pro omni servicio ad nos pertinente duodecim denarios, medietatem ad Pent' et aliam medietatem ad festum [**f. 215ᵛ**] sancti Martini in yeme. Predictus autem Henricus et heredes sui vel quicumque in predicta terra manserit sex solidos in obitu suo pauperibus domus nostre nomine testamenti fideliter persolvent. Nos vero predictum toftum cum pertinentiis predicto Henrico warantizabimus quamdiu carta donator(is) quam inde habemus nobis illud warantizare poterit. In cuius rei testimonium huic scripto sigillum nostrum apposuimus. Et in illius rei testimonium ego predictus Henricus huic scripto sigillum meum apposui.

The land was given to the hospital by Robert de Anford the younger in *c*.1230 × 1245 (R616).

**R619.** Acknowledgement of receipt, with recital, by Robert son of Ranulf of Broomfleet, of the deed of Robert, rector, and the brethren of the hospital, granting him the toft in North Cave between the toft of William Bou(er) and the toft of Henry the skinner, in length from the road called Eastholme Gate to Milnebeck, paying 12*d.* annually and a portion of chattels as an obituary payment [1250 × 1265]

*Dimissio terre in Northecave.*
Sciant omnes presentes et futuri quod ego Robertus filius Ranulfi de Brungelflete recepi cartam hospitalis sancti Leonardi Ebor' in hec verba: Omnibus cristi fidelibus ad quos presens scriptum pevenerit, Robertus rector et fratres hospitalis sancti Petri Ebor' salutem. Noverit universitas vestra nos concessisse et hac carta nostra confirmasse Roberto filio Ranulfi de Brungelflete unum toftum cum pertinenciis suis in Northcava, illud scilicet quod iacet inter toftum Willelmi Bou[er] et toftum Henrici pelliperii, sicut se extendit in longitudine a via que vocatur Estholmgate usque ad rivulum qui vocatur Milnebec, tenendum et habendum predicto Roberto et heredibus suis vel assignatis suis predictum toftum cum omnibus pertinenciis suis asiamentis et libertatibus suis infra villam et extra libere integre et quiete, reddendo inde nobis annuatim pro omni servicio ad nos pertinente duodecim denarios, medietatem ad Pent' et medietatem ad festum sancti Martini in yeme. Predictus vero Robertus et heredes sui vel assignati sui vel quicumque in predicta terra manserint vel dictam terram tenuerint portionem catallorum ipsos in obitu contingentem pauperibus domus nostre nomine testamenti fideliter persolvent. Hoc autem fideliter faciendum pro se et suis tactis sacrosanctis iuravit predictus Robertus et affidavit. Nos vero predictum toftum cum pertinenciis predicto Roberto et heredibus suis vel suis assignatis warantizabimus quamdiu carta donatoris quam inde habemus nobis illud warantizare poterit. In cuius rei testimonium huic scripto sigillum nostrum apposuimus. Hiis testibus, Petro filio Petri, Radulfo Foliot, Rogero filio Willelmi Russel, Iohanne Tothe, Petro clerico de Brungelflet, Henrico del Flet, Simone filio Roberti de Cava et multis aliis. In cuius rei testimonium ego predictus Robertus huic scripto sigillum meum apposui.

The date range is given by the extreme dates for Robert as master. An almost identical grant of the same land was made to William son of Ranulf before the same witnesses (R620). Robert son of David of North Cave's grant of this land to the hospital is attested by all the witnesses to the present deed (R615).

**R620.** Acknowledgement of receipt, with recital, by William son of Ranulf of Broomfleet, of the deed of Robert, rector, and the brethren of the hospital, granting him the property described in R619, paying 12*d.* annually and a portion of chattels as an obituary payment [1250 × 1265]

*Carta Willelmi filii Ranulfi de Brungerflete de terra sibi dimissa per hospitale in Northcave.*
Sciant omnes presentes et futuri quod ego Willelmus filius Ranulfi de Brungelflete recepi cartam hospitalis Ebor' in hec verba de quodam tofto. Omnibus cristi fidelibus hoc scriptum audituris Robertus rector et fratres hospitalis sancti Leonardi Ebor' salutem. Noverit universitas vestra nos concessisse et hac carta nostra confirmasse Willelmo filio Ranulfi de Brungelflet unum toftum cum pertinenciis suis in North-cava, illud scilicet toftum quod iacet inter toftum Willelmi Bou(er) et toftum Henrici pelliperii, sicut se extendit in longitudine a via que vocatur Estholmgata usque ad rivulum qui vocatur Milnebec, habendum et tenendum predicto Willelmo et here-dibus suis vel assignatis suis exceptis iudeis et viris religiosis aliis a nobis predictum toftum cum omnibus pertinenciis suis aisiamentis et libertatibus suis infra villam et extra libere integre et quiete, reddendo inde nobis annuatim pro omni servicio ad nos pertinente duodecim denarios, medietatem ad Pent' et medietatem ad festum sancti Martini in yeme. Predictus vero Willelmus et heredes sui vel assignati sui vel quicumque in predicta terra manserint vel dictam terram tenuerint portionem catallorum ipsos in obitu contingentem pauperibus domus nostre nomine testamenti fideliter persolvent. Hoc autem fideliter faciendum tactis sacrosanctis iuravit predictus Willelmus pro se et suis et affidavit. Nos vero predictum toftum cum pertinenciis suis predicto Willelmo et heredibus suis vel assignatis suis warantizabimus quamdiu carta donatoris quam inde habemus nobis illud warantizare poterit. In cuius rei testimonium huic scripto sigillum nostrum apposuimus. Hiis testibus, Petro filio Petri, Radulfo Foliot, Rogero filio Willelmi Russel', Iohanne Tothe, Petro clerico de Brungelflet', Henrico del Flet', Simone filio Roberti de Cava et multis aliis.

See the note to R619.

**R621.** Chirograph (*scriptum cirograffatum*) witnessing that whereas there had been disagreement between the master and brethren of the hospital of St Leonard, York, and John son of Hugh de Cave, parson of the church of Northburg, concerning a certain portion of chattels of Hugh de Cave, brother of the said John de Cave who is Hugh's heir, which is due to the hospital from the tenement which Hugh held in Northcave of the hospital's fee, it had been agreed as follows. The master and brethren and their successors have granted to John, his heirs and assigns, who will hold the tenement, that John and his heirs will pay ½*m.* as an obituary payment, and John binds himself and his heirs and assigns to the payment of ½*m.* whenever the holder of the tenement dies. Alternate seals. This for the souls of John and his ancestors. 8 July 1301.

*De dimidia marca solvenda in obitu pro terra in Northcave.*

Dat' apud Ebor' die sabbati prox' post festum translationis sancti Thome martiris, anno domini millesimo CCC^mo i°.

In 1295 Hugh of Hotham gave property in Hotham and Cave to John of Cave, priest, by deed dated at Narborough (*Northbury*), in Leicestershire (Hall, *South Cave*, pp. 102–3, citing Coram Rege, 26 Edw. I, Trinity, m. 36). John of Cave, parson of Narborough, paid £100 for property in Hotham in 1300, and £40 for a rent of 5m. 16d. and certain homages and services in North Cave in 1303 (*YF*, 1272–1300, p. 152; ibid., 1300–1314, p. 35). In 1321 John of Cave, parson of Narborough, was being impleaded concerning tenements in Narborough and villages nearby (*CalPat*, 1317–1321, p. 609).

**R622.** Gift and confirmation to the hospital by Roger son of Nigel of all land it holds of his fee in North Cave, being a toft of his own gift and another toft which Walter Talun his man gave [authentic ?]

PRINTED: *EYC*, II, no. 1124, where dated 1148 × 1156.

**[f. 216ʳ]** *Henricus[51] filius Nigelli de duobus toftis in Northecave.*
Notum sit omnibus videntibus et audientibus litteras has quod ego Rogerus filius Nigelli concessi et dedi et hac carta mea confirmavi deo et pauperibus hospitalis beati Petri Ebor' totam terram quam habent de feudo meo in Northkave, scilicet ex propria donatione mea unum toftum et aliud[52] toftum quod Walterus Talun homo meus dedit eis, liberam et quietam et immunem ab omni humano servicio sicut puram et perpetuam elemosinam preter orationes pauperum. Hanc vero elemosinam ego et heredes mei warentizabimus predictis pauperibus contra omnes homines ut simus participes elemosinarum et orationum pauperum eiusdem domus dei. Hiis testibus, Radulfo sacerdote, Willelmo diacono, Reginaldo Ruffo, Petro filio Willelmi, Willelmo filio Chnut, Roberto et Turstino filiis Langus, Sampsone filio Toke, Ricardo filio Ailmer.

Clay assumed the grantor to be Roger Hay (*EYF*, p. 40), but Roger Hay does not otherwise appear as son of Nigel, and this gift, unlike Roger Hay's grant of the mill of North Cave, was not confirmed by Thomas Hay. Roger de Mowbray, son of Nigel d'Aubigny, had interests in South Cave, and possibly in North Cave, but does not occur as Roger son of Nigel. A deed of Osbert Salvain concerning Cuckney (Notts.) given in 1135 × 1143 is witnessed by Ilbert de Lacy and R. son of Nigel, though Clay read the text differently: 'witnessed by Ilbert de Lasci and R[alph] his [Osbert's] own son'. The actual reading is apparently *dominus Ilbertus de Lasci. et. R. fil' ni'g. et cetera.* (Nostell cartulary, f. 53ᵛ; 'Ctl. Nostell', no. 398; *EYC*, XII, 99). Archbishop Theobald's confirmation of 1154 includes a *mansura* of land in Cave held of Roger de Mowbray (C194 [*EYC*, I, no. 185]), but this was probably the property described in later confirmations as being in *Marcacava*, i.e. South Cave (HN: South Cave). Farrer's suggested dating is insecure. It is presumably based on the confirmation in 1157 by Adrian IV of two *mansa* in North Cave, which are not included in the confirmation of 1148. But the deed is very formulaic for the mid-twelfth century, and the warranty clause is of a type unusual in deeds of that period. Walter Talun and the witnesses are otherwise

---

51 sic.
52 MS: *alium.*

unknown. *Tocca prepositus*, who attests Robert Hay's grant of the mill of North Cave (R598), may have been father of Sampson. Robert son of Toke held 2 bv. in [South] Cave in *c.*1170 × 1184 (*Mowbray Charters*, no. 343). Talun occurs as a surname in North Cave deeds in the thirteenth century (R603, R611). Nevertheless the authenticity of this deed is somewhat doubtful and its approximate date has not been ascertained.

## *Northeduffelde* [North Duffield]

For the rather complex tenurial history of North Duffield, see *VCH Yorks ER*, III, 91–101. The hospital's holdings in North Duffield are noticed only by these three deeds.

**R623.** Gift to the hospital by John Flambard of his capital messuage in North Duffield and all pasture and liberty of 1 bv. of the donor's land in the same vill [*c.*1215 × *c.*1245]

[f. 217<sup>r</sup>] *Iohannes Flambarde de capital(i) mesuagio suo in Northduffeld'.*
Omnibus cristi fidelibus ad quos presens scriptum pervenerit Iohannes Flambard' salutem in domino. Noveritis me dedisse concessisse et presenti carta mea confirmasse deo et sancto Leonardo Ebor' et magistro fratribus et sororibus ibidem deo servientibus totum meum capitale mesuagium in villa de Northeduffelde quod incipit a tofto Hugonis de Ganth et durat in longitudine usque ad viam versus occidentem et in latitudine a tofto Willelmi Franchomo[1] usque ad Puddiglane, et totam pasturam et libertatem unius bovate terre mee in eadem villa, in puram et perpetuam elemosinam sine ullo retenemento, pro salute anime mee et antecessorum meorum, cum omnibus libertatibus aisiamentis ad predictum mesuagium et ad predictam pasturam et libertatem infra villam de Norduffeld' et extra pertinentibus. Et ego Iohannes Flambard' et heredes mei predictum mesuagium predictam pasturam et libertatem predictis magistro fratribus et sororibus contra omnes homines et feminas imperpetuum warantizabimus defendemus et aquietabimus. In huius rei testimonio huic scripto signum meum apposui. Hiis testibus, Willelmo filio Hosberti, Ricardo de Nevill', Henrico de Hardnest, Iohanne filio Alani, Willelmo de Menethorp', Willelmo filio Willelmi, Hugone filio Haund' de Northduffeld' et multis aliis.

John Flambard made a fine with Walter Russell in 1218, whereby it was agreed John would hold 2 bv. in North Duffield of Walter for 2*s.* annually, for which privilege John gave 6*s.* (*YF*, 1218–1231, p. 5). These were possibly the 2 bv. referred to in R624. Whether John Flambard can be identified with the man of that name who had interests in Great Langton through his wife Exclamode in 1223, and who was living in 1246, has not been established (ibid., 1218–1231, pp. 47–48; 1232–1246, p. 150). The first witness to the present deed, as William son of Osbert of Skipwith, gave land in Skipwith to Selby Abbey in 1190 × 1227[2] (*EYC*, IX, no. 68).

**R624.** Gift to the hospital by John Flambard of land in North Duffield, and all service with profits and escheats which can come from those 4 a. which Alexander the chaplain held of him in *Blaketoft* [*c.*1218 × 1248]

*Iohannes Flambarde de pluribus in North Duffelde.*
Omnibus hominibus has litteras visuris vel audituris Iohannes Flambard salutem. Noverit universitas vestra me dedisse concessisse et hac presenti carta mea confirmasse deo et sancto Leonardo Ebor' et fratribus et sororibus ibidem deo servientibus in puram et perpetuam elemosinam duas acras et dimidiam terre in territorio de Norduffelde que iacent inter terram Iordani de Menethorp' et terram Thome de

---

[1]   i.e. Freeman.
[2]   Witnessed by John of Birkin.

Nevill' super Hungerhill', et illam terram in Thirspittes que pertinet meis duabus bovatis terre in eodem territorio, et unam acram et unam rodam terre, scilicet dimidiam acram in nova mora versus occidentem et unam selionem in Neubroc et unum wandail iuxta Neubrocsic et unam rodam ad Stub et unam rodam iuxta terram Iordani militis versus occident(em) et unam selionem ad Vhelbrigge iuxta terram dicti Iordani et unam acram prati in Lokincroft, et totum pratum et totam pasturam que pertinent meis duabus bovatis terre de Holbaggeflet usque ad Waterhuses et totam partem pertin(entem) meis duabus bovatis terre in Rainis versus aquilonem itineris, preter dimidiam acram quam Robertus filius Suayn tenuit, et totum servicium cum exitibus et excaetis que poterunt evenire de illis iiii[or] acris terre quas Alexander capellanus tenuit de me in Blaketoft', tenend(a) et habend(a) in puram et perpetuam elemosinam pro salute animarum antecessorum meorum cum omnibus libertatibus aisiamentis et pertinenciis suis ubique imperpetuum. Et sciendum est quod ego Iohannes Flambard' et heredes mei warantizabimus defendemus et adquietabimus omnes dictas terras cum pertinenciis predictis fratribus et sororibus domus sancti Leonardi contra omnes homines imperpetuum. Hiis testibus, Galfrido de Rukford', domino Willelmo de Dayvill', Alexandro de Santon', Rogero fratre suo, Rogero de Dayvill', domino Radulfo capellano magistri tunc, domino Michaele le[3] Segherstaine, magistro Iohanne de Gaytigton', Radulfo fratre suo, Petro de Faxflete, Adam clerico et multis aliis.

Flambard probably acquired the 2 bv. mentioned here in 1218 (R623n). The first witness, Geoffrey of Rufforth, died in 1246 × 1248. Sir William de Daiville last occurs in 1231, and was dead in 1251. Alexander of Sancton succeeded his father William in 1208 × 1218, and was living in 1252 × 1255 (FNs). Jordan of Menthorpe, named here in an abutment, gave a toft in Menthorpe to Selby Abbey in 1190 × 1227[2] (EYC, IX, no. 69). It was said in 1274–75 that Jordan of Menthorpe had paid a bribe to Giles of Goxhill (sheriff 1268–69) after his indictment at the sheriff's tourn (YQW, p. 105). The seventh witness was apparently lord of [Kirby] Sigston (NR). Michael son of Michael held ¼ k.f. in Sigston of the bishop of Durham in 1208 × 1210 (Bk of Fees, p. 24). Some details of his descendants are given in VCH Yorks NR, I, 405–6, and Brown, 'Heraldic Glass', pp. 139–44.

**R625.** Acknowledgement of receipt, with recital, by Ranulf of Faxfleet, of the deed of master Hugh, rector, and the brethren of the hospital, by which they confirmed the conveyance which John Flambard made to Ranulf of lands and rents in North Duffield, Ranulf paying the hospital 12d. annually, and ½m. for the portion of chattels due as an obituary payment [1238 × 1245]

*Transcriptum confirmationis Ranulfi de Faxeflete de terris et redditibus in Northduffeld'.*
Sciant omnes presentes quod ego Ranulfus de Faxeflete recepi cartam hospitalis sancti Leonardi in hec verba: Omnibus cristi fidelibus ad quos presens scriptum pervenerit, magister Hugo rector et fratres hospitalis sancti Leonardi Ebor' salutem. Noverit universitas vestra nos ratam et gratam habere donationem quam Iohannes Flambarde fecit Ranulfo de Faxeflete de quibusdam terris et redditibus cum omnibus suis pertinenciis in villa de Northeduffelde, tenend(a) et habend(a) predicto Ranulfo et heredibus suis prout carta dicti Iohannis quam idem Ranulfus inde habet testatur, reddendo inde nobis annuatim pro omni servicio ad nos pertinente xii[cim] denarios,

---

[3] sic.

medietatem ad Pent' et medietatem ad festum sancti Martini in yeme. Predictus vero Ranulfus et heredes sui vel quicumque dictam terram tenuerint pro portione catallorum eos in obitu contingent(e) dimidiam marcam argenti pauperibus domus nostre nomine testamenti fideliter persolvent. Hoc autem fideliter faciendum pro se et suis tactis sacrosanctis iuravit predictus Ranulfus et affidavit. Nos vero huic scripto sigillum nostrum in testimonium apposuimus. Hiis testibus, domino Radulfo persona de Neut', magistro Nicholao de London', Iohanne rectore ecclesie sancte Margarete Ebor', fratre Roberto celer(ario), fratre W. subceler(ario), fratre Ricardo, fratre Stephano de celar(io) et aliis. In cuius rei testimonium ego Ranulfus huic scripto sigillum meum apposui.

This deed was given between the institution of Ralph of Geddington as rector of Newton-on-Ouse in 1238 and the death of rector Hugh in 1245. William of Bowes, chaplain, who was instituted to St Margaret in Walmgate, York, at the presentation of the hospital, on 30 October 1227[4] (*Reg. Gray*, p. 18), was presumably the predecessor of John. Nicholas of London can probably be identified with Nicholas son of Josce of London, clerk, who was presented to a mediety of the church of Cotgrave (co. Notts.) by the prior and convent of Lenton Priory (co. Notts.) in 1238 (*Reg. Gray*, p. 82). Nicholas of London attests as a clerk *c.*1230 × *c.*1245 (C630 [Cott., f. 123$^v$]); without title and as *magister* in 1238 × 1245 (R590; M: Beningbrough [*MA*, III, 557, no. 36]); and as *magister* in 1239 × 1244 (C377 [Cott., f. 73$^v$]). In December 1241, described as clerk, he was acting as proctor for the hospital (C292 [Cott., f. 59$^r$]). He attested several deeds concerning the vicars choral of York, including examples of 1250 and 1269 or later,[5] where he is described as *magister*, and January 1259[/60], where he appears without title (*CVC*, I, nos 169, 170, 373).

---

4    The date given is 3 kal. November, thirteenth year, which indicates 1228, according to Raine's table of the archbishop's pontifical years (*Reg. Gray*, pp. xxxvii–xxxviii). But the deed appears at the start of the entry for the thirteenth year, so almost certainly belongs to 1227.
5    Walter de Stokes, who attested as mayor, is unlikely to have held that office before 1269.

## *Naburn'*

In 1086 there was a manor of 2 ct. in Naburn held by the king, and another estate of 4 ct. held by Robert de Tosny. Robert de Tosny's estate passed to the Palmes family, who in the later thirteenth century held of Watervill, who held of Ros. The smaller estate was held by the Mansel family, who held of Malebisse, who held of the honour of Eye in Suffolk (*KI*, pp. 62–63; *VCH Yorks ER*, III, 77).

Naburn is not mentioned in the papal confirmations, nor in the extents of the later thirteenth century. The four Naburn deeds which follow appear to represent two separate sales of *c.*1210 × *c.*1230, each of 4 a. meadow, one by Richard Mansel and the other by Robert Vilers. The hospital had land and tenements in Naburn and Fulford worth £2 yearly in 1535 (R905), which included 'a few acres of meadow in Naburn ings, granted by the Crown to George Darcy in 1545' (*VCH Yorks ER*, III, 78).[1] In 1550, Sir George Darcy and Dorothy his wife paid 12s. for licence to grant 8 a. meadow in Naburn and Fulford, then in the tenure of John Good, late belonging to St Leonard's, to John Eyre, citizen and mercer of London (*CalPat*, 1549–1551, p. 228).

The first three Naburn deeds and rubrics (R626–R628) are in the later form of the main hand [A-2]. The decorated capitals are uniform with others in the volume. The final deed in the Naburn section (R629) is in hand B, and has no rubric or initial capital, though space has been left for them.

As well as their land in Naburn, the MANSEL family held land in Birdforth of Malebisse, who held of the honour of Eye (*VCH Yorks NR*, II, 16–17). Richard Mansel gave the hospital a toft and croft with 1 a. in Birdforth in 1209 × 1212 (M: Birdforth [MS Dods. 120b, f. 62$^r$]). In 1218–19 there was a plea of novel disseisin against Richard Mansel for a free tenement in Birdforth, which was found to have been given to Richard's brother Robert by Henry Mansel some time beforehand (*Yorkshire Eyre Rolls*, no. 100). By the middle of the century Richard Mansel was heavily indebted, and the grants of land in Naburn he made to the Templars in 1240 and 1241 (*YF*, 1232–1246, pp. 82, 110),[2] to the archbishop of York in or before 1235 (*Reg. Gray*, p. 69), to the hospital in 1214 × 1231 (R626), and to St Andrew's Priory in York (Anon., 'Yorkshire Deeds', *YAJ*, XVII, 103–4) were undoubtedly intended to raise money. Richard Mansel was described as *miles* in a deed made before July 1246[3] (ibid., 104–5). In 1247 Richard Mansel made a fine with Richard son of Richard Mansel, apparently his son, by which he gave Richard son of Richard the manor of Naburn. Richard son of Richard acquitted Richard of £100 in Judaism. The manor of Birdforth was to remain to Richard for his life, but he was not to alienate or pledge any part of the manor so that it would pass entire to Richard son of Richard on his death (*YF*, 1246–1272, p. 4). Richard Mansel, knight, of Birdforth, gave to John Mansel his [younger] son a carucate called *Fulmose*, in Naburn (Anon., 'Yorkshire Deeds', *YAJ*, XVII, 105). This was presumably before the fine of 1261 by which Richard Mansel gave a messuage and 3 ct. in Birdforth and *Fulmos* to John son of Richard Mansel (*YF*, 1246–1272, pp. 123–24). In 1273 Amice, widow of Richard Mansel, brought a writ of account against Belya, widow of Mansel [recte Manser, a Jew] of York (*Cal. Jewish Plea Rolls*, II, p. 80). The younger Richard appears to have been succeeded by

---

[1]   Citing ERRO, DDPA/7/115, 129; i.e. Palmes of Naburn papers, now at Hull History Centre. The collection includes Naburn deeds of the thirteenth century.

[2]   See also MS Dods. 129, f. 29$^r$, for an abstract of a deed belonging to these transactions.

[3]   When Hugh of Selby, a witness, was dead (ML).

his son Edmund, who in 1277, as Edmund son of Richard son of Richard, claimed two parts of the manor of Birdforth against John Mansel (*VCH Yorks NR*, II, 17, citing De Banco R. 19, m. 24). Richard Mansel, who in 1280 gave 52*s.* 4*d.* rent in Hutton Sessay (*Heton*) and Birdforth to William of Upsall and Maud his wife in exchange for property in Sessay, was perhaps a younger brother of Edmund[4] (*YF*, 1272–1300, p. 48). In 1284–85 John Mansel held land in Birdforth of Edmund Mansel, who held of Richard Malebisse. Edmund Mansel also held of Malebisse in Naburn. In both places Malebisse held of the earl of Cornwall as of the honour of Eye (*KI*, pp. 63, 94). Edmund Mansel made a grant in Naburn in 1295, and issued a licence to dig turves in Fulmose in Naburn in 1300 (Anon., 'Yorkshire Deeds', *YAJ*, XVII, 106). In 1301 John Mansel gave the manor of Birdforth to Richard Mansel, who regranted it to John Mansel, to be held of Richard, with reversion to Richard and his heirs (*YF*, 1300–1314, pp. 11–12). John Mansel of Birdforth owed Roger Carlton, merchant of York, £24 in 1295 (PRO, C 241/35). John Mansel of Birdforth, and Richard his son owed Nicholas de Langton 46*s.* 8*d.* in 1305 (PRO, C 241/79). In 1316 John Mansel was named as one of the three lords of Birdforth (*KI*, p. 323).

**R626.** Gift to the hospital by Richard Mansel of 4 a. in the meadow of Naburn, in *Brinedale*, next to the hospital's meadow on the north side [1214 × 1231, hand A-2]

**[f. 218ᵛ]** *Carta Ricardi Maunsell' de iiii. acris prati in Naburn'.*
Omnibus cristi fidelibus ad quos presens scriptum pervenerit, Ricardo Mansell' salutem. Noverit universitas vestra me caritatis intuitu dedisse concessisse et presenti carta mea confirmasse deo et pauperibus hospitalis sancti Petri Ebor' quatuor acras prati in prato de Naburn', scilicet in Brinedale, illas videlicet que sunt proximo adiacentes prato predictorum pauperum ex parte aquilonali, tenendas et habendas predictis pauperibus de me et heredibus meis in puram et perpetuam elemosinam, libere integre et quiete ab omni servicio et exactione sicut aliqua elemosina liberius et melius teneri potest et haberi cum libero introitu et exitu ad fenum cariandum cum eis placuerit. Ego autem et heredes mei predictas quatuor acras prati cum perti-nenciis suis memoratis pauperibus warantizabimus adquietabimus et defendemus in omnibus et contra omnes gentes imperpetuum. In huius autem rei robur et testimo-nium huic scripto sigillum meum apposui. Hiis testibus, Iohanne Malebis', Willelmo Paumes, Iohanne de Fuleford', Thoma de Fuleford' clerico, Roberto Blundo de Fule-ford', Ricardo Walensi, Roberto Bustard', Henrico Bustard', Alexandro de Laceles de Eskerig', Petro de Seleby, Henrico Pincerna, Iohanne de Rawude, Petro de Knapeton' et multis aliis.

It is probable that the quitclaim by Pictavin son of Ellis to rector Hugh (R629) was issued at about the same time as the present deed. The first witness John Malebisse, of whom Mansel held his property in Naburn, was lord of Acaster Malbis, and indicates 1209 × 1231 (FN). The second witness can be identified as the William Palmes who held ¾ k.f. in North Dalton and Naburn in 1242–43 (*Bk of Fees*, p. 1101). Alexander de Lascelles does not appear in Clay's account of the family, which held Escrick of

---

4   He is perhaps to be indentified with the Richard Mansel of Hutton Sessay (*Heton*) who gave land
    in Sessay and Hutton to Ellen his daughter in 1293–94 (A2A: D AY 1/265; ibid. 2/32 [Carlisle RO,
    Aglionby papers, which contain several other references to members of the Mansel family]).

the honour of Richmond and St Mary's, York (*EYC*, v, 182–85; see also *VCH Yorks ER*, iii, 20; *CP*, vii, 444–46).

**R627.** Confirmation to the hospital by William de Vilers of 4 a. in the meadow of Naburn given by Robert de Vilers, the grantor's uncle [*c*.1210 × *c*.1230, hand A-2]

COPIES: *b* Rawl., f. 218ᵛ; *c* MS Dods. 7, f. 103ᵛ, differences as noted, further minor variations of spelling.

*Carta Willelmi de Vilers de iiii. acris prati de Naburn' predict(is).⁵*
Omnibus presentes litteras visuris vel audituris Willelmus de Vilerers⁶ salutem. Noverit universitas vestra me pietatis et caritatis intuitu concessisse et hac mea presenti carta confirmasse deo et pauperibus hospitalis beati⁷ Petri Ebor' quatuor acras prati continuas in prato de Naburn', quas Robertus de Vileres avunculus meus dedit deo et pauperibus predicti hospitalis in puram et perpetuam elemosinam, et carta sua confirmavit, ita quod ego⁸ et heredes mei predictas quatuor acras prati cum omnibus suis pertinenciis deo et predictis pauperibus warantizare aquietare et defendere contra omnes homines imperpetuum. Testibus, Willelmo filio Radulfi, Ricardo Maunsel, Ricardo de Fulefort', Thoma de Fulefort', magistris Laurencio de Wilton', Willelmo de Torinton', Henrico de Swine, Roberto Guer', Henrico capellano, Paulino de Lilling', Rogero Calvo, Willelmo Haket, Ilgero de Hemelesia et multis aliis.

Robert de Vilers' gift has the same witnesses and was given on the same occasion (R628). The origin of the Vilers interest in Naburn has not been ascertained. The witness LAURENCE OF WILTON appears variously as clerk and master. He attested as Laurence the clerk of Wilton in 1206 (*Ctl. Bridlington*, p. 251) and as Laurence of Wilton in 1205 × 1213⁹ (*Ctl. Bridlington*, p. 244), 1217 × 1220¹⁰ and March 1221 (*Reg. Gray*, pp. 139n, 141n, 279). In 1204 × 1209 he attested with Robert Waleys, sheriff of Yorkshire, once as clerk and once as master (*Ctl. Byland*, nos 188, 236). On one occasion he witnessed as Laurence of Wilton, parson of Goxhill (Lincs.), and in 1219, as Laurence the clerk of Wilton, made an agreement with Bridlington Priory concerning the churches of Goxhill and [South] Ferriby (Lincs.), whereby he undertook to pay the priory 13*m*. annually, and gave up pasture in Goxhill (*Ctl. Bridlington*, pp. 349, 442). Laurence of Wilton, clerk, gave land in Fossgate, York, to William Burgman; an endorsement refers to him as master Laurence Wilton (*CVC*, i, no. 101). Master Laurence, clerk, who attested deeds to Byland in 1193 × 1219 was probably the same man (*Ctl. Byland*, nos 598, 611).

Master William of Thornton may have been dead in 1229, when the archbishop instituted Hugh de Foston, clerk, to a mediety of the church of Hutton [Bushel], in the vale of Pickering, which master William de Thorinton held, at the presentation of the abbot and convent of Whitby. If so, William of Thornton, who was named in an

---

5   *c* has rubric *Carta Willelmi de Vilares*.
6   *b*: *Wileres*.
7   *c*: *sancti*.
8   *c* has . . . *ita quod ego Iohannes* (sic) *et heredes mei* . . . .
9   Whilst Brian de Lisle was steward of Knaresborough (FN) and before the death of William de Percy of Bolton Percy (*EYC*, xi, 107).
10   When Hamo was dean of York.

act of the archbishop in 1251 and was an executor of William of Widdingdon, must have been another man (*Reg. Gray*, pp. 31, 223n, 264).

Master Henry of Swine, who attested in 1194 ('Ctl. Meaux', no. 355), may possibly have been a successor to Robert and Philip, who were named as masters of Swine [Priory] earlier in the century (Burton, *Monastic Order*, p. 171). 'Brother Peter, master and warden' of Swine occurs in 1231 (PRO, JUST 1/1042, mm. 7d, 8).[11]

**R628.** Gift to the hospital by Robert de Vilers of 4 a. lying together in the meadow of Naburn [*c.*1210 × *c.*1230, hand A-2]

COPIES: *b* Rawl., f. 218$^v$; *c* MS Dods. 7, f. 103$^v$, differences as noted, with further minor variations of spelling.

*Carta Roberti de Vilers de iiii$^{or}$ acris prati in Naburn'.*[12]
Omnibus presentes litteras visuris vel audituris Robertus de Vileres salutem. Noverit universitas vestra me caritatis et pietatis intuitu concessisse et dedisse et hac mea presenti carta confirmasse deo et pauperibus hospitalis beati Petri Ebor' iiii$^{or}$ acras prati continue iacentes in prato de Naburn' cum omnibus pertinenciis suis, in puram et perpetuam elemosinam liberam solutam et quietam ab omni servicio et exactione seculari, sicut ulla elemosina liberius et melius dari potest, ita quod ego et heredes mei predictas quatuor acras cum omnibus pertinenciis suis debemus warantizare defendere et aquietare predictis pauperibus imperpetuum contra omnes homines. Hiis[13] testibus, Willelmo filio Radulfi, Ricardo Maunsel, Ricardo de Fulefort', Thoma de Fulefort', magistris[14] Laurencio de Wilton', Willelmo de Torenton', Henrico de Swine, Roberto Guer, Henrico capellano, Paulino de Lilling', Rogero Calvo, Willelmo Haket, Ilgero de Hemeleseya et multis aliis.

See R627.

**R629.** Quitclaim to master Hugh and the brethren of the hospital by Pictavin, son of Ellis, Jew of Lincoln, of all claim in 4 a. in the meadow of Naburn, which the brethren bought from Richard Mansel, arising from any debts which Richard or his heirs owed to Pictavin [1214 × 1231, hand B]

Omnibus[15] visuris vel audituris litteras istas Pictau(in) filius Elye iud(eus) Lincoln' salutem. Noverit universitas vestra quod quietum clamavi magistro Hugoni et fratribus hospitalis sancti Petri Ebor quatuor acras prati in prato de Naburn' quas emerunt de Ricardo Maunsell' de omnibus debitis et demandis que unquam predictus Ricardus vel heredes sui michi vel heredibus meis debuerunt a principio mundi usque ad finem. Et in huius rei testimonium hui scripto litteram meam Hebraicam apposui.

It is likely that this deed was issued at about the same time as Richard's sale of the 4 a. to the hospital (R626).

[11]   AALT, IMG_1210 and IMG _1267.
[12]   *c* has rubric *Carta Roberti de Vileres.*
[13]   *b*: *Hiis* omitted.
[14]   *c*: *magistro.*
[15]   No rubric; first letter omitted and space left for decorated capital.

## *Octon'*

Domesday lists two holdings in Octon. The king had 4 ct. in *Fornetorp* and Octon; the count of Mortain held 14 ct. in Octon. In 1284–85 there were said to be 14 ct. in Octon, comprising 12 ct. held by Marmaduke of Thwing of the Mauley fee as 1 k.f., and 2 ct. held jointly by Walter de Bukden, Henry de Rouceby, William son of Helen and John of Octon for 20s. in lieu of archery service (*KI*, p. 57). As Marmaduke of Thwing was the successor to John of Octon, and Mauley succeeded to the Fossard fee, we might expect John of Octon's ancestor William son of Robert of Octon to have been the tenant of 1 k.f. in Octon of Fossard in 1166, but there is no trace of such a tenancy in the Fossard *carta* (*EYC*, II, no. 1003).[1] For the holdings of religious houses other than the hospital in Octon, and the subsequent history of the manor, see *VCH Yorks ER*, II, 326–27.

A bovate in *Occatuna* was included in the papal confirmations to the hospital of 1157 and 1173, but not that of 1148 (C178–C180 [*EYC*, I, nos 179, 186, 197]). A bovate with a toft of annual value 5s. given by Robert of Octon was confirmed by Archbishop Theobald in 1154 (C194 [*EYC*, I, no. 185]). Robert of Octon's gift can therefore be assigned to 1148 × 1154. His son William issued a confirmation in c.1175 × 1194 (R630), and within the same limits of date gave the hospital an additional 5 a. (R631). John son of William of Octon confirmed the gifts of his father and grandfather. He also granted the hospital a villein (R632) and a toft (R633). John son of John of Harpham gave a toft and a croft in c.1206 × c.1220 (R634). Three deeds of the later thirteenth and early fourteenth century show the hospital's interest in its tenants' conveyances (R635–R637). Agatha 'late wife of Robert de Rouceby' was found at an inquisition after her death in 1341 to have held a messuage in Octon, of the inheritance of her husband, of the hospital, by service of 2s. annually (*CalInqPM*, VIII, no. 312). No mention of Octon is made in the *Valor Ecclesiasticus*, or the account of 1542.

The OCTON family held of Fossard and Aumale in the twelfth century. Robert of Octon attested a deed of William Fossard in '1154 × 1160' (*EYC*, II, no. 1118). William earl of Aumale gave to Robert of Octon, his man, all the land of *Holmet*,[2] probably at about the same time (Octon deeds, no. 6).[3] According to the chronicle of Meaux,

1   Farrer suggested that Octon may have been held of William Fossard by William son of Godfrey '[of Harpham ?]' as 1 k.f. in 1166, but elsewhere he says that it formed part of the 2 k.f. held by Durand son of William 'of Butterwick' [recte of Hotham] (*EYC*, II, 331, 374, 378). Neither proposition seems likely. Although the Harpham family appear to have held in Octon, there is no record of William son of Godfrey of Harpham. No evidence has been found to show the Butterwick or Hotham families had interests in Octon.
2   For the location of *Holmet* see p. 717 below.
3   In 1578 excerpts were made from the charters of John Lumley, Baron Lumley, of Lumley castle in Durham, which included evidences inherited from the Thwing and Octon families. The following are those concerning Octon, given in full from MS Dods. 20. Additional details in square brackets are taken from BL, MS Harley 1985, ff. 269–93, which was apparently drawn from the same source (*Cat. Harleian; SC, loc. cit.*). They are cited here as 'Octon deeds'.
[f. 127ᵛ] [1] Ego Marmaducus filius Roberti de Thweng dedi Iohanni filio Iohannis de Oketon et Alicie sorori mee et heredibus et cet'.
[f. 128ᵛ] [2] Ego Marmaducus de Thwenge dedi domino Roberto Constabulario de Flaynburgh' consanguineo meo manerium meum de Oketon et manerium meum de Holme in Holdernes et cet'. Dat' anno regni regis Edwardi filii regis Edwardi 13. [1319–20]
[3] Ego Iohannis de Oketon dedi Marmaduco filio domini Marmaduci de Thwenge totum manerium meum de Oketon et totum manerium meum de Holme, una cum terra que domina Huguelina que

the abbey acquired the site of its grange in Octon in the time of Adam, the first abbot (1151–1160), from Henry, son of Robert of Octon. Robert of Octon had been sheriff of Yorkshire, says the chronicle,[4] and later became a monk at Meaux. Henry had 60*m*. from the monks on setting out for Jerusalem, in exchange for 2½ ct. in Octon, 2 ct. of which were to be held of Godfrey of Harpham and the remainder of Henry's brother William. William confirmed the land, with pasture for 500 sheep in the common pasture of Octon, and exchanged acre for acre the land which his father

fuit uxor domini Roberti de Thwenge tenet in dotem in Holme et in Oketon et cet'. [Testibus, Richardo de Twenge, Willelmo de Hassethorpe, Galfrido Auguilum militibus, sine dat'.]

[4] Iohannes de Oketon et Alicia uxor eius dant plenam seisinam domino Marmaduco filio domini Marmaduci de Thwenge de toto manerio de Lund' et cet'. Dat' apud Ebor' anno domini 1284.

[5] Ego Marmaducus de Thwenge dedi Willelmo de Thwenge filio et heredi meo manerium meum de Oketon et cet'. Reddendo inde annuatim pro me domine Alicie de sancto Mauro 15 libras et cet'. Dat' anno 13.E.2 domini 1319.

[f. 133$^v$] [6] Willelmus Albermarlie comes dapifero et vicecom(iti) omnibusque baronibus suis francis et anglis salutem. Sciatis me concessisse Rodberto de Octona homini meo totam terram de Holmet etc. Testibus, Alano de Moncels, Willelmo de Albemarle et cet'.

[7] Domine Hugeline quondam uxori domini Iohannis de Octon, Iohannes de Octon filius et heres domini Iohannis de Octon salutem. Precipio vos quatinus sitis attendens domino Marmaduco de Thwenge nepoti meo de terris que apud Holme in Holdernes et apud Octon tenetis nomine dotis. Sciatis namque me domino Marmaduco de Thwenge nepoti meo pro me et heredibus suis totum ius meum resignasse et concessisse in eisdem et cet'. Dat' apud Ebor' anno domini 1284.

[8] Ego Iohannes de Oketon dedi Marmaduco filio domini Marmaduci de Thwenge totum manerium meum de Holme, una cum terra que domina Huguelina que fuit uxor domini Roberti de Thwenge tenet in dotem in Holm' et in Oketon et cet'. Testibus, Ricardo de Thweng, Willelmo de Hassethorpe, Galfrido Aguylon militibus et cet'.

[9] Ego Iohannes de Oketon dedi Marmaduco filio domini Marmaduci de Thwenge terram in territorio de Rottesle et cet'. Reddendo inde mihi et Alicie uxori mee et heredibus de nobis legitime exeuntibus quatuor marcas. Et si sine herede de nobis exeuntibus in fata decesserimus, predicta tenementa dicto Marmaduco et heredibus suis remaneant imperpetuum et cet'. Testibus, Ricardo de Thwenge milite et cet'.

[10] Iohannes de Oketon condit testamentum suum anno domini 1271 fatetur [MS: *fabetur*] se olim fuisse senescallum hospitii domini Hugonis Bygod, et dat terras pro anima dicti Hugonis et pro anima domini Willelmi de Fortibus quondam comitis Albemarlie [et domini Iohannis Maunsell etc]. Ibi facit mentionem [Cecilie filie sue,] Alicie uxoris sue et Alicie sororis sue, et Roberti filii sui et Amandi de Rue generis sui et Gilberti de Aton generis sui, Agnete filie sue, Mariorie filie sue, Lucie filie sue, et Emme filie sue [et domine Iohanne consanguinee sue unam marcam]. Dat terras Gilberto de Aton' et uxori sue Lucie. Item dat Ydonie sorori sue unam marcam. Item dat Nicholao fratri suo 10 libras, Emma filia sua fuit tunc innupta. Executores fuerunt Iohannes et Robertus filii sui. Item dat domine Dionisie amite sue unam marcam.

[11] Carta Iohannis filii et heredis domini Iohannis de Okenton, in qua facta est mentio Alicie matris sue et Alicie uxoris sue et cet'. Testibus domino Marmaduco de Thwenge, domino Roberto filio suo militibus et cet'.

[12] Ego Iohannes filius Iohannis de Okenton assignavi Henricum de Rouceby ad seisinam nomine meo tradendam Marmaduco filio Marmaduci de Thwenge, de maneriis meis de Okenton et Holm' in Holdernessia, et de terris meis in Swauethorpe, que tenementa dictus Marmaducus filius Marmaduci habet de dono meo in villis predictis et cet'. Dat' apud Ebor' anno 12.Ed' primi 1284.

[13] Anno domini 1284. Ego Iohannes de Okenton condo testamentum meum. Lego Alicie uxori mee et cet'. Item lego domino Marmaduco de Thwenge avunculo meo omnes balistas meas. Item lego Iohanni de Monceux nepoti meo et cet'. Item lego Cicilie sorori mee moniali de Wykeham quinque marcas. Ibi facit mentionem Ywaini de Thwenge cui accommodavit pecuniam quando ivit versus Walliam. Item constituo executorem meum principalem dominum Marmaducum de Thwenge heredem meum. Item lego corpus meum sepeliendum in ecclesia conventuali sancti Andree Ebor' in Fiskergate ante altare sancte Marie et cet'.

[14] Ego Alicia quondam uxor domini Iohannis de Octon in viduitate mea remisi domino Marmaduco de Thwenge iuniori totum clameum meum in manerio de Lund et cet. [Testibus Willelmo Constabulario milite.] Dat' anno domini 1284.

4   Green found no other evidence for him as sheriff (Green, *Sheriffs*, p. 90).

## OCTON

ROBERT OF OCTON,
tenant of William de
Aumale, occs c.1155

WILLIAM OF OCTON  HENRY OF OCTON  MABEL = JORDAN BRITO  Unnamed nun
of Wykeham

SIR JOHN OF OCTON I, succ.   WILLIAM OF OCTON    Unnamed nun
by 1194, dead in 1221              of Wykeham

SIR JOHN OF OCTON II,         ROBERT OF THWING,
succ. by 1221, living 1235        living 1246

(2) HUGELINA, remar. = SIR JOHN OF OCTON III, = (1) ALICE OF MARMADUKE OF
Robert of Thwing  succ. by 1250, sheriff of THWING THWING II, succ.
before 1280, living  Yorks 1260–61, 1265–66,    by 1251, died 1284
1290     d. c.1274

SIR JOHN OF = ALICE, remar.  ROBERT, d.s.p. by 1287  MARMADUKE
OCTON IV, succ. Ralph de St- MARGERY, dead in 1287, had issue OF THWING III
c.1274,  Maur by 1289, John, Beatrix, both d.s.p. by 1287
died 1284  living 1321  AGNES, wife of Amandus of Routh
         LUCY, wife of Ralph de Lelley
ALICE, d.s.p.   EMMA, wife of Ingram de
by 1287    Monceaux, had issue John
        CECILY, a nun of Wykeham

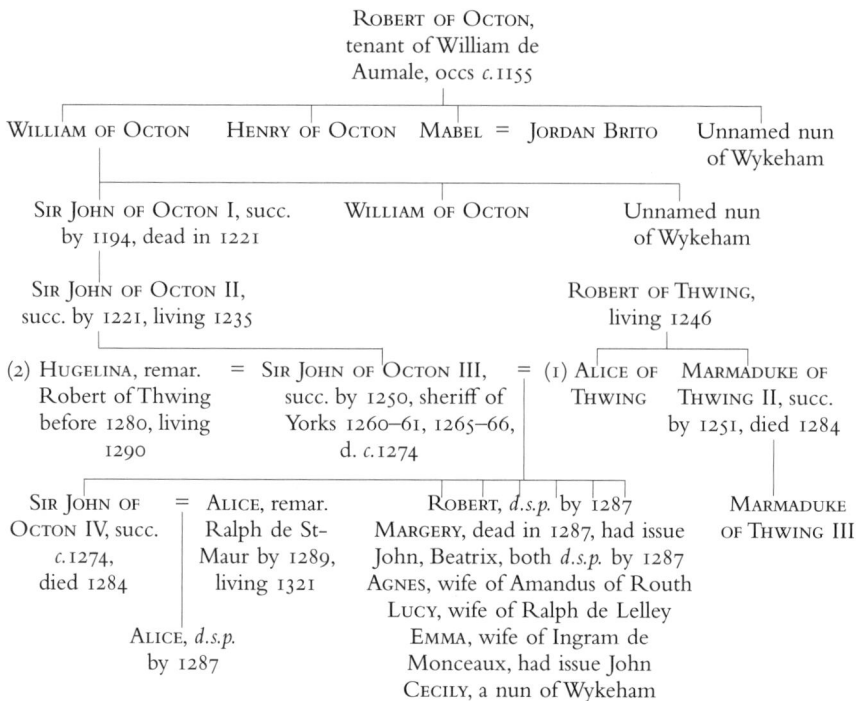

had given to the Hospitallers. A further 2 bv. in Octon were bought from Mabel, sister of William and Henry, for 5m. (*Chron. Meaux*, I, 102–3).[5] The grange of Octon was confirmed to Meaux by Pope Alexander III in 1172 (*EYC*, III, no. 1391).

It is suggested above that Robert of Octon's gift to the hospital of 1 bv. in Octon was made in 1148 × 1154. The confirmations made by William son of Robert of Octon (to which he added first 2 a. and later 5 a. of his own gift), and by John son of William of Octon are difficult to date accurately, but prove the descent from Robert (R630–R632). William son of Robert of Octon was a benefactor of the monastery of Wykeham, to which he gave, with his nephews William and Robert as brethren of the monastery, ½ ct. in Octon, from the carucate which his father Robert had previously given to Jordan Brito in marriage with William's sister Mabel (*EYC*, II, no. 1065). This gift too was confirmed by John son of William of Octon (*EYC*, II, no. 1070). William of Octon also gave to Wykeham, with his sister, 13 a. in his culture at Westcotes, and 13 a. in his culture where the grange of the nuns was sited, with

5 Elsewhere in the chronicle it is stated that Sir Robert of Octon, who lived in the time of Adam the first abbot, had three daughters. One, named Aubrey, he gave in marriage to Sir Hugelin of Etton with the land he had in Skerne. Another was wife to William Duayd (stated in an interlineation in one version of the chronicle to have been the parents of John of Octon), and the third was wife to Godfrey of Harpham. Hugelin lost the land when he lost the king's favour, and it was given to Odard de Mansel, who was grandfather of Thomas of Etton the elder (*Chron. Meaux*, I, 316–17). In 1270 × 1280, John of Octon claimed five tofts, 4 ct. and 5 bv. land in Skerne which Sir Robert of Octon, his ancestor, had given with his daughter Aubrey in marriage to Hugelin of Etton. John quitclaimed the land for 50m. (ibid., II, 155; cf. *EYC*, IX, 192; *EYF*, p. 25; Bilson, 'Gilling Castle', pp. 107–9).

further land in East and West Hovetland, with pasture for 300 sheep, in exchange for the land which Godfrey of Harpham gave with his two sisters. William also gave 5 a. with his daughter, next to the 6 a. which Godfrey of Harpham gave with his daughter (Burton transcripts 1, f. 167$^v$, p. 282, B14 N44, cited *Monasticon Eboracense*, p. 256). It was probably the same William of Octon who gave 1 bv. in Octon, which he had bought, to his nephew John of Octon, to be held of the Hospitallers (*EYC*, II, no. 1068).

John son of William of Octon had succeeded by May 1194, when he quitclaimed to the monks of Meaux all right in the wall of their grange in Octon, and in the sheepfolds outside their gate. John's brother William joined in the quitclaim ('Ctl. Meaux', no. 355; *Chron. Meaux*, I, 230). John son of William of Octon confirmed the gifts which his predecessors had made to Bridlington Priory of Hallytreeholme, Thornholme, Brackenholme, *Nepeholme*, and Hempholme (all par. Leven) with two fisheries in the [river] Hull, half the marsh of *Witheland*, and free passage from the bridge of *Miclene* to Hallytreeholme through *Miclene* Fleet in 1185 × 1207[6] (*EYC*, III, no. 1410). In 1198 × 1226[7] Sir[8] John of Octon and Ellis, prior of Bridlington, issued reciprocal deeds whereby John granted the priory a marsh near Hallytreeholme and fisheries in the river Hull in return for a chaplain to celebrate divine service at Hallytreeholme. William, brother of Sir John of Octon, attested the prior's deed (*YD*, I, no. 209; *Ctl. Bridlington*, p. 305). John of Octon gave all the marsh and all the firm ground between *Mikelnfled* and the new fosse in the length of the Hull, and all the new fosse the canons had made, by a deed of uncertain date witnessed by William of Octon and J[ohn] of Octon (*Ctl. Bridlington*, p. 305). This gift was included in a general confirmation by William de Forz, earl of Aumale, in 1214 × 1239,[9] where the land is described as being in Hallytreeholme (ibid., p. 343). In *c*.1180 × 1210 John son of William of Octon was licensed by Adam, parson of Thwing, to hold divine service, performed by the chaplain of Thwing, in the chapel of St Michael in Octon, in consideration of the gift of 2 bv. in Octon (*EYC*, II, no. 1069). John of Octon was a knight on a grand assize in 1207 (*EYC*, III, 70) and was named as a pledge in 1208 (Stenton, *Pleas*, IV, nos 3418, 3428). It is uncertain whether John of Octon, who was attorney for Alice de Amundeville in a plea concerning ½ k.f. in Winthorpe (Kilnwick) in 1200–01, was the same man (*CRR*, I, 309, 317; ibid., 1201–1203, p. 42).

The first John of Octon was dead by Easter term 1221, when the abbot of Meaux claimed warranty for pasture for 500 sheep from John of Octon, son and heir of John of Octon (*CRR*, 1221–1222, pp. 56, 179). The claim was unsuccessful, and Richard abbot of Meaux quitclaimed to John [II] son of John of Octon all right in pasture for 500 sheep in Octon, saving the pasture belonging to the 30 bv. held by the monks in Octon, and made a fine to the same effect in 1222 ('Ctl. Meaux', no. 357; *YF*, 1218–1231, p. 45). John [II] was a benefactor of Nunkeeling, to which he gave 2 bv. in Octon (Burton transcripts 1, f. 109$^r$, p. 165, B7 N38)[10] and turbary in Holme, both of which gifts were confirmed by his son and grandson.[11] In 1231 John of Octon was one of four knights to choose twelve (*YF*, 1218–1231, p. 158n), and in 1233 John

---

6    Dated by Farrer 1175 × 1190. Robert Constable, who succeeded his father in 1185 or later and was dead in 1207 (*EYC*, XII, 145–46), and Richard his brother are the first witnesses.
7    Ellis became prior in 1198 × 1200 and last occurs in 1210. His successor does not occur until 1226.
8    So styled in the prior's deed, but not his own.
9    The date range is that of the earl's marriage (*CP*, I, 355), as his confirmation was for the health of his soul and that of his wife Avelina.
10   Attested by Sir Anselm de St-Quintin, William son of Robert of Octon, John his brother, and others named; cited *Monasticon Eboracense*, p. 386.
11   For these confirmations, and the gift in Holme, see below.

son of John of Octon, William of Arundel and Sybil his wife claimed against Ann, Sybil and Joan, daughters of John Mauleverer, land in Bursea (in Holme on Spalding Moor), as their reasonable share in the heredity of William Foliot, who was father of Sybil, and grandfather of John, Ann, Sybil and Joan (*CRR*, 1233–1237, no. 759).[12] Sir John of Octon attested in 1235 (MS Dods. 7, f. 258ᵛ).

There are no closely datable references to John of Octon between 1235 and 1250,[13] and it is probable that the death of John II and the succession of his son John III can be placed between these dates. Arrangements for the marriage of John [III] were put in place in or after 1246.[14] In 1253 John of Octon was granted exemption for life from being put on assizes, juries, or recognitions, and from being made forester or verderer (*CalPat*, 1247–1258, p. 192), and in 1260 he was granted free warren in all his demesne lands in Holme,[15] Octon, Baggaby [Bottom], Helperthorpe, Rotsea and Easthorp, co. York (*CalCh*, 1257–1300, p. 29). As John of Octon, knight, he granted the manor of Baggaby, which was held of Ros, to Hugh of Bilbrough. The gift was confirmed by John son of John of Octon, and Bilbrough subsequently granted the manor to the priory of Warter (Warter cartulary, f. 32ʳ).[16] Sir John of Octon attested many deeds as steward of St Mary's Abbey in York, including examples of 1254, 1255[/56], 1256 × 1258, 1257, and 1259 (St Mary A1, ff. 136ʳ, 140ᵛ, 232ʳ⁻ᵛ, 275ʳ⁻ᵛ, 278ᵛ–279ʳ). In October 1255 he was appointed with two monks of St Mary to take custody of the abbey, which had fallen into debt (*CalPat*, 1247–1258, p. 428). He left lands in his will for the soul of Sir Hugh Bigod (d. 1266)[17] saying he had once been his household steward (Octon deeds, no. 10). He was sheriff of Yorkshire in 1260–61 and 1265–66 and was a prominent servant of the king in Yorkshire during the disturbances of the 1260s, when he served as constable of Scarborough castle (*CalPat*, *CloseR*, passim). He occurs as steward of the bishop of Durham in 1266 (Holford, 'Office-Holders', p. 166), and was a justice in the visitation of 1268–72 (*General Eyre*, pp. 137–39). He was associated with Edmund 'Crouchback', Henry III's second son, earl of Leicester and earl of Lancaster,[18] particularly in 1270–71, immediately before the earl's departure for the Holy Land, witnessing several of his deeds (*CalCh*, 1257–1300, pp. 135, 161–62; *CalPat*, 1281–1292, p. 174; *CP*, VII, 382). In that year Octon loaned the earl £300 on the security of his manor of Easingwold, and was one of those who received a loan of 1000*m*. from the king's brother, Richard, 'king of the Romans', for the use of Edmund (*CalCh*, 1257–1300, pp. 162; *CalPat*, 1266–1272, p. 566). He acted as the earl's steward in Yorkshire (*YQW*, p. 40),[19] probably in connection with the mortgage. He continued to receive commissions of various kinds after the accession of Edward I, the

---

[12]  By a deed of uncertain date John, son and heir of John of Octon, knight (*militis*) gave to Nunkeeling the homage and service of 8*s*. from John son of Robert de Hoton and his heirs, for 2 bv. in Sunderlandwick (near Driffield), which William Foliot, once his ancestor, had bought from the nuns, and which had descended to John as one of William's heirs (MS Dods. 7, f. 262ᵛ; noted *EYC*, II, no. 682n).

[13]  In that year a feodary of serjeantries included 2 bv. in Octon held by John of Octon of Anketin Mallory and Sarah his wife (*Bk of Fees*, p. 1201).

[14]  See below.

[15]  Identified as Holme on the Wold at *YQW*, p. 181, but see p. 717 below.

[16]  According to a narrative history of Warter Priory, John Thorpe, the 11th prior [1280–1314], bought the manor and the field of Baggaby from Hugh of Bilbrough. A carucate in Baggaby was confirmed to the priory by William de Ros after June 1285, when he succeeded to the family estates (*MA*, VI, 299–300; *CP*, XI, 96).

[17]  For Hugh Bigod [III], son of Hugh Bigod [II], earl of Norfolk, see *ODNB*.

[18]  For Prince Edmund see *ODNB* and *CP*, VII, 378–87.

[19]  Crouchback is conflated with Edmund, earl of Cornwall in *YQW*, index. Crouchback is called 'earl of Derby' in proceedings of 1279–81 (*YQW*, p. 150). He had received the forfeit lands of Robert de Ferrers, earl of Derby, in 1266, but rarely, if ever, used the title himself (*CP*, IV, 200–3). The evidence

last of these being issued on 3 June 1274 (*CalPat*, 1272–1281, pp. 9, 50–51, 66; *CalIn-qMisc*, 1219–1307, no. 964). He died at about that time. There were many complaints about his conduct in the hundred rolls of 1274–75, where he is described as formerly sheriff [of Yorkshire] and also as steward of the bishop of Durham, Robert [Stichill].[20] Amongst other charges, he had taken money from many men to release them from knighthood 'but because he is dead, it is not mentioned here' (*YQW*, pp. 31, 69, 79 and passim). The identity of John III's first wife, and mother of his son and heir John IV, is shown by an abstract of a deed made in 1246 or later,[21] by which Marmaduke [II] son of Robert of Thwing gave lands to John son of John of Octon and Alice his (Marmaduke's) sister (Octon deeds, no. 1).[22] John of Octon [III] mentions his wife Alice in his will of 1271 (Octon deeds, no. 10), but if she was then living she must have died soon afterwards, as his widow was named Hugelina. John of Octon [IV] granted a life annuity of 13½m. to Hugelina of Thwing, who had claimed nine tofts and 15 bv. land in Octon from him in 1280 (*YF*, 1272–1300, p. 59).

John of Octon [IV] gave his manors of Holme and Octon to Marmaduke son of Marmaduke of Thwing, with the [reversion of the] land which Lady Hugelina, who had been wife of Sir Robert of Thwing,[23] was holding in dower in Holme and Octon (Octon deeds, no. 3). This grant was made at the same time as, or slightly before, the deed of attorney to deliver seisin of 1284, and the notification by John of Octon [IV], son and heir of Sir John of Octon, to Lady Hugelina, formerly wife of Sir John of Octon, stating that he had resigned his interest in Holme in Holderness and in Octon to Marmaduke of Thwing, his *nepos*, on whom she should attend concerning the lands she held in those places by way of dower, also issued in 1284 (Octon deeds, nos 7, 12).

John of Octon IV, the eldest son of John of Octon III, was probably the John son of John of Octon who was amongst the men in the munition of Scarborough Castle who were granted protection in December 1264 (*CalPat*, 1258–1266, p. 391), though it is unlikely he was then more than eighteen years old. John of Octon was

for Ormrod's statement that John of Octon served as steward to Richard, earl of Cornwall (father of Edmund), is unclear (Ormrod, *Sheriffs*, p. 58).

[20] He does not attest any surviving Durham episcopal acta (*EEA*, XXIX, passim).

[21] 1246 is the earliest date for the succession of Marmaduke II son of Robert of Thwing (*CP*, XII (1), 737–38).

[22] John [IV], son and heir of Sir John of Octon, named both his wife and his mother as Alice (Octon Deeds, no. 11). John of Octon [IV] mentions his uncle Sir Marmaduke of Thwing in his will of 1284 (Octon deeds, no. 13), so it is clear that it was John of Octon III who was married to Alice of Thwing, and not John IV. As Marmaduke of Thwing II was betrothed to Lucy de Brus by 1243, being then under the age of twenty (*CRR*, 1243–1245, no. 752), and held lands in 1251 (*Ctl. Gisborough*, no. 868), he was born in the period c.1223 × 1230. John of Octon IV's widow Alice was still living in 1319.

[23] Vincent says Hugelina was wife of the Robert of Thwing 'perhaps an illegitimate son of Sir Robert [III]', who was a household knight of Henry III from 1262, and participated in negotiations with the Scots (*ODNB*, s.n. Robert of Thwing), but no evidence to support this statement has been found. Robert of Thwing, the eldest son of Marmaduke of Thwing [II], who predeceased his father, had been married or betrothed by December 1265 to Alice, daughter of Robert de Merlay, then aged eight. But a little over two years later, in February 1268, Alice was dead. In 1278 or before Robert married a lady whose identity is not known, who was mother to his heir the 'notorious lady' Lucy of Thwing, born on 24 March 1279 (*EYC*, IX, 31; ibid., XI, 206; *CP*, XII (1), 739 and n). It is unclear which Robert of Thwing performed service in Wales for the bishop of Durham in August 1282 (*CP*, XII (1), 739; *Parl. Writs*, I, 228, 235; cf. *CalCl*, 1279–1288, p. 188). It seems most likely that Robert son of Marmaduke of Thwing was then dead, for it was Marmaduke son of Marmaduke of Thwing who performed service on behalf of his father, by the king's grace, in August 1282 (*Parl. Writs*, I, 229b, 242). Sir Richard of Thwing, knight, attested acta of the bishop of Durham in 1267 and 1261 × 1274 (*EEA*, XXIX, nos 133, 161).

said to hold 1 k.f. in Octon of Mauley in 1279 (*YI*, 1, 197). As Sir John of Octon, son and heir of the late Sir John of Octon, he quitclaimed to Edmund ['Crouchback'], son of King Henry, the manor of Easingwold, having received the £300 due (PRO, DL 25/2478 [Duchy of Lancaster deeds]; *Honor of Pickering*, II, 48). In quo warranto proceedings of 1279–81 he claimed free warren in his demesne lands, citing the grant of Henry III to John his father (*YQW*, pp. 181–82). John of Octon was granted protection in June 1283 until the following November, as he was going beyond seas (*CalPat*, 1281–1292, p. 68). His will, written in 1284, mentioned his wife Alice, his uncle Sir Marmaduke of Thwing, to whom he left all his crossbows, his *nepos* John de Monceux, and his sister Cecily, a nun of Wykeham. His body was to be buried in the conventual church of St Andrew in Fishergate [York]. John died the same year and was survived by his wife (Octon deeds, nos 13, 14). Almost all his lands passed to his first cousin, Marmaduke [III] son of Marmaduke of Thwing, named in his will as chief executor and heir.[24] Marmaduke had no legal claim to be considered John's 'right heir', but matters were arranged by several feoffments, some dated 1284, so that the manors of Octon, Holme, and Lund, and lands in Rotsea and Swaythorpe, passed to him (Octon deeds, nos 7, 8, 9, 12, 14). Amandus of Routh (*Ruda*) and Agnes his wife, Ralph de Lelley and Lucy his wife, and Ingram de Monceaux and Emma his wife claimed tenements in Baggaby [Bottom] and Easthorpe in Easter term, 1287, as the right heirs of John son of John of Octon. Agnes, Lucy, and Emma were his surviving sisters (Warter cartulary, ff. 32ᵛ–33ʳ).[25]

John's wife Alice may have been a member of the Cam family, of Kirby Cam, now Kirby Cane, in Norfolk.[26] In 1276–78 justices were appointed to take assizes of mort d'ancestor arraigned by John of Octon and Alice his wife against Thomas Charles and Joan his wife,[27] regarding land in Croxton, co. Camb., and Frettenham and *Maydeneton*,[28] in Norfolk. The resulting inquisition in Norfolk found that a messuage and other property had previously been held by Walter de Kam (*Rep. Dep. Keeper*, XLVI (1885), App. 2, 164; ibid., XLVII (1886), App., 202).[29] Alice also succeeded Walter de Cam in Rutland. The prior of Newstead (Lincs.) appointed a clerk to the church of Little Casterton, in Rutland, late in 1282, but after disputes in the king's and bishop's courts the subsequent presentation by Sir John of Octon and Alice his wife was upheld and their candidate instituted in the second half of 1283 (*Reg. Sutton*, II, 34–36). The previous presentation, disputed by Richard of Casterton and Richard de Deyn', had been made in 1263 by Walter de Came (*Rot. Gravesend*, p. 103). Alice married as her second husband Ralph de St-Maur. In 1289 the couple claimed from Marmaduke of Thwing a third part of two parts of the manor of *Hulmo*, a third part of the manors of Octon and Swaythorpe, a third part of 1 bv. in Helperthorpe, and a third part of 6 bv. in Rotsea, as the dower of Alice by the endowment of John of Octon, her first husband. It was agreed that Marmaduke would pay £15 15s. 8d.

---

[24] John calls Marmaduke *nepos* (Octon deeds, no. 7) but as it is clear that Marmaduke was the son of Marmaduke of Thwing II by his wife the heiress Lucy de Brus (*CP*, XII (1), 739–41), nephew in its strict meaning is not intended.

[25] The plea mentions other kin of John of Octon IV, then deceased, namely his daughter Alice, brother Robert, and sister Margery, as shown in the table.

[26] For this manor and family, see Blomefield, *Norfolk*, VIII, 28–29.

[27] Some notes on the Charles family, and their interests in Croxton, are given at *VCH Cambs*, v, 37–38.

[28] Mayton Hall in Frettenham.

[29] 'In the sixth of that king [Edward I] it was found that Walter de Kam, a long time before his death, had enfeoffed William Charles of a messuage, 70 a. land, an acre and half of meadow, and 20s. rent per ann. in Fretenham and Maindenton, so that Thomas Charles and Joan his wife who were impleaded by John de Oketon and Alice his wife were amerced' (Blomefield, *Norfolk*, X, 418).

annually for the life of Alice. On the same date a similar claim was made against the prior of Warter, for a third part of the manor of Baggaby [Bottom], but no details of the settlement are recorded (*YF*, 1272–1300, pp. 87–88). In 1299 the corn in the common fields of Easthorpe belonging to the dowers of the ladies Alice of Octon and the relict of Sir Gilbert of Louth, knight, deceased (*defunctorum*), had been taken into custody (*Reg. Romeyn*, II, 323). This appears to show that Alice was dead in that year, but it is clear she was living many years later. In 1312 Nicholas son of Gilbert of Louth sold to Geoffrey of Cave, for 100m., the reversion of four tofts and 10 bv. land in Easthorpe near Londesborough, which Alice, widow of John of Octon, was holding in dower (*YF*, 1300–1314, no. 494), and in 1319 Marmaduke of Thwing enfeoffed William his son and heir with the manor of Octon, reserving the above-noted rent to Lady Alice de St-Maur (Octon deeds, no. 5). In 1321, Alice, late the wife of Ralph de St-Maur was named as the tenant of lands in Thingden, co. Northampton (*CalCl*, 1318–1323, p. 289). In 1343–44 John de St-Maur, possibly a descendant of Ralph and Alice, sold his interest in Mayton (Blomefield, *Norfolk*, X, 418).

In the survey of 1284–85 Marmaduke of Thwing is shown as the tenant of 1 k.f. comprising 12 ct. in Octon, i.e. the fee held in 1279 by John of Octon; though John of Octon is still named as one of the tenants of the 2 ct. in Octon held by serjeantry (*KI*, p. 57). Marmaduke of Thwing received a grant of free warren in 1292 in all the demesne lands of his manors of Thwing, *Lyum*,[30] Kilton, *Morsum*,[31] Thorp,[32] Holme in Holderness, Octon, Rotsea, and Lund, co. York (*CalCh*, 1257–1300, p. 428). He was named as lord of Octon and Swaythorpe in 1316 (*KI*, p. 311).

The location of *Holme* has been the subject of confusion. The gift of land in *Holmet* by William earl of Aumale to Robert of Octon in the mid-twelfth century, known only from an abbreviated abstract made in the late sixteenth century, is noted above. This has been identified as Holmpton (Dalton, *Yorkshire*, p. 153n, citing English, 'Counts of Aumale', App. A, no. 11). If *Holmet'* were an accurate rendition of the original deed Holmpton would seem the most likely location, but as no subsequent interest of the Octon or Thwing families can be traced there, the reading is doubtful.[33] John of Octon, son and heir of John of Octon, knight (*militis*), confirmed 2 bv. in Octon, and turbary in *Holem* to Nunkeeling, of the gift of his late father (MS Dods. 7, f. 256v). In 1274 × 1284[34] John of Octon son and heir of Sir John of Octon, formerly justice (*iusticiarii*) of the king, confirmed this gift, which had been made by his grandfather, and confirmed by his father, describing the turbary as lying in '*Holme in parochia de Leven*' (ibid., f. 258v).[35] The grant of free warren to John of Octon of 1260 included his demesne lands in Holme. The manor was called 'Holme in Holderness' when Marmaduke of Thwing had his grant of free warren in 1292, and also at the inquisition following the death of Marmaduke of Thwing in 1323 where it was stated to be held of Beverley Minster for 13s. 4d. annually (*CalInqPM*, VI, no. 407). The Beverley Chapter Act book notes the acknowledgment made in 1309 by Sir Marmaduke of

---

30  'perhaps this is Upleatham' (*KI*, p. 125n).
31  Great Moorsholm (ibid.).
32  Kilton Thorpe (ibid., p. 132n).
33  For Holmpton, see Poulson, *Holderness*, II, 388–92; *VCH Yorks ER*, V, 47–54.
34  The date is after the death of John of Octon the justice, and before the death in 1284 of Sir Marmaduke of Thwing, who attests with his brother Sir Richard of Thwing (FN).
35  Also at Burton transcripts 3, f. 54r, p. 81, B7 N37. Burton identified the place as 'Holme in Holderness, near Pagula, alias Paul-Holme', despite noting that Holme is described as being in the parish of Leven (*Monasticon Eboracense*, p. 386).

Thwing that he held his capital manor of Holme 'in the parish of Leven' of the chapter for 1*m.* annually (*Beverley Act Bk,* I, 239).[36]

An inquisition held in 1328 as to whether there ought to be a ferry over the water of Hull from Godalehouses to Rotsea found that there had been a common ferry from time immemorial, which went by the way lying by the paths of Brandesburton to le Bergh, thence to Octonholme, thence to Godalehouses, over the water of Hull to Rotsea and thence to Hutton by Cranswick. It was maintained by the lord of Octonholme. William of Thwing and Isabel his mother, who held the manor of Octonholme, had taken away the ferry boat some months previously (Flower, *Public Works,* II, 308–9). When the manor was sold by the Lumley family in 1577, and on its subsequent sale in 1588, it was called 'Hempholme, otherwise Hemphowe, otherwise Octonholme' (*YFTP,* II, 109; ibid., III, 93; see also *VCH Yorks ER,* VII, 300). These references show that the manor of Holme was centred on the hamlet of Hempreeholme by the fourteenth century, though the provision of a chaplain to serve Hallytreeholme in the early thirteenth century suggests the manorhouse may then have been a mile to the north.

The superior interest of Godfrey of HARPHAM in the holdings of Henry son of Robert of Octon in Octon noticed in the Meaux chronicle has been mentioned above. But Godfrey is not named in the Fossard carta of 1166, and there is no evidence of a Harpham mesne tenancy in the 1 k.f. held by the Octon family and by their successors the Thwing family of Peter de Mauley in the thirteenth century. Apart from this difficulty, and the unexplained connection with a branch of the St-Quintin family, the descent of the Harpham family from the later twelfth century until the early years of the fourteenth century appears straightforward. Walter *de Harpenna,* who rendered account in Yorkshire and Northumberland for £11 6s. 8d. for 12 ct. of land in 1130 (*PR,* 31 Hen. I, p. 25) may have been an ancestor of the family. Godfrey of Harpham was amerced for forest trespass in 1175–76 (*PR,* 22 Hen. II, p. 117). He gave a rent of 12*d.* annually, from an unspecified location, to Thornton Abbey (Lincs.) which was included in the general confirmation of Richard I in 1190 (*EYC,* III, no. 1312). He witnessed a deed of William earl of Aumale made before August 1179[37] (*EYC,* III, no. 1405), and with John of Harpham attested a deed of Anselm de Stuteville in 1172 × 1199 (*EYC,* IX, no. 64). Godfrey of Harpham witnessed deeds of Robert Talun in the second half of the twelfth century, once with his brother Adam of Harpham (*Ctl. Bridlington,* pp. 165–66). He attested the gift of John son of John, vintner, of Beverley, to Rievaulx, made *c.*1167 × 1189[38] (*Ctl. Rievaulx,* no. 135). With his son John, Godfrey witnessed a deed of William Ingram to Lady Alice de Stuteville, sister of Anselm de Stuteville, presumably after Anselm's death in 1194 × 1199[39] (*Ctl. Gisborough,* II, 283n). John of Harpham confirmed to the nuns of Wykeham the gifts of land and pasture in the field of Octon made by Godfrey his father, as his father's deed specified (MS Dods. 7, f. 295[r]). Godfrey of Harpham's benefactions to Wykeham

---

[36]  The Octon family held of both Aumale and Beverley Minster in par. Leven. Hallytreeholme was held of Aumale, as is shown by the confirmation to Bridlington by William de Forz of John of Octon's gift there, noted above. It is unclear whether Beverley Minster held Hempholme by gift of Aumale, or as appurtenant to their manor of Leven, held by the archbishop in 1086.

[37]  When the earl died (*CP,* I, 353).

[38]  Included in the general confirmation of Richard I dated 17 September 1189. It is also included in the fabricated amplification of Henry II's general confirmation, apparently from 1155 × 1157, but not in the original version of this charter or Pope Alexander's confirmations of 1160 and 1167 × 1169 (*Ctl. Rievaulx,* nos 172, 197, 212, 250, 252).

[39]  For Anselm de Stuteville, see *EYC,* IX, 28–29.

# HARPHAM

WALTER DE HARPENNA,
occs 1130

| GODFREY OF HARPHAM, occs *temp.* Henry II and Richard, retired to Meaux by 1201 | ADAM OF HARPHAM | Two unnamed nuns of Wykeham |

| JOHN OF HARPHAM I, succ. by 1201, dead in 1206 | = | SYBIL, accused of death of her husband in 1206, a fugitive in 1208 | Unnamed nun of Wykeham |

JOHN OF HARPHAM II,   =   GUNDREDA,
succ. by 1208, dead          living 1246
in 1226

ANSELM OF HARPHAM,
occs 1237–72, dead in 1281

WILLIAM OF HARPHAM,
succ. by 1281, occs 1310

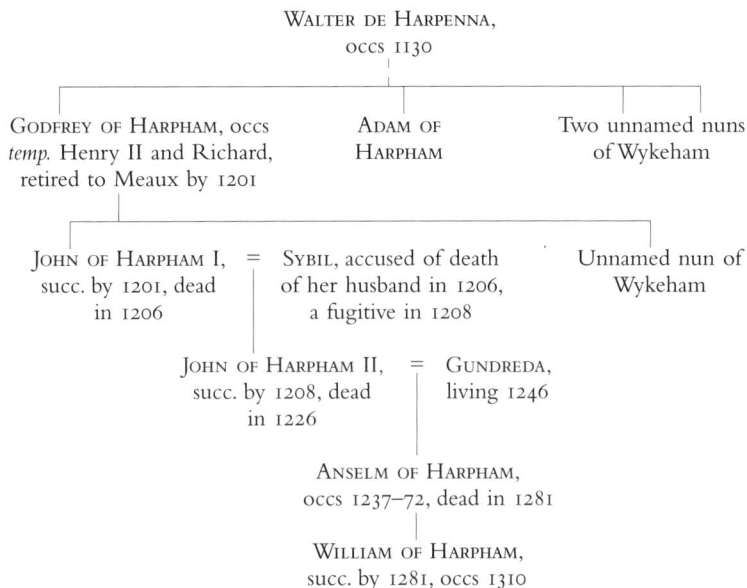

were mentioned in a deed of William of Octon, and included land he had given with his daughter, and with two of his sisters (Burton transcripts 1, f. 167ᵛ, p. 282, B14 N44, cited *Monasticon Eboracense*, p. 256; cf. *EYC*, 11, no. 1070). The Meaux chronicle states that service for 2 ct. of the 2½ ct. in Octon which the monks acquired from Henry son of Robert of Octon in the time of Abbot Adam (1151–1160) was owed to Godfrey of Harpham, who later confirmed the gift, and gave another 1 ct. in Octon. The monks were to do the forinsec service for ten years and pay 8s. annually, which rent was released to them in the time of Abbot Richard (1221–1235). The chronicle claims that Godfrey later became a novice at Meaux, and quitclaimed the land on which its grange was built (*Chron. Meaux*, 1, 102–3; *EYC*, 11, no. 1064). In the time of Abbot Alexander (1197–1210), when Godfrey of Harpham was dead, his son John received the fraternity of the abbey, and gave all the movable goods which pertained to his part, and confirmed everything the monks held of his fee. But after John's death his son John could not carry out the gift, and a long dispute followed, which was resolved in the time of Abbot Richard (*Chron. Meaux*, 1, 321, 429–30), doubtless by the final concord of 1222 between Richard, abbot of Meaux and John 'of Barpham', whereby John quitclaimed 3 ct. in Octon to the abbey and was thereby received into the benefactions and prayers of the church (*YF*, 1218–1231, p. 46).

In 1201 there was a case in the king's court concerning two bonds John of Harpham had made to Jewish moneylenders, one for £60 and the other for £30 (*CRR*, 1, 389–91). In 1203 William de Rochesford rendered account of £100 and two palfreys for licence to agree with John of Harpham concerning a breach of the peace, and John of Harpham separately accounted for an amercement of 3m. (*PR*, 5 John, pp. 213, 217). The first John of Harpham was dead in Michaelmas term, 1206, when a summons was issued concerning his death (*CRR*, 1205–1206, p. 267). His goods and chattels were seized in that year until Sybil his widow, and the men of his daughter[40] belonging to Harpham made fine for 60m. for the debt owing by those men to the Crown (PR, 8 John, p. 208; RFine, p. 351). In September 1206 Sybil, who had been wife of John of Harpham, made a fine with John son of John [of Harpham] concerning her dower, whereby she released her claim in 1 ct. in Ruston Parva (Rouston) in exchange for ½ ct. in Rolston (Rolinstun),[41] and all the land in Thwing which John, husband of Sybil, used to hold there, to be held of John son of John (PF John, p. 107). In 1208 John of Harpham accounted for 50m. for having his mother's dower, she having fled after being accused of the death of John of Harpham, formerly her husband (RFine, p. 423).[42]

It was presumably the younger John whose homage and service for a tenement in Harpham was included in an undated deed of Agnes, daughter of Sir Roger de Stuteville, giving to her son Alexander de St-Quintin all her lands in Harpham, Burton Agnes, Thornholme and Gransmoor (both par. Burton Agnes), and other property, with reversion to William and Anselm de St-Quintin, brothers of Alexander, and their heirs respectively (HHC: U DDSQ/12/1[a]).[43] John son of John of Harpham was named as the tenant of William de Muletorp[44] in the 2 ct. in Octon held by serjeanty in 1226 × 1228 (Bk of Fees, p. 357), but early in 1226 he was dead, when Gundreda his widow claimed as dower the third parts of 2 bv. in Ruston Parva (Rouston), a toft in Thwing, and a number of rents in the same place, from several defendants (CRR, 1225–1226, nos 1970, 2635).[45] The abbot of Meaux did not immediately hear of his death, as he made Thomas Burri his attorney in a plea against John of Harpham early in 1228. The case remained without day as John had died (ibid., 1227–1230, nos 399, 480). Gundreda of Harpham was living in 1246, when she called to warrant Walter of Pickering and Agnes his wife concerning 3 bv. and a third part of 1 bv. in Rolston (YF, 1232–1246, p. 159).[46]

The grant by John son of John of Harpham to Bridlington Priory of a moiety of the church of All Saints of Thwing can therefore be dated 1206 × 1226. The descent from John son of John is shown by subsequent deeds of confirmation. In 1239 × 1254[47] Anselm of Harpham, son of John of the same, issued a quitclaim in the moiety of the church of Thwing given by his father, and in May 1302, after an unsuccessful action to recover the advowson, William son and heir of Sir Anselm of Harpham, son and heir of Sir John of the same, issued a similiar quitclaim (Ctl. Bridlington,

---

[40]  'Sibilla que fuit uxor Iohannis de Herpham et homines filie eius . . .' in RFine, and similarly in PR, 8 John, but 'homines filii eius' in PR, 9 John, p. 68.

[41]  There can be little doubt that this is the correct identification. The land was to be held for the service pertaining to it, where 48 ct. made a fee. This was the normal reckoning in Holderness. The form Rolinstun is unlikely for Ruston Parva or Ruston (NR). Gundreda of Harpham had an interest in Rolston in 1246. The Harpham family's interest in Rolston was possibly, like its interest in Harpham, an undertenancy of St-Quintin. Herbert de St-Quintin was named as lord of Rolston in 1316 (KI, p. 303; see also VCH Yorks ER, VII, 313).

[42]  These entries are somewhat difficult to interpret. It is hard to see how the elder John's 'daughter's men', could be holding in Harpham. Perhaps the entry in PR, 9 John (see n. 40 above) is accurate and corrects those made the previous year.

[43]  Papers of St Quintin family of Harpham and Scampston.

[44]  Mowthorpe, par. Terrington. William's interests in Octon and Mowthorpe were inherited by his daughter Sarah, wife of Anketin Mallory (Bk of Fees, p. 1354; VCH Yorks NR, II, 204).

[45]  Gundreda was a name used by the descendants of Roger de Stuteville, including a daughter and a granddaughter. The granddaughter was a sister of Alexander de St-Quintin of Harpham, mentioned as domina Gundreda in his will of 1257, who may perhaps have been the wife of John of Harpham (EYC, IX, 33–34; Brown, 'Harpham Wills', p. 71).

[46]  William of Pickering was named as a tenant in Rolston in a feodary of 'the latter part of the reign of Henry III' (KI, p. 371).

[47]  Witnessed by Henry, vicar of Scalby, who held the vicarage during this period (Fasti Parochiales, III, 74).

pp. 172–73; MS Dods. 7, f. 264ᵛ). Anselm of Harpham may have been underage at his father's death, as his first dated occurrence is in 1237. In that year Hugh de Capella and Joan his wife claimed from Anselm son of John of Harpham the custody of the land of Geoffrey of Carthorpe in Carthorpe, as the right of Joan, of whom Geoffrey had held his land by knight service (*YF*, 1232–1246, p. 47). In 1242–43 it was said that Anselm of Harpham's holdings of Brus comprised ½ k.f., less 1 ct., in Foxholes, and 3 ct., apparently in Harpham, where 8 ct. made a fee (*Bk of Fees*, p. 1098). In the same period Anselm was impleaded by Alexander de St-Quintin for an undefined trespass, and himself impleaded Thomas son of Augustin for breaking his mill and carrying off fish from his pond in Harpham (*CRR*, 1242–1243, nos 2366, 2493). Alexander de St-Quintin and Anselm of Harpham were amongst the recognitors in a case of 1250 (ibid., 1249–1250, no. 2002). In 1259 Robert of Everingham, who had received 1½ ct. in Foxholes from his father Robert of Everingham, agreed to acquit John of Langtoft, clerk, to whom he had given the land, of the scutage due to Anselm of Harpham (*YF*, 1246–1272, p. 110). Anselm of Harpham was appointed in February 1260 with John of Octon and two others to inquire into the persons who came armed to the castle of Scarborough, and into trespasses against Gilbert de Gant, the king's constable of that castle (*CalPat*, 1258–1266, p. 65). After the battle of Evesham in 1265 and the restoration of royal government his land was seized into the hand of Sir Peter de Brus, as he had been with the rebel Sir John de Eyville with horses and arms at Richmond, and at the burning of Raskelf and *Wervelton*.[48] His land was assessed at 20m. annual value, comprising 15m. in Harpham, held of William de St-Quintin, and 5m. in Thwing, held of Sir Peter de Brus (*CalInqMisc*, 1219–1307, pp. 186–87, 286). Anselm of Harpham was a party to fines in Thwing in 1268 (*YF*, 1246–1272, pp. 149–50) and was apparently living in 1272, when his holdings of [?] 1 ct. 2 bv. in Harpham, and 3½ ct. [in Thwing ?] were listed in the inquisition following the death of Peter de Brus III (*CalInqPM*, I, no. 800; *YI*, I, 139).[49]

William of Harpham had succeeded his father Anselm by 1281, when ½ k.f. held by him was assigned to the share of Margaret de Ros, one of the coheirs of Peter de Brus III (*CalCl*, 1279–1288, p. 106). In 1284–85 Robert de Acklam[50] held 2 ct. in Foxholes of William of Harpham, who held of the Lady [Percy] of Kildale [who held of Brus] who held of the king. A further 1½ ct. in Foxholes was held by Robert le Despenser of William of Harpham. In Thwing William son of Anselm of Harpham held 3 ct. 2 bv. of Brus, who held of the king (*KI*, pp. 53, 56).

A series of deeds of the late thirteenth and early fourteenth centuries show that William of Harpham was then assigning property to members of the St-Quintin family, but the deeds give no indication of any relationship. On 28 April 1297 Herbert de St-Quintin gave to his kinsman Sir William de St-Quintin a messuage and 4 bv.

---

[48] For the rebel John de Eyville, see *ODNB*, s.n. Deyville and De Ville, 'John Deyville', passim. Eyville was ordered by the short-lived Montfort government to take the castle of Richmond from Guichard de Charrun in April 1265 (*CloseR*, 1264–1268, pp. 101–02, 113). *Wervelton* is probably Whorlton (NR), a castle held by the Meynell family.

[49] The two printed calendars vary somewhat: the original is very faded and mutilated.

[50] Robert was apparently son and heir of Nicholas de Acklam, who had a writ of consanguinity concerning 4 bv. in Ganton in April 1249 (*CalFine Hen. III*, 33/164). Robert son of Nicholas de Acklam and Richard of Thwing had a grant of free warren in Newton [Mulgrave] in Whitby Strand in 1261 (*CalCh*, 1257–1300, p. 37). Robert de Acklam held 4 ct. land in Newton [Mulgrave] by knight's service, of Mauley, in 1279. Ralph of Thwing and Robert de Acklam were joint undertenants in Newton Mulgrave in 1284–85, as were Richard of Thwing and Robert de Acklam in 1302–3 (*VCH Yorks NR*, II, 396; *YI*, I, 193). Sir Robert de Acklam was a witness in 1310 and 1311 (*Ctl. Whitby*, p. 391n), and was named as lord of Foxholes and joint lord of Ganton in 1316 (*KI*, p. 312).

in Harpham which he had from William son of Anselm of Harpham, which William held of Sir William (HHC: U DDSQ/12/1[g]); and on 8 June 1297 William son of Sir Anselm of Harpham gave to Sir William de St-Quintin a capital messuage in Harpham, except the third part which Maud of Routh (*Ruda*)[51] had in dower, with other property in Harpham (HHC: U DDSQ/5/1). But not all the Harpham land went to the St-Quintins. In 1308 William son of Sir Anselm of Harpham, knight, gave to Sir Anselm the chaplain of the same all his land in *le Morecroft* (Collier, 'Scampston Docs', p. 32); and in 1310 he granted to William son of Mauger de Erghum and Eustacia his wife the homage and service of Sir Robert de Acklam, knight, due from Robert's tenement in Foxholes, which Acklam had been accustomed to do for the grantor and his predecessors (MS Dods. 7, ff. 228ᵛ–229ʳ).

In 1447, William son of Anthony de St-Quintin, lord of Harpham, showed some confusion when he confirmed a quitclaim of William son of Sir Anselm of Harpham in 1¾ bv. in Harpham to St Mary's Abbey, calling the grantor 'William son of Sir Anselm de St-Quintin, formerly lord of Harpham, my predecessor (*antecessor meus*)' (MS Dods. 7, f. 228ʳ⁻ᵛ). But Sir Anselm of Harpham was not the same person as Anselm de St-Quintin, who was a son of Herbert de St-Quintin and Agnes his wife (*EYC*, IX, 32).[52]

**R630.** Confirmation to the hospital, by William son of Robert of Octon, of his father's gift of 1 bv. in Octon with a toft. Also gift of 2 a. in the same vill [*c.*1175 × 1194]

COPIES: *b* Rawl., f. 219ʳ; *c* MS Dods. 7, f. 274ᵛ; *d* Burton transcripts 2, f. 84ᵛ, p. 135, B17 N32, differences as noted with further minor variations of spelling. PRINTED: *EYC*, II, no. 1066, from *b*, where dated *c.*1175 × 1185.

**[f. 219ʳ]** *Carta Willelmi de Ochetun de una bovata cum uno tofto et ii. acris terre in eadem villa.*[53]
Universis filiis sancte matris ecclesie Willelmus filius Rodberti de Ochetuna salutem. Notum sit vobis me concessisse et dedisse et presenti carta confirmasse deo et pauperibus hospitalis sancti Petri Ebor'[54] unam bovatam terre in Ocheton' cum tofto, quam scilicet bovatam pater meus prius eis dederat cum plenaria communione ad omnia aisiamenta que ad eandem villam pertinent. Et preterea dedi eis in aumentum elemosine patris mei duas acras terre in eadem villa, unam iuxta Stodfalde conterminam terre fratrum de Meusle ad occidentalem partem vie, alteram in Padocdailes iuxta terram hospitalis Ierosolime. Hec predicta concessi et dedi eis in puram et perpetuam elemosinam, tenenda de me et heredibus meis libere et quiete ab omni seculari servicio preter orationes pauperum. Ego autem et heredes mei hanc elemosinam eis contra omnes homines warentizabimus. Hiis testibus, Radulfo presbitero, Turstino clerico, Willelmo filio Thome, Martino Malherba, Nicholao de Buggetorpe, Hugone fratre eius, Alexandro Rudibac, Godefrido de Ochet(on).

William son of Robert of Octon was dead in 1194 (FN). Although Ralph the priest

51  She was presumably the widow of Sir Anselm of Harpham.
52  For the descent from Sir Anselm de St-Quintin, see Clay, *Dugdale's Visitation*, III, 185.
53  *c* has rubric *Carta Willelmi filii Rodberti de Ochetunia.*
54  *c: Ebor'* omitted.

and Martin Mala Herba attested hospital deeds before *c.*1171 (R452, R683), the presence of Nicholas of Bugthorpe and Hugh his brother suggests a date after *c.*1180.[55]

**R631.** Confirmation to the hospital by William son of Robert of Octon of 1 bv. in Octon with a toft, which his father gave previously. Also gift of 5 a. in addition [*c.*1175 × 1194]

COPIES: *b* Rawl., f. 219ʳ; *c* Burton transcripts 2, f. 84ᵛ, p. 135, B17 N31. PRINTED: *EYC*, II, no. 1067, from *b*, where dated *c.*1175 × 1185.

*Willelmus filius Roberti de Oketon' de una bovata et v. acris terre in Oketon'.*
Universis sancte matris ecclesie filiis, Willelmus filius Rodberti de Ochetona[56] salutem. Notum sit vobis me concessisse et dedisse et presenti carta confirmasse deo et pauperibus hospitalis sancti Petri Ebor' unam bovatam terre in Ochet' cum tofto, quam scilicet bovatam pater meus prius eis dederat cum plenaria communione ad omnia aisiamenta que ad eandem villam pertinent. Et preterea dedi eis in augmentum elemosine patris mei quinque acras terre in eadem villa, duas acras et dimidiam in Padocdeiles iuxta terram hospitalis Ierosol' et unam acram et dimidiam super buttas et unam iuxta Stodfalde conterminam terre fratrum de Meus ad occidentalem partem vie. Hec predicta concessi et dedi eis in puram et perpetuam elemosinam, tenenda de me et heredibus meis libere et quiete ab omni seculari servicio preter orationes pauperum. Ego autem et heredes mei hanc elemosinam eis contra omnes homines warentizabimus. Hiis testibus, Rogerio presbitero, Simone presbitero, Willelmo presbitero,[57] Adam clerico de Cliveland', Rogerio Pictavensi, Gaufrido clerico, Martino Malaherba, Everardo clerico, Willelmo clerico,[58] Uctredo Malherba, Ricardo clerico de Neut' et Waltero filio eius, Henrico[59] de Burt', Randulfo de Ochet' et multis aliis.

A similar range of date to R630 is probable.

**R632.** Confirmation and quitclaim to the hospital by John son of William of Octon of 1 bv. in Octon, with a toft, which Robert, John's grandfather, had given before, and 5 a. land in the same vill, which William, John's father, had given. Also grant of Robert son of Fulk and his children [*c.*1182 × 1198]

COPIES: *b* Rawl., f. 219ʳ; *c* MS Dods. 7, f. 288ᵛ; *d* Burton transcripts 2, f. 80ʳ, p. 126, B12 N69, differences as noted, with further minor variations of spelling. NOTED: Drake, *Eboracum*, p. 334, via Torre's collections.

*Carta Iohannis de Ochetona de una bovata terre et v. acris et de quietum clam(atione) Roberti filii Fulconis et suorum.*[60]
Universis sancte matris ecclesie filiis, Iohannes filius Willelmi de Ochetona salutem. Notum sit vobis me concessisse et dedisse et presenti carta confirmasse deo et

---

[55] Details for Nicholas of Bugthorpe, whose widow was living in 1227 (R4) will be provided with the York deeds.
[56] *de Ochetona* omitted by Farrer, but present in Rawl. and Burton.
[57] *c: Rogero, Simone, Willelmo presbyteris.*
[58] *c: Everardo, Willelmo clericis.*
[59] *c: Heru'.*
[60] *c* has rubric *Carta Iohannis filii Willelmi de Ochetuna.*

pauperibus hospitalis sancti Petri Ebor'[61] unam bovatam terre in Ochet' cum tofto, quam scilicet bovatam Robertus avus meus prius eis dederat cum plenaria commun- ione ad omnia aisiamenta que ad eandem villam pertinent, et quinque acras terre in eadem villa quas Willelmus pater meus eis dederat et confirmaverat, duas acras et dimidiam in Padochedeiles iuxta terram hospitalis Ierosol' et unam acram et dimidiam super Buttas et unam iuxta Stodfalde conterminam terre fratrum[62] de Meaus ad occidentalem partem vie. Et preterea dedi eis in puram et perpetuam elemosinam Robertum filium Fulconis et omnes liberos eius et quietos clamavi imperpetuum de me et heredibus meis. Hanc vero elemosinam ego et heredes mei predictis pauperibus contra omnes homines warentizabimus ut simus participes orationum que in eadem domo fient imperpetuum. Hiis testibus, Willelmo de Ettona, Iohanne Arundell', Radulfo filio Radulfi, Thoma filio Radulfi de Chelingtorp', Henrico de Gaumet(on), fratre Hugone de Munchanesi, fratre Baldewino de Hudernessa, Willelmo filio Thome, Roberto capellano, Willelmo capellano, Iohanne capellano, Andrea capellano, Martino Malaherba, Galfrido clerico.

Martin Malaherba and Geoffrey the clerk (of the hospital), who witness R631 and R632, attested in c.1173 × 1177 (R153, R154) and c.1170 × c.1190 (R117, R432). William of Etton and Ralph son of Ralph witnessed Stuteville deeds in 1191 × 1194 and 1189 × 1192 (*EYC*, IX, nos 29, 71).[63] Ralph son of Ralph was probably the man of that name of the Grimthorpe family, which held in Etton. He was dead in 1198 (*EYC*, I, no. 449n). Thomas of Kellythorpe first becomes visible in 1182, and was apparently dead in 1198 (FN).

**R633.** Gift to the hospital by John son of William of Octon of a toft in Octon, being that which Reginald son of Godwin used to have. The gift was confirmed by John's brother W[illiam] [c.1180 × c.1215]

COPIES: *b* Rawl., f. 219ʳ; *c* MS Dods. 7, f. 127ᵛ; differences as noted with further minor variations of spelling.

*Iohannes filius Willelmi de uno tofto in Oketon'.*[64]
Sciant presentes et futuri litteras has visuri vel audituri quod ego Iohannes filius Willelmi de Ocketon' dedi deo et pauperibus hospitalis sancti Petri Ebor' toftum quoddam in Ocketon', illud scilicet quod Reginaldus filius Godwini aliquando habebat,[65] et ut prefati pauperes illud habeant in puram et perpetuam elemosinam solutam et liberam et quietam ab omni seculari servicio. Hanc vero donationem concessit frater meus W[illelmus] eisdem pauperibus et suo sigillo confirmavit. Hiis testibus, Iohanne capellano hospitalis, Willelmo filio Segerit,[66] Thoma filio Rankelli, W. fratre ipsius, Iohanne filio Suani, Iohanne filio Oseberti, W. Warewyk, Iohanne filio Lamberti et multis aliis.

---

[61]  *c, d: Eboraci.*
[62]  *d: firmam.*
[63]  In his account of the Etton family, Bilson mentions a deed by which Thomas son of Geoffrey of Etton gave William, son of his first wife, 1 bv. in Gilling, and places him as a younger brother to Thomas son of Thomas son of Geoffrey (Bilson, 'Gilling Castle', p. 109). But it would be unexpected to find a younger son of the Etton family leading the witness list, before Thomas of Kellythorpe who held 1 k.f. in Etton of Fossard (FN), so it is possible that some revision to Bilson's account is required.
[64]  *c* has rubric *Carta Iohannis filii Willelmi de Ocketun.*
[65]  *b: habebant.*
[66]  *b: Segeru'.*

John of Octon released to the monks of Meaux all disputes with them in May 1194, his brother William joining in the deed (FN).

**R634.** Gift to the hospital by John son of John of Harpham of all that toft and croft in Octon which is between the toft and croft of Robert Sot and the toft and croft of Gedefrid son of Horm, and also all that intake in Octon, which is between the intake of John of Octon and the boundary between Octon and Thwing [c.1206 × c.1220]

*Iohannes filius Iohannis de Harpham de terra in Oketon' et ovena.*
Sciant omnes presentes et futuri quod ego Iohannes filius Iohannis de Harpam dedi et concessi et hac presenti carta mea confirmavi, pro anima patris mei et animabus ante-cessorum et successorum meorum, totum illud toftum et croftum cum pertinenciis suis in villa de Oketon' quod iacet inter toftum et croftum Roberti Sot' ex una parte et toftum et croftum Gedefridi filii Horm ex alia parte, et preterea totum illud ofnam in territorio de Oketon', quod iacet inter ovenam Iohannis de Oketon' et divisam inter Oketon' et Theweng', deo et pauperibus hospitalis beati Petri Ebor', scilicet tenendum totum predictum tenementum cum pertinenciis cum communa et aisia-mentis predicte ville predictis pauperibus in puram et perpetuam elemosinam liberam et quietam ab omnibus **[f. 219ᵛ]** serviciis et auxiliis et exactionibus secularibus sicut ulla elemosina liberius dari potest, ita quod ego et heredes mei totam predictam donationem et concessionem predictis pauperibus warantizabimus adquietabimus et defendemus imperpetuum contra omnes homines. Hiis testibus, Willelmo persona de Neuton', Ricardo capellano de Oketon', Iohanne de Oketon', Gaufrido clerico de Theweng', Waltero de Wartre, Rogero fratre eius, Reginaldo de Wyverthorp', Ranulfo de Boitorp', fratre Roberto capellano, Thoma celerario, Girardo, Godefrido, Waltero et aliis fratribus predicti hospitalis, Willelmo, Petro, Lamberto et aliis capellanis suis, Thoma de Langwad', Willelmo de Notingham, Rogero de Derby cleric(is), Malgero marescaldo, Ingulfo, Waltero, servientibus et multis aliis.

The five brethren and three chaplains attesting were witnesses to a deed of c.1210 × 1217 (R490). Thomas de Langwath is usually described as master after c.1220. The donor succeeded his father in 1206 or shortly before, and was dead in 1226. The first witness may have been priest of Wold Newton, but the list of incumbents starts only at the end of the thirteenth century (*Fasti Parochiales*, III, 93–94).

**R635.** Conveyance by Christiana de Scardeburgh, in her widowhood, to Emma her daughter, of one messuage and 1 bv. of land in the vill and field of Octon, which John Tubbyng, Christiana the grantor, and Isabel the grantor's sister formerly had by gift of Ellen widow of Robert de Wincton, to be held of the master of the house of St Leonard, York, paying the master 2s. yearly by equal portions at Pentecost and St Martin in winter for all services. Warranty and sealing clauses. 11 November 1322.

*Cristiana de Scardeburgh' de uno mesuagio et una bovata terre in villa et campo de Octon'.*

Hiis testibus, Willelmo de Redenesse, Iohanne Wartre de Swathorp', magistro Iohanne Forte de Tweng', Thoma de Hunkelby de eadem, Roberto de Malton', Roberto Suart de Octon', Willelmo Squier clerico et aliis. Dat' apud Thweng' die sancti Martini in yeme anno domini millesimo CCCᵐᵒ vicesimo secundo.

**R636.** Conveyance by John Westiby of Thweng to Walter Adam of Neuton and Emma his wife of one messuage and 1 bv. of land in the vill and field of Octon, which the grantor had by gift of Emma Blake, to hold to Walter and Emma and the legitimate heirs of their bodies, of the master of the hospital of St Leonard, York, paying the master 2s. annually by equal portions at Pentecost and St Martin in winter for all service. Warranty. Remainder, if no legitimate heirs of the bodies of Walter and Emma, to William Blake of Scardeburgh and John his brother, and their heirs and assigns. Sealing clause. 12 January 1328[/29]

*Octon' pro hospitali sancti Leonardi de Ebor'.*

Hiis testibus, Marmeduco de Garton' de Thweng', Roberto atte Crose, Marmeduco de Hunkelby, Thoma de Hunkelby de eadem,[67] Iohanne de Wartre de Swathorp', Willelmo fratre eiusdem Iohannis et multis aliis. Dat' apud Octon' duodecimo die ianuarii anno domini millesimo trecentesimo vicesimo octavo.

**R637.** Bond to the hospital made by Henry de Rouceby, living in Octon, to pay the hospital 12d. annual rent for a toft and croft in Octon, which he bought from Alice of Hallytreeholme, which Alice held before of the hospital for the said annual rent. Also ½m. as an obituary payment [c.1274 × 1284, probably c.1276 × c.1280]

*Annuus redditus de Okton' xii.d.*
Sciant presentes et futuri quod ego Henricus de Rouceby manens in Oketon' obligavi me et heredes meos ac assignatos magistro et fratribus hospitalis sancti Petri Ebor' ac eorum successoribus in duodecim denar(iis) annui redditus pro quodam tofto et crofto in villa de Oketon', que emi de Alicia de Halytreholme et que eadem Alicia prius tenuit de predicto hospitali pro predicto annuo redditu duodecim denariorum, quod quidem toftum cum crofto iidem predicti magister et fratres antedicti hospitalis michi et heredibus meis pro predicto annuo redditu concesserunt imperpetuum, habend(um) et de eisdem tenend(um), solvend(o) eisdem annuatim ad duos terminos, scilicet sex denarios ad Pent' et sex denarios ad festum sancti Martini in yeme. Necnon et in dimidia marca argenti de me et heredibus meis ac assignatis aut a quocumque vel quibuscumque qui in dicto tenemento manserit vel manserint, quocienscumque contigerit aliquem nostrum vel eorum in eodem tenemento infatum decedere nomine testamenti pro portione catallorum nobis vel eis in obitu contingentium sine aliqua controversia percipienda, ita quod non liceat michi vel heredibus meis seu assignatis aut illis qui in dicto tenemento manebunt testamentum condere nec executoribus nostris vel suis aliquam administrationem de bonis nostris vel suis possidere donec predicto magistro et fratribus dicti hospitalis de predicto annuo redditu xii.d. et portione dimidie marce plenarie fuerit satisfactum. Nec liceat predictis magistro et fratribus aliquam exactionem aliam servitutem consuetudinem demandam sectam curiarum seu aliquam maiorem quantitatem **[f. 220ʳ]** pecunie quam predictum annuum redditum duodecim denariorum et dimidiam marcam t(antu)m pro portione de predicto tenemento aut de me predicto Henrico vel aliquo heredum meorum vel assignatorum aut a quocumque qui in dicto tenemento manserit exigere vel vendicare usque ad finem mundi. Et ut hoc presens scriptum robur imperpetuum optineat

---

[67] sic.

firmitatis tam sigillum dicti Henrici quam sigillum commune dicti hospitalis huic scripto ad modum cirographi confecto alternatim in testimonium sunt appensa. Hiis testibus, dominis Marmeduco de Thweng, Roberto et Marmaduco filiis eius, Ricardo de Tweng', Galfrido Agillyon', Iohanne de Oketon', militibus, Roberto de Ackelom', Willelmo Danyell', Iohanne de Crauncewyk', Nicholao de Crosseby, Willelmo de Beaumes et aliis.

Rouceby was named in 1284–85 as one of the tenants of the 2 ct. in Octon held by serjeantry (*KI*, p. 57). As all the attestations of Nicholas de Crosby which can be accurately dated belong to 1276–80 (FN), the sixth witness is probably Sir John of Octon IV, who succeeded in 1274–75 and was dead in 1284 (FN). The first witness is Marmaduke of THWING II, son of Robert of Thwing who was living in 1246. Marmaduke was first named in 1243, when he was under age. He was holding land in 1251, and received a grant of free warren in 1257. He was a royal knight banneret in 1260 and 1261, and died in 1284. Marmaduke's eldest son Robert died at about the same time, or slightly before, leaving an infant daughter Lucy, who inherited the estates of her grandmother Lucy de Brus, wife of Marmaduke of Thwing II. The heir to the Thwing estates was Marmaduke II's second son Marmaduke III (*CP*, XII (1), 737–40; *Ctl. Gisborough*, II, 100n–102n; *CRR*, 1243–1245, no. 752; Octon deeds, no. 13). The connection of Sir Richard of Thwing, who occurs in 1261–82 (Moor, *Knights*, s.n. Thwenge), to the main line of the family is shown by a deed of 1274 × 1284,[68] attested by Marmaduke [II] of Thwing and Richard of Thwing his brother, knights (MS Dods. 7, f. 258ᵛ).

[68] See p. 717, n. 34 above.

## *Overhemelsay*[1] [Upper Helmsley, NR]

## [Eastby, in Embsay, WR]

**R638.** Gift to the hospital by Walter son of Helto, of 3½ a. in Eastby comprising 2 a. in *Bouflat*, 1 a. in Hard Ings and above *Redingam* and the wide selion of *Stainbricge* which divides two carucates of land. Also gift of the ½ a. which Walter son of Golle gave to Henry Forte with his daughter, and the messuage belonging to the ½ a. [*c*.1200 × 1219]

[**f. 220ᵛ**] *Walterus filius Helte de Hemelsay de iii. acris et dimid(ia) in eadem villa que innovatur per aliam.*
Sciant qui sunt et qui venturi sunt quod ego Walterus filius Helte dedi et concessi et hac carta mea confirmavi deo et hospitali sancti Leonardi Ebor', in pura et perpetua elemosina pro anima patris mei et matris mee et antecessorum meorum et propria salute, tres acras terre et dimidiam acram terre in Estby, scilicet duas acras terre in Bouflat et unam acram terre in Hardenges et supra Redi(n)gam[2] et latum sultum[3] de Stainbricge qui dividit duas carrucatas terre. Preterea dedi eidem domui sancti Leonardi dimidiam acram terre quam Walterus filius Golle dedit Henrico Forte cum filia sua et mesuagium illius dimidie acre, tenend(a) libere et quiete et pacifice cum omnibus communibus aisiamentis ad prefatam pertinentibus terram. Hiis testibus, Willelmo de Mart(on'), Rog' Te(m)p(est'), Iohanne de Halt(on'), Hugone filio Iohannis, Willelmo filio Edwardi, Roberto le Maz.

The rubric's addition of *de Hemelsay* to the name of the donor doubtless follows an endorsement, and is presumably a mistake for one of the medieval spellings of Embsay. Walter son of Helto issued another deed to the same effect, with different witnesses, in *c*.1214 × *c*.1230 (M: Eastby [Burton transcripts 1, f. 180ʳ, p. 307, B11 N8]). This is presumably the additional deed referred to in the rubric, and as it is not included in the Rawlinson volume we must assume this information too was contained in an endorsement. John son of Walter son of Helto surrendered the vill of Eastby to his lord William de Forz, earl of Aumale, who subsequently confirmed it to Bolton Priory (*EYC*, vii, no. 42). William of Marton occurs in 1192, 1203, 1206 and 1212 (ibid., 234–35). Roger Tempest occurs in 1192 and 1209, and was probably dead by Michaelmas 1219 (ibid., 245). The last witness was doubtless Robert *le macun*, who attests deeds of the honour of Skipton of similar date (ibid., nos 143, 152, 153). He can probably be identified with Robert *cementario de Skipton* (ibid., nos 158, 175), and may have been an ancestor of Henry the mason, who held 2 ct. of the honour in 1287 (ibid., 283–84).

---

[1] *in Northryddyng'* has been added in the margin, by a hand possibly of the mid-fifteenth century which has made a similar annotation to the Stockton heading on f. 228ʳ.
[2] *Riding* in B11 N8.
[3] *selionem* in B11 N8.

# [Upper Helmsley, NR]

In addition to the present section of the cartulary, there was originally another entitled 'Helmsley', which occupied f. 191 in the East Riding division (R769–R772), and was removed after Dodsworth made his abstracts and the Contents List was compiled. However, the separation appears to have been an artificial one, as the hospital's holdings were, as far as can be ascertained, entirely in Upper Helmsley.

In 1086 Nigel [Fossard] held 4 ct. of the count of Mortain in *Hamelsech* (Upper Helmsley), and the archbishop held 4 ct. and 2 bv. in *alia Hamelsech* (Gate Helmsley), both places being in the Domesday wapentake of Bulmer. The archbishop's land later formed part of the prebend of Osbaldwick. In an extent of this prebend made in 1294, 32 bv. were said to be held in service in [Gate] Helmsley (*YMF*, II, 64; Bishop, 'Prebends', p. 10). The returns of 1284–85 for Bulmer, in the North Riding, are very incomplete, and include no mention of either Helmsley, but the returns for Ouse and Derwent wapentake in the East Riding include 6 bv. in *Hemelsay* held by Walter de Hemelsay of the heirs of Chamberlain of North Duffield, of the heirs of Percy, of the king (*KI*, pp. 60, 109). Bulmer is not included in the feodary of 1302–03, and neither Helmsley is listed in the wapentake of Bulmer in the *Nomina Villarum* of 1316, though John of Helmsley is named as lord of Helmsley in Ouse and Derwent wapentake (ibid., p. 319). In 1316 an inquisition was taken concerning those who held of the king in Bulmer in 1300 and 1303, which says that Ranulf de Neville held *Over Hemylsey* of Peter de Mauley (to whom the Fossard fee had passed), and he of the king. Gate Helmsley is not mentioned (ibid., p. 379).

The deed by which Nigel d'Aubigny, repenting his sins and preparing for death, restored 2 ct. in [Upper] Helmsley to the sustenance of the 'poor brethren near that church' (i.e. York Minster) in 1109 × 1114 (R769 and n), provides the earliest evidence for the hospital's existence and its territorial possessions. There is no indication as to how the hospital initially acquired the land. It seems most likely that it was originally given, with the church, by Nigel Fossard, who was named as the tenant of [Upper] Helmsley in 1086. He made a grant of this type in favour of Ramsey Abbey in the late eleventh century, which included the church of Bramham, land for two ploughs, and various tithes. Similarly St Mary's, York, in '*c.*1100 × *c.*1115', received from him the churches of Doncaster and St Crux in York, with other property (*EYC*, II, nos 1001–02). The difficulties which Nigel Fossard's son Robert appears to have had in gaining seisin of his lands in 1130 and before[4] may have encouraged the hospital to prefer to remember Nigel d'Aubigny as their benefactor. The papal confirmation of 1148 notes the grant of 2 ct. and the church of [Upper] Helmsley but does not name the grantor (C178 [*EYC*, I, no. 179]). Those of 1157 and 1173 say the grant was made by Nigel d'Aubigny (C179–C180 [*EYC*, I, nos 186, 197]). The gift of 2 ct. made by Nigel d'Aubigny, with other doubtful benefactions, is included in a supposed confirmation of Henry I, which was probably drawn up early in the reign of Henry II (R1). A confirmation by Henry II, issued in 1155 × 1170, included '2 ct. in Helmsley, and the church of the same vill' (C10 [*EYC*, I, no. 175]).[5] Ralph son of Wimund gave the *mansio* of the priest in Helmsley in *c.*1150 × 1177 (R770).

---

4  For the few details available, see *EYC*, II, 326–27.

5  Page's statement that Roger de Mowbray was identified as the grantor of the church of [Upper] Helmsley in this confirmation is unsafe, as it depends on a particular interpretation of the punctuation (*VCH Yorks NR*, II, 143).

By the early thirteenth century the hospital's 2 ct. were held by Roger Gernun and
Maud his wife at fee-farm of the hospital, and in 1214 × c.1220 Hugh, rector of the
hospital, confirmed the land to William son of Roger Gernun (R771–R772). In 1214
× 1234 William son of R[oger] Gernon, at the urging of his mother Maud, confirmed
the intakes of the 2 ct. to his brother Paulinus (R640). It was perhaps this land, now
specified as a toft with 2 bv., which Walter son of Paulinus son of Maud Gernun
conveyed to Michael de Burton, formerly chaplain of the hospital, who gave it to
the hospital in c.1260 × c.1290 (R641). William son of Thomas Gernun gave 'Michael
of the hospital' a selion in Upper Helmsley in c.1240 × c.1275 (R639). Neither the
extents of the later thirteenth century nor the *Valor Ecclesiasticus* make reference to
the hospital's land in Helmsley. It is questionable whether the hospital retained the
church of Helmsley, as it does not appear amongst its possessions after the twelfth
century. A rent in Helmsley, formerly belonging to the hospital, was mentioned in
1542 (*Dissolved Houses*, IV, 226). Further details of the manor of Upper Helmsley are
included in the account of the parish in *VCH Yorks NR*, II, 141–43.

**R639.** Gift to Michael of the hospital of York by William son of Thomas Gernun of
Helmsley, of a selion of land in the field of Upper Helmsley, in The Braces,
paying the grantor ½d. annually at Helmsley [c.1240 × c.1275]

*Willelmus Gernun de una selione iacente in The Braces contin(enti) i. acra et dimid(ia).*
Sciant omnes presentes et futuri quod ego Willelmus filius Thome Gernun de Hemelesheia concessi dedi et hac presenti carta mea confirmavi Michaeli de hospitali Ebor'
unam selionem terre in campo de superiori Hemelesheia iacentem in The Braces,
habendam et tenendam eidem Michaeli et quibusdam assignatis suis vel cuicumque
dare vendere vel assignare voluerit libere integre et quiete, reddendo inde annuatim
michi et heredibus meis pro omni servicio exactione consuetudine et secta curie
unum obulum die Pent' vel infra septimanam Pent' apud Hemelesh' per se vel per
attorn(atum) suum. Ego autem et heredes mei predictam selionem terre predicto
Michaeli et assignatis suis warantizabimus adquietabimus et defendemus in omnibus et
contra omnes homines imperpetuum. In huius rei robur et testimonium huic scripto
sigillum meum apposui. Hiis testibus, Willelmo de Kelingthorp, Willelmo Toroldby,
Stephano de Shuptona, Ricardo filio Radulfi, Stephano de Hundemanby, Benedicto
de Hewrth', Thoma filio Roberti de eadem, Waltero Bret, Roberto Gernun, Waltero
Lesquier, Roberto de Wilberfosse, Henrico Gernun et aliis.

Michael 'of the hospital' can probably be identified with Michael de Burton, who as a
former chaplain of the hospital gave it land in Helmsley (R641). He witnessed deeds
from c.1230, and in c.1260 × c.1280 appeared in deeds apparently acting as a trustee
for the hospital (FN). Benedict of Heworth witnessed several Heslington deeds in
c.1250 × c.1265 (R516, R526, R534, R540).

**R640.** Confirmation by William Gernun of Upper Helmsley, at the petition of his
mother Maud, to his brother Paulinus, of all intakes in the field of Upper
Helmsley, which belong to 2 ct. land, which R[oger] Gernun, the grantor's
father, held of the hospital by hereditary right, and which Maud the grantor's
mother, in widowhood, gave to Paulinus her son for his homage and service;
also the toft which belonged to Ingulf; paying the grantor 12d. annually [1214
× 1234]

*Confirmatio de Overhemelsay.*

Universis hoc presens scriptum audientibus et videntibus Willelmus Gernun de Huverhemelsai, salutem eternam in domino. Noverit universitas vestra me consilio et petitione Matildis matris mee concessisse et hac presenti carta mea confirmasse Paulino fratri meo omnes ofnames in campo de Hoverhemelsay, quas dicta Matildis mater mea in sua libera viduitate dedit dicto Paulino filio suo in dicto campo, pro homagio et servicio suo, q(ue) pertinent ad duas carrucatas terre quas pater meus R[ogeru]s Gernun tenuit in dicta villa de hospitali sancti Leonardi de Ebor' et de fratribus ibidem deo servientibus iure hereditario, tenendas et habendas cum omnibus libertatibus et aisiamentis ad predictam villam pertinentibus in omnibus locis sine aliqua diminutione, et cum tofto quod fuit Iggolf, libere honorifice pacifice et quiete, illi et heredibus suis de me et heredibus meis in feudo et hereditate, reddendo annuatim dicto Willelmo Gernun et heredibus suis duodecim denarios argenti, scilicet vi. denarios ad Pent' et vi.d. ad festum sancti Martini in yeme, pro omnibus actionibus et consuetudinibus et omnibus demandis ad prefatum Willelmum et ad heredes suos pertinentibus. Scilicet tres acras iuxta Grengat que vocatur Croft, et dimidiam acram ad stocis Osberti versus occidentem, et ad Toflandes iiii$^{or}$ acras et dimidiam, et ad Forinsec' stoc(is) iuxta boscum versus occidentem duas acras, et ad stocis propinquior Netherhemelsai tres acras, et ad Prestestocis tres acras, et ad Gateland' tres percatas, et ad Sunnmeland' dimidiam acram, et duas gaires ad Meirebal', et duas ad Uhol riding', et unam ad Stainbrig'. Et ut ista carta rata et sine dolo permaneat uterque Matild(is) et Willelmus Gernun hoc scriptum sigillis suis corroboraverunt. Hiis testibus, Rainero persona de Hemels', Ranulfo de Wilberfosse, Illgero[6] de Hemels', Waltero suo filio, Willelmo de Waritil, Roberto Guer,[7] Hugone de Aubur', Odone de Rupe, Waltero filio Ricardi de Butare et multis aliis.

In 1214 × *c*.1220 rector Hugh confirmed to William Gernun the 2 ct. in Helmsley, previously held by William's father Roger and Maud his wife (R771). Rainer, or Reginald, parson of [Upper] Helmsley, who attested a deed in the first quarter of the thirteenth century (C344 [Cott., f. 66$^v$]), was a predecessor of Ralph, who occurs in 1234 (C103 [Cott., f. 15$^r$]). Ilger of Helmsley and Robert Guer attested Naburn deeds of *c*.1210 × *c*.1230 (R627–R628).

**R641.** Gift and quitclaim to the hospital by Michael de Burton, formerly chaplain of the hospital, of a toft with 2 bv. land in Upper Helmsley, which 2 bv. he had by gift of Walter son of Paulinus son of Maud Gernun of Upper Helmsley. The toft lies between the toft of John Gernun and the toft which the donor gave to Walter son of Walter son of Ilger [*c*.1260 × *c*.1290]

*De uno tofto et duabus bovatis terre in Overhemelsay.*

Sciant presentes et futuri quod ego Michael de Burton', quondam capellanus hospitalis sancti Petri Ebor', dedi concessi quietum clamavi et hac carta mea presenti confirmavi deo magistro et fratribus et pauperibus hospitalis sancti Petri Ebor', unum toftum cum duabus bovatis terre in villa et in territorio Superioris Hemelsey, quas quidem duas bovatas terre habui ex concessione et donatione Walteri filii Paulini filii Matild(is) Gernun de predicta Hemelsey, et iacet predictum toftum inter toftum Iohannis Gernun et toftum quod dedi Waltero filio Walteri filii Ilgeri, tenend(a) et

---

[6]  MS: *Ill'g.*
[7]  MS: *Suer.*

habend(a) predictis magistro fratribus et pauperibus hospitalis antedicti et eorum successoribus universis, predictum toftum et duas bovatas terre antedictas, cum omnibus pertinenciis suis libertatibus et aisiamentis infra villam et extra, in liberam puram et perpetuam elemosinam sicut aliqua elemosina liberius et melius dari potest et haberi imperpetuum. Ego vero predictus Michael et heredes mei predictum toftum cum dictis duabus bovatis terre et cum omnibus pertinenciis suis libertatibus et aisiamentis pretitulat' magistro fratribus pauperibus predicti hospitalis et eorum successoribus universis contra omnes homines warantizabimus acquietabimus et defendemus imperpetuum. In cuius rei testimonium huic scripto [**f. 221ʳ**] sigillum meum apposui. Hiis testibus, Waltero de Emelsey, Willelmo de Killington', Iohanne Ramkille, Iohanne Gernun, Henrico Gernun, Stephano de Hounemanby, Thoma de Wilberfosse et aliis.

The date range is given by the likely period for Michael de Burton as 'former chaplain'. Walter son of Walter son of Ilger can probably be identified with Walter son of Walter of Helmsley, who with Henry Gernun attested a deed of 1267 × 1286 (R782).

# *Pons Belli anglice Staineford' brig'*
# [Stamford Bridge]

In 1086 William de Percy held the manor of Catton, assessed at 12 ct., which included Stamford Bridge, of Hugh earl of Chester. Clay suggested that Alan de Percy's grant of facilities at the mills of Stamford might indicate that the tenancy in chief had passed to Percy at an early date (*EYC*, II, 196; *EYC*, XI, 334). In the division of the Percy fee made in 1175 half of Stamford Bridge was assigned to the earl of Warwick, and half to Jocelin de Louvain (*EYC*, XI, no. 89).

Alan de Percy's grant of right to use his mills of Stamford Bridge in *c.*1130 × *c.*1136 (R642) is amongst the earliest of the hospital's deeds. The benefaction was confirmed on two occasions by William de Percy, Alan's son (R643, R784). A further confirmation by Richard de Percy [grandson of William de Percy] restricted the hospital's use of the mill to 200 quarters of grain annually (R644), and suggests some tension as to the previous level of use. The hospital made an agreement in 1204 × 1217 allowing Gilbert son of Geoffrey use of the barn, or house, in Stamford Bridge after the brethren had removed their corn each year until the autumn following (R647).

The use of the mill of Stamford Bridge free from multure, given by Alan de Percy and his son, together with a *mansura* in the vill, was included in the papal confirmations of 1148, 1157 and 1173 (C178–C180 [*EYC*, I, nos 179, 186, 197]). In the last quarter of the twelfth century, Ilger son of Ascur gave 3 a. in Stamford Bridge to the hospital, and on a different occasion another 4 a. (R645, R646). No mention was made of Stamford Bridge in the hospital's extents of the late thirteenth century, nor in the *Valor Ecclesiasticus*, but a rent there was included in the account of 1542 (*Dissolved Houses*, IV, 226).

**R642.** Grant to the hospital by Alan de Percy of right to mill all its corn without multure at his mills, which are at Stamford Bridge [*c.*1130 × 1136]

COPIES: *b* Rawl., f. 221ᵛ; *c* PRO, C53/80, Charter Roll, 22 Edw. I, m. 9 (royal inspeximus and confirmation of 16 June 1294); differences as noted, with further minor variations of spelling. PRINTED: *MA1*, II, 394, from *c*, abbreviated; *MA*, VI, 612, no. 14, from *MA1*; *EYC*, II, no. 908, from *b* and *c*, where dated *c.*1130 × 1135; ibid., XI, no. 7 (witnesses only), dated similarly. NOTED: *CalCh*, 1257–1300, p. 441, no. 13.

[f. 221ᵛ] *Alanus de Perceio de multura annone hospital(is) ad Pontem Belli.*
Alanus de Perceio omnibus hominibus suis et amicis et omnibus fidelibus cristi salutem. Sciatis quod concessi et dedi imperpetuum pauperibus hospitalis sancti Petri Ebor' molere totum bladum suum sine omni multura ad mea molendina que sunt ad Pontem Belli, pro salute anime mee et pro remissione peccatorum meorum et omnium antecessorum meorum, ut sim particeps[1] omnium beneficiorum que in illa sancta domo fiunt die ac nocte. Quare volo et firmiter precipio quatinus libere et quiete et sine omni impedimento et sine omni terreno lucro et premio statim molant cum venerint [statim][2] post annonam que super molendinum iam posita fuerit. Testibus, Roberto filio Fulconis et Iohanne Arundel et Bainardo dapifero et

---

[1]   *b, c*: sic, not *simus participes* as in *EYC*.
[2]   *c* only.

Galeberto[3] de Arches et Golleno[4] filio Odonis et Galtero de Perceio et Raven de Cattuna. Valete.

Alan de Percy's gift to the hospital of 2 bv. in Dalton (par. Topcliffe), with confirmation of a further 2 bv., is witnessed by Lefwin the priest, followed by the seven witnesses to the present deed, so was apparently made on the same occassion (M: Dalton [*EYC*, XI, no. 6]). It has generally been accepted that Alan de Percy, whose last dated occurrence is in 1130 (*PR*, 31 Hen. I, p. 25), was dead by the end of the reign of Henry I. King Stephen's general confirmation to Whitby Abbey, given at York apparently in February 1136,[5] includes the gifts of 'William de Percy, and Alan his son, and William son of Alan', and is attested by W[illiam] de Percy (*EYC*, II, no. 868; *Regesta*, III, no. 942). King Stephen's confirmation to Bridlington, also given at York and probably at the same time,[6] notes that 'Emma wife of Alan de Percy gave 1 ct. land, with the consent of her son William, in [Wold] Newton', as its last clause, suggesting that her gift was made immediately before the king's confirmation[7] (*EYC*, II, no. 1144; *Regesta*, III, no. 119). Although Wold Newton was part of Emma's maritagium (*EYC*, XI, no. 8n), it is unlikely her gift would have been recorded in such terms during her husband's lifetime. William de Percy was the last witness to one of the king's charters to Winchester given at Westminster at Easter 1136 (*Regesta*, III, no. 944). Thus it seems clear that Alan had at the very least resigned his fee in favour of his son by early in 1136, though Farrer's view was that 'Alan's death . . . can only with certainty be stated to have occurred before the summer of 1138', when his son William was, according to John of Hexham, amongst the leaders of the Yorkshire forces at the battle of the Standard (*EYC*, II, nos 970n, 1144n; John of Hexham, *Historia regum*, II, 294).

Alan's grant to the hospital of the use of the mills of Stamford Bridge, and his son William's confirmation of the grant made by his father *in vita sua* (R643), are in very similar terms. The first witness to William's deed is Gilbert the canon, who is followed by all seven witnesses to Alan's deed, ordered differently. This suggests that Alan's deed was drawn up very shortly before his death, and William's immediately thereafter.

**R643.** Confirmation to the hospital by William de Percy of his father Alan's grant (R642) [1130 × *c*.1136]

COPIES: *b* Rawl., f. 221[v]; *c* PRO, C53/80, Charter Roll, 22 Edw. I, m. 9 (royal inspeximus and confirmation of 16 June 1294); minor differences of spelling. PRINTED: *EYC*, II, no. 909, from *b* and *c*, where dated *c*.1130 × 1138. CALENDAR: *CalCh*, 1257–1300, p. 441, no. 14, from *c*. NOTED: *EYC*, XI, no. 7n.

*Willelmus de Perceio de Ponte Belli.*
Willelmus de Perceio omnibus hominibus suis et amicis salutem. Sciatis quod do et

---

3    *c: Gilberto.*

4    *c: Goseleno.*

5    So dated in *EYC* and *Regesta*. For the king's itinerary early in 1136 see *Regesta*, III, p. xl; *EYC*, II, 213–14. Of the five witnesses all except Percy attested the king's confirmation to Beverley Minster which is explicitly dated 1135[/36] (*EYC*, I, no. 99; *Regesta*, III, no. 99).

6    Dated 1135 × 1139 in *EYC* and *Regesta*. The three witnesses attested Stephen's charter to Beverley. However, the king may have been in York in February 1138, during which month he visited Northumberland and southern Scotland (*Regesta*, III, p. xl).

7    Or perhaps added in a later amplification. The absence of witnesses from William de Percy's confirmation of his mother's gift is also suggestive of falsification (*Ctl. Bridlington*, p. 72).

confirmo in perpetuam elemosinam pauperibus hospitalis sancti Petri Ebor' molere totum suum bladum sine omni multura ad mea molendina que sunt ad Pontem Belli, pro salute anime mee, et pro remissione peccatorum meorum et omnium antecessorum meorum, et ut sim particeps omnium beneficiorum que in illa sancta domo fiunt die ac nocte, ita libere et quiete quemadmodum pater meus Alanus eis in vita sua pro salute anime sue sine omni multura dederat, et ita ut sine impedimento statim post annonam que super molendinum iam posita fuerit cum venerint molant. Teste Gileberto canonico et Gileberto de Arches et Rotberto filio Fulconis et Raven de Cattun et Iohanne Arundel et Bainardo dapifero et Goeslino filio Odonis et Waltero de Perci. Valete.

**R644.** Grant to the hospital by Richard de Percy of right to mill 200 quarters of wheat annually, to the use of the hospital, without multure, at his mills at Stamford Bridge [1222 × 1234, possibly 1222 × 1229]

*Ricardus de Perci de CC. quarteriis bladi molendis apud Pontem Belli.*
Omnibus cristi fidelibus ad quos presens scriptum pervenerit Ricardus de Perci eternam in domino salutem. Noverit universitas vestra me caritatis et pietatis intuitu et pro salute anime mee et animarum antecessorum et successorum meorum, dedisse concessisse et presenti carta mea confirmasse deo et pauperibus hospitalis sancti Petri Ebor' molere annuatim ducentas quarteria bladi ad usus dictorum pauperum sine aliqua multura ad molendina mea que sunt ad Pontem Belli, in puram et perpetuam elemosinam, libere et quiete ab omni servicio et exactione preter orationes pauperum, ita ut sine omni occasione molant cum venerint post annonam que super molendina iam posita fuerit. Ego autem et heredes mei predictam elemosinam dictis pauperibus imperpetuum warantizabimus. In huius autem rei robur et testimonium huic scripto sigillum meum apposui. Hiis testibus, domino Iohanne abbate de Fontibus, domino Stephano abbate de Sellay, domino Roberto de Percy, domino Willelmo de Flayneburg' constabulario, Daniele Teutonico, magistro Osberto de Semar, Roberto de Schegnes, magistro Lamberto, Radulfo de Fontibus capellano, Radulfo de Gaitington'.

The grantor was Richard de Percy, son of Agnes de Percy and Jocelin de Louvain, who died 'at an advanced age' in 1241 × 1244 (*EYC*, XI, 7, 77; *CP*, X, 449–52). The extreme dates for Stephen [of Eston], abbot of Sallay, who occurs in 1225 and 1233, are 1219–1240.[8] But if we accept the brief account of his career in the President's book of Fountains, which states he was abbot of Sallay for ten years, and McNulty's proposition that he had been succeeded as cellarer of Fountains in 1223, the extreme dates for his tenure may be stated as 1222–1234 (McNulty, 'Stephen of Eston', passim; Clay, 'Early Abbots', pp. 40–41). The narrower range of date depends on the identification of the third witness as Robert de Percy II of the Bolton Percy family, who died in or before 1229 (*EYC*, XI, 108). This is probable, as the Bolton Percy family had an interest in Stamford Bridge (*EYC*, XI, 109; *KI*, p. 61).

---

[8] The earliest date for a deed witnessed by Abbot Richard, a predecessor of Stephen, is provided by another witness, Robert, prior of Bolton, who succeeded after February 1219 (*Ctl. Sallay*, no. 534n). The death of John de Lacy, earl of Lincoln, in July 1240 provides the latest date for a deed given by Abbot Walter, Stephen's successor (*Ctl. Sallay*, no. 208; *CP*, VII, 679). A deed of William, earl Warenne, who died in May 1240, attested by Abbot Walter, provides further evidence for Walter's succession in or before 1240 (*EYC*, VIII, 25, 235–36). Stephen occurs as abbot of Newminster in 1241.

**R645.** Gift to the hospital by Ilger son of Ascur of Stamford Bridge of 3 a. in the fields of Stamford Bridge [*c.*1175 × 1192]

PRINTED: *EYC*, II, no. 912, where dated 1170 × 1181.

*Ilgerus filius Asceri de iii. acris cum communi pastura in Pontem Belli.*
Notum sit omnibus videntibus et audientibus litteras istas quod ego Ilgerus filius Asceri de Ponte Belli et heredes mei concessimus et dedimus et hac presenti carta nostra confirmavimus deo et hospitalis pauperibus beati Petri Ebor' tres acras terre in campis de Ponte Belli, liberas et quietas et immunes ab omni humano servicio, in puram et perpetuam elemosinam, et communem pasturam eiusdem ville cum omnibus asiamentis ad eandem pertinentibus. Et contra omnes homines predictam elemosinam warentizabimus. Hanc vero elemosinam dedimus predictis pauperibus pro salute animarum nostrarum ut simus participes omnium beneficiorum que fiunt in illa sancta domo dei. Hiis testibus, Ranulfo clerico de Bringenhala, Pagano de Cattun, Gerardo de Sexdecim Vallibus, Gaufrido de sancto Petro, Iheremia et Ysaia fil(iis) Ilgeri de Cattun, Waltero de Cu(m)tona, Gervasio homine H., Henrico Pusaz, Radulfo de Labara, Suartgero de Ponte Belli, Rogero de Middeltun et multis aliis.

It is difficult to assign secure limits of date to this deed and the similar grant immediately following. Farrer's suggestion that the donor was possibly the Percy tenant Ilger son of Roer, Ascer being his mother's name, was not accepted by Clay (*EYC*, II, 251; ibid., XI, 225n). The first witness had an interest in Brignall church for a considerable period. In 1157 × 1183 William de Vescy granted the church of Brignall to Ranulf the clerk (C126 [*EYC*, V, no. 388]). In 1214 or later Ranulf the clerk of Brignall acknowledged the pension of 4s. he had been accustomed to pay to the hospital for the church of Brignall in the time of master Swain, rector of the hospital, and which he would pay each year during his lifetime (C122, C124 [Cott., f. 18ʳ]). Thomas son of Roger, clerk, was admitted to the church on the presentation of the hospital in 1241 (C121 [Cott., f. 18ʳ]). In 1246, Thomas, parson of Brignall, successor of one Ranulf living in the time of King John, recovered common pasture in Brignall (*EYC*, V, 334, citing Farrer's Honors and Knights' Fees MS, from Assize Roll 1045, m. 18). The second witness, Pain of Catton, was dead in 1192. Geoffrey de St-Pierre was a benefactor of Byland, to which he gave 2 bv. in Scrayingham with his body at an unknown date (*Ctl. Byland*, no. 1162). It is likely that Jeremy and Isaiah were sons of Ilger the priest of Catton, who died in 1175 × 1181 (FN).

**R646.** Gift to the hospital by Ilger son of Ascur of 4 a. in the fields of Stamford Bridge [*c.*1175 × *c.*1200]

PRINTED: *EYC*, II, no. 911, where dated 1170 × 1181.

*Ilgerus filius Ascur' de iiii. acris terre in Ponte Belli.*
Sciant omnes videntes et audientes litteras has quod ego Ilgerus filius Ascur' concessi et dedi et presenti carta confirmavi deo et pauperibus hospitalis sancti Petri Ebor' iiiiᵒʳ acras terre in campis de Ponte Belli, liberas et quietas ab omni servicio plenarias in pascuis et in omnibus libertatibus in puram et perpetuam elemosinam. Hanc vero elemosinam ego et heredes mei warentizabimus predictis pauperibus contra omnes homines ut simus participes orationum que in eadem domo fient imperpetuum. Hiis testibus, Gaufrido de Percy, Hugone capellano, Ricardo capellano, Willelmo capellano, Bartholomeo de Gairegrave, Gaufrido filio Sunnive, Laurencio diacono, Waltero

de Beverlaco, Waltero de Wiverthelaia, Iohanne de Spotford', Gileberto filio Martini, Pagano filio Alui, Arnaldo filio Torfini.

Geoffrey de Percy occurs as steward to Jocelin de Louvain in *c.* 1174 (*EYC*, XI, no. 68), and as rector of Gargrave in the 1170s and 1180s. His last appearance as rector is in 1189. The evidence for Robert de Percy, who occurs as parson or rector of Gargrave in 1214 ('R.') and 1219 or later,[9] is difficult to interpret. In 1226 the vicarage, to which he was said to have been instituted by Archbishop G[eoffrey] on the presentation of Agnes de Percy, who died in 1201 × 1204, was confirmed to him (*Ctl. Furness*, II, 313; *Fasti Parochiales*, IV, 42, 45–46). Bartholomew of Gargrave witnessed deeds of Agnes de Percy in '? 1189' and 1180 × 1204, and occurs with Geoffrey de Percy and his son Walter in 1176 × 1184 (C522 [*EYC*, I, no. 231; ibid., XI, no. 76]; *EYC*, XI, nos 77, 138). Walter of Beverley witnessed a deed of Henry du Puiset in 1182 × 1211 (*EYC*, XI, no. 254), and a deed of Adeliza de Percy given in 1167 or later[10] (M: Collingham [*EYC*, XI, no. 297]).

**R647.** Agreement between master Ralph, rector, and the brethren of the hospital, and Gilbert son of Geoffrey of Stamford Bridge. The master and brethren have demised to Gilbert and his heirs the land with a house which the hospital has in Stamford Bridge, next to the churchyard towards the south. Gilbert and his heirs will prepare and maintain the house at their own expense, suitable and convenient for the reception and storage of the hospital's corn. And after the brethren have taken away their corn Gilbert will have the house until the following autum. Gilbert will pay the hospital 1 *lb.* cumin annually [1204 × 1217]

*Cirograph(um) inter hospitale et Gillebertum filium Gaufridi de Ponte Belli.*
Hec est conventio facta inter magistrum Radulfum rectorem et fratres hospitalis sancti Petri Ebor' ex una parte et Gillebertum filium Gaufridi de Ponte Belli ex altera parte, quod predicti magister et fratres dimiserunt predicto Gilleberto et heredibus suis illam terram cum domo et cum pertinenciis quam ipsum hospitale habet in Ponte Belli iuxta [f. 222ʳ] cimiterium versus meridiem, ita quod Gillebertus et heredes eius parabunt propriis sumptibus et sustinobunt predictam domum quod sit competens et conveniens predictis fratribus ad bladum predicti hospitalis suscipiendum et servandum sine aliquo impedimento qua(cumque)[11] est eis opus domo predicta. Et qu(ando) fratres predicti absportaverint totum bladum suum Gillebertus habebit domum predictam usque ad autumpnum sequentem singulis annis ut predivisum est. Et pro predicta terra et domo sic habenda reddent predictus Gillebertus et heredes eius predicto hospitali unam libram cimini annuatim ad festum sancti Martini in yeme. Et hoc legitime servandum pro se et pro heredibus suis affidavit predictus Gillebertus et sigillo suo confirmavit. Et ad huius rei certitudinem magister et fratres huic scripto sigillum suum apposuerunt. Hiis testibus, Thoma celerario, Willelmo Balki, Alano de Cnapetoft', Girardo, Waltero de Stoketon', Willelmo de Hecke, Ricardo de Wakefeud', Gamello, fratribus predicti hospitali, Willelmo, Petro, Lamberto capellanis, Thoma, Willelmo diacono, Malgero marescallo, Hingolfo, Ricardo, Waltero, Eustachio, Radulfo de Celabria, Ernufo servientibus et multis aliis.

The date range is the period for Ralph as rector.

---

9  It is unclear on what basis dates of '*c.* 1190', '*c.* 1200' and '*c.* 1188 × 1216' were assigned to deeds in the Furness coucher attested by Robert as rector.
10  Clay gives '1167 × *c.* 1175', but his *terminus ad quem* is on unspecified paleographical grounds.
11  MS: *q'ᵃ*.

# *Queldryk* [Wheldrake]

Much of the land in Wheldrake was acquired in the early thirteenth century or before by the monks of Fountains, who established a grange there (*VCH Yorks ER*, III, 122–23). In 1346 William Darell was said to hold 1 ct. in Wheldrake (*Feudal Aids*, VI, 222). According to an inquisition of 1364, it was during the mastership of Thomas Brembre (1349–1361) that the hospital was 'charged with' William Darell and his wife, in return for their lands in Wheldrake (*CalInqMisc*, 1348–1377, p. 202). An extensive series of deeds commencing in 1368, by which the hospital acquired the Darell manor in Wheldrake and then assigned it to Fountains Abbey in exchange for a rent of 16m., were copied into a cartulary of Fountains, and are noted below. The rent was still being paid in 1535. In that year the annual value of Fountains' possessions in Wheldrake was assessed at £104 16s. 6d., and amongst the expenses of the hospital was the sum of 11s. 4d. for the annual obit for William Darell (*MA*, v, 311–12; R905).

The hospital also acquired Darell's property in Gillygate, York. On 28 September 1368 William Darell of Wheldrake assigned to Sirs William Garland and Thomas Hillington, vicars choral of York, the tenement in Gillygate he had by feoffment of master William Langton, formerly advocate of the court of York. The grantees assigned the tenement to Alan Head, warden of the hospital, William Ireland, chaplain, and Richard Garton, clerk of the hospital, on 31 May 1381 (C605, C606 [Cott., ff. 118ᵛ–119ʳ]).

The deeds concerning the hospital's acquisition of the rent of 16m. in Wheldrake, as contained in the cartulary of Fountains (*Ctl. Fountains*, pp. 836–39), may be summarised as follows:

(i) 12 October 1368. Grant by William son of Thomas Darell of Wheldrake to Sir William Garlands of Malton and Thomas Hillington, vicars choral of York, of all his lands and tenements etc. in Wheldrake.

(ii) 24 October 1375. Grant by William Garlands of Malton and Thomas Hillington, vicars choral of York, to Walter Nafferton, rector of the churches of St Margaret and St Mary in Walmgate, York, Robert Friseton, rector of the church of Helagh, Thomas Kyrkby, vicar choral of York, John Brawby senior, Hugh Catall, William Ireland, Hugh Borton, chaplains, and Roger Allerthorp, barker, of all the lands etc. in Wheldrake which they had by grant and feoffment of William son of Thomas Darell of Wheldrake.

(iii) 3 November 1375. Release and quitclaim by William son of Thomas Darell of Wheldrake, to the grantees named in (ii), of the premises in Wheldrake.

(iv) 1 April 1379. Grant by Walter Nafferton and the other grantees in (ii), except Robert Friseton, to Richard Ravenser, archdeacon of Lincoln, John Ravenser, parson of the church of Algarkirk (Lincs.), and John Waltham, canon of Hereford, of the premises in Wheldrake.

(v) 13 May 1379. Inquisition *ad quod damnum* taken at Wheldrake, before William Mirfield, escheator in Yorkshire, by oath of William Paumes of Naburn and his fellows, who say it is not to the damage of the king or others if he should grant to Richard Ravenser, archdeacon of Lincoln, John Ravenser, parson of the church of Algarkirk, and John Waltham, canon of Hereford, licence to grant to the abbot and convent of Fountains certain lands etc. in Wheldrake, to the value of 16m. annually, so that the said abbot and convent may be able to grant 16m. yearly to the master and brethren of St Leonard's Hospital, York, to be received from the lands etc., aforesaid, for certain burdens in the said hospital, to be borne by the said master and brethren according to the ordinance of the said archdeacon, John and John, namely that manor of Wheldrake, described as in R648. The lands etc. are held of the abbot and convent of Fountains by knight service and by service of rendering to them and their successors 12*d*. annually. The abbot and convent hold of Henry Percy, earl of Northumberland, in pure and perpetual alms, and they are worth by the year in all issues according to the true value 16*m*. sterling, and there remain to the said archdeacon, John and John, beyond the said donation, divers lands and tenements in the city of York and the vill of Beverley and in Lund-on-Wold worth yearly £40 sterling, held of diverse lords by various services, sufficient to the customs and services etc.

(vi) 23 April 1380. Licence by Richard II (for 20*m*. paid) for the alienation of the above premises to the abbot and convent, and for the grant by them to the master and brethren of the hospital of St Leonard, York, of 16*m*. annually for certain burdens in the said hospital according to the ordinance of the above-named archdeacon, John Ravenser, and John Waltham.

(vii) 14 August 1382. Licence by Henry Percy, earl of Northumberland, to the abbot and convent of Fountains, to acquire the manor of Wheldrake, formerly William Darell's, from the above-named Richard, John and John.

(viii) 1382–83. Similar licence by Adam Bekwith and Elizabeth his wife.

(ix) 28 August 1383. Appointment by the said archdeacon, John and John, of attorneys to deliver seisin.

(x) 1 September 1383. Appointment by the abbot and convent of Fountains of attorneys to receive seisin.

(xi) 28 August 1383. Grant by the above-named archdeacon, John and John, to the abbot and convent of Fountains of the manor of Wheldrake.

(xii) 4 October 1383. Counterpart to R648.

(xiii) 30 August 1383. The abbot and convent of Fountains admit they owe the master and brethren of the hospital of St Leonard, York, 1000*m*., to be paid at Easter next.

(xiv) 30 September 1383. Notification by the master and brethren of the hospital of St Leonard, York, that if the abbot and convent paid the agreed 16*m*. annually, their recognisance in 1000*m*. would be void, otherwise to remain in force.

(xv) 5 October 1383. Release by the master and brethren of the hospital of St Leonard, York, to the abbot and convent of Fountains, of the aforesaid sum of 1000*m*.

The original of another deed pertaining to this transaction survives. It is a tripartite indenture of 14 September 1382, witnessing that Richard Ravenser, archdeacon of Lincoln, John Ravenser, parson of Algarkirk, and John Waltham, canon of Hereford, assigned to the abbot and convent of Fountains the manor of Wheldrake, formerly William Darell's (described as in R648) on condition of payment by Fountains to the hospital of St Leonard, York, of 16*m*. annually (*Bodleian Charters*, p. 689).

The Torre charters included a further deed, apparently dated 26 September 1380, which laid down the use to be made of the 16*m*. rent for Wheldrake from Fountains. 6*m*. was to be used *in subsidium cuiusdam elemosinarie* providing a loaf of bread every Thursday for each poor person (*pauper*) in the hospital, 'of the same value and weight as those they were accustomed to get'. From the remaining 10*m*., each brother applying was to have 6*s*. 8*d*. at Pentecost. Under the same reference, Torre noted what was apparently a different deed by which the master Sir Richard Ravenser, archdeacon of Lincoln, and the brethren bound themselves to hold three obits annually, at their own expense. The first was to be held on the day of Richard [Ravenser]'s death; the second for Edward III on the day of St Alban the martyr (22 June); and the third for the same king's mother Isabel and his wife Philippa on the octave of the assumption of the blessed Mary (22 August).[12] Each brother attending one of the obits was to have 6*d.*, each sister present in church 4*d.*, three secular chaplains *in dicto hospitali celebrantibus* 3*d.*, choristers present 1*d.*, deacons and subdeacons ministrating at mass 2*d.* each, sacrists ringing the bells 3*d.*, and the *pauperibus* 5*s.* divided between them at the discretion of the warden (*guardiani*) (Bodl., MS Top. Yorks. b. 14, f. 227ʳ, p. 450, B10 N53).[13]

**R648.** Indenture by which the abbot and convent of Fountains granted to the master and brethren of the hospital of St Leonard, York, and their successors, by licence of King Richard II, an annual rent of 16*m.* from all the manor with appurtenances in Queldryk, which formerly belonged to William Darell, and from eight messuages, nineteen tofts, 180 a. land, 14 a. meadow, 14 a. wood, 100 a. moor, 6*s.* 1*d.* rent, and the rent of a pair of gloves, in Queldrik, which the abbot and convent have by feoffment of Sirs Richard de Ravenser, archdeacon of Lincoln, John de Waltham, canon of the cathedral church of Herford, and John de Ravenser, parson of the church of Algarkirk, and from all other lands and tenements of the abbot and convent in Queldryk, to be paid at the feasts of Pentecost and St Martin in winter by equal portions, the first term of payment starting next St Martin in winter, for certain charges in the hospital supported by the master and brethren, according to the order of the said Sirs Richard, John and John. Right of distraint in the premises for the rent, arrears, and expenses if the rent is wholly or partly in arrears for forty days. And if sufficient distraint cannot be taken in the said premises, then the master and brothers may distrain in the abbot and convent's manor of Thorp Undir Wod. If the rent or any part is in arrears for fifty days, then for each occasion a penalty of 40*s.* would be paid for the fabric of the church of the hospital. Right of distraint for this penalty. The master and brethren have granted that if any part of the premises is recovered by any heir of William Darell, or by any just and ancient title, the abbot and convent taking all customary delays, and straightaway after the summons warning the master and brethren, so that the abbot and convent defend the plea according to the order and counsel of the master and brethren, then the rent should cease by proportion equivalent to the part so recovered. The parties have affixed their communal seals to alternate parts of the indenture. No witnesses. 4 October 1383 [hand A-2]

COPIES: *b* Rawl., f. 222ᵛ; *c* BL, MS Addit. 18276 (Fountains cartulary, Davis, no. 422), f. 191ʳ⁻ᵛ, not collated. CALENDAR: *Ctl. Fountains*, p. 839.

[f. 222ᵛ] *Carta abbatis et conventus de Fontibus de quodam annuo redditu xvi. marcarum in Queldryk' facta magistro et fratribus hospitalis sancti Leonardi per licencia metuendissimi domini regis Ricardi secundi etc.*

Dat' Ebor' iiii^to die mensis octobris anno domini millesimo trescentesimo octogesimo tertio, et regni regis Ricardi secundi post conquestum supradicti septimo.

Sir Richard Ravenser was master of the hospital when this deed was made, but as usual is described as archdeacon of Lincoln.

---

12   Edward III died on 21 June 1377; Philippa died shortly before 14 August 1369; Queen Isabella died on 23 August 1358.
13   Burton makes only a brief note of the deed (Burton transcripts 5, f. 84ᵛ, p. 160).

*Ruhthorp' al' dict' Thorpe in Strata*
[Thorpe le Street, par. Market Weighton]

For Thorpe le Street, otherwise Rudthorpe or Ructhorp, where Gilbert Tison held a manor of 3 ct. in 1086, and for the branch of the Salvain family which held 3 ct. there in 1254, see *EYC*, XII, 109–12. A messuage or cottage with two crofts in Thorpe le Street, now or late in the occupation of William Palmer, formerly belonging to the hospital of St Leonard in York, was amongst property assigned by the Crown by letters patent of 16 July 1563 (A2A: YM/FD/1;[1] *CalPat*, 1560–1563, p. 576).

**R649.** Gift to the hospital by William Salvain of a toft in Ruhthorp, which Walter Urri held, and which lies next to the road on the west side opposite the chapel [*c.*1200 × 1219]

COPIES: *b* Rawl., f. 223[r]; *c* Hull History Centre, U DDEV/xi/25/1 (Constable Maxwell of Everingham papers), copy possibly of seventeenth century date, deemed 'unfit for production', November 2010. PRINTED: *EYC*, XII, no. 84, where dated *c.*1190 × *c.*1210, from *b*.

**[f. 223[r]]** *Willelmus Salvain de uno tofto in Ruhthorp' aliter dict' Thorp' in Strata.*
Omnibus sancte matris ecclesie filiis cartam istam visuris et audituris Willelmus Salvein salutem. Noveritis me pro salute anime mee et omnium antecessorum et heredum et successorum meorum dedisse concessisse et hac presenti carta mea confirmasse deo et pauperibus hospitalis beati Petri Ebor' unum toftum apud Ruhthorp', quod Walterus Urri tenuit et quod iacet propinquius vie iuxta ipsam viam ex parte occidentali ex opposito capelle, scilicet tenendum et habendum cum liberis pertinenciis suis predictis pauperibus in puram et perpetuam elemosinam libere et quiete sicut ulla elemosina liberius potest dari, ut omnes antecessores et heredes et successores mei et ego simus participes omnium orationum elemosinarum et aliorum beneficiorum que fiunt vel facienda sunt in prefato domo dei. Et ego et heredes mei warantizabimus predictam donationem et concessionem predictis pauperibus contra omnes homines imperpetuum. Hiis testibus, magistro Waltero canonico Ebor' ecclesie, Ricardo, Petro, Ada, Roberto, capellanis, Roberto Luvel,[2] Gileberto de Bernerthorp', Thoma de Languath, Galfrido, Paulino, clericis, Waltero de Alredale, Rogero Treuweluve, Roberto Wirlepipin,[3] Willelmo et multis aliis.

The first witness was master Walter of Wisbech, prebendary of Givendale, some 7 m. north of Thorpe le Street. He occurs as a canon of York in 1206[/07] (*Ctl. Rievaulx*, no. 363) and 1204 × 1214[4] (*YMF*, I, no. 31), and was archdeacon of the East Riding by April 1219 (FN). Peter, Adam, Robert chaplains, and Thomas de Langwath attested a deed of 1206 (R463).

1  Borthwick, Yarburgh muniments.
2  *c*: *Lincel* (according to catalogue entry).
3  *c*: *Roger Wirlepipin* (catalogue entry).
4  Whilst Simon de Apulia was dean, and Ralph was rector of the hospital. See Carpenter, 'Paulinus', p. 17n for the revision to Clay's dating.

## *Ristun* [Long Riston]

For Long Riston, see Poulson, *Holderness*, I, 341–48; *VCH Yorks ER*, VII, 340–49. In 1086, in the fee of Drogo de Bevrere, there were two manors of 3 ct. altogether, then held by Gerbod, in [Long] Riston, and also 2 ct. 6 bv. soke of Hornsea. The vill was held by the Scures family of the Aumale barony of Holderness until the 1270s. There is no evidence that the hospital held anything in Riston beyond the acre given by Robert de Scures in the mid-twelfth century, which does not appear in the papal confirmations. The hospital's toft in Riston was mentioned in a deed of 1337 (A2A: SpSt/4/11/82/22).[1] In 1609, a cottage formerly belonging to the hospital in Riston was granted to Edward Bates and Henry Elwes (*VCH Yorks ER*, VII, 346, citing PRO, C 66/1800, no. 7).

Poulson gave a pedigree of SCURES based largely on the details given in the chronicle of Meaux and entries in the Dodsworth manuscripts which he did not identify (Poulson, *Holderness*, I, 341–44). Farrer and Clay also gave accounts (*EYC*, III, 64; *EYF*, pp. 82–83). Both Loyd and Clay suggested that the family took its name from Écuires, by Montreuil-sur-Mer. The first husband of Adeliza, mother of Stephen, count of Aumale, was Enguerrand count of Ponthieu, to whose fee Écuires belonged, and it is possible that the counts of Ponthieu were in possession of Aumale in the first half of the eleventh century (*ANF*, p. 97). Anschetil de Scures was named in the Lindsey survey of 1115 as holding 6½ bv. in Hackthorn, co. Lincoln, of Stephen of Aumale (*LDLS*, p. 239), but no subsequent trace can be found of this interest. Anschetil's wife was Emma, whose death on 2 June was recorded in the twelfth-century obit book of Lincoln Cathedral (Gerald of Wales, *Opera*, VII, 157). Anschetil was dead in 1130, when Alan de Scures was pardoned 75s. of the old pleas of Holderness, and rendered account of £15 for the dower of his wife (*PR*, 31 Hen. I, p. 26). Alan de Scures follows Alan de Percy and Richard de Verli in the witness list of a grant by Archbishop Thomas II or Thurstan made in 1109 × c.1136 (*EEA*, V, no. 26). The descent of Robert de Scures, the hospital's benefactor, from Anschetil and Alan is shown by the confirmation by William de Scures to the priory of Bridlington of 2 bv. in Acklam (ER), which Robert his brother gave to the same church, in exchange for [4 bv.] land in Riston which Anschetil his (William's) grandfather gave, and also confirming the demesne toft of Alan de Scures, his (William's) father, in Acklam. The Acklam land was held of the Chamberlain's fee, and was confirmed to Bridlington by S[tephen] son of Herbert the Chamberlain (*Ctl. Bridlington*, pp. 225–26; *EYC*, II, nos 825n, 827). Robert de Scures attested deeds to Newhouse Abbey concerning the church of Halton, and Cabourne (all Lincs.) in 1143 × 1148[2] (*Danelaw Docs*, nos 255, 281) and in 1148 × 1158[3] attested the 'foundation charter' of that abbey (*MA*, VI, 865). He gave ½ ct. in Skillington (Lincs.) to Nun Cotham, with the agreement of his brother and heir William. Adam, abbot of Meaux (1151–1160) was a witness. It is unclear whether William de Scures' gift of the same land to Nun Cotham, dated 21 September 1160, was made before or afterwards (Nun Cotham cartulary, f. 13ᵛ). Robert had been

---

[1]   WYAS, Bradford, Spencer-Stanhope papers.

[2]   The Melrose chronicle tells us *s.a.* 1143 *Ordo premonstratensis venit ad Neus* (*Chron. Melrose*, p. 34). The deeds are addressed to Bishop Alexander of Lincoln, who died in February 1148.

[3]   Addressed to Robert, bishop of Lincoln, whose episcopate lasted from 1148 until 1166. The deed appears to have been issued during the lifetime of Ranulf de Bayeux, who was dead at Michaelmas 1158, when Hugh de Bayeux accounted for 20m. in Lincolnshire (Sanders, *English Baronies*, p. 88; *PR*, 2–4 Hen. II, p. 137).

## SCURES OF RISTON

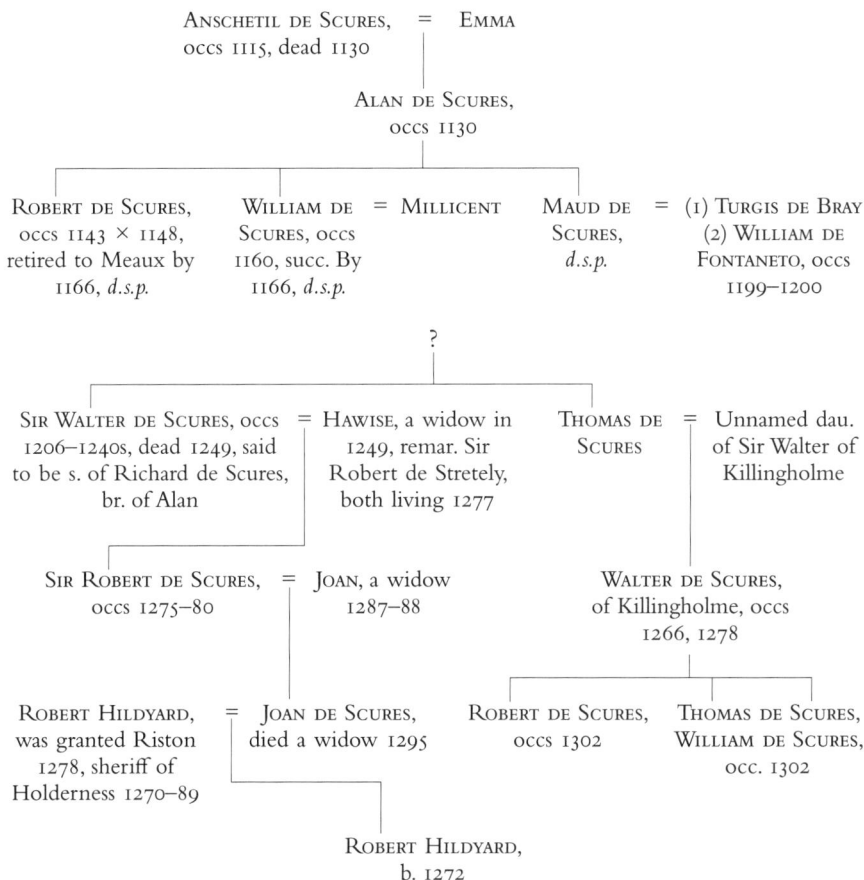

ANSCHETIL DE SCURES, = EMMA
occs 1115, dead 1130

ALAN DE SCURES,
occs 1130

| ROBERT DE SCURES, occs 1143 × 1148, retired to Meaux by 1166, *d.s.p.* | WILLIAM DE SCURES, occs 1160, succ. By 1166, *d.s.p.* | = | MILLICENT | MAUD DE SCURES, *d.s.p.* | = | (1) TURGIS DE BRAY (2) WILLIAM DE FONTANETO, occs 1199–1200 |

?

| SIR WALTER DE SCURES, occs 1206–1240s, dead 1249, said to be s. of Richard de Scures, br. of Alan | = | HAWISE, a widow in 1249, remar. Sir Robert de Stretely, both living 1277 | THOMAS DE SCURES | = | Unnamed dau. of Sir Walter of Killingholme |

| SIR ROBERT DE SCURES, occs 1275–80 | = | JOAN, a widow 1287–88 | WALTER DE SCURES, of Killingholme, occs 1266, 1278 |

| ROBERT HILDYARD, was granted Riston 1278, sheriff of Holderness 1270–89 | = | JOAN DE SCURES, died a widow 1295 | ROBERT DE SCURES, occs 1302 | THOMAS DE SCURES, WILLIAM DE SCURES, occ. 1302 |

ROBERT HILDYARD,
b. 1272

succeeded by his brother William in 1166, when the latter held 1 k.f. of Stephen son of Herbert the Chamberlain of old feoffment (*EYC*, II, no. 825) and ½ k.f. of Archbishop Roger, which lay in Skillington and Woolsthorpe, Lincs. (*EYC*, I, no. 38 and n). It can be deduced that William also held 1 k.f. of Aumale, in Long Riston, Tunstall, Flinton, Fitling, Humbleton and Cowden Parva.[4] In 1154 × 1181[5] Stephen son of Herbert the Chamberlain confirmed the grant of the church of Acklam which William de Scures had made to Thornton Abbey (*EYC*, I, no. 32). This grant, and William's further grants of the vill and church of Humbleton, 13¼ bv. land in Flinton, and 7*s.* rent in the same place, were included in Richard I's general confirmation to the abbey of 1190 (*EYC*, III, no. 1312).[6] The deed by which William de Scures gave

4    There is no 1166 return for Aumale. Farrer's conjectural list of Holderness fees has Scures holding ½ k.f. (*EYC*, III, 34). But Robert Hildyard, who inherited the Scures fee in Holderness, was said to hold 1 k.f. in [Long] Riston, Tunstall, Flinton, Fitling and Cowden Parva in 1284–85. Robert de Scures had interests in all these places earlier in the century (*KI*, pp. 75, 371–77).
5    The period for Archbishop Roger, to whom the confirmation is addressed.
6    The identity of Nicholas de Scures, who was said to have given the mill, five tofts, and 4 bv. land in Acklam to Thornton Abbey, has not been established. The abbey gave the property to Bridlington in

the church of Humbleton was exhibited in 1308 (*Reg. Greenfield*, v, 223). In or before
1173[7] Henry II confirmed to St Mary's Abbey 2 bv. land and pasture in Acklam given
by William de Scures (*EYC*, II, no. 824).[8] William de Scures, with the support of his
wife Millicent, restored to the church of Hornsea, and St Mary's Abbey, the church
of [Long] Riston, which he had ascertained his father had built to the detriment of
the mother church of Hornsea (*EYC*, III, no. 1348).

According to the chronicle of Meaux, it was in the time of Abbot Adam (1151–
1160) that Robert de Scures gave the abbey 1 ct. land between Leven and Burshill,
where the monks' manor of Heigholme was established. The gift was made *cum se ipso*,
and Robert entered the monastery as a novice, becoming only the second monk to
die during his novitiate. '[Heig]holme, between Leven and Burshill' was included in
Alexander III's confirmation of 1172 ('Ctl. Meaux', no. 4). This land was mentioned
in 1187, when Meaux paid 60s. for a quitclaim by Osbert son of Godfrey and Ralph
of Flinton for 1 ct. land in [Heig]holme, formerly belonging to Alan de Scures, after
an assize of mort d'ancestor (*EYC*, III, no. 1351). The chronicle goes on to say that
Robert was succeeded by his brother William, who confirmed his grant, and died
without heir of his body, his interests passing to his sister Maud, wife of Turgis de
Bray. Maud and Turgis confirmed the gift of Heigholme. Elsewhere the chronicle
states that Turgis de Bray and William de Fontaneto, and Maud de Scures *uxor eorum*
confirmed 'the great dike, now called *Wythedyk*, from the bridge of Routh (*Rude*)
to the yard (*curtem*) of the abbey,' with other property belonging to the territory of
Riston (*Chron. Meaux*, I, 96, 304). Charter evidence provides support for this account,
and shows that Robert and William had a sister Maud, but does not prove that it
was the same Maud who was wife to Bray and Fontaneto. The deeds of Robert
de Scures giving [Heig]holme, and the confirmation by William his brother, are
noted in the Meaux register. There were also confirmations by Hawise, countess, and
Baldwin de Béthune, earl of Aumale (Meaux register, f. 13ᵛ). Maud de Scures, without
specifying her marital status, confirmed the gift of [Heig]holme between Leven and
Burshill made by her brother Robert de Scures (*EYC*, III, no. 1350). Turgis de Bray
and Maud de Scures, his wife, confirmed a ditch from Turkhill to Brackenholme
[in Leven], made for 'our souls and the souls of Alan de Scures and Robert and
William', by a deed witnessed by Henry de Scures ('Ctl. Meaux', no. 232; cf. Meaux
register, f. 14ᵛ). Thomas Burton noted a deed of Turgis de Bray and Maud de Scures
his wife confirming and quitclaiming the gift of Robert de Scures of the whole of
[Heig]holme, but Maud's relationship to Robert is not stated. There are also notes
of confirmations by William de Fontaneto, William de Scures, and Robert de Scures,
knight (Meaux register, f. 14ʳ). William de Fontaneto and Maud de Scures together
confirmed the great ditch to Meaux (Meaux register, f. 14ᵛ). The entry in the pipe
roll of 1199, and the corresponding fine of 1200, by which William *de Funtenay* and
Maud his wife quitclaimed their right in the advowson of the church of Riston to
Robert, abbot of St Mary's, for 10m., shows that Maud was a successor to William
de Scures (*PR*, 1 John, p. 123; *PF John*, p. 4). Turgis de Bray, Henry de Scures, and
Maud de Scures are the fourth, eleventh and thirteenth witnesses respectively to a
deed dated '*c.* 1160 × *c.* 1180' by Clay (*EYC*, XI, no. 279).

---

1233 × 1259 (*Ctl. Bridlington*, p. 226; dating from the extreme limits for Robert as abbot of Thornton
(*Heads*, II, 469)).

7   No *dei gratia*.

8   William's deed of gift was catalogued by Torre in the 1670s or 1680s, but it was not printed by Drake
or copied by Burton (Bodl., MS Top. Yorks. b. 14 (Torre's catalogue), f. 243ʳ, p. 73 [old], p. 482 [Burton],
B19 N38).

The chronicle's account of the subsequent descent, *quorum quidem genealogia in scriptis sic legitur exarata*, states that as Maud died without heir of her body, the lordship of Riston passed to Walter de Scures, son of Richard de Scures, Richard being Maud's paternal uncle. Richard de Scures was a son of Anschetil de Scures, and brother to Alan. Walter de Scures was father of Robert de Scures, who gave to Robert Hildyard the elder his interest in Riston (*Chron. Meaux*, I, 97–98).

Despite the detailed and coherent nature of this account, it is difficult to accept in its entirety. Whilst it is not chronologically impossible for Walter de Scures, who died in 1241 × 1249, and whose widow was living as late as 1277, to have been a grandson of Anschetil de Scures, who was dead in 1130, it is unlikely, and supporting evidence is wanting. Anschetil's wife was named Emma, and Richard's mother was Juetta de Verli, who survived her Scures husband. There is no charter evidence to show the relationship of Richard de Scures, who occurs in Lincolnshire from the middle of the twelfth century, with Anschetil de Scures. Nor is there anything to show Richard's relationship with Walter de Scures, who occurs from the early thirteenth century.

Richard de Scures attested Simon son of William [de Kyme]'s foundation charter of Bullington Priory (Lincs.) which has been assigned to *c*.1155 and was certainly given in the period 1148 × 1166[9] (*Gilbertine Charters*, p. 91). On 10 November 1160 Richard de Scures confirmed the gift which his mother Juetta made to Nun Cotham of all her land in Keelby, in return for 30*s*. annually and ½ ct. in Skillington. If the nuns could not warrant the land in Skillington they would pay a further 10*s*. If Richard took a wife, and she survived him, but he had no heir by her, then they would pay her the rent by way of dower. If Richard and his wife died without a son or daughter for an heir, Nun Cotham would have the land. He and his wife were to be buried at Nun Cotham (Nun Cotham cartulary, f. 14[v]). The gift of the land in Skillington to Nun Cotham by William and Robert de Scures has been noted above. The subsequent acquisition of this land by Richard provides good evidence that they were close kinsmen, as does the statement of 1238 × 1241 that the master of Cotham held ½ k.f.[10] in Keelby of Walter de Scures (*Bk of Fees*, p. 1476). The identity of Richard's mother Juetta is shown by the general confirmation to Nun Cotham made in 1159 × 1181 by Pope Alexander III, which includes 4½ bv. in Keelby given by Juetta de Verli, with the consent of Richard de Scures her son and heir (*MA*, v, 676). A confirmation by Robert, bishop of Lincoln, includes 4 bv. in Keelby given by Gilbert de Scures, with the agreement of his mother Juetta de Verli, who had given it before (Nun Cotham cartulary, f. 13[v]). At a date unknown the chapter of Lincoln issued a notification that Richard de Scures, in chapter, had confirmed the grant made by his mother of the church of Keelby to Nun Cotham (ibid., f. 11[v]). Richard de Scures is the second witness to a deed to Nun Cotham made *c*.1160 × *c*.1183[11] (*Danelaw Docs*, no. 425).

Walter de Scures occurs in 1206, when he accounted in Lincolnshire for ½*m*. for not prosecuting a plea (*PR*, 8 John, p. 102). Whether this was the same man who attested a Killingholme deed of '*c*.1185' is open to question (*Danelaw Docs*, no. 294). In 1211 Walter de Scures rendered account of 10*m*. for having seisin of ½ k.f. in Skillington and Woolsthorpe[12] (*PR*, 13 John, pp. 34, 61), presumably as the successor to Maud de Scures and her second husband William de Fontenay. Walter is named in the survey of 1212 as the archbishop's tenant of ½ k.f. in the two places, owed scutage for

[9]   Attested by Robert [de Chesney] bishop of Lincoln.
[10]   recte ½ ct. ?
[11]   Attested by Ralph, subdean.
[12]   *Scalton* [identified as Scawton, NR] *et Wulstorp*.

½ k.f. held of the archbishop in 1214, and in 1242–43 was said to hold ½ k.f. in Skillingon of the archbishop (*Bk of Fees*, pp. 183, 1050; *Red Bk*, pp. 491, 495; *PR*, 16 John, p. 69).[13] Walter de Scures attested a deed of Baldwin de Béthune earl of Aumale, in favour of Meaux, in 1195 × 1212[14] (MS Dods. 7, f. 232v), and two deeds made by William de Forz, earl of Aumale, to the hospital, in 1214 × 1231 (R581, R582). He witnessed a Riston deed with Thomas his brother (A2A: SpSt/4/11/82/19). As a knight he witnessed a deed of Fulk Basset, provost of Beverley, to Ellerton Priory, in 1228 × 1234[15] (Burton transcripts 2, f. 120ʳ, p. 204, B29 N22). He attested again as a knight in 1241 × 1251;[16] Thomas de Scures occurs further down the witness list (A2A: SpSt/4/11/7/1). Walter was doubtless dead in 1249, when Dame Hawise de Scures [his widow], let a toft with a croft in Eske, near Beverley (*Esc*), which Alan of Holderness held, for seven years (*Cat. Anc. Deeds*, IV, A.6755). Walter's heir was his son Robert. In or after 1249[17] Sir Robert, son of Walter de Scures, confirmed the grant of lands in his fee in Riston made by Sir Andrew Fauconberg to Nunkeeling (Poulson, *Holderness*, I, 377; MS Dods. 7, f. 247ʳ). Robert son of Walter de Scures sold to Richard son of Peter de Bernville the service from a messuage and 5 ct. in Leavening, and, by another deed, the advowson of the church of Acklam (MS Dods. 95, f. 13r, citing Kirkham cartulary, f. 55). In a Holderness feodary of 'the latter part of the reign of Henry III', R[obert] de Scures was said to hold 6 ct. in [Long] Riston (*KI*, p. 372). Sir Robert de Scures, knight, confirmed a grant in Skillington of land 'adjoining the court of Sir Robert de Scures' to the dean and chapter of Lincoln in 1254 × 1258 or 1272 × 1274[18] (*Reg. Antiquissimum*, VII, nos 2136–37). According to Poulson's pedigree, Sir Robert's heir was his daughter Joan, wife of Robert Hildyard. Though Joan is not described as Robert's daughter in deeds, the relationship seems the most likely explanation of the transactions of the 1270s, particularly as Robert Scures' widow was also named Joan. The marriage had no doubt fallen to Hildyard as a result of his tenure of the shrievalty of Holderness under the king in 1270–89 (FN: Holderness Sheriffs). In October 1275 Sir Robert de Scures, son of Walter de Scures, granted to Robert Hildyard and his wife Joan the reversion of the manor of Riston in Holderness, then held in dower by his (Robert de Scures') mother Hawise, for 10*m.* annually. Before November 1277 Hawise and her then husband Sir Robert de Stretely had issued a quitclaim in the property (A2A: DDRI/22/2–4;[19] A2A: SpSt/5/4/3/1; Poulson, *Holderness*, I, 342);[20] and in October 1277 they attorned Peter Miller of Riston to deliver seisin of all the tenements they held by way of dower in Riston, which had belonged to Walter de Scures, formerly Hawise's husband (MS Dods. 94, f. 91ᵛ). In 1278 Robert de Scures entered a fine by which he granted to Robert Hildyard and Joan his wife the manor of Riston in Holderness, at a yearly rent of 1*d.*

---

[13]   The undated archiepiscopal feodary, which has Walter holding 1 k.f. in Skillington, is presumably in error (*KI*, p. 395).

[14]   The period for Baldwin de Béthune as earl (*CP*, I, 354).

[15]   With Roger de Lisle, dean, and master John Romeyn, subdean.

[16]   Also attested by Sir Henry [le Moigne], steward, [of William de Forz III], which William succeeded in 1241 (*EYC*, VII, 22, 83–84); and by William Anglicus, sheriff [of Holderness], who had been succeeded in that office by 1251 (FN: Holderness sheriffs).

[17]   Attested by William of Calverley, rector of Beeford, who was instituted in 1249 (*Reg. Gray*, p. 106).

[18]   Sir Robert's confirmation is attested by the same five witnesses as the grant, which was made to Sir Richard, dean, and the chapter of Lincoln. Richard of Gravesend (preferred by Major) was dean 1254–1258, and Richard de Mepham was dean 1272–1274. The first witness, Savaric vicar of Skillington, occurs in 1250 (*Reg. Antiquissimum*, VII, no. 2146), and survived until shortly before 8 October, 1275, when his successor was presented (*Rot. Gravesend*, p. 66).

[19]   ERA, Bethell of Rise Park papers.

[20]   Poulson's reference (*MA1*, II, 922) is incorrect.

(*YF*, 1272–1300, p. 13); and in 1280 Sir Robert de Scures granted to Robert Hildyard and his heirs the service that Peter of Goxhill did for his manor of Cowden Parva (Poulson, *Holderness*, I, 369). In 1284–85 Robert Hildyard held 48 ct. land, or 1 k.f., in [Long] Riston, Tunstall, Flinton, Fitling, and Cowden Parva (*KI*, p. 75). In 1286 a licence was issued for the alienation in mortmain to the Templars of a group of benefactions, including 70 a. land and pasture for 180 sheep in Skirlington, and 7s. rent in *Flete*, near Metheringham (Lincs.), by Robert de Scures (*CalPat*, 1281–1292, p. 244) though this is not good evidence Robert was then still living. Robert was dead in November 1287 × November 1288 when his widow Joan de Scures issued a deed of attorney to receive seisin of land in Sutton from Robert Hildyard. Hildyard had assigned her a messuage and 2 bv. land in Wawne (*Waghene*), and ½ bv. in Sutton [in Holderness] as dower in the land which had belonged to her husband Robert de Scures in Holderness (MS Dods. 139, f. 52ᵛ).

Joan, widow of Robert Hildyard, died shortly before 25 December 1295. The inquisition after her death found she had property in Riston including a capital messuage worth 20s. annually, sixteen tofts, 12½ bv. land, and two windmills, held of the Aumale barony of Holderness; and 120 a. and pasture for 1000 sheep in Sutton in Holderness held of John of Sutton. The property was found to have been purchased by her late husband, Joan holding for life by feoffment. Robert Hildyard, son of Robert and Joan, was the next heir, aged twenty-three. There was no inquisition as to any lands held outside Yorkshire (*YI*, III, 26–27; *CalInqPM*, III, no. 332).

Sir Walter de Scures of Killingholme, Lincs., may have been a son of Thomas, the above-mentioned brother of Sir Walter de Scures of Riston. An inquisition of 1266 found that Walter de Scures and others had been with Baldwin Wake and John de Eyville at the sack of Lincoln and the assault on the castle, and were then at Ely [i.e. continuing in rebellion]. Walter's lands at Killingholme and Goxhill were said to be worth 20s. a year (*CalInqMisc*, 1219–1307, p. 107). Describing himself as Walter de Scures son of Thomas de Scures, he gave the moiety of lands he had inherited in Killingholme to Thornton Abbey, which lands the abbey had held previously by demise of his [maternal] grandfather [Sir] Walter [of Killingholme].[21] His co-parcener was William son of William de Wylgeby, whose mother was another daughter of Sir Walter of Killingholme, and who refers to Walter de Scures as a knight (*CalCh*, 1300–1326, pp. 13–14). Sir Walter de Scures attested a gift to Thornton in 1278 (ibid., p. 11). An extent of the honour of Richmond, probably made in 1280 or 1281, states that Walter de Scures and his parceners held 1 k.f. in Killingholme (*CalInqPM*, II, 218). A complaint was made in 1302 that Robert son of Walter de Scures, Thomas and William his brothers, and others named had carried away goods at Halton, Lincs. (*CalPat*, 1301–1307, p. 84). In 1303 it was said that Robert de Scures and four others were tenants of 2½ k.f. in Killingholme, which the earl marshall formerly held (*Feudal Aids*, III, 157).

Another branch of the family held in Faldingworth, Lincs. In 1242–43 Robert de Scures was said to hold ¼ k.f. in Faldingworth of the earl of Salisbury (*Bk of Fees*, pp. 1066, 1073). Robert made a fine concerning 29 a. in Faldingworth in 1245 (*Lincs. Fines*, II, 29). In 1303, Ralph de Scures held ¼ k.f. in Faldingworth, which Robert de Scures formerly held, of [William] Longespee, earl of Salisbury (*Feudal Aids*, III, 136). In 1331 the ¼ k.f. was held by Alan de Scures (*CalInqPM*, VII, 233).

---

[21] For Sir Walter, see Moor, *Knights*, s.n. Kilingholm.

**R650.** Gift to the hospital by Robert de Scures, with the consent of William his brother, of 1 a. in [Long] Riston, for the erection of a building, with common pasture [*c.*1150 × 1166]

COPIES: *b* Rawl., f. 223ᵛ; *c* MS Dods. 7, f. 243ᵛ, differences as noted, with further minor differences of spelling. PRINTED: *EYC*, III, no. 1346, from *b*, where dated *c.*1145 × 1166. NOTED: Poulson, *Holderness*, I, 342, from *b*.

**[f. 223ᵛ]** *Robertus de Scures de una acra in R(istun).*[22]
Sciant omnes legentes et audientes has litteras me Rodbertum de Scures dedisse et presenti carta confirmasse in perpetuam elemosinam hospitali sancti Petri Ebor'[23] unam acram terre in territorio de Ristun, liberam et quietam ab omni servicio et consuetudine ad edificium faciendum et ibidem habere communem pasturam, Willemo fratre meo concedente, pro anima patris sui et antecessorum suorum. Testibus, Nicholao sacerdote, Ricardo de Warhsand',[24] Roberto de Scirlaga, Baldewino de Haitefelde, Stephano de Fitlyng', Willelmo fratre suo, Gileberto coco, Waltero filio Willelmi milite,[25] Ricardo filio Aichus, Baldewino rufo, Simone filio Nicholai.[26]

Five of the witnesses, including Nicholas the priest, attested R[obert] de Scures' gift of 2 bv. in Riston to Gilbert the cook (*EYC*, III, no. 1345), but it is difficult to assign definite dates to any of them. The explicit agreement of the donor's brother suggests a date not far removed from Robert and William de Scures' grants to Nun Cotham of 1151 × 1160 and 1160 mentioned above.

---

[22]  *c* has rubric *Carta Rodberti de Scures.*
[23]  *c: Eboraci.*
[24]  *c: Warsande.*
[25]  *b: milit'.*
[26]  *c: Medlai.*

# *Schirlyngton'* [Skirlington]

For Skirlington, which lay in the Aumale fee of Holderness, see Poulson, *Holderness*, I, 177–82; *VCH Yorks ER*, VII, 208–9. In 1086 there were 5 ct. soke of Hornsea in Skirlington, in the fee of Drogo de Bevrere. In 1284–85 the prior of Bridlington had 5 ct. in Skirlington and Arram, and in the undated feodary of the latter part of the reign of Henry III it was said that there were 2 ct. in Arram and 3 ct. in Skirlington (*KI*, pp. 75, 372).

The hospital's property in Skirlington appears to have been restricted to the annual thrave of wheat and the 3 a. land detailed in the three deeds which follow. Ralph son of Gilbert of Skirlington confirmed the thrave, which was originally granted by his parents, in *c.*1210 × *c.*1214 (R651). In 1214 × 1245 he gave a toft of 3 a., which was promptly let at fee-farm by the master for 2*s.* annually (R652, R653). A rent of 2*s.* in Skirlington paid to the hospital by Bridlington Priory was noted in a memorandum in the cartulary of Bridlington, and was still being paid at the Dissolution (*Ctl. Bridlington*, p. 322; Purvis, 'Monastic Rentals', p. 23). The rent doubtless originated in an assignment of the toft to the priory, but details of the transaction have not survived. The rent does not appear in the extents of the later thirteenth century nor the *Valor Ecclesiasticus*, but the post-Dissolution accounts include a rent in Skirlington (*Dissolved Houses*, IV, 226).

Farrer gives a brief note on the SKIRLINGTON family (*EYC*, III, 116). In 1180 × 1189[1] Gilbert of Skirlington attested a deed of William de Mandeville, earl of Essex (*EYC*, III, no. 1311). With his wife Emma, Gilbert made a quitclaim to William of Thorpe in 1182 × 1199[2] (*Ctl. Bridlington*, pp. 313–14). Gilbert of Skirlington's debt to the Crown of ½m. for a default first appears in 1190 and was paid in 1196 (*PR*, passim). Gilbert's wife was Emma or Emeline, daughter of Simon, who after her husband's death confirmed her father's gift of 1 ct. in Skirlington to Bridlington, and quitclaimed the rent of 5*s.* due on the property. Ralph, son of Gilbert of Skirlington and Emeline, issued a similar quitclaim on the same occasion (*Ctl. Bridlington*, p. 313). This may have been the land mentioned in a grant to the canons by William earl of York in '1147 × 1154'[3] of liberty in 3 ct. 5 bv. in his fee, including 1 ct. in Skirlington, 'for repair of an injury which he had done to them' (*EYC*, III, no. 1306). On 17 February 1228[/29] Ralph of Skirlington, son of Gilbert of Skirlington, confirmed property in Skirlington to Bridlington (*Ctl. Bridlington*, p. 316), and in 1232 Ralph of Skirlington made a fine with the prior of Bridlington confirming his gift of 10 bv. in Skirlington and agreeing to warrant another 14 bv. there (*YF*, 1232–1246, p. 4). Ralph of Skirlington, son of Gilbert of Skirlington, confirmed a grant of John, prior of Newburgh, in 1228 × 1232[4] (*Ctl. Bridlington*, p. 319). According to the chronicle of Meaux, Ralph married one Ernburgh, and by her had four daughters and coheirs named Marjorie, Beatrix, Cecilia and Alice (*Chron. Meaux*, I, 370; ibid., II, 102).

---

[1] Between the marriage in 1180 of William de Mandeville to Hawise, daughter and heir of William earl of Aumale, by which he acquired his interests in Holderness, and Mandeville's death in 1189 (*CP*, V, 118–19).

[2] After the death of Peter de Fauconberg, who was living in 1182, and before the death of Stephen, brother of Walter de Fauconberg (*EYC*, III, 48–49).

[3] As Aumale styles himself earl of York, the confirmation was almost certainly made in the reign of Stephen. The injury to the priory was doubtless the earl's occupation and fortification of the site of *c.*1143 (John of Hexham, *Historia regum*, II, 315).

[4] The earliest date for Prior John is 1228. The grant was included in the fine of 1232.

**R651.** Confirmation to the hospital by Ralph son of Gilbert of Skirlington of the grant in alms which his father and mother Emeline gave, being a thrave of wheat every year from his land of Skirlington, whosoever shall hold the land. Also a thrave every year [from every plough] ploughing, according to the custom of the country [*c.*1210 × *c.*1214]

[**f. 224ʳ**] *Radulfus filius Gilleberti de Schirlington' de una trava frumenti annuatim reddenda preter travas assisas.*
Omnibus has litteras visuris vel audituris Radulfus filius Gilleberti de Schirlington' salutem. Noverit universitas vestra me intui(tu) caritatis et pietatis concessisse et hac presenti carta mea confirmasse deo et pauperibus hospitalis beati Petri Ebor' in puram et perpetuam elemosinam elemosinam quam pater meus Gill(ebertus) et mater mea Emelina dederunt et concesserunt predictis pauperibus, scilicet unam travam frumenti singulis annis imperpetuum, percipiendam de terra mea de Schirlington', quicumque ipsam terram tenuerit. Et preterea travam singulis annis in predicta terra [de qualibet caruca]⁵ arante reddendam, scilicet secundum consuetudinem patrie. Hanc autem concessionem feci pro anima mea et pro animabus omnium antecessorum et successorum et beneficiorum nostrorum, ut simus participes omnium bonorum que fiunt vel fient in prefata domo dei imperpetuum. Hiis testibus, fratre Roberto capellano, Girardo, Waltero et aliis fratribus predicti hospitalis, Willelmo, Petro, Lamberto et aliis capellanis predicti hospitalis, Thoma de Langwath', Willelmo de Notyngham, Rogero de Derby et aliis clericis predicti hospitalis, Waltero de Alredale, Ingulfo, Ricardo fratre eius, Malgero marescaldo et aliis servientibus predicti hospitalis et multis aliis.

Thomas de Langwath usually attested as master after *c.*1220; Girard, Ingulf, and Mauger do not attest after Thomas de Langwath became master. Mauger attested only in the time of rector Ralph; Lambert attested as chaplain in *c.*1200 × *c.*1220; Walter of Allerdale indicates *c.*1210 × *c.*1235. All the witnesses to the present deed, with the exception of brother chaplain Robert and Walter of Allerdale, attested a deed of *c.*1200 × 1214 (R792).

**R652.** Gift to the hospital by Ralph son of Gilbert of Skirlington of a toft in Skirlington containing 3 a. land, being the toft which Michael Darci formerly held, which lies next to the toft of the prior of Bridlington on the west side [1214 × 1245]

*Radulfus filius Gilberti de Scirlington' de uno tofto et iii. acris in eadem villa.*
Omnibus cristi fidelibus ad quos presens scriptum pervenerit, Radulfus filius Gileberti de Scirlington' salutem. Noverit universitas vestra me caritatis intuitu et pro salute anime mee dedisse concessisse et hac presenti carta mea confirmasse deo et pauperibus hospitalis sancti Petri Ebor' unum toftum in Scirlingtona continens tres acras terre, videlicet illud toftum quod Michael Darci aliquando tenuit, et iacet iuxta toftum prioris de Bridlington' ex parte occidentali, tenendum et habendum predictis pauperibus de me et heredibus meis in puram et perpetuam elemosinam cum omnibus pertinenciis suis aisiamentis et libertatibus suis infra villam et extra cum libero introitu et exitu libere integre et quiete ab omni seculari servicio et exactione, sicut aliqua elemosina liberius et melius teneri potest et haberi. Ego autem et heredes predictum toftum cum pertinenciis predictis pauperibus warantizabimus adquietabimus et

⁵ Supplied.

defendemus in omnibus et contra omnes homines imperpetuum. Hoc pro me et heredibus meis tactis sacrosanctis iuravi et affidavi. In huius rei testimonium istud scriptum consignavi. Hiis testibus, Stephano clerico, Iohanne de Rednesse, Roberto fratre suo, Stephano filio Benedicti, Henr(ico) nigro, Stephano filio [Roberti]⁶ de Drenghou et multis aliis.

As the donor and the four leading witnesses attested the hospital's grant of the same land (R653) the same occasion is indicated. Michael Darci (*Aceciî*) had a grant of 2 bv. in Skirlington from Newburgh Priory in 1256 × 1262⁷ (*Ctl. Bridlington*, p. 318). Henry *dictus Niger* of Wilsthorpe made a quitclaim of lands in Wilsthorpe and Arram in Holderness (par. Atwick) to the priory of Bridlington (*Ctl. Bridlington*, p. 31). Stephen son of Benedict of Owstwick had interests in Skirlington (*Ctl. Bridlington*, p. 317). John and Robert of Reedness attested several deeds belonging to Bridlington Priory (*Ctl. Bridlington*, passim). Stephen son of Robert of Dringhoe (*Dring'*) attested a quitclaim to Bridlington made by Alan Burdoun of Winkton and Isabel his wife (*Ctl. Bridlington*, p. 325).

**R653.** Acknowledgement of receipt, with recital, by William son of Peter of Atwick, of the deed of master H[ugh], rector, and the brethren of the hospital, granting him a toft in Skirlington containing 3 a., specified as in R652, paying 2s. annually, and a portion of chattels as an obituary payment [1214 × 1245]

*Willelmus filius Petri testificat se suscepisse cartam hospitalis de uno tofto in Schirlington'.*
Sciant presentes et futuri quod ego Willelmus filius Petri de Attingwihc cartam hospitalis sancti Petri Ebor' suscepi in hec verba: Omnibus cristi fidelibus ad quos presens scriptum pervenerit magister H[ugo] rector et fratres hospitalis sancti Petri Ebor' salutem. Noverit universitas vestra nos concessisse et presenti carta nostra confirmasse Willelmo filio Petri de Attingwhic unum toftum in Scirlingtona continens tres acras terre, videlicet illud toftum quod Mich(ael) Darci aliquando tenuit et iacet iuxta toftum prioris de Bridlingtona ex parte occident(ali), tenendum et habendum predictum toftum cum pertinenciis suis aisiamentis et libertatibus suis infra villam et extra cum libero introitu et exitu sibi et heredibus vel assignatis suis exceptis iudeis et viris religiosis aliis a nobis libere integre et quiete ab omni servicio et exactione, reddendo inde nobis annuatim duos solidos pro omni servicio ad nos pertinente, medietatem ad Pent' et aliam medietatem ad festum sancti Martini in yeme. Et in obitu suo et heredum vel assignatorum suorum in eadem terra manentium portionem catallorum suorum eos contingentem in obitu suo pauperibus domus nostre nomine testamenti fideliter persolvent. Hoc autem fideliter observandum tactis sacrosanctis pro se et heredibus suis iuravit et affidavit. Nos autem predictam terram predicto Willelmo et heredibus vel assignatis suis warantizabimus quamdiu carta donatoris quam inde habemus nobis illam warantizare poterit. In huius rei testimonium istud scriptum consignavimus. Hiis testibus, Radulfo filio Gilberti de Scirlington', Stephano clerico, Iohanne de Redenese, Roberto fratre suo, Stephano filio Benedicti et multis aliis. In huius robur et testimonium huic scripto sigillum meum apposui.

The date range is the period for Hugh as rector. See the note to R652.

⁶   MS: *Stephano filio de Drenghou*; but see the note to the deed.
⁷   When R[ichard] was prior.

## Swauethorp'
## [Swaythorpe]

In 1086, Odo the crossbowman held 9 ct. in Swaythorpe, a lost vill near Thwing. The survey of 1284–85 includes 9 ct. in Swaythorpe in the Chauncy fee, but does not name the tenant. In 1316 Marmaduke of Thwing was lord of the vill, which he had been given by John of Octon IV c.1284 (KI, pp. 57, 311; FN: Octon). The Thwing estate in Swaythorpe passed with other Thwing lands to the Lumley family, and thence to Sir Thomas Heneage in 1579 (VCH Yorks ER, II, 253, 255). Robert of Warter gave the hospital a toft and croft in Swaythorpe in c.1160 × c.1185 (R654); and Walter of Warter, possibly his son, gave a toft in c.1200 × c.1220 (R655). We can surmise that these were the tenements granted out at fee-farm by rector Hugh in c.1232 × 1245 and rector Roger in 1276 × 1280 (R658, R659). There is no trace of Swaythorpe in the extents of the later thirteenth century, the Valor Ecclesiasticus, or the post-Dissolution accounts.

Robert of WARTER, possibly the hospital's benefactor, attested in 1148 × 1189[1] (Ctl. Bridlington, p. 166). It is uncertain whether he is to be identified with Robert son of Osmund of Warter, or with Robert son of Nigel of Warter, whose gifts of land in Warter to Meaux were placed in the time of Abbot Adam (1151–1160) and Abbot Philip (1160–1182) respectively by Abbot Burton (Chron. Meaux, I, 101, 173; EYC, x, nos 89–94). Alice of Swaythorpe, widow of Robert of Warter, gave land in Little Kelk to Robert Talun, which was confirmed by her son Walter, son of Robert of Warter, on the same occasion (Ctl. Bridlington, p. 164). Walter of Warter and Roger of Warter attested a deed of William of Octon possibly made in or before 1194[2] (EYC, II, no. 1068). Walter son of Robert of Warter witnessed a deed of John son of William of Octon in 1185 × 1207[3] (EYC, III, no. 1410). Roger of Warter and Walter his brother attested a deed of uncertain date belonging to Marton, near Bridlington (Ctl. Bridlington, p. 34). In 1206 a fine was made between Richard of Bossall and Maud his wife, and Roger of Warter and Maud his wife, whereby Roger and Maud recognised 2 bv. in Ganton to be the right of Maud, wife of Richard, in return for 2m. (PF John, p. 102).

**R654.** Gift to the hospital by Robert of Warter of a toft and croft in Swaythorpe [c.1160 × c.1185]

**[f. 225ʳ]** *Robertus de Wartria de uno tofto in Swauethorp'.*
Notum sit omnibus sancte matris ecclesie filiis tam futuris quam presentibus quod ego Robertus de Wartre et heredes mei concessimus et dedimus deo et pauperibus hospitalis sancti Petri Ebor' unum toftum et unum croftum in Suatorp' in puram et perpetuam elemosinam liberam et solutam et quietam ab omni humano servicio preter orationes pauperum, quam elemosinam predictis pauperibus contra omnes homines warentizabimus. Hiis testibus, Radulfo presbitero, Nicholao presbitero.

The suggested limits of date depend on the priests attesting. They were the leading witnesses to deeds of c.1160 × 1185 (R487) and c.1160 × c.1171 (R683).

[1] The period for G[regory], prior of Bridlington, who also attested.
[2] When William son of Robert of Octon was dead.
[3] For the date, see FN: Octon.

**R655.** Gift to the hospital by Walter of Warter of a toft in the vill of Swaythorpe, 16 perches in length and 6 perches in width, being that which Ranulf the clerk held, with common of pasture, waters, roads, and paths [*c.*1200 × *c.*1220]

PRINTED: *EYC*, II, no. 850, where dated 1190 × 1210.

*Walterus de Wartria de uno tofto in Swauethorp'.*
Omnibus has litteras visuris vel audituris Walterus de Wartre salutem. Noverit universitas vestra me dedisse et concessisse et hac presenti carta mea confirmasse deo et pauperibus hospitalis beati Petri Ebor' unum toftum in villa de Suauethorp', quod est in longitudine xvi. perticatarum et in latitudine vi. perticatarum, scilicet quod Ranulfus clericus tenuit cum communione predicte ville, scilicet in pasturis in aquis in viis in semitis in omnibus libertatibus et aisiamentis ad predictam villam de Suauetorp' pertinentibus infra villam et extra pro salute anime mee et animarum antecessorum et successorum meorum in puram et perpetuam elemosinam libere honorifice et quiete ab omni servicio et exactione sicut ulla elemosina liberius dari potest. Et ego predictus Walterus et heredes mei warantizabimus et adquietabimus predictis pauperibus predictum toftum contra omnes homines imperpetuum. Hiis testibus, Hereberto, Suano, Anketino, Reginaldo, Simone, Willelmo, fratribus, T[homa] de Languad', Rogero, Eustachio, Willelmo, Simone, clericis, Ingolfo, Waltero, Ricardo, Bernardo, Arnaldo, Petro servientibus et multis aliis.

Herbert indicates *c.*1200 × *c.*1230; Thomas de Langwath was usually called 'master' after *c.*1220; Richard the serjeant attested within *c.*1200–*c.*1220, and not after Langwath gained the title master.

# [Snapethorpe, in Kexbrough, WR]

The location of Jordan Foliot's grant (R656) is not immediately obvious. Farrer followed the cartularist and printed the deed with others belonging to Swaythorpe, but revised his identification to Snapethorpe (Wakefield) when he came to discuss the Foliot fee (*EYC*, III, 219n). But as the deed is attested by three important Lacy tenants, and was confirmed by Henry de Lacy, we can be sure that the land lay in the Lacy fee, which Snapethorpe (Wakefield), did not. For this reason Michelmore suggested that the place was Snapethorpe in Kexbrough township, Kexbrough being in the fee of Ilbert de Lacy in 1086 (*WYAS*, p. 305). Foliot held in Cudworth and Shafton, both some 6 m. east of Kexbrough (*EYC*, III, 221–22), but no further evidence to show his interest in Kexbrough or Snapethorpe has been found.[4]

No mention of Snapethorpe is made in the papal confirmation of 1148, but those of 1157 and 1173 include land in Snapethorpe (*Sneiptorp*, *Sneipetorp*) which Jordan Foliot gave (C178–C180 [*EYC*, I, nos 179, 186, 197]). The gift is also included in Henry de Lacy's amplified confirmation, probably dating originally from 1148 × 1155, as 'land in Snapethorp (*Snaipethorp*), which pays 5s., by the gift of Jordan Foliot' (R121). Snapethorp is not mentioned in the extents of the later thirteenth century, the *Valor Ecclesiasticus*, or the post-Dissolution accounts for the hospital.

---

4   Purdy names Foliot as a demesne tenant in Swaythorpe and cannot have seen Farrer's emendation (*VCH Yorks ER*, II, 255).

**R656.** Gift to the hospital by Jordan Foliot and his heirs of Leveric of Snapethorpe, and all the land which Leveric holds in Snapethorpe, with the toft and croft. This gift they gave towards payment of 7s. which Jordan's father William and brother Richard gave to the hospital each year [1148 × 1156]

PRINTED: *EYC*, II, no. 849, where dated 1160 × 1170.

*Iordanus Foliotth de manumissione Leuerici de Swauethorp' et de terra eiusdem.*
Sciant omnes videntes et audientes litteras has quod ego Iordanus Foliotth et heredes mei concessimus et dedimus et hac presenti carta confirmavimus deo et pauperibus hospitalis sancti Petri Ebor' Leuericum de Snaipetorp', et totam terram suam quam tenet de nobis in Snapethorp', cum tofto et crofto, plenariam in bosco et plano et terra arabili in pratis et pascuis et in aquis in viis et in semitis et in omnibus aisiamentis que ad prefatam terram pertinent in puram et perpetuam elemosinam solutam liberam et quietam et immunem ab omnibus geldis et consuetudinibus et exactionibus et auxiliis et ab omni humano et seculari servicio preter orationes pauperum, quam elemosinam warentizabimus et tuebimur contra omnes homines. Hanc autem elemosinam dedimus ad persolvendum septem solidos quos pater meus Willelmus et Ricardus frater meus singulis annis pauperibus prefati hospitalis dederunt. Istam vero elemosinam fecimus pro salute animarum nostrarum et omnium antecessorum nostrorum et heredum, ut simus participes omnium beneficiorum et orationum que fiunt vel facienda sunt in illa sancta domo dei tam in vita quam in morte nostra. Isti sunt testes, Henricus frater meus, Adam filius Petri, Umfridus de Ruhala, Willelmus de Insula, Simon Scutarius de Pontefracto, Suanus prepositus, Godwinus prepositus et plures alii.

There seems no reason to assign a date later than 1156, which is indicated as a *terminus ad quem* by the papal confirmation. For the grantor and his family, see *EYC*, III, 219–20; *EYF*, pp. 33–35.

**R657.** Acknowledgement of receipt, with recital, by Adam son of Alexander of Snapethorpe, of the deed of his father Alexander son of Robert son of Ranulf, granting Adam all his land in Snapethorp, which Alexander held of the hospital, except the toft with houses between the land of the hospital and the land of the Templars, and except an acre of land in two parts of the field, to hold to Adam and the heirs of his body by Custance his wife, paying Alexander 1d. and the hospital 4s. 8d. annually, and a portion of chattels as an obituary payment as other tenants of the hospital customarily do [c.1230 × c.1255]

*De terra in Suathorp'.*
Sciant omnes presentes et futuri quod ego Adam filius Alexandri de Snethorp'[5] recepi cartam Alexandri patris mei in hiis verbis: Sciant omnes presentes et futuri quod ego Alexander filius Roberti filii Ran(ulfi) dedi concessi et hac carta mea confirmavi Ade filio meo et heredi totam terram meam in Snaipethorp' quam tenui de magistro et fratribus hospitalis sancti Petri Ebor' sine ullo retenemento excepto tofto cum domibus iacent(e) inter terram dicti hospitalis et terram Templariorum et excepta una acra terre in duabus partibus campi iacente, tenend(um) et habend(um) sibi et heredibus suis de Custancia uxore sua procreatis totum predictum tenementum cum omnibus pertinenciis suis aisiamentis et libertatibus suis infra villam et extra de

---

5   MS: *Suethorp'*.

me imperpetuum, reddendo inde annuatim michi pro omni servicio et exactione unum denarium in festo sancti Martini, et magistro et fratribus hospitalis sancti Petri Ebor' pro omni servicio ad nos pertinen(te) iiii°ʳ solidos et octo denarios, medietatem ad festum sancti Martini in yeme et medietatem ad Pent', et portionem catallorum ipsum vel suos in obitu contingentem secundum consuetudinem aliorum tenentium dicti hospitalis. Ego autem dictus Alexander totum predictum tenementum cum suis pertinenciis dicto Ade et heredibus suis warantizabo sicut dominus meus magister hospitalis et fratres michi warantizaverunt vel warantizabunt. In huius autem rei robur et testimonium huic scripto sigillum meum apposui. Hiis testibus, et cetera. Et ne tempore succedente possit collusio fieri inter me et Alexandrum patrem meum vel aliq(uem) aliu(m) in preiudicium hospitalis. Huic scripto sigillum meum apposui et illud eidem hospitali dedi, obligando me et heredes meos ad omnia prescripta fideliter facienda. Hiis testibus, Henrico de Munketon' capellano, Petro de Thornhou(er), Thoma ianitore, Hugone socio suo, Petro Franceis, Rogero carpentario, Willelmo carpentario et multis aliis.

The forms *Snethorp* and *Snaipethorp* rule out Swaythorpe, so it is likely this deed belongs to the same place as R656. Most of those attesting appear sporadically in the hospital's deeds. Peter de Thornhouer attested in *c.*1235 × *c.*1260 (R491). Roger the carpenter, Hugh and Thomas the door keepers are amongst the witnesses to a deed concerning property in Blake Street, York, made in the mid-thirteenth century (C468 [Cott., f. 88ʳ⁻ᵛ]). Lemer the carpenter, Roger his brother, and Peter Franceys witnessed York deeds of 1238 × 1245 (C395, C744 [Cott., ff. 75ᵛ, 148ʳ]). Roger the carpenter, brother of Lemer the carpenter, was a tenant of property in Blake Street, which he gave to Michael, chaplain of the hospital (C454–C456 [Cott., f. 86ʳ⁻ᵛ]).

# [Swaythorpe resumes]

**R658.** Chirograph of grant at fee-farm by Roger, rector of the hospital, and the brethren, to Simon son of Alan of Swaythorpe of a toft and croft in Swaythorpe, which Simon's father once held of the hospital, paying 12*d.* annually, and a portion of chattels as an obituary payment [1276 × 1280]

*Copia carte de terra in Swauethorp' dimissa ad firmam.*
Omnibus ad quos presens scriptum pervenerit, rector Rogerus hospitalis beati Petri Ebor' et fratres eiusdem domus salutem in domino. Noveritis nos dedisse concessisse et hac presenti carta nostra confirmasse Simoni filio Alani de Swauthorp' quoddam toftum cum crofto in villa de Swauethorp' quod pater dicti Simonis quondam de nobis [**f. 225ᵛ**] tenuit, tenendum et habendum predicto Simoni et heredibus suis de nobis et successoribus nostris libere quiete integre ac pacifice imperpetuum, ita videlicet quod nec dictus Simon nec ipsius heredes dictum toftum cum crofto sine assensu nostro alicui dare vendere valeant vel assignare, reddendo inde annuatim nobis et successoribus nostris duodecim denarios argenti, videlicet medietatem ad festum Pent' et medietatem ad festum sancti Martini in yeme pro omnibus serviciis secularibus et demand(is). Nos vero et successores nostri dictum toftum cum crofto prefato Simoni et heredibus suis contra omnes homines warentizabimus acquietabimus et defendemus quamdiu carta donatoris nostri quam inde habemus nobis poterit illud warantizare. Idem vero Simon et heredes sui ac quicumque dictum toftum tenuerint seu manserint in eodem portionem catallorum suorum ipsos in obitu suo contin-

gentem pauperibus domus nostre nomine testamenti fideliter relinquent. In cuius rei testimonium sigillum commune domus nostre et sigillum dicti Simonis huic scripto cirograffato alternatim apponuntur. Hiis testibus, Henrico de Rouceby, Waltero de Garton', Willelmo filio Thome, Roberto fratre eius de Tueng', Willelmo Crosseman, Nicholao de Crosseby, Willelmo de Warter de Suauthorp' et aliis.

The date range is the period for Roger of Malton as rector.

**R659.** Acknowledgement of receipt, with recital, by William son of Stephen of Swaythorpe, of the deed of master Hugh and the brethren of the hospital granting him a toft in Swaythorpe which Ranulf the clerk held, with common of the vill, paying 1*lb.* pepper annually, and ½*m.* as an obituary payment [*c.*1232 × 1245]

*Transcript(um) Willelmi filii Stephani de tofto in Swauethorp'.*
Sciant omnes presentes et futuri quod ego Willelmus filius Stephani de Swauethorp' suscepi cartam hospitalis sancti Petri in hec verba: Omnibus cristi fidelibus ad quos presens scriptum pervenerit magister Hugo rector et fratres hospitalis sancti Leonardi Ebor' salutem. Noverit universitas vestra nos concessisse et hac carta nostra confirmasse Willelmo filio Stephani de Swauethorp' unum toftum in Swauetorp' quod Ranulfus clericus tenuit, tenendum et habendum illi et here(dibus) in feodo et hereditate libere et honorifice et quiete imperpetuum ab omni servicio et exactione ad nos pertinente, cum communione predicte ville de Swauethorp', videlicet in pasturis in aquis in viis in semitis et in omnibus aliis libertatibus et aisiamentis ad predictum toftum pertinentibus infra villam et extra, reddendo inde annuatim nobis pro omni servicio ad nos pertinente unam libram piperis in festo sancti Martini in yeme. Predictus vero Willelmus et heredes sui vel quicumque in predicta terra manserint vel predictam terram tenuerint pro portione catallorum suorum ipsos contingente in obitu pauperibus domus nostre dimidiam marcam argenti nomine testamenti fideliter persolvent. Hanc autem terram de nobis tenebunt predictus Willelmus et heredes sui quamdiu se legaliter erga nos habuerint. Et predictam firmam et predictum censum bene et plenarie fideliter et sine fraude persolverint. In huius autem rei robur et testimonium huic scripto sigillum nostrum apposuimus. Hiis testibus, fratre Roberto de Colingham, Iohanne de Notingham et aliis. In cuius rei testimonium huic scripto ego Willelmus sigillum meum apposui. Hiis testibus, Petro Franceis, Willelmo de Creik, Willelmo Scot, Ranulfo de Heselington', Iohanne ianitore et multis aliis.

Franceys, Crayke, Scot and Heslington attest in *c.*1214 × 1238 (R414), with Henry *ianitor*, rather than John *ianitor*. John of Nottingham, brother chaplain, indicates *c.*1232 × *c.*1245; Robert of Collingham indicates *c.*1214 × *c.*1245. Rector Hugh died in 1245.

# Seteryngton' [Settrington]

For Settrington, in the Bigod fee, see *EYC*, I, 494–95. The following deed appears to be the only evidence for the hospital interest in Settrington.

**R660.** Gift to the hospital by Alfred son of William of Settrington of a toft in Settrington, 4 perches in width and 12 in length [1157 × 1187]

PRINTED: *EYC*, I, no. 625, where dated 1180 × 1185 or *c.*1185 × 1208.

**[f. 226ʳ]** *Amfridus¹ filius Willelmi de i. tofto in Seterington'*.
Notum sit omnibus videntibus et audientibus litteras has quod ego Alfredus filius Willelmi de Seteringtona et heredes mei concessimus et dedimus deo et pauperibus hospitalis beati Petri Ebor' unum toftum in Seterington iiiiᵒʳ perticatas continens² in se latitudinis et xii. longitudinis in puram et perpetuam elemosinam liberum et quietum et solutum ab omnibus geldis et consuetudinibus. Hanc vero elemosinam confirmavimus predictis pauperibus et contra omnes homines warentizabimus ut simus participes omnium beneficiorum et orationum que fiunt in illa sancta domo dei tam in vita quam in morte. Hiis testibus, Roberto de Morevilla, fratre Gileberto de Loncastr', Willelmo Pictavense, Waltero filio Alani de Folifait, Ricardo Malherbe, Martino fratre eius, Toke fabro, Helia nepote magistri Suani,³ Rogero et Willelmo clericis hospitalis.

The range of date is given by the mastership of Swain. Everard son of Alfred held a tenement in Settrington in 1208 (*PF John*, p. 142).

---

¹   sic.
²   MS: *continent'*.
³   Farrer gives the alternative reading *Helia nepote magistri, Suain,* . . . .

## *Stillingflete* [Stillingfleet]

For Stillingfleet, see *VCH Yorks ER*, III, 101–12. According to the Domesday summary, the king held 2 bv., Erneis [de Burun] 2 ct., and Hugh son of Baldric 1½ ct. in 1086. There were also 2 bv. soke of Count Alan's manor of [Gate] Fulford. By the end of the twelfth century the hospital held 2 bv. in Stillingfleet in chief. Comparison of the Domesday tenants in Stillingfleet with those of the survey of 1284–85 (*KI*, p. 65), show this was the 2 bv. held by the king in 1086, but the hospital's benefactor is unknown. According to a doubtful deed in the Selby Coucher, master Paulinus granted 2 bv. in Stillingfleet to Henry son of William for 8*s.* annually in 1194 × 1202 (R811). For 6*m.*, Henry son of William of Leeds sold to John son of Daniel 2 bv. in Stillingfleet which Paulinus of Leeds, rector of the hospital, had given him. John was attorned by Henry to pay the hospital 8*s.* annually, and ½*lb.* of cumin to Henry's heirs at Stillingfleet (*Ctl. Selby*, no. 594). This was done in *c.*1200 × *c.*1220, without the consent of the hospital, which made an attempt to recover the land (R662–R664). This does not appear to have been successful, and later the tenancy was split into moieties. Richard son of John son of Daniel of York quitclaimed to Selby 1 bv. in Stillingfleet, which he had held of Henry son of William of Leeds, with an assart, and a rent of 6*d.* for a windmill (*Ctl. Selby*, no. 595). Richard son of John's conveyance to Selby was apparently in exchange for land in Acaster, which he sold to Robert of Stopham and Hawise his wife in 1221 × 1237.[1] In addition to the rent on the land at Acaster, Robert and Hawise agreed to acquit the abbey of an annual rent to the hospital of 4*s.* for 1 bv. land, a toft and a croft, and 6*d.* rent from a windmill in Stillingfleet (*Ctl. Selby*, nos 568–69). In 1284–85 the abbot of Selby had 1 bv. in Stillingfleet, and Warin le Calfherd 1 bv., both holding of the hospital (*KI*, p. 65). In 1287, the hospital's rents in Heworth [?] and Stillingfleet were said to be worth 33*s.* 4*d.* annually (R903). A rent in Stillingfleet, formerly belonging to the hospital, was mentioned in 1542 (*Dissolved Houses*, IV, 226).

**R661.** Agreement between the hospital and Lambert son of Hubert the smith of *Elflee*, whereby Lambert will pay to the hospital 2*s.* annually for the windmill of Stillingfleet whilst the land which John son of Daniel held in Stillingfleet was out of the hands of the hospital. When the land comes into the hospital's hands Lambert will pay 5*s.* annually [*c.*1210 × *c.*1220]

**[f. 226ᵛ]** *Lambertus filius Hugonis[2] fabr(i) de Elflee de ii.s. annuis de molendino ad ventum de Stillingflete.*

Hec est conventio facta inter magistrum et fratres hospitalis sancti Petri Ebor' ex una parte et Lambertum filium Huberti fabri de Elflee ex altera, quod dictus Lambertus singulis annis solvet dictis magistro et fratribus de molendino ad ventum de Stiflingflete duos solidos, videlicet medietatem ad Pent' et medietatem ad festum sancti Martini, quamdiu terra quam Iohannes filius Daniel' tenuit in Stiflingflete fuerit extra manum magistri et fratrum predictorum. Cum autem in manum eorundem venerit solvet predictus Lambertus et heredes sui imperpetuum de predicto molendino quinque solidos annuos medietatem ad Pent' et medietatem ad festum sancti Martini. Hec autem pro se et heredibus suis iuravit predictus Lambertus et affidavit et in super utraque pars huic scripto sigillum suum apposuit. Testibus, Willelmo, Roberto,

---

[1]   The period for Abbot Richard of Selby.
[2]   sic, i.e. not as in the body of the deed.

Bernardo, Rogero fratribus et capellanis hospitalis, Radulpho de Fontibus, Thoma de Langwath', Roberto de Stowa, Henrico de Cava et multis aliis.

Bernard and Robert of Stowe indicate *c.*1210 × *c.*1230; Thomas de Langwath usually attested as master after *c.*1220.

**R662.** Notification by Henry of Leeds that without the consent of the hospital he had sold to John son of Daniel of York the land of Stillingfleet which he had formerly held of the hospital [*c.*1200 × *c.*1220]

*Confessio Henrici de Ledes de vendicione terre de Stiflingflete.*
Omnibus presentes litteras visuris vel audituris, Henricus de Ledes salutem. Noverit universitas vestra me sine assensu et consensu magistri et fratrum hospitalis sancti Petri Ebor', immo eis invitis et reclamantibus, vendidisse Iohanni filio Daniel' de Ebor' terram de Stiflingflete quam aliquando de eis tenui. Ut autem hec rei veritas posteris innotescat, huic scripto sigillum meum apponere dignum duxi. Valete.

**R663.** Quitclaim by John, nephew of Thomas son of Herbert of York, to the hospital, of all right and claim he had in 2 bv. which Henry of Leeds holds of it in Stillingfleet. In return the hospital gave him the land in Ousegate [York] which Thomas son of Herbert formerly held of it, paying 1*m.* annually [*c.*1200 × *c.*1220]

*Quieta clamatio Iohannis nepotis Thome filii Herberti de ii. bovatis terre quas Henricus de Ledes tenet in Stivelingflete pro terra in Usegate quam Thomas filius Herberti aliquando tenuit, tenend(a) per firmam unius marce annue.*
Sciant omnes presentes et futuri quod ego Iohannes nepos Thome filii Herberti de Ebor' abiuravi et quietum clamavi et hac presenti carta mea confirmavi deo et hospitali sancti Petri Ebor' imperpetuum totum ius et clam(eum) quod habui versus predictam domum de duabus bovatis terre quas Henricus de Ledes tenet in Stivelingflete de magistro et fratribus predicti hospitalis. Et pro predicta quieta clamatione et abiurat(ione) concesserunt michi predicti fratres et carta sua confirmaverunt illa terram in Usegate quam Thomas filius Herberti aliquando de eis tenuit, scilicet tenend(am) michi et heredibus meis, in feodo et hereditate, pro una marca argenti annuatim sibi reddenda, medietate ad Pent' et medietate ad festum sancti Martini, quamdiu ego et heredes mei nos legitime habuerimus versus predictam domum et firmam predictam bene persolverimus. Hanc vero quietam clamationem ego et heredes mei warantizabimus predicto hospitali imperpetuum contra omnes homines sine impedimento et retenemento. Hiis testibus, Gerardo, Suano, Astino, Herberto, Leomar' et aliis fratribus predicti hospitalis, Willelmo, Petro, Iohanne, Petro, Waltero capellanis, Thoma de Languath, Eustach(io), Rogerio, Willelmo de Notingh(am), clericis, Ingolfo, Waltero nepote Mathei clerici thesaur(arii), Rogerio de Hustwaite et multis aliis.

Thomas de Langwath is usually called master after *c.*1220; brother Gerard did not attest after he had gained the title, and William of Nottingham once or twice only. Ingulf implies *c.*1200 × *c.*1220; Herbert *c.*1200 × *c.*1230.

**R664.** Release and quitclaim to the hospital by Henry of Leeds of the land he formerly held in Stillingfleet [*c.*1210 × *c.*1220]

*Resignatio Henrici de Ledes terre de Stifl'*.

Omnibus sancte matris ecclesie filiis ad quos presentes littere pervenerint, Henricus de Ledes salutem. Noverit universitas vestra me reddidisse resignasse et quietam clamasse magistro et fratribus hospitalis[3] sancti Petri Ebor' totam terram quam de illis aliquando tenui in Stiflingflete cum omnibus suis pertinenciis et quicquid iuris vel clamii in illa habui vel habere potui eisdem remisisse, et pro me et pro heredibus meis imperpetuum iurasse et affidasse quod numquam de predicta terra prenominat(is) magistro et fratribus controversia movebimus. Predictam autem resignationem et quiet' clamat' presenti carta sigillo meo confirmat(ionis) corroborare dignum duxi. Testibus, Roberto capellano, Girardo, Anketino, Thoma celler(ario), Waltero, Henrico, et aliis fratribus hospitalis, Petro, Willelmo, Rogero, Ricardo capellanis, Anketino de Esingwalde, Thoma de Langwath, Roberto de Stowa, Waltero de Alredale, Ricardo, Malgero, Roberto et multis aliis.

Thomas de Langwath is usually called master after *c.*1220; Gerard had ceased to attest by the time he gained the title. Robert of Stowe attested within *c.*1210–*c.*1230; Thomas the cellarer and Mauger *c.*1200–*c.*1220. Anketin of Easingwold attested a deed in 1204 × 1214, probably 1212 × 1214 (C88 [*EYC*, VI, no. 53]).

---

3   MS: *hospitalis* repeated.

## Skirpenbec [Skirpenbeck]

The Domesday schedule of the land of Odo the crossbowman includes 5 ct. 6 bv. in Skirpenbeck. In the summary Odo was said to hold 9 ct. in Skirpenbeck, of which the count of Mortain had 3 ct. 2 bv. No details for Skirpenbeck were given in the survey of 1284–85; but in 1302–03 there were 5 ct. 3 bv. in the Chauncy fee in Skirpenbeck, held by ten lay tenants. No monastic tenancies were noted (*KI*, p. 274).

By time of the Lindsey survey Odo the crossbowman's lands in Yorkshire and Lincolnshire had passed to Amfrey and Alfred de CHAUNCY (*EYC*, II, 175–76).[1] Amfrey was succeeded by Walter de Chauncy, who accounted in 1130 for £15 for the right to marry a wife of his own choice (*PR*, 31 Hen. I, p. 26). With the consent of his son and heir Alfred, Walter de Chauncy gave the advowson of the church of Skirpenbeck, with parts of his demesne there, to Whitby Abbey in the mid-twelfth century (*EYC*, II, nos 828–29). Walter was dead in 1161, when Alfred de Chauncy paid 12*m*. into the exchequer (*PR*, 7 Hen. II, p. 36).[2] Alfred was dead in 1165, when Amfrey de Chauncy owed 66s. 8d. and Simon de Chauncy the same amount (*PR*, 11 Hen. II, p. 50). In 1166 Amfrey held 5 k.f. in chief in Yorkshire, and Simon the same in Lincolnshire (*Red Bk*, pp. 378, 426). As Amfrey confirmed the church of Skirpenbeck to Whitby *sicut enim in carta patris mei*, and confirmed his father's gift to William de Fublet, it is clear he was a son of Walter and a brother of Alfred (*EYC*, II, nos 830–33). Farrer postulated that Simon was another brother, and that Amfrey and Simon had divided the fee (*EYC*, II, 176).

The monks of Byland already had sheepfolds in Skirpenbeck in or before 1181,[3] the latest date for Amfrey de Chauncy's gift of scattered plots containing a total of 72 a. and pasture for 400 sheep (*EYC*, II, no. 838). In 1177 × 1186[4] Amfrey de Chauncy made a gift of land in Skirpenbeck to the canons of St Peter, York (*EYC*, II, nos 840–44, 846). In the year to Michaelmas 1191 Amfrey made a payment towards the Welsh scutage, and at Michaelmas 1192 the sheriff accounted for the farm of Skirpenbeck *que fuit Ansfredi de Canci* for half a year (*PR*, 3&4 Ric. I, pp. 72, 218, 223). Amfrey must have died at about Easter 1192.[5]

Amfrey de Chauncy gave the hospital 1 ct. in Skirpenbeck in 1186 × 1189 (R665). The hospital promptly demised the land to Josce the Jew of York (R666), presumably to raise ready money. This was before March 1190, when Josce, the most prominent of the York Jews, died in the mass-suicide and massacre at York Castle.[6] The property of the dead Jews was seized by the Crown, and in 1194 the sheriff accounted for 20s. for 1 ct. in Skirpenbeck for half a year (*PR*, 6 Ric. I, p. 12). 40s. continued to be paid annually to the Crown until 1199, when Paulinus, master of the hospital of York, accounted for 15*m*. for having seisin of 1 ct. in Skirpenbeck 'which Josce the Jew held of him' together with a rent of 6d. in York (*PR*, passim; 1 John, p. 53). In 1199 × 1201 the hospital granted the carucate at fee-farm to Byland, at a rent of 2*m*. annually (R667). £20 was to be paid by the hospital to the monks if the land could not be guaranteed to them (R812). Nevertheless a carucate in Skirpenbeck was included in

[1] *EYC*, II, 175–77; *EYF*, pp. 15–17, and Sanders, *English Baronies*, pp. 78–79 give details of the Chauncy descent.
[2] No evidence for Sander's statement that Walter died *c.*1130 (Sanders, *English Baronies*, p. 78) has been discovered.
[3] Addressed to the archbishop of York, and attested by Robert the dean.
[4] Attested by Guy, master of schools, and Robert dean.
[5] Farrer, followed by Clay, assigned the death of Amfrey to 'before 1190' for reasons unstated.
[6] For Josce, see Davies, 'Jews of York', passim; Dobson, *Jews of York*, esp. pp. 12–13, 28.

the confirmation of Innocent III of 1204 (C182 [*Letters Innoc. III*, no. 562]). The land subsequently passed to master John Romeyn, subdean of York, to whom Hugh, rector of the hospital issued a quitclaim in the 2*m*. annual rent in 1228 × 1242 (R813). In 1249 Romeyn, by then archdeacon of Richmond, gave this and other property to Easby Abbey (*EYC*, II, 182; Easby cartulary, ff. 253$^v$–259$^r$).

**R665.** Gift to the hospital by Amfrey de Chauncey of 1 ct. in Skirpenbeck with four tofts and crofts, three tofts being in the vill next to the toft of William son of Hugh, and the fourth next to the toft of Ralph Burdun [1186 × 1189]

COPIES: *b* Rawl., f. 227$^r$; *c* Easby cartulary, f. 253$^v$, slightly abbreviated, no witnesses.
PRINTED: *EYC*, II, no. 839, from *c*, where dated 1160 × *c*.1180.

[**f. 227$^r$**] *Amfridus de Canceio de una carucata terre in villa de Scerpenbec' cum iiii$^{or}$ toftis.*[7] Omnibus sancte matris ecclesie filiis tam presentibus quam futuris litteras has visuris vel audituris, Amfridus de Canceio salutem. Universitati vestre notificetur me concessisse et dedisse et presenti carta mea confirmasse deo et beato Petro et sustentamento pauperum hospitalis sancti Petri Ebor' unam carrucatam terre in Scerpenbehc cum iiii$^{or}$ toftis et croftis, et in villa prenominata tria tofta iuxta toftum Willelmi filii Hugonis et quartum iuxta toftum Radulfi Burdun plenariam infra villam et extra, in viis et semitis in pratis et pascuis et aquis et in omnibus aisiamentis et libertatibus que ad eandem terram pertinent absque ullo retenemento, in puram et perpetuam elemosinam liberam et quietam et solutam et immunem ab omnibus geldis et consuetudinibus et auxiliis et exactionibus et ab omni humano et seculari servicio et etiam forensi servicio regis, et quam warentizabo et heredes mei post me imperpetuum ab omni servicio erga regem et omnes alios homines qui possunt mori. Et hoc eis affidavi tenend(um) et warentizand(um). Hiis testibus, Huberto decano, Hamone cantore et capitulo sancti Petri, Reinerio vicecomite et comitatu.

Hubert Walter succeeded as dean in 1186 and retained the dignity until he was elected bishop of Salisbury in 1189. Rainer of Waxham was undersheriff of Yorkshire whilst Ranulf de Glanville was sheriff, between 1175 and 1189 (*EYC*, I, no. 337n).

**R666.** It was inquired of the master of the hospital by Robert Ros, William de Aubeny, Simon de Kyme, and Thomas de Moulton, then justices itinerant of King John, how he holds a carucate in Skirpenbeck which Josce the Jew of York had held. He answered that Josce held through the hospital, and that the carucate was given to the hospital by Amfrey de Chauncy before Josce held, and the master showed the deed of Amfrey. When the Jew was dead, the carucate was taken into the hand of King Richard with other land of Josce. Afterwards, when Sir G[eoffrey] FitzPeter and Benedict Thalemunt were sent by the king to dispose of the lands of the Jews of York, the master redeemed the deed of the land as his right, by 15*m*. paid to King Richard, and the land was quit and this was enrolled in the roll at the exchequer in London. Afterwards, when other justices, Adam de Port, Simon of Pattishall, Ralph Hareng, Robert de Percy, Henry of Northampton, and Geoffrey de Lisle, came, it was recognised that the master and brethren owned the land. This was asserted by Robert de Percy, one of the justices [1213]

---

7    *c* has rubric *Amfr(idu)s de Chanceyo de i. carucata terre et iiii$^{or}$ toftis hospitali beati Leonardi Ebor'.*

*Qualit(er) resid(uum) negotium coram iusticiariis ultimo itinerantibus super carrucata terre de Scerpenbec'.*

Requisitus magister hospitalis sancti Petri Ebor' a Roberto de Ros, Willelmo de Albeni, Simone de Kime, Thoma de Muleton' tunc iusticiariis domini regis Iohannis itinerantibus quomodo teneret unam carrucatam terre in Scerpingbec quam Ioceus iudens Ebor' tenuerat. Respondit quod Ioceus per hospitale tenuit et quod illa carrucata terre data fuit hosp(itali) ab Amfredo de Canceio in puram et perpetuam elemosinam priusquam Ioceus illam habuisset, et inde cartam Amfredi ostendit magister hospitalis. Mortuo autem iudeo seisita fuit illa carrucata cum aliis terris quas Ioceus tenuerat in manu domini regis Ricardi. Postea cum missi essent a domino regi G[alfridus] filius Petri, et Benedictus Thalemunt iudeus ut disponerent de terris iudeorum Ebor', magister hospitalis redemit cartam terre predictam sicut ius suum per xv. marcas domino regi Ricardi datis, et quieta clamata est illa carrucata dicto hospitali. Et hoc inrotulatum est in rotulo Lond' ad scaccarium. Postea vero in adventu aliorum iusticiariorum, scilicet Ada de Port', Simon' de Patesshill', Radulfo Harang', Roberto de Perceio, Henrico de Nor'hat', Godfrido de Insula, mota questione de predicta carrucata terre et recognita predicta veritate possiderunt magister et fratres dicti hospitalis predictam carrucatam terre in pace. Huius autem rei perhibet testimonium Roberti de Perci qui tunc fuit unus iusticiariorum.

Benedict de Talemunt was one of the first four justices of the Jews recorded in 1198 (*Select Pleas, Starrs*, p. xx). Port, Pattishall and the other justices were in Yorkshire in the second half of 1208 (*General Eyre*, p. 68). On 25 February 1213 King John appointed Robert de Percy sheriff of Yorkshire, and on the same day issued a notification that he was sending Ros, Aubigny, Kyme and Moulton to investigate complaints against the sheriffs of Lincolnshire and Yorkshire and their officers, but there was no general eyre in that year (*RPat*, p. 97; *General Eyre*, p. 71).

**R667.** Agreement in chirograph form between the monks of Byland and the hospital, made in the time of Hamo, abbot of Byland, and master Paulinus, proctor of the hospital. Master Paulinus and the brethren have granted to the abbot and convent the carucate which they have in Skirpenbeck by gift of Amfrey de Chauncy, and by confirmation of King John, to be held of the hospital, paying *2m.* annually [27 May 1199 × 4 March 1201]

COPIES: *b* Rawl., f. 227ʳ; *c* Easby cartulary, ff. 254ᵛ–255ʳ, no witnesses. NOTED: Byland cartulary, f. 115ʳ (old f. 221ʳ) *C(art)a cy(rographata) fratrum hospitalis sancti Petri Ebor' de una carucata terre in Skirpenbek' quam habuerunt ex dono Amphridi de Cauncy reddendo eis duas marcas annuatim.* CALENDAR: *Ctl. Byland*, no. 1154 from *c*.

*Cyrograph' inter abbatem de Belland' et hospitale de ii. marcis annuis pro Scerpinbec.*[8]
Hec est conventio inter monachos sancte Marie de Bella Landa et conventum fratrum hospitalis sancti Petri Ebor' tempore Hamonis abbatis de Bellalanda et magistri Paulini procuratoris predicti hospitalis. Magister Paulinus et predicti fratres communi consilio et assensu dimiserunt et concesserunt et presenti scripto confirmaverunt abbati de Bella Landa et conventui domus eiusdem illam carrucatam terre quam habuerunt in territorio de Scerpingbec ex donatione Amnfridi de Kanci et ex confirmatione regis Iohannis, tenendam de fratribus predicti hospitalis proprie libere solute et quiete ab

---

[8]    *c* has rubric *Magister hospitalis sancti Leonardi et conventus de eadem terra monachis Bellelande.*

omni terreno servicio et exactione seculari excepta regia exactione cum toftis et
croftis et cum omnibus pertinenciis suis et libertatibus et aisiamentis infra villam et
extra sine ullo retenemento, scilicet in terra et aqua in bosco et plano in pratis et
pasturis in viis et semitis et in omnibus aliis aisiamentis imperpetuum pro duabus
marcis argenti predictis fratribus annuatim solvendis, scilicet una marca ad festum
sancti Martini et una marca ad Pent'. Et predicti fratres warantizabunt predictam
terram cum pertinenciis omnibus prefatis monachis contra omnes homines imperpetuum, sicut sibi ipsis eam liberius poterunt warantizare. Et ne tempore succedente
possit aliqu(is) ab alterutra parte hec conventio infringi, predicti monachi et fratres
hospitalis hoc cirographum inter se inde fecerunt et utriusque partis sigill(is) appensis
roboraverunt,[9] et in capitulo utriusque domus recitari fecerunt. Hiis testibus, Simone
decano Ebor', Reginaldo precentore, Hamone thesaur(ario) et capitulo sancti Petri,
Stephano celerario, Anketino, Suano, Gamello et aliis fratribus predicti hospitalis.

This agreement was drawn up between the accession of King John and the death of
Reginald the precentor, which occurred before 4 March 1201. It is curious that the
confirmation by King John, if it ever existed, has not been preserved in the cartularies
of the hospital, Byland, or Easby, nor in the charter rolls, which begin in July 1199,
some six weeks after John's coronation.

[9] *b*: *et utriusque . . . roboraverunt* repeated.

## *Stokton'*[1] [Stockton on the Forest, NR]

For Stockton on the Forest, see *VCH Yorks NR*, II, 190–93. In 1086 the archbishop held 3 ct. and Count Alan 3 ct. in Stockton. The archbishop's land later became part of the prebend of Bugthorpe (*YMF*, II, 15). 3 ct. in Stockton were confirmed to the hospital by Eugenius III in 1148. The land in Stockton was not included in the confirmations of 1157 or 1173, but was noticed in that of 1204 (C178–C180, C182 [*EYC*, I, nos 179, 186, 197; *Letters Innoc. III*, no. 562]). The hospital appears to have originally acquired the land at a rent of 20s. annually from Thomas Guacelinus, who held of Mowbray, in *c.*1138 × 1148 (R814). The land was presumably part of Mowbray's fee of the honour of Richmond. The relationship, if any, between Thomas Guacelinus and Geoffrey son of Reiner, who gave what must have been the same 3 ct. to the hospital in *c.*1160 × 1171 (R668), and gave a toft in *c.*1170 × 1184 (R669), is not known. In 1218 justices were appointed to hold an assize of novel disseisin which Thomas de Normanville arraigned against the master of the hospital and Roger de Stapleton concerning Thomas' free tenement in Stockton (*PatentR*, 1216–1225, pp. 174–75). Page gives details of the subsequent tenants, but the hospital's interest cannot be discerned, and by 1303 the land was said to be in the Mauley fee (*VCH Yorks NR*, II, 191). Stockton does not appear in the extents of the later thirteenth century, the *Valor Ecclesiasticus*, or the account of 1542.

**R668.** Gift to the hospital by Geoffrey son of Reiner of 3 ct. in Stockton [*c.*1160 × 1171]

ORIGINAL: *a* YAS, MD59/1/77/2, formerly MD59/21/Misc (part), 16 cm. (wide) × 10 cm., bottom turn-up, slit for seal tag, seal gone. Medieval endorsements: *H(ec) est karta Gaufridi filii Reineri de Stocatuna*; *script'*; numeral not visible. COPY: *b* Rawl., f. 228ʳ. PRINTED: *EYC*, IV, no. 120, from *b*, where dated '*ante* 1175'. FACSIMILE: Plate IX.

**[f. 228ʳ]** *Hec est carta Gaufridi filii Reineri de Stocatuna.*
Notum sit omnibus videntibus et audientibus litteras has quod ego Gaufridus filius Reinerii concessi et dedi deo et pauperibus hospitalis beati Petri Ebor' tres carrucatas terre in Stocatuna cum omnibus que ad eandem terram pertinent in liberam et puram et perpetuam elemosinam quietam et solutam ab omni seculari servicio et consuetudine preter forense servicium, quam videlicet terram ego warentizabo predictis pauperibus contra omnes homines. Hanc elemosinam dedi prenominatis pauperibus pro anima patris mei et matris mee et omnium antecessorum meorum ut simus[2] participes omnium bonorum que fiunt in illa sancta domo in vita et in morte. His testibus, magistro Benedicto cementario, Willelmo albo, Gerardo de Lundoniis, Hugone cementario, Lamberto filio Osmundi, Ingeram filio magistri Benedicti, Osberto cementario, Ketello Westmering, Radulfo presbitero, Petro clerico de Biri, Rogero Nicher et Osberto filius[3] eius, Gerardo filio Pagani, Lamberto filio Reginaldi, Helya de Waddewrthe, Mildret de Midlinctun', Willelmus de Uckerbi, Alanus Bigot de Bartun, Alanus filius Elinant de Barton, Ricardus filius Toraldi de Latu(n),

---

[1]  *in Northryddyng'* has been added in the margin, by a hand possibly of the mid-fifteenth century, which has made a similar annotation to the Over Helmsley heading on f. 220ᵛ.

[2]  *b: scimus.*

[3]  *a*: sic, using the usual 'arabic 9' symbol for *us*. The possibility that *filiis* was intended ought not perhaps to be ruled out, but the scribe's lack of attention to the cases of witness names favours *filius*.

Willelmus de Cutuna filius Iichel, Ricardus de Brettevill', Elinant de Crachale, Alanus
de Kerrecan, Willelmus filius Eldredi.[4]

The witness Meldred of Middleton [Tyas] died in 1168 × 1175 (*EYC*, IV, 142). At
Michaelmas 1168 Alan son of Elinand [of Barton, some 6 m. south west of Darlington]
owed 20*m*. for the fine of his land in Yorkshire (*PR*, 14 Hen. II, p. 87; ibid., 15 Hen. II,
p. 35). In the account of Michaelmas 1171 Robert son of Elinand owed 40 hawks
for the fine of the land which Alan his brother had held (*PR*, 17 Hen. II, p. 73). This
suggests Alan was only in possession *c*. 1167–1171 (*EYC*, V, 102).

**R669.** Gift to the hospital by Geoffrey son of Reiner of a toft in Stockton surrounded
by a ditch [*c*. 1170 × 1184]

ORIGINAL: *a* YAS, MD 59/1/77/1, formerly MD 59/21/Misc (part), 10–11 cm. (wide)
× 17–19 cm., no turn-up, two slits for seal tag (gone), 4 mm. apart and not vertically
aligned. Medieval endorsements: *Galfri' fil' Reiner' de i. tofto in Stoketon'*; *script'*; numeral
not visible. COPY: *b* Rawl., f. 228[r]. PRINTED: *EYC*, IV, no. 121, from *b*, where dated *c*. 1174
× *c*. 1181. FACSIMILE: Plate X.

*Galfridus filius Reineri de uno tofto in Stoketon'.*
Notum sit omnibus videntebus et audientibus literas has quod ego Gaufridus filius
Reinerii et heredes mei concessimus et dedimus deo et pauperibus hospitalis beati
Petri Eboraci unum toftum in Stoket' ex omni parte fossato circumdatum in puram
et perpetuam elemosinam, ut simus[5] participes orationum et elemosinarum que in
doma[6] prefata fiunt. His testibus, Radulfo de Val' eo tempore vic(ecomite), Roberto
filio Radulfi, Torphino de Manefeld, Akaris de Halnathebi, Alano clerico de Sindarebi,
Alano Soldan, Alinad filio Akaris, Rogero filio Fromundi, Valtero de Stoket', Willelmo
filio Meldred', Roberto filio Elinand.

The witness Ralph de Valognes was sheriff of Richmond. A deed of 1174 × 1181 was
sworn in his hand in the court of Richmond (*EYC*, IV, no. 93), and he attested two
deeds of 1156 × 1181[7] as sheriff (*EYC*, V, nos 284–85). His predecessor as sheriff,
Wigan son of Cades, attested in 1159 × 1171 (*EYC*, V, 357). Robert son of Ralph [of
Middleham] succeeded his father in 1168 or later and died in 1184 or 1185 (*EYC*, V,
302); William son of Meldred [of Middleton Tyas] succeeded in 1168 or later, and was
dead in 1184 (*EYC*, IV, 142); Robert son of Elinand succeeded his brother in 1170–1 or
shortly before (FN). Acaris of Halnaby and Halnath his son attested a deed of '*c*. 1190
× *c*. 1192' (*EYC*, V, no. 184B).

---

4   *a*: sic, switches to nominative witness.
5   *b*: *scimus*.
6   *b*: *domo*.
7   Witnessed by Alan son of Brian [of Bedale], implying 1156 × 1188 (*EYC*, V, 201–3), and addressed to
    the archbishop of York.

# *Southecave* [South Cave]

For South Cave, see *VCH Yorks ER*, IV, 37–59. In 1086 Robert Malet held 24 ct. in [South] Cave and 7 ct. 2 bv. in another [North] Cave. Much of this land passed, with other Malet holdings, to Nigel d'Aubigny, father of Roger de Mowbray (*EYC*, III, 454–57; *Mowbray Charters*, p. xxiv). Roger de Mowbray made benefactions in [South] Cave to York Minster, and possibly to the prior and monks of Durham (*EYC*, III, 434). He also gave ½ ct. and 5 a. in [South]¹ Cave to the monks of Byland (*EYC*, III, nos 1827–28).

The *mansura* which the hospital held of Roger de Mowbray in Cave was confirmed by Archbishop Theobald in 1154 (C194 [*EYC*, I, no. 185]). A *mansum* in *Marcacava* (South Cave)² was included in the papal confirmations to the hospital of 1157 and 1173 (C179, C180 [*EYC*, I, nos 186, 197]). But Roger de Mowbray's deed of gift of 32 a. in [South] Cave, which was confirmed by his son Nigel on the same occasion, was given *c.*1160 × Sept. 1182 (R670), so either refers to different land or was made retrospectively. Alexander of Sancton gave 1½ a. in the meadow of South Cave in 1208 × 1249 (R675). William de Daiville gave 8 bv. in [South] Cave in 1208 × 1214 (R673), and his son Roger de Eyville gave a small piece of salt meadow in *c.*1270 × *c.*1285 (R672). In 1297, Walter of Langton, master of the hospital, claimed a messuage in South Cave against Margaret daughter of John Haldayne (Baildon, *Monastic Notes*, I, 247). In 1385 the then master, Richard Ravenser, claimed against John Garpe, clerk, a messuage in Ellerker, which is close to South Cave (ibid., I, 249). South Cave is not mentioned in the hospital's extents and rentals of the late thirteenth century, nor the *Valor Ecclesiasticus*. The post-Dissolution accounts indicate that part of the hospital's property in South Cave was included in the manor of Broomfleet (*Dissolved Houses*, IV, 224, 226).

Benefactions to the hospital of land in South Cave were made by three successive generations of the DAIVILLE family (R672–R674). In the twelfth century the name was usually given as 'de Daiville' or similarly, but during the thirteenth century it became 'de Eyville' or 'Deyville' (*CP*, IV, 130n). The family's interests in South Cave originated in '*c.*1170 × 1184', when Roger de Mowbray gave all his remaining demesne in [South] Cave, after the enfeoffment of Nicholas de Bellun and Robert le Norreis, to Roger de Daiville, as ½ k.f. (*Mowbray Charters*, no. 360). In the 1180s Roger de Mowbray ordered Roger de Daiville and other tenants of his demesne to cease withholding the ninth sheaf from the hospital (C335 [*Mowbray Charters*, no. 315]). William de Daiville and Roger de Daiville appear as brothers (*Mowbray Charters*, nos 343, 349), and as William also appears as brother to Robert de Daiville (ibid., nos 70, 307) Greenway postulated that William and Roger were younger brothers to the Robert de Daiville who held 4 k.f. of old feoffment and 1 k.f. of new

---

¹ It is unclear why Farrer, followed by Greenway and Burton, assigned this gift to North rather than South Cave. Both of Mowbray's deeds relating to the gift refer to *Cava*, though Burton calendars this as 'North Cave' (*Mowbray Charters*, nos 41, 62; *Ctl. Byland*, nos 153–54; cf. *VCH Yorks ER*, IV, 47). Most of the Byland entry is missing from the *Valor Ecclesiasticus* (op. cit., V, 93), but a post-Dissolution account shows that it had a tenement in South Cave at farm for 13*s.* 4*d.* annually. North Cave is not mentioned (*MA*, V, 355; *Dissolved Houses*, IV, 188). In the mid-thirteenth century the abbot of Byland granted ½ ct. and 5 a. in *Cava* to Simon son of Simon *de Cave* for a rent of 1*m.* (Byland cartulary, f. 22/124ʳ; *Ctl. Byland*, no. 155, where both place and personal names are calendared as 'North Cave').

² For the identification of *Marcacava* with South Cave, which rests on the market held there, see *PN YorksER*, p. 223; cf. *EYC*, III, no. 1825.

feoffment of Mowbray in 1166 (ibid., no. 360n).[3] Roger de Daiville was the leading lay witness to Thomas Hay's confirmation to the hospital of property in North Cave (R600), and attested William de Mowbray's confirmation to the hospital made in 1194 × 1201[4] (*CalCh*, 1257–1300, p. 442, no. 20).

Roger was probably dead in 1204, when William de Daiville was a juror in a plea concerning land in Sancton (Stenton, *Pleas*, III, no. 909). In or before 1208,[5] William son of Roger de Daiville granted 7 bv. in *Esebi*, with lordship of a further 3 bv. there, and land in *Birchau*,[6] to Fountains Abbey in exchange for £10 and 6 ct. in Sancton (*Ctl. Fountains*, p. 101). In 1208 × 1214 William de Daiville gave the hospital 8 bv. in Cave for his own soul and that of his father Roger (R673). In 1218–19 he withdrew a plea of novel disseisin against Roger of Cave concerning a tenement in Cave (*Yorkshire Eyre Rolls*, no. 347). He occurs as a knight in Yorkshire in 1223 and 1224 (*CRR*, 1223–1224, nos 1148, 2142), and in 1225 was impleaded by Denise, widow of Geoffrey de Bellun, for her right in dower in 5 bv. in Cave (ibid., 1225–1226, nos 385, 482). In 1231, William de Eyville made a fine concerning 2 bv. in Cave (*YF*, 1218–1231, pp. 150–51).

In the cartulary of Fountains Abbey is a copy of a deed by which a member of the Mowbray family gave in frank-marriage to William de Daiville, with Maud his aunt (*patrua*) and to William's heirs by Maud, 1 ct. in Nutwith [near Aldburgh, Masham, NR] (*Ctl. Fountains*, p. 18). Mowbray's first name has been omitted by the copyist. Lancaster suggested the deed belonged to William de Mowbray, who was son of Nigel de Mowbray I, had seisin of his lands in 1194, and died in 1223–24 (*CP*, IX, 373–74). If so, William de Daiville's wife Maud was a daughter of Roger de Mowbray I, and probably illegitimate, as chronological considerations make it unlikely she was a daughter of Roger's wife Alice de Gant.[7] But it is more likely that the grant in frank-marriage was made by William de Mowbray's eldest son Nigel de Mowbray II, who held the Mowbray fee between 1223 and 1230 (*CP*, IX, 375), which would make Maud a sister of William de Mowbray and a daughter of Nigel de Mowbray I.[8] William de Daiville, by the consent and wish of Maud de Mowbray his wife gave to Geoffrey de Lund 1 bv. in Nutwith in the territory of [Grewel]thorp. He made another grant in Nutwith to Walter de Thorp (*Ctl. Fountains*, pp. 346–47). Walter of Hedon claimed 5 bv. in Nutwith against William de Eyville and Maud his wife in 1230. Walter quitclaimed his right for 4½m. (*YF*, 1218–1231, p. 126; *CRR*, 1227–1230, no. 2480; ibid., 1230–1232, nos 19, 79). William de Daiville of Cave and Maud his wife gave the monks of Fountains a culture called *Hedunridding* beside the vill of *Thorp in Kirkebysiria* [Grewelthorpe] (*Ctl. Fountains*, p. 19). A quitclaim in the property in *Esebi* and *Birchau* was issued by Maud, widow of William de Daiville of

---

3  For the antecedents and descendants of Robert de Daiville, of Egmanton (Notts.) and Adlingfleet (WR), see FN; *CP*, IV, 130–34; *YF*, 1246–1272, p. 57n; *EYC*, IX, 98, 222–23; *EYF*, pp. 23–24; De Ville, 'Deyville', passim.

4  After Mowbray had seisin of his lands in 1194, and before the death of the witness Geoffrey Haget in 1199 × 1201 (FN).

5  The deeds are witnessed by Alan son of Ellis of Hammerton, who was probably dead in that year (FN).

6  Stated by Lancaster to be lost places adjacent to Baldersby, near Thirsk, par. Topcliffe (cf. *EYC*, XI, 48, 261).

7  Roger de Mowbray and Alice de Gant married in 1141 × 1143, and their sons Nigel and Robert appear to have been born in the 1140s. Alice probably died 1176 × c.1181 (*CP*, IX, 372; *Mowbray Charters*, pp. xxv–xxvi, xxviii–xxix, xxxii).

8  De Ville's assertion that the marriage took place 'by 1180' cannot be accepted (De Ville, 'Deyville', p. 17). The source of the statement in Keats-Rohan, *Domesday Descendants*, s.n. de Moubrai, that Roger had an (unnamed) daughter who married William de Daiville, is unclear.

## DAIVILLE OF SOUTH CAVE

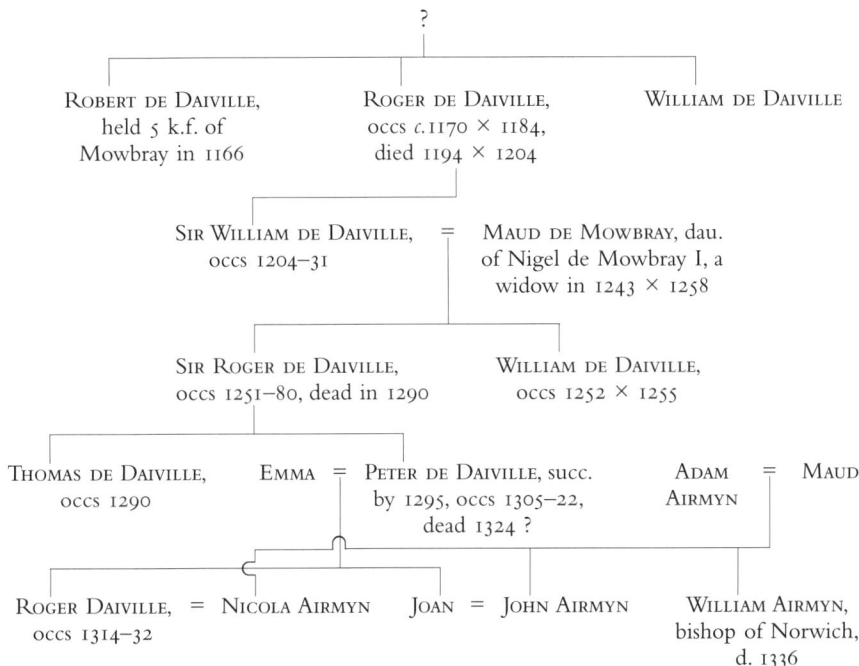

?

ROBERT DE DAIVILLE, held 5 k.f. of Mowbray in 1166 | ROGER DE DAIVILLE, occs *c.*1170 × 1184, died 1194 × 1204 | WILLIAM DE DAIVILLE

SIR WILLIAM DE DAIVILLE, occs 1204–31 = MAUD DE MOWBRAY, dau. of Nigel de Mowbray I, a widow in 1243 × 1258

SIR ROGER DE DAIVILLE, occs 1251–80, dead in 1290 | WILLIAM DE DAIVILLE, occs 1252 × 1255

THOMAS DE DAIVILLE, occs 1290 | EMMA = PETER DE DAIVILLE, succ. by 1295, occs 1305–22, dead 1324 ? | ADAM AIRMYN = MAUD

ROGER DAIVILLE, occs 1314–32 = NICOLA AIRMYN | JOAN = JOHN AIRMYN | WILLIAM AIRMYN, bishop of Norwich, d. 1336

Cave, in 1243 × 1258.[9] By another deed, before the same witnesses, and described similarly, she confirmed the culture called *Hedunridding* to the monks (*Ctl. Fountains*, pp. 19, 101).

William was succeeded by his son Roger. Roger de Daiville was named in fines concerning South Cave in 1251 and 1252 (*YF*, 1246–1272, pp. 53, 87), and in 1252 × 1255 witnessed, with his brother William, a quitclaim in South Cave (*YMF*, II, no. 56). In June 1253 Roger de Eyville of South Cave was granted exemption for life from being put on assizes, juries and recognitions (*CalPat*, 1247–1258, p. 195); and in the same year he assigned to the Templars the market and fair in South Cave which he held by the king's grant (*Cat. Anc. Deeds*, III, D.141). In 1274–75 Roger de Daiville claimed to have the assize of bread and ale in South Cave, as also did the Templars (*YQW*, p. 101). Roger de Eyville, son of Sir William de Eyville, knight, gave the hospital salt meadow [in South Cave ?] in *c.*1270 × *c.*1285 (R672). In 1280 Roger de Eyville confirmed a toft and 2 bv. in South Cave to the Templars at an annual rent of 7*s.*, for 60*m.* (*YF*, 1272–1300, pp. 38–39).

Roger was presumably dead in February 1290, when a commission of oyer and terminer was issued touching an appeal by Thomas son of Roger de Eyville of

9   Witnessed by Peter de Daiville, then bailiff of Ripon. Peter de Daiville occurs as bailiff of Ripon shortly after June 1250, 1247 × 1252 (with Stephen, abbot of Fountains), 1254, 1255 and March 1256[/57] (*Ctl. Fountains*, pp. 94, 144, 349, 570, 666, 707, 763). Warin was bailiff at Christmas 1242 (*Mem. Ripon*, IV, 72–73), and John de Tocotes in May 1258 (*Ctl. Fountains*, p. 544). De Ville's statements that Peter de Daiville was bailiff of Ripon in 1220, and held South Cave *c.*1220, are doubtful (De Ville, 'Deyville', pp. 3, 17). No evidence has been found to show the bailiff was a member of the branch of the family which held in South Cave.

South Cave against brother Robert de Halton, master of the bailiwick of the Temple in Yorkshire, and several others, for the death of Thomas's brother William (*CalPat*, 1281–1292, p. 344). In 1293 a pardon was issued to master Thomas of Burland, canon of Lincoln, for abetting Thomas de Eyville to appeal brother Robert de Halton of the Templars for the death of William de Eyville at Cave, of which abetting master Thomas had been convicted at Nottingham (*CalPat*, 1292–1301, p. 6).

Peter de Eyville had succeeded by 1295 (R674). In 1296 Peter, son of Roger de Eyville of Cave, made a fine with master Thomas of Burland[10] concerning the manor of Burland [in Eastrington] (*YF*, 1272–1300, p. 116). In Hilary term 1305 Peter de Eyville claimed 1 ct. in Nutwith from the abbot of Fountains, claiming that the abbot had no entry except by a lease which William de Eyville, Peter's grandfather, made to Abbot William,[11] for a term now past. The abbot produced William and Maud's deed concerning Hedunriding, but Peter claimed this related to different land. It seems Peter later accepted the abbot's claim, for in 1310 Peter de Eyville of Cave quitclaimed to the abbot all right in 1 ct. in Masham, in a place called Hedunriding (*Ctl. Fountains*, pp. 19–20). In 1308 Peter de Eyville had a grant of free warren in South Cave, Burland and Spaldington, and in 1314 he was granted a weekly market in South Cave, and an annual fair (*CalCh*, 1300–1326, pp. 121, 237). The lords of South Cave in 1316 were named as Peter de Eyville and Alexander of Cave. Peter de Eyville, Alexander of Cave, and John son of John of Cave, were lords of South Cliff with North Cliff (*KI*, p. 309).

In 1313–14 William Airmyn, clerk,[12] issued a deed noting that Sir Peter de Eyville, knight, lord of South Cave, had undertaken that Roger, Peter's eldest son, would marry Nicola, William's sister (MS Dods. 68, f. 52ʳ).[13] It was doubtless in connection with this marriage that Peter de Eyville, knight, acknowledged that he owed William Airmyn, clerk, 500*m*., in June 1314. There were further acknowledgements of debt between the pair, including statements of debts owed by Airmyn to Eyville (*CalCl*, 1313–1318, pp. 99, 103, 209, 335; ibid., 1318–1323, p. 129). Early in 1319 Roger son of Peter de Eyville, knight, granted to William Airmyn, clerk, £10 of the yearly rent of £20 which Peter had given to Roger and his wife Nicola and their heirs, to be received from Peter's manor of South Cave. Roger came into chancery with Peter his father and acknowledged the deed (*CalCl*, 1318–1323, p. 127). It is stated in an Airmyn pedigree that Joan, daughter of an unnamed Daiville, was married to John Airmyn, brother of William Airmyn, sometime bishop of Norwich, and was living as his widow in 1337 (*Lincs. Pedigrees*, I, 38).

In January 1322 a licence in mortmain was issued for the alienation by Peter de Eyville of a messuage, 2 bv. land, and 17*s*. 8*d*. rent in Howden, Burland, Portington and Eastrington for a chaplain to celebrate divine service for Peter, Emma his wife, master Thomas of Burland, and the ancestors and successors of Peter and Emma (*CalPat*, 1321–1324, p. 46). Sir Peter de Eyville attested an Owsthorpe (near Eastrington) deed in May 1322 (Anon., 'Yorkshire Deeds', *YAJ*, XVII, 107). In 1323 Roger de Eyville and Nicola his wife were granted a pardon for acquiring without licence for their lives a messuage, 19 tofts, a mill, 24 bv. and 3 a. land, 90 a. meadow, and 52*s*. 4*d*. rent in South

---

[10] For Burland, see Emden, *Oxford*, s.n. Birland. He was apparently a relative of the Daivilles of South Cave, but the exact connection has not been established.

[11] It is doubtful whether the lease, if it existed, was made to Abbot William. William de Daiville was dead before William of Allerton became abbot in 1252, and it is improbable that the lease dated from the rule of the previous Abbot William in *c*.1180–1190.

[12] For the career of William Airmyn (d. 1336), bishop of Norwich, see *ODNB*.

[13] Dodsworth's abbreviation of a deed then belonging to Thomas Danby of South Cave, *armiger*. Other fourteenth century Eyville deeds are also noted, but in very abbreviated form.

Cave, from John de Mowbray, who held them in chief, subject to rendering Mowbray £22 annually (*CalPat*, 1321–1324, p. 296). In 1324 William de Moreby, living in Cavil (near Eastrington) granted a messuage in Cavil to Roger son of Sir Peter de Eyville, knight, for the lifetime of the grantor (*YD*, x, no. 118). Sir Roger de Eyville attested North Cliff deeds in 1331, and a Cavil deed in 1332 (*YD*, VII, nos 264, 266; ibid., x, no. 119).

The ARAINES family, members of which witnessed hospital deeds belonging to North and South Cave (R599, R673), held of the earl of Aumale in Holderness, and probably took their name from Airaines, dép. Somme, some 20 m. north west of Amiens.[14] The Meaux chronicle, after noting a benefaction of William de Araines, gives a short note on his descendants. In the time of Abbot Alexander (1197–1210), it states, William de Araines, with the consent of his sons and heirs, by several feoffments, gave Meaux 4 bv. 12 a. land, and 1 bv. meadow in West [Little] Hatfield, with specified rights of pasture, and sold 3 bv. in Seaton to the monks for 40*m.*, which they paid to free him from his debts to Jews. Some of the land was sold by the monks to recoup the outlay, and the remainder was let at farm in the time of Abbot Hugh (1210–1220). William, who was lord of West Hatfield, had sons Arnold, Thomas and Bernard. He was succeeded by Arnold, who confirmed his father's gifts, and died without heir of his body. Thomas, Arnold's brother, was next heir, and gave Meaux 2 bv. from ½ ct. which he had received from his father William, which were alienated by Abbot Hugh.[15] Thomas also died without heir of his body, and was succeeded by Bernard his brother, who was succeeded in turn by his son Thomas. In the time of Abbot Roger (1286–1310), Thomas issued a confirmation of all the abbey's lands in West Hatfield (*Chron. Meaux*, I, 306–08; ibid., II, 219). The chronicle's account is in accord with surviving documentary references.

Thomas de Araines attested two deeds of William, earl of Aumale, dated by Farrer '1150 × 1160' and '1149–50' (*EYC*, III, nos 1352, 1379). Arnald de Araines attested a act of Archbishop Henry in 1151 × 1153, and a deed of Robert Escrop of '1156 × 1184' (*EEA*, v, no. 129; *EYC*, II, nos 1108, 1216). The connection of Thomas and Arnald with William de Araines, who attested a North Cave deed in 1190 × 1212 (R599), is unknown. In 1202 an agreement was made between the dean and chapter of York and St Andrew's Priory in York whereby 2 ct. in Cave were assigned to St Andrew's, one of which was held by William de Araines by hereditary right at an annual rent of 16s. 8d. (*MA*, VI, 962). In 1205 William de Araines gave 1*m.* in Yorkshire for a plea to be held in the king's court (*RFine*, p. 254). He appears as a knight in Yorkshire in 1208 (*CRR*, 1207–1209, pp. 140, 162). Arnold de Araines [II] first occurs in 1208 × 1214 (R673). In October 1217 he had returned to allegiance, and the sheriff was ordered to restore his property (*RClose*, I, 337b). He attested a Marton deed assigned to the abbacy of Richard (1221–1235) ('Ctl. Meaux', no. 264; *Chron. Meaux*, I, 415). Arnold de Araines confirmed to Meaux the gift of 2 bv. in West Hatfield made by his brother Thomas. Abbot Hugh (1210–1220) alienated the land, describing it as the gift

---

[14] Some references to the family were collected by A.S. Ellis, and published in 1898 (Ellis, 'De Araines'). Stephen, count of Aumale, issued a deed giving the church of Airaines to the priory of St Martin de Champs in Paris, which was witnessed by the treasurer of Amiens, Warner de Arenis (*CalDocsFr*, p. 459). No connection has been discovered with the Araines of Whittonstall and Newlands in Northumberland, who were tenants of Balliol, and descended from Bernard de Araines who occurs early in the thirteenth century. This family also held in Mixbury, Oxfordshire (*Hist. Northumberland*, VI, 177, 187; *CRR*, 1207–1209, p. 71; *RChart*, p. 88; Stenton, *Pleas*, I, no. 3395; *VCH Oxon*, VI, 253).

[15] The text of Abbot Hugh's deed survives ('Ctl. Meaux', no. 243, and see below).

of Thomas son of William de Araines ('Ctl. Meaux', no. 243; Meaux register, f. 17$^r$).
In 1224 Arnald de Araines was called to warrant 3 bv. land in Seaton[16] as the son and
heir of William de Araines, who had given the property to Meaux. In 1226 a final
concord between Ernald and the abbot settled the matter (*YF*, 1218–1231, p. 95 and
n; *Chron. Meaux*, I, 423; *CRR*, 1223–1224, nos 2420, 2574, 2585). Arnulf de Araines was
a juror in 1228 ('Ctl. Meaux', no. 216). In 1229 and 1230 Andrew de Fauconberg was
suing Ernald de Araines for 1*m.* in the king's court (*CRR*, 1227–1230, nos 1573, 2152,
2739). Ernald was dead in 1231, when his widow Agnes attorned her father, Rannulf
of Faxfleet, in her plea of dower against Thomas de Araines, Bernard his brother, and
William de Rue. When the plea came to be heard, Agnes claimed a third part of 1 ct.
in Drewton and 1 ct. in Kettlethorpe from 'Thomas son of William', a third part of
½ ct. in Hatfield from 'Bernard son of William', and a third part of various property
in Hatfield from William de Rue.[17] Thomas claimed that Ernald had never been seised
of the land, as it had been dower of Ernald's mother Eleanor. Rue called Bernard de
Araines to warrant, who warranted, and called Thomas son of William to warrant,
both for Rue's land and his own (PRO, JUST 1/1042 [Assize Roll], m. 3–3d).[18] This
shows that Thomas de Araines was William's son and heir, but there is scant evidence
for his tenure.

In 1231, Bernard de Araines and Helen his wife gave 2*m.* for licence to agree
with the prior of Byland concerning ½ ct. in Sutton[-under-Whitestonecliffe] (PRO,
JUST 1/1042, m. 5);[19] and in 1240, with the consent of Helen his wife, probably
a daughter of Geoffrey de Coigners,[20] Bernard de Araines gave ½ ct. in Sutton to
Byland Abbey. He made a fine with the abbot of Byland concerning the same ½ ct.,
described as 'in Gildusdale' in 1248. Thomas son of Bernard subsequently issued a
quitclaim (*Ctl. Byland*, nos 1018–23). Bernard was surety for Stephen de Barkedal in
1252 (*YF*, 1246–1272, p. 96n). He occurs as coroner in Holderness in 1257 (English,
*Holderness*, p. 78, citing 'the 1257 assize roll'[21]) and was a surety in Holderness in 1264
(*YD*, VIII, no. 214). In 1268 he was appointed with Thomas de Leleie to keep the
wapentakes and bailiwicks of Holderness, and to safely store their issues, until the
king had made an award concerning the disputes of Amice, countess of Devon, and
Isabel, countess of Aumale (*CalPat*, 1266–1272, p. 296). A feodary of Holderness made
'during the latter part of the reign of Henry III' shows that Bernard de Araines then
held 3 ct. in Little Hatfield (*KI*, p. 371). Another feodary showing the Holderness
fees held in dower by the countess of Aumale, copied in 1290, but compiled before
that date, noted 3 ct. in Hatfield, where 48 ct. make a fee, held by Bernard de Araines
(*CalCl*, 1288–1296, p. 148).

Bernard de Araines last occurs in November 1278 × November 1279, when he
attested an agreement concerning [Long] Riston (MS Dods. 139, f. 40$^v$). Thomas
de Araines had almost certainly succeeded in 1279 × 1281 when he was named as
a juror in quo warranto proceedings (*YQW*, pp. 122, 137, 157). In February 1281
Thomas de Araines and William de Araines witnessed an Easthorpe (ER) deed (*YD*,
IX, no. 141). In 1284–85 Thomas de Araines held 3 ct. in Little Hatfield of the king,

---

[16]  Identified by Parker as Seaton Ross, but presumably Seaton near Little Hatfield.
[17]  This was presumably William of Routh (*Ruda*), knight, who acquired 5 bv. in West Hatfield from
William de Araines and 3 bv. in the same place from Thomas his son, part of which land was given to
the abbey in the time of Abbot Richard (1221–1235), subject to an annual rent of ½*lb.* wax payable to
Thomas de Araines (*Chron. Meaux*, I, 422).
[18]  AALT, IMG_1200, IMG_1259.
[19]  AALT, IMG_1204.
[20]  So described in the rubric but not the deed itself.
[21]  Presumably PRO, JUST 1/1109 (Yorkshire eyre, 1257).

1 ct. in Kettlethorpe (in North Cave) of the Templars, who held of York Minster, and another 1 ct. there directly of the Minster (*KI*, pp. 75, 92). He was a juror in two Holderness inquisitions of 1287, and in 1288 was referred to as Thomas de Araines of Drewton. He again occurs as a juror in 1289, 1296, 1303 and 1305 (*YI*, II, 58, 59, 69, 81, 84; ibid., III, 42; IV, 49, 67). Thomas de Araines was said to hold 2 ct. of the manor of Market Weighton, with the members, in 1302–03 and in 1316 was named as the lord of Drewton (*KI*, pp. 261, 309). In 1318 the pope reserved to William Darrayns, called 'of Drewton', M.A., of the diocese of York, a benefice of value 20*m.* in the gift of the abbot and convent of Whitby, notwithstanding that he already held the rectory of St Nicholas, Beverley (*CalPapalL*, 1305–1342, p. 174). William Darrayns of Drewton made a fine in 1339 (*YF*, 1327–1347, p. 133).

Members of the SANCTON family witnessed hospital deeds pertaining to North and South Cave, and Alexander of Sancton gave the hospital 1½ a. meadow in South Cave in 1208 × 1249 (R675). It is frequently difficult to identify members of the Sancton family with certainty in twelfth and thirteenth century documents, and the following notes must be regarded as provisional, pending a more thorough examination of the Watton deeds transcribed by John Burton and other material. The names Alexander, William and Peter occur more than once, and there were at least two families, probably linked, which used the cognomen. The shared interests of the Sancton and Anlaby families in Sancton and its church (*EYC*, XII, 26–27), suggest a division between coheirs during the second half of the twelfth century, but details remain elusive. Clay gives several references for the ANLABY family, and states that William of Anlaby was 'probably the William son of Peter de Santon who owed half a mark in 1195 for licence to make an agreement'. He occurs both as William son of Peter[22] and William of Anlaby in 1203 in a dispute with William son of Alexander [of Sancton] concerning the advowson of the church of Sancton. William of Anlaby had three sons, Peter, Thomas, and William (*EYC*, XII, 25–28). In 1204 Thomas son of Gerold claimed his father had been seised at the time of his death with ½ ct. in Anlaby, of which William son of Peter was disseising him. Judgment was given in favour of William. On the same day the court heard a similar claim made by the same Thomas against William son of Alexander [of Sancton] concerning ½ ct. in Sancton. Again Thomas lost his case (Stenton, *Pleas*, III, nos 963–64). William son of Peter was presumably dead in February 1204[/05] when Peter son of William of Anlaby settled a dispute concerning 34 bv. in Anlaby (*EYC*, XII, no. 1). Peter of Sancton, a knight, was a recognitor in 1220 (*CRR*, 1220, p. 255). A narrative account preserved by Dodsworth states that Peter son of William of Anlaby died at about the time his brother William son of William of Anlaby murdered the husband of his sister Avice, an event which appears to have taken place in 1233. Peter's heir was said to be his son John, then aged five (*EYC*, XII, 25).

Clay's account of the descendants of Alexander son of William of Sancton was written with slight reference to his notes on Anlaby, and some of the evidence he cites may belong to that family (*EYC*, XII, 75–78).[23] Alexander son of William of Sancton gave land called Hessleskew in Sancton to Watton Priory in *c.*1155 × *c.*1180 (*EYC*, XII, no. 54). As Alexander of Sancton he restored ½ ct. in Sancton to his kinsman William son of John (ibid., no. 55). Alexander of Sancton and William his son

[22] Not to be confused with William son of Peter of Goodmanham, for whom see FN: Hay.
[23] In particular it seems at least possible that Peter of Sancton, who attested in the third quarter of the twelfth century, was the father of William of Anlaby (*EYC*, XII, 75).

attested a deed of William son of Godfrey Talun, probably given in or before 1196[24] (Burton transcripts 3, f. 15ᵛ, p. 4, B7 N34). Alexander of Sancton may have been dead in 1195, when Peter son of Alexander was a pledge for Alan son of Alexander (*PR*, 7 Ric. I, p. 94). The assize of mort d'ancestor of 1204, to establish if Gerold father of Thomas was seised in demesne as of fee of ½ ct. land in Sancton on the day that he died, of which land Thomas accused William son of Alexander of disseising him, has been mentioned above. William Constable, son of Robert Constable, granted to William son of Alexander of Sancton certain rights in Holme [on Spalding Moor] appurtenant to Sancton's ½ k.f. in Sancton, in 1211 or before,[25] by a deed attested by Peter of Sancton, Alan his brother and others (*EYC*, XII, no. 56). William son of Alexander of Sancton gave Watton all his land in *Haldeherghes*, which was probably in Sancton[26] (Burton transcripts 1, f. 162ᵛ, p. 272, B8 N53).[27] William son of Alexander of Sancton, Peter and Robert the parson his brothers, and William son of Peter of Sancton, attested an agreement between Watton Priory and William son of Gilbert of Dalton (MS Dods. 7, f. 298ᵛ); William son of Alexander of Sancton, Peter, Robert the parson, and Alan, his brothers, with Alexander son of William of Sancton, attested a deed of Adam son of Arnald of Sunderlandwick to Watton (ibid., f. 354ᵛ). William of Sancton, Peter son of Alexander of Sancton, William son of Peter of Sancton and Alan son of Alexander of Sancton were amongst the witnesses to a Rotsea deed given in the late twelfth century (ibid., f. 322ᵛ). William of Sancton and Peter of Sancton his brother occur on several occasions, including proceedings or deeds of 1198, 1199, 1202 and 1207. In 1206 William of Sancton was a knight on the business of the king's court in Yorkshire (*EYC*, XII, 76), and in 1208 William son of Alexander claimed he had been disseised of his common wood of Holme belonging to his tenement in Sancton (*CRR*, 1207–1209, p. 264).

Records from 1218–19 show that William of Sancton had been succeeded by his son Alexander by 1218 at the latest. Alexander of Sancton occurs in 1228 and 1231 (*EYC*, XII, 77). Gundreth, widow of William of Sancton, gave 14 bv. in Cave to the Templars in 1226, and can probably be identified with Gundreda de Daiville, who confirmed 1 ct. land in South Cave to Alexander of Sancton in 1231, to be held of the Templars (*YF*, 1218–1231, pp. 94, 140). The land of Gundreda [in Sancton] is mentioned as an abutment in a deed of Alexander son of William of Sancton made in 1218 or before (*EYC*, XII, no. 59). Alexander son of William of Sancton gave a rent of 8s. from 1 ct. in Sancton, held by Alexander Burdun, to Watton in 1217 × 1220[28] (Burton transcripts 2, f. 129ʳ, p. 222, B25 N7).[29] It was probably this Alexander son of William of Sancton who gave ½ ct. in Houghton (*Houetona*) [in Sancton], which Alan of Sancton his uncle (*avunculus*) had held, to Watton (Burton transcripts 2, f. 47ᵛ, p. 66, B12 N27).[30] He attested as a knight on several occasions (Burton transcripts 2, f. 47ᵛ, p. 66, B12 N38; ibid. 3, f. 15ʳ, p. 3, B7 N22, B7 N25; *YD*, VI, nos 318–21, 323–25). He occurs with his brother Roger in *c.* 1218 × 1248 (R624), in or after 1246 (*YMF*, I, no. 41), and in or before 1249 (R675). He last occurs in 1252 × 1255, when as Alexander son of William of Sancton he made a quitclaim to York Minster, attested by Roger of Sancton, presumably his brother, and Peter his (Roger's) son (*YMF*, II, no. 56). Roger

---

24  Attested by Roger Hay, who was dead in that year (FN).
25  Witnessed by Jordan of Bugthorpe, who was dead in that year (FN).
26  For Alderges, see *EYC*, XII, 22n; *PN YorksER*, p. 230.
27  Cited *Monasticon Eboracense*, p. 416.
28  Attested by H[amo] dean of York.
29  Cited *Monasticon Eboracense*, p. 415.
30  Cited *Monasticon Eboracense*, p. 414.

of Sancton 'in South Cave' and Peter his son attested a North Cave deed in or after 1252[31] (MS Dods. 7, f. 335ᵛ).

Alexander was apparently succeeded by Richard son of Alexander of Sancton, who confirmed his father's grant of the advowson of a moiety of Sancton church to Watton Priory (*EYC*, xii, no. 63). Peter son of Alexander of Sancton, who was party to a fine concerning land in Cave in 1249 (*YF*, 1246–1272, p. 10), was involved in litigation against Nicholas, formerly bishop of Durham, in 1249–50 (*CRR*, 1249–1250, nos 983, 2104). He attested a deed concerning Kilnwick (*YD*, vi, no. 312), and may have predeceased Richard, or been a younger brother to him.

**R670.** Gift to the hospital by Roger de Mowbray of 32 a. meadow in Cave and Swain son of Dune in Thirsk with his toft and croft and 2 bv., which Roger gave before to Warin the viol player for his service. Warin will hold the land of the hospital for his life, paying 1*lb.* pepper annually [*c.*1160 × 1182]

PRINTED: *Mowbray Charters*, no. 308, where dated *c.*1160 × September 1182.

**[f. 228ᵛ]** *Carta Rogeri de Molbrai de terra Warini Vielatoris.*
Universis filiis sancte matris ecclesie Rogerus de Molbrai salutem. Notum sit vobis me et heredes meos dedisse et presenti carta confirmasse deo et pauperibus hospitalis sancti Petri Ebor' triginta duas acras prati in Cava, et Suanum filium Dune in Tresco, et toftum suum et croftum et duas bovatas terre plenar(ie) in omnibus in liberam et puram et perpetuam elemosinam, que scilicet prius dederamus Warino Vielatori pro servicio suo. Cuius etiam petitione et concessu predictis dei pauperibus hec in puram et perpetuam elemosinam dedimus. Et predictus Warinus hanc elemosinam tenebit in vita sua de prefatis pauperibus reddendo eis annuatim unam libram piperis. Hiis testibus, Roberto de Molbrai, Hugone Malabissa, Adam Luvel, Rodberto de Bucei, Herberto filio Ricardi, Nicholao de Bellun, Willelmo de Daivilla, Radulfo de Beuuer, Rodberto de Tresco, Rogero fratre archid(iaconi), Willelmo de Tichehil, Hugone filio Lewini.

Greenway states that Nicholas de Bellun first occurs in Mowbray deeds after *c.*1160 (*Mowbray Charters*, no. 343n). William of Tickhill was dead at Michaelmas 1182 (*PR*, 28 Hen. II, p. 46). Mowbray made several benefactions of property in Thirsk to the hospital (M: Thirsk [*Mowbray Charters*, nos 296, 311–12]). 'A messuage in Thirsk' is included in the papal confirmations of 1148, 1157, and 1173 (C178–C180 [*EYC*, i, nos 179, 186, 197]).

**R671.** Gift [confirmation] to the hospital by Nigel de Mowbray of the property described in R670 [*c.*1160 × Sept. 1182]

COPIES: *b* Rawl., f. 228ᵛ; *c* Burton transcripts 3, f. 118ʳ, p. 209, B18 N11, slightly abbreviated, all witnesses given. PRINTED: *Mowbray Charters*, no. 309, from *b*, where dated *c.*1160 × September 1182. NOTED: Drake, *Eboracum*, p. 335, via Torre's collections.

*Carta Nigelli de Molbrai de terra Warini Vielatoris.*
Universis filiis sancte matris ecclesie Nigellus de Molbrai salutem. Notum sit vobis me et heredes meos dedisse et presenti carta confirmasse deo et pauperibus hospitalis

---

[31] A deed of German son of Roger Hay.

sancti Petri Ebor' triginta duas acras prati in Cava et Suanum filium Dune in Tresco et croftum suum et toftum[32] et duas bovatas terre plenarie in omnibus in liberam et puram et perpetuam elemosinam, que scilicet pater meus prius dederat Warino Vielatori pro servicio suo. Cuius etiam petitione et concessu predictis dei pauperibus hec in puram et perpetuam elemosinam dedimus. Hiis testibus, Rodberto de Molbrai, Hugone Malabissa, Adam Luuel, Rodberto de Bucei, Herberto filio Ricardi, Nicholao de Bellun, Willelmo de Daivilla, Radulfo de Beuuer, Rogero fratre archid(iaconi), Willelmo de Tichehil, Hugone filio Lewini.

The same witnesses and occasion as R670.

**R672.** Gift to the hospital by Roger de Eyville, son of Sir William de Eyville knight, of 2 a. 1 r. salt meadow, with the base [?] in Mickledales, between Bagfleet and Colcroft, in width between the hospital's meadow and the meadow which John de Foro of Cave held of the nuns of Wilberfoss, and in length from Mickledike to the north [c.1270 × c.1285, probably 1276 × 1280]

*De ii. acris et una roda prati salsi cum fundo.*
Omnibus cristi fidelibus hoc scriptum visuris vel audituris Rogerus de Eyvile filius domini Willelmi de Eyvile militis eternam in domino salutem. Noverit universitas vestra me caritatis intuitu et pro salute anime mee antecessorum et successorum meorum concessisse et dedisse et hac presenti carta confirmasse magistro et fratribus hospitalis beati Petri Ebor' duas acras et unam rodam prati salsi cum fundo in Mikeldales, inter Bagflete et Colcroft', quod iacet in latitudine inter pratum dicti hospitalis et pratum quod Iohannes de Foro de Cave tenuit de monialibus de Wilberfosse, et extendit se in longitudine a Mikeldik' usque ad umbram, tenendum et habendum totum predictum pratum cum fundo dictis magistro et fratribus et eorum successoribus in liberam puram et perpetuam elemosinam, sicut aliqua elemosina liberius et melius teneri potest et haberi. Et ego siquidem predictus Rogerus de Eyvile et heredes mei totum predictum pratum cum fundo prefat(is) magistro et fratribus et eorum successoribus contra omnes homines warantizabimus acquietabimus et defendemus imperpetuum. In cuius rei testimonium huic scripto sigillum meum apposui. Hiis testibus, Petro de Santon', Roberto filio Custancie de Cave, Waltero dicto mercatore de Malton', Nicholao de Crosseby, Willelmo de Beaumes et aliis.

The majority of deeds attested by Nicholas de Crosby, sometimes described as 'of Kilham', can be accurately dated, and all of these belong to 1276–1280, the period for Roger of Malton as rector (R119, R493, R594, R658, C313, C472, C497, C909, C910, C914 [Cott., ff. 60ᵛ, 89ʳ, 94ʳ, 186ʳ⁻ᵛ]). In a deed of 1276 × 1280 he is described as steward of the hospital (C498 [Cott., f. 94ʳ⁻ᵛ]). He occurs on several occasions with Walter the mercer of Malton and William Beaumes, including four examples from the rectorship of Roger of Malton (R287, C313, C911, C912 [Cott., ff. 60ᵛ, 186ʳ⁻ᵛ]). It is probable that Crosby's stewardship and attestations are limited to the rectorship of Roger of Malton, but the wider date range of c.1270 × c.1285 has been ascribed. Roger de Eyville was dead in 1290 (FN).

Smith identified Bagfleet as Bagletts, in South Cave (*PN YorksER*, p. 223). The Templars held a mill at Bagfleet in 1185 (Lees, *Templars*, p. 131). In 1371 Bagfleet was described as lying between Ellerker and Cave (Flower, *Public Works*, II, 341). A fine

---

[32]   *c: toftum suum et croftum.*

concerning 60 a. land and 60 a. of meadow in South Cave, called Bagfleet, was made in 1416–17 (Hall, *South Cave*, p. 11). Reference was made to 'a pasture called Bagfleet' in 1466 (*North Country Wills*, I, 54).

**R673.** Gift by William de Daiville, for the health of his soul and that of his father Roger de Daiville, to the hospital, of 8 bv. with eight tofts belonging in [South] Cave, which Hugh Pluket, William son of Gregory, William ad Fontem, William son of Meriet, Hugh his brother, Ranulf son of Simon, Tocke son of William, and Thole the provost held, and also all Bagfleet, to hold with tofts and crofts and the men living in the lands. The men living in the lands will render a portion of chattels as an obituary payment. No religious man or magnate should have entry or access to any of the donors' tenements in Cave or Bagfleet without the consent of the hospital. The hospital will receive the body of the donor and his heirs for burial, and those belonging to them, and do for them just as they do for the most distinguished of their brethren [1208 × 1214]

*Willelmus de Daivill' de viii. bovatis terre et viii. toftis in Cava, conced(ere) etiam hospitali partem catallorum tam eum quam homines suos contingentem obligavit, et se hoc instr(ument)o fratribus hospitalis que sine eorum consensu nullus religiosus vel potens ingress(um) habebit ad aliquod tenementum suum.*

Sciant omnes presentes et futuri quod ego Willelmus de Daivile, pro salute anime mee et Rogeri de Daivile patris mei et omnium antecessorum et heredum et successorum nostrorum, dedi concessi et hac presenti carta mea confirmavi deo et beato Petro et pauperibus hospitalis beati Petri Ebor' in puram et perpetuam elemosinam octo bovatas terre cum octo toftis ad eas pertinentibus in territorio de Cave cum omnibus pertinenciis suis, unde Hugo Pluket tenuit unam bovatam cum crofto et Willelmus filius Gregorii tenuit aliam bovatam et Willelmus ad Fontem tenuit terciam et Willelmus filius Meriet tenuit quartam et Hugo frater eius tenuit quintam et Ranulfus filius Simonis tenuit sextam et Tocke filius Willelmi tenuit septimam et Thoue prepositus tenuit octavam bovatam, et preterea totum Baggeflete cum pertinenciis suis, scilicet tenendum et habendum totum predictum tenementum cum toftis et croftis et cum hominibus in ipsis terris manentibus, et cum omnibus ad ipsos homines et ad ipsas terras pertinentibus infra villas et extra libere integre honorifice et quiete ab omni servicio et ab omni exactione, sicut ulla elemosina liberius et melius potest dari, ita quod in obitu suo reddent omnes homines manentes in terris predictis suam portionem catallorum suorum pauperibus predicti hospitalis. Et est sciendum quod bene volumus et firmiter et libere concessimus dedimus et presenti carta nostra confirmavimus predictis pauperibus imperpetuum ut nullus religiosus vel aliquis potens habeat ingressum vel accessum ad aliq(uod) ten(ementum) nost(ru)m de Cave vel de Baggeflete preter assensum magistri et fratrum predicti hospitalis. Et in obitu meo et heredum meorum recipient nos magister et fratres predicte domus dei ad sepulturam suam cum hiis que ad nos spectant, et facient pro nobis sicut pro excellenciori fratrum suorum imperpetuum. Et ego predictus Willelmus de Daivile et heredes mei warantizabimus adquietabimus et defendemus tota predicta tenementa cum omnibus pertinenciis suis et cum prefat' concessionibus predictis pauperibus imperpetuum sicut ulla elemosina [**f. 229ʳ**] liberius et melius potest warantizari adquietari et defendi contra omnes homines ut participes simus omnium bonorum que fiunt vel facienda sunt in predicta domo dei. Hiis testibus, domino S[imone] decano, H[amone] thesaurario, magistro Greg(orio) et pluribus aliis de capitulo Ebor' ecclesie, Hugone capellano decani et aliis vicariis prefate ecclesie, Iohanne de Daivile,

Ernulfo de Arains, Rogero de Cundi, Simone filio Galfridi de Cave, Willelmo clerico, Silvestro de Cave, Rogero de Kent, Viel filio Bereng', Rogero de Cave, Thoma de Languat, Willelmo de Notigh(am), Hugone de Graha(m) et multis aliis.

Simon de Apulia as dean indicates 1194 × 1214; Hamo as treasurer 1197 × 1218. Ernulf de Araines succeeded his father William in or after 1208 (FN). The first lay witness was probably John de Daiville of Adlingfleet, apparently a cousin of the donor. John de Daiville had confirmation of his father's lands in 1185 × 1191 (*EYC*, IX, no. 137; *Mowbray Charters*, no. 361), and was living in 1228. By 1242–43 he had been succeeded by [his son] Robert de Daiville, who then held 2½ k.f. of Mowbray in Yorkshire (*CP*, IV, 131; *Bk of Fees*, p. 1097).

**R674.** Grant and quitclaim to the hospital by Peter de Eyville of South Cave, of all right he had in the presentation of two poor infirm people to two beds in the infirmary of the hospital; and also in the demand to have two oxen with or without a yoke, from the hospital, for the use of his ploughs at South Cave every second, third, or fourth year, or at any other time, by reason of the ninth sheaf of all types of corn in his demesne in the same vill which the hospital ought to have, or for any other reason. Also licence to the hospital to collect the ninth sheaf of all types of corn within his demesne in South Cave, which previously were demesne of Sir Roger de Mowbray [May 1295].
[Endorsed:] note of reading and enrolment on 16 May 1295 at York, before the justices assigned to determine a certain trespass made by Eyville on Langton.

*De terra in Southecave.*
Pateat universis per presentes quod ego Petrus de Eyvill' de Suthcave pro me et heredibus meis concessi remisi et imperpetuum quiet'clamavi domino Waltero de Langeton' magistro hospitalis sancti Leonardi Ebor' fratribus sororibus et pauperibus eiusdem hospitalis et eorum successoribus totum ius et clam(eum) quod habui vel aliquo modo habere potui in presentatione duorum pauperum infirmorum ad duo lecta in infirmaria eiusdem hospitalis habenda, et etiam in petitione habendi duos boves cum uno iugo vel sine iugo ad usum carucarum mearum de Southcave a predicto magistro seu hospitali suo predicto quolibet secundo tercio vel iiii° anno vel aliquo alio tempore percipiend(os) ratione none garbe singulorum bladi generum domini-corum meorum in eadem villa, quam iidem magister et fratres singulis annis ibidem percipere et habere debent et percipere et habere consueverunt, seu aliqua alia ratione proposita vel non proposita. Quare volo et concedo pro me heredibus et assignatis meis quod predicti magister et fratres sorores et pauperes eiusdem hospitalis et eorum successores imperpetuum sint immunes de receptione singulorum pauperum ad aliqua lecta in infirmaria aut alibi infra hospitale predictum per presentationem meam seu heredum meorum, et etiam de eorundem sustentacione omnimoda, necnon et a solu-tione duorum boum predictorum, et ab omni alio onere servicio terreno et seculari actione ratione none garbe predicte aut aliqua alia causa seu contractu, ita quod nec ego nec heredes mei aliquid iuris vel clam(eum) in presentatione duorum hominum ad lecta predicta seu in peticione duorum boum ad[33] carucas meas ut predictum est aliqua ratione de cetero vendicare vel exigere poterimus imperpetuum. Volo etiam et pro me et heredibus et assignatis meis concedo quod predicti magister et fratres et eorum successores per suos ministros quoscumque imperpetuum libere nonam garbam omnis generis bladi eorundem magistri et fratrum infra omnes dominicas

[33] MS: *ad* repeated.

terras in villa de Southcave que aliquando fuerunt dominice terre domini Rogeri de Moubrai sicut et ubi percipere colligere et adunare plenius consueverunt, percipere colligere et adunare possint et ad utilitatem eorundem magistri et fratrum absque perturbatione seu inquietatione mei heredum vel assignatorum meorum seu ministrorum nostrorum quorumcumque quo voluerint cariare et in usus eiusdem hospitalis pro libito convertere. In cuius rei testimonium presentibus sigillum meum apposui. Hiis testibus, dominis Hugone de Cressingham et Iohanne de Lythegraynes domini regis Angl(ie) iusticiariis, domino Iohanne Byron tunc vicecomite Ebor', Franco le Tyays, Petro Becard' milit(ibus), Iohanne de Barton', Alexandro de Cave, Galfrido de Hert'pole, Iohanne de Tilton', Roberto de Sexdecim Vallibus et aliis.

Istud scriptum lectum fuit et irrotulatum coram dominis Hugone de Cressingham et Iohanne de Lithegreynes iusticiariis domini regis ad audiendam et terminandam quandam transgressionem domino Waltero de Langeton magistro hospitalis sancti Leonardi Ebor' per Petrum de Eyvill' factam assignatis apud Ebor' in hospital(i) predicto die lune prox' post festum ascentionis domini, anno regni regis E(dwardi) xxiii°.

In April 1295 Cressingham and Lythegreynes had a commision of oyer and terminer, on complaint by Walter of Langton, king's clerk and master of the hospital, that Peter de Eyville, John of Cave, and John de Eyville carried away crops and goods of the hospital at North Cave (*CalPat*, 1292–1301, p. 160).

**R675.** Gift to the hospital by Alexander of Sancton of 1½ a. in the meadow of South Cave, on the west side of *Schelflet*, being the 1½ a. which belong to the 2 bv. of land which William the miller once held [1208 × 1249]

*Alexander de Santona de una acra prati in Suthcava.*
Sciant presentes et futuri quod ego Alexander de Santona caritatis intuitu et pro salute anime mee et animarum antecessorum et successorum meorum dedi concessi et presenti carta mea confirmavi deo et pauperibus hospitalis sancti Petri Ebor' unam acram et dimidiam prati in prato de Suthcava ex parte occident(ali) de Schelflet, scilicet illam acram et dimidiam que pertinent ad illas duas bovatas terre quas Willelmus molendinarius aliquando tenuit, tenend(as) et habend(as) predictis pauperibus in puram et perpetuam elemosinam libere integre et quiete ab omni servicio et exactione sicut aliqua elemosina liberius et melius teneri potest et haberi. Ego autem et heredes mei predictam pratam predictis pauperibus warantizabimus adquietabimus et defendemus in omnibus et contra omnes homines imperpetuum. In huius rei robur et testimonium huic scripto sigillum meum apposui. Hiis testibus, Willelmo de Ayvilla, Rogero de Santona, Rogero de Ayvilla, Ranulfo de Faxflet, Laurencio de eadem villa, Alexandro de Brungelflete, Willelmo filio Osberti, Alfredo de Brungelflet et multis aliis.

Alexander of Sancton succeeded his father in 1208 × 1218. William de Eyville was living in 1231 but had been succeeded by his son Roger by 1251 (FNs). Ranulf of Faxfleet had his lands in North Duffield confirmed by the hospital in 1238 × 1245 (R625). William son of Osbert and Alfred of Broomfleet are the final witnesses to a deed concerning Hotham made in *c*.1214 × 1223 (R766). In May 1249 a fine was made between John son of Richard of Cave, claimant, and Alexander of Sancton, who had been called to warrant by Peter son of Alexander, concerning 2 bv. land in South Cave, excepting a toft and 1½ a. meadow, and also by William, master of St Leonard's, concerning 1½ a. meadow in South Cave (*YF*, 1246–1272, p. 10).

## *Skelton iuxta Houeden'* [Skelton]

In 1086 there were 3 ct. 2 bv. in Skelton, a berewick of the bishop of Durham's manor of Howden. In 1284–85 it was assessed at 3 ct. (*KI*, p. 70). The hospital acquired two dwellings in Skelton from the bishop of Durham in the third quarter of the twelfth century, in exchange for a dwelling in York (R677, R678). The hospital also had 2 bv. in Skelton, which were the gift of Adam son of Richer (R676). Skelton does not appear in the papal confirmations to the hospital, the late-thirteenth-century extents, the *Valor Ecclesiasticus*, or the account of 1542. The three Skelton deeds, and their rubrics, have been added at a later date by the cartularist (hand A-2). The decorated initial capitals are uniform in style with the rest of the volume.

A note has been added after the Skelton deeds:
Sunt etiam ibidem tria tofta et tria crofta cum pertinenciis iacentia ad finem borialem predicte ville, que dudum fuerunt nisi tantum due mansure, que iacent in longitudine ab Usa ab occidente usque ad finem et coniunctionem longi crofti et curti ad orientem, et in latitudine inter toftum ibidem modo vastum sed dudum edificat(um) et crofti domini episcopi Dunolmens(is) ad boream. Et aliud toftum modo ibidem vastum, sed dudum edificat(um) eiusdem episcopi cum crofto ad austrum etc. Sunt etiam ibidem due bovate terre. Et [*ends,* hand E]

**R676.** Gift to the hospital by Adam son of Richer of 2 bv. in Skelton. While he lives, the donor will do the service to the lord of the land, and afterwards his heir will do it [*c.*1160 × *c.*1190, hand A-2]

PRINTED: *EYC*, II, no. 982, where dated 1175 × 1185.

**[f. 229ᵛ]** *Carta Ade filii Richeri de ii. bovatis terre in Skeltuna iuxta Houeden'.*[1]
Notum sit tam presentibus quam futuris sancte matris ecclesie filiis quod ego Adam filius Richeri dedi in elemosinam hospitali sancti Petri Ebor' duas bovatas terre in Skeltune liberas et quietas ab omni servicio pro anima patris mei et salute anime mee et corporis. Et ego faciam servicium apud dominum eiusdem terre dum vixero et heres meus post me. Testibus, Ada de Estpatric, Willelmo Albo clerico, Roberto filio Bernardi.

The donor and the witnesses are obscure, and it is unclear why Farrer proposed a narrow range of date. William *Albus* witnessed a deed of Hugh du Puiset, bishop of Durham, in *c.*1174 × 1183 (*EEA*, XXIV, no. 102).

**R677.** Gift to the hospital by Hugh, bishop of Durham, of two dwellings in Skelton, from the Ouse as far as the 'old water', and fishery of the same vill in the Ouse with common pasture, without injury to the men of the vill. For which master Robert, warden of the hospital, with consent of his brethren, gave a dwelling in Fishergate [York] which Genebois, by leave of Sir Roger de Mowbray, gave to the hospital [1154 × 1164, hand A-2]

---

[1]   Here and in R686 a pilcrow, or paragraph mark, in blue ink, perhaps that of the capitals, has been inserted between the text and the rubric, as if to separate them or to fill excessive blank space.

PRINTED: *EYC*, II, no. 981, where dated 1155 × 1165; *EEA*, XXIV, no. 171, where dated 1154 × 1173.

*Carta Hugonis episcopi Dunelmensis de ii. mansuris in Sektuna² iuxta Houedon' et cetera.*
Hugo dei gratia Dunelmensis episcopus omnibus sancte matris ecclesie filiis et universis hominibus suis salutem. Sciatis nos concessisse et hac presenti carta nostra confirmasse deo et pauperibus hospitalis sancti Petri Ebor' duas mansuras in Skeltuna continuas ab Usa usque ad veterem aquam et piscariam eiusdem ville in Usa et communem pasturam sine gravamine hominum illius ville liberas et immunes et quietas ab omni geldo et consuetudine et omni exactione et ab omni humano servicio. Quapropter magister Robertus custos supradicti hospitalis consilio et assensu fratrum suorum concessit et dedit deo et sancto Cutheberto et nobis [et] successoribus nostris imperpetuum illam mansuram in Fiscaria gata³ quam Genebois, concessione domini Rogeri de Molbray, dedit hospitali sancti Petri in puram et perpetuam elemosinam. Cuius rei hii sunt testes, Galterus monachus, Robertus de Fribois, Ricardus dapifer, Iohannes clericus nepos prioris, Helyas diaconus, Hugo clericus nepos vicecomitis, Hugo Rom, Lewinus filius Turwif, Baldawinus qui habet uxorem Iohannis de Walamira, Gamellus de Bugatorp, Nicholaus de porta sancti Petri, Haldanus Wala.

The date range is given by the consecration of Hugh du Puiset in Rome on 20 December 1153, and the latest likely date for Robert as master of the hospital. Greenway assigns Roger de Mowbray's deed confirming Genebois' gift in Fishergate to the hospital to *c.*1147 × 1165 (C607 [*Mowbray Charters*, no. 304; *EYC*, I, no. 332]). The land in Fishergate does not appear in the papal confirmations.

**R678.** Surrender to the hospital by Hugh, bishop of Durham, of two dwellings in Skelton, from the Ouse as far as the 'old water', and fishery of the same vill in the Ouse, with common pasture, without damage to the men of the vill, which he and his predecessors gave and confirmed by their charters [1192 × 3 March 1195; probably late February × 3 March 1195, hand A-2]

PRINTED: *EYC*, II, no. 983, where dated 1189 × 1190; *EEA*, XXIV, no. 172, where dated '1192 × 3 March 1195, probably late'.

*Carta Hugonis Dunolm' episcopi de ii. mansuris in Skelton' iuxta Houeden'.*
Hugo dei gratia Dunelm' episcopus omnibus sancte matris ecclesie filiis ad quos presens carta pervenerit salutem. Sciatis nos pro amore dei et salute anime nostre reddidisse deo et hospitali sancti Petri in Ebor' duas mansuras in Scheltona contiguas ab Husa usque ad veterem aquam, et piscariam eiusdem ville in Husa et communem pasturam sine gravamine hominum eiusdem ville, quas predecessores nostri et nos eis dederamus et cartis nostris confirmaveramus in puram et perpetuam elemosinam ita libere et quiete sicut carte nostre quas inde habent testantur. Testibus hiis, Bertramno priore Dunel(mens)i, Bucardo thesaurario Ebor', Willelmo subdecano Lincoln', Willelmo archidiacono Dunel', magistro Ricardo de Coldingham, Henrico de Puteaco, Roberto de Mara et multis aliis.

---

² sic.
³ MS: *grata*.

The grantor Hugh, bishop of Durham, died on 3 March 1195. Smith points out the similarity of the witness list to that of Bishop Hugh's deathbed act for Roger parson of Howden (*EEA*, xxiv, no. 71). His statement that the witness William de Blois was not subdean of Lincoln earlier than 1192 is apparently based on the presumption that his predecessor in that office, Wimar, cannot have resigned it before that year, as the archdeaconry of Northampton, Wimar's subsequent office, was not vacant. Smith's proposition that the witness list is truncated seems unlikely, as the deed is in the hand of the main cartularist, and it does not otherwise appear abbreviated.

## *Thorpe in Strata* [Thorpe le Street]

[**f. 230ʳ**] *Quer' cartas de Thorp' in Strata supra in Rugthorp'.*

## *Thwenge* [Thwing]

For Thwing, which was land of the king in 1086, and was given to Robert de Brus by Henry I, see *VCH Yorks ER*, II, 324–31. The following deed appears to be the only notice of the hospital's property in Thwing prior to the account of 1542, which recorded a rent there (*Dissolved Houses*, IV, 226).

**R679.** Gift to the hospital by Simon son of Ascelin de Merston of a toft in Thwing, between the donor's toft and the toft of Godfrey Pulein [1194 × *c.*1220]

PRINTED: *EYC*, II, no. 761, where dated 1190 × 1210.

*Carta Simonis filii Acelini de Merston' de uno tofto in Thweng'.*
Sciant omnes presentes et futuri quod ego Simon filius Acelini de Merston' dedi et concessi et hac presenti carta mea confirmavi deo et hospitali sancti Petri Ebor' et fratribus hospitalis ipsius ibidem deo servientibus pro salute anime mee et antecessorum et successorum meorum unum toftum in Thueng' sicut divise proportant inter toftum meum et toftum Godefridi Pulein, scilicet tenend(um) et habend(um) predicte domui imperpetuum cum omnibus liberis pertinenciis suis infra villam et extra libere integre honorifice et quiete ab omni servicio et ab omni exactione sicut ulla elemosina liberior potest dari. Et ego predictus Simon et heredes mei warantizabimus predictum toftum predicto hospitali imperpetuum sine retenemento contra omnes homines pro fraternitate ipsius domus. Hiis testibus, Stephano celerario, Anketino, Suano, Willelmo Balki et aliis fratribus ipsius domus, Alexandro de Thueng', Willelmo filio Walteri, Adam Minet, Waltero filio Oseberti, Helia filio Malgeri, Thoma de Langwath et multis aliis.

Thomas de Langwath usually attests as master after *c.*1220. Stephen became cellarer in 1194 or later and does not occur with Langwath as master.

## *Wilbirfosse* [Wilberfoss]

For Wilberfoss, the territory of which lay within the Percy manor and soke of Catton in 1086, see *VCH Yorks ER*, III, 190–97. Two bovates in Wilberfoss were confirmed to the hospital in 1148, 1157 and 1173, but the name of the donor is not given (C178–C180 [*EYC*, I, nos 179, 186, 197]). Osbert son of Ulger [of Wilberfoss] confirmed the gift of 2 bv., without naming the original donor, and gave further property in Wilberfoss in *c.*1160 × *c.*1171 (R683). In *c.*1170 × *c.*1200 Osbert son of Ulger made three small additional gifts (R680–R682). Thomas son of Robert Burdun of Kexby gave 7 a. and a toft in Wilberfoss in 1267 × 1286 (R782). Wilberfoss is not mentioned in the extents of the later thirteenth century, or the *Valor Ecclesiasticus*, but a rent there was included in the post-Dissolution accounts (*Dissolved Houses*, IV, 226).

Osbert son of Ulger of WILBERFOSS was a benefactor of Wilberfoss Priory. His gift of 'all the land with the meadow belonging to his carucate of Derwent next to Catton', was amongst the gifts confirmed by Henry II in 1174–75[1] (*CalPat*, 1461–1467, pp. 341–42); and was perhaps the property described as 6 a. in Wilberfoss confirmed by his son Ilger of Wilberfoss in 1235 (*YF*, 1232–1246, p. 37). Ilger son of Osbert of Wilberfoss also confirmed to the nuns 1 a. which Bertram held of him, at an uncertain date (MS Dods. 7, f. 360[r]). Osbert son of Ulger gave 4 bv. in Wilberfoss to Warter Priory, which William *cognomento monachus*, parson of the church of Warter, and Geoffrey his son after him held of Osbert's father. The gift was confirmed by Ilger son of Osbert, who also exchanged various tenements in Wilberfoss for 1 bv. in Wilberfoss which Reginald son of Alger held previously of the canons (Warter cartulary, f. 87[r]). Ilger son of Osbert was a defendant in a case of novel disseisin in Wilberfoss in 1228 (*PatentR*, 1225–1232, p. 208). Ilger of Wilberfoss, Ilger of Catton and others issued a quitclaim to Richard de Percy in *c.*1220 × 1240[2] for common in Lund *subtus Brek* (*Ctl. Percy*, no. 264). According to Glover's pedigree of the Wilberfoss family, Ilger of Wilberfoss married Margaret, daughter of William son of Philip de Kyme, lord of Wilberfoss, but the evidence on which this claim rests is not given, nor is it certain that Ilger was the ancestor of the Wilberfoss family (*Glover's Visitation*, p. 158). William son of Simon of Wilberfoss held 9 bv. in Wilberfoss of William de Kyme in 1260 (*CalInqPM*, I, 131), and in 1284–85 the many tenancies in Wilberfoss included 2 bv. held by Robert son of Simon of Wilberfoss, and 2 bv. held by Letia of Wilberfoss, on behalf of her son and ward John (*KI*, p. 87).

**R680.** Gift to the hospital by Osbert son of Ulger of 2 a. in Wilberfoss [*c.*1180 × *c.*1200]

PRINTED: *EYC*, II, no. 913, where dated *c.*1180 × 1193.

**[f. 231[r]]** *Carta Osberti filii Ulgeri de Wilberfossa de duabus acris terre in eadem.*
Sciant universi fideles qui viderint et audierint has litteras quod ego Osbertus filius Ulgeri dei amore dedi pauperibus hospitalis beati Petri Ebor' duas acras terre continuas in Wilburfossa in puram et perpetuam elemosinam liberas et quietas et immunes ab

---

[1]   Witnessed by William son of Aldelin, steward, implying 1174 or later, and John, dean of Salisbury, implying 1175 or before.
[2]   Confirmed by Christiana, prioress of Wilberfoss, who occurs in 1231 and 1235, and had been succeeded in 1240.

omni seculari servicio preter orationes pauperum, et communem pasturam eiusdem ville, quam videlicet elemosinam predicti fratres imperpetuum tenebunt, sicut aliquam elemosinam liberius et honorificentius in domo sua possident. Hanc vero elemosinam ego Osbertus et heredes mei contra omnes homines predictis pauperibus warentizabimus. Hiis testibus, Simone capellano de sancto Clemente, Willelmo diacono, Everardo clerico, Dolfino de Wilburfosse, Everardo de Canteb', Henrico de Quenebi, Ernaldo filio Leuus, Radulfo Fin, Reinero filio Herberti, Willelmo nepote Ernaldi, Ricardo de Hedun et multis aliis.

Only approximate limits of date can be deduced from the donor and witnesses. Everard the clerk attested in *c.*1170 × *c.*1190 (R117, R432), and *c.*1175 × 1194 (R631), and was presumably a different man from Everard the clerk who witnesses in 1219 × 1246 (R292, R293). Ernald son of Levus occurs in 1181 × 1198 (C460 [*EYC*, I, no. 253]) and 1204 (Stenton, *Pleas*, III, no. 1000). Ralph Fin witnessed in 1178 × 1181[3] (*EYC*, I, no. 160); *c.*1190 × *c.*1202 (R159, R165, R183); and *c.*1185 × 1207[4] (*EYC*, I, no. 557).

**R681.** Gift to the hospital by Osbert son of Ulger and his heirs of 5 a. in Wilberfoss, comprising 4 a. in the fields and 1 a. in a toft [*c.*1170 × *c.*1190]

*Osbertus filius Ulgeri de quinque acris terre in Wilburfossa.*
Sciant omnes qui viderint vel audierint litteras has quod ego Osbertus filius Ulgeri et heredes mei concessimus et dedimus deo et pauperibus hospitalis sancti Petri Ebor' quinque acras terre in Wilburfossa, quatuor in camp(is) et unam in tofto cum plenaria communione et omnibus aisiamentis in omnibus que ad eandem villam pertinent, in puram et liberam et perpetuam elemosinam, quietam et immunem ab omni humana consuetudine et auxilio preter orationes pauperum cristi. Hiis testibus, Petro filio Grente, Pagano de Kattona, Henrico de Beningburga, Willelmo de Wilburfossa, Ricardo de Kelca, Roberto filio Oreni, Roberto filio Hugonis.

Clay gives some details for the first witness, Peter son of Grente, who with another held 1 k.f. fee of Percy, and with two others 1 k.f. of Amfrey de Chauncy, in 1166. He is named in the partition of the Percy lands of 1175, and is described in an attestation to a deed of Amfrey de Chauncy as Peter son of Grente of [Full] Sutton. He was living in 1184 and 1196, but had been succeeded by his son Everard by 1201 (*EYC*, XI, 254–55). With his sons Everard and William he attested a deed of 1161 × 1192[5] (*Ctl. Fountains*, p. 318). The attestation of Henry of Beningbrough suggests *c.*1160 × *c.*1187 (M: Beningbrough). Pain of Catton was probably dead in 1192 (FN).

**R682.** Gift to the hospital by Osbert son of Ulger and his heirs, of the property described in R681, with the addition of a *pertica* of land, and also a toft in the vill next to the way out towards the gill [*c.*1170 × 1190]

---

3  During the archiepiscopate of Roger, and whilst Hamo was precentor.
4  The *terminus a quo* is not easy to fix. Amongst those named Fulk of Rufforth died in 1214 × 1217; Alan of Knapton in 1207 or before; Adam son of Alan of Knapton in 1226 × 1229; and Robert de Wivelestorp in 1214 (FNs).
5  The extreme dates for Amfrey de Chauncy, who also attests (*EYC*, II, 176; FN).

*Carta Osberti filii Ulgeri⁶ de v. acris et uno tofto in Wilburfosse.*
Sciant omnes qui viderint vel audierint litteras has quod ego Osbertus filius Ulgeri
et heredes mei concessimus et dedimus deo et pauperibus hospitalis sancti Petri Ebor'
quinque acras terre in Wilburfosse, iiii°ʳ in campis et unam in tofto, cum una pertica
terre, et preterea unum toftum in eadem villa iuxta exitum versus torrentum, scilicet
quicquid ibi habeo, cum plenaria communione et omnibus aisiamentis in omnibus que
ad eandem villam pertinent, in puram et liberam et perpetuam elemosinam quietas et
immunes ab omni humana consuetudine et auxilio preter orationes pauperum. Hiis
testibus, Petro filio Grent, Pagano de Cattona, Henrico de Beningburg, Willelmo de
Wilberfossa, Ricardo de Celca, Orein filio Hugonis, Roberto.

It is likely that the names of the final two witnesses are more correctly given in R681,
where they are more in keeping with the witness clause as a whole.

**R683.**   Grant at fee-farm to the hospital by Osbert son of Ulger of a croft in Wilberfoss 4 perches wide and 1 furlong long, and [confirmation ?] of 2 bv. in the
same vill, paying 2s. for all service [*c.*1160 × *c.*1171]

PRINTED: *EYC*, II, no. 914, where dated *c.*1180 × 1193.

*Osbertus filius Ulgeri de uno tofto et ii. bovatis terre de Wilberfossa.*
Sciant universi fideles qui viderint vel audierint has litteras quod ego Osbertus
filius Ulgeri dei amore dedi pauperibus hospitalis beati Petri Ebor' unum croftum
in Wilburfos in latitudine iiii. pertic(atas), in longitudine i. quadragenam, in puram
et perpetuam elemosinam, quietam et immunem ab omni humana exigencia preter
preces⁷ in domino, quam videlicet elemosinam imperpetuum predicti fratres
tenebunt, sicut aliquam elemosinam liberius et honorificentius in domo sua possident. Preter hoc concessi eisdem pauperibus in prenominata villa iiᵃˢ bovatas terre
cum omnibus pertinenciis suis, tenend(a) de me et heredibus meis in feudi firma
annuatim pro ipsa terra michi et heredibus meis ii.s. pro omni servicio quod ad me
et heredes meos inde pertinet persolvendo, et pro ea forense faciendo servicium. Hanc
autem firmam predicti pauperes michi et heredibus meis in duobus terminis anni
persolvent, videlicet xii.d. ad Pent' et xii. denarios ad festum sancti Martini. Hii sunt
testes, Radulfus presbiter, Nicholaus presbiter, Petrus presbiter de Biria, Willelmus
miles de Wilburfosse, Willelmus de Sancta Lege, Paganus de Catt(on), Alfredus forestarius, Robertus de Argent', Stephanus de Hupt', Walterus Engain, Willelmus Tuschet
et Simon frater eius, Willelmus de Pisa, Martinus Mal' herba, Robertus carpentar(ius),
Simon de Catt', Henricus garcifer, Rand(ulfus) de Glairu(i)ll'.

The use of *concessi* rather than *dedi* for the grant of the 2 bv. indicates this land was
confirmed rather than given, so the date is not necessarily before the confirmation
of 2 bv. in Wilberfoss by Eugenius III in 1148 (C178 [*EYC*, I, no. 179]). The survival
of Ilger, son of Osbert son of Ulger, until at least 1235 renders a date much before
*c.*1150 improbable. It seems unlikely that the witness William de St-Éloi, who first
occurs in 1148 × 1156, survived into the 1170s (FN).
      Peter clerk *de Biria* attested several deeds to the hospital. He perhaps took his
name from Bury St Edmunds, which occurs as *Biri* in the late twelfth century. In

---

⁶   MS: *Ulgi.*
⁷   MS: *preces* repeated.

1150 × 1157 he witnessed with Ralph the priest and Martin Mala Herba (M: Crosby
[Burton transcripts 2, f. 79ʳ, p. 124, B12 N25; ibid., f. 82ᵛ, p. 131, B6 N19]), and in 1148
× 1157, as Peter, chaplain *de Biri*, he witnessed with Martin Mala Herba (M: Pickhill
[Burton transcripts 2, f. 79ᵛ, p. 125, B12 N36]). He attested with Ralph the priest in
*c.*1160 × 1171 (R668); with Nicholas the priest in *c.*1150 × *c.*1180 (M: Heworth [MS
Dods. 120b, f. 55ʳ]); and with Ralph, chaplain, Nicholas, chaplain, and Martin Mala
Herba in *c.*1160 × 1181 (R152).

**R684.** Conveyance by Aubrey, formerly daughter of Thomas Queneld of Neuton
super Derwynt, to Alan de Stanewegs of Wilbirfosse and Helewise his wife,
of 1 a. with appurtenances in the field of Wilbirfosse lying above le Bergh,
as it lies in length from the common pasture called le Ragrene towards the
east as far as the common moor towards the west, and in width between the
lands which formerly belonged to Adam de Wilton on both sides, to hold of
the chief lords of the fee, for the due services. Warranty and sealing clauses.
30 April 1360.

*Albreda quondam filia Thome Queneld' de Neuton' de una acra terre.*

Hiis testibus, Willelmo de Botelrie, Iohanne de Greygnesby, Willelmo de Catton',
Roberto de Catton', Nicholao de Catton', Iohanne filio Iacobi de Neuton', Iohanne
Burdon', Henrico filio Mariot', Petro de Brouneflete et aliis. Dat' apud Wilburfosse
die iovis proxima ante festum apostolorum Philippi et Iacobi anno domini millesimo
trescentesimo sexagesimo.

**R685.** Grant by Alan de Stanewegs of Wilbirfosse to Thomas de Stanewegs of
Wilbirfosse of 1 a. above le Bergh with appurtenances, in the west field of
Wilberfosse, in a selion in length from the common pasture called le Ragrene
towards the east to the common moor towards the west, and in width between
the lands which once belonged to Adam de Wilton on both sides, which
land the grantor formerly held by the gift and feoffment of Aubrey, formerly
daughter of Thomas Queneld of Neuton super Derwent, as the deed of feoffment made to him shows, to hold of the chief lords of the fee by the due
services. Warranty and sealing clauses. 16 July 1364.

*Alanus de Stanewegs de una acra terre* **[f. 231ᵛ]**

Hiis testibus, Willelmo del Botelrie, Iohanne de Beverley, Iohanne de Graynesby,
Willelmo de Catton', Nicholao de Catton', Roberto de Catton', Iohanne filio Iacobi
de Neuton', Iohanne Burdon', Henrico filio Mariote, Petro de Brouneflete et aliis.
Dat' apud Wilberfosse die martis prox' ante festum sancte Margarete virginis, anno
domini millesimo trescentesimo sexagesimo quarto.

## *Wyghton'* [Market Weighton]

The medieval forms of the place names Weeton (ER), Weeton (WR), Little Weighton, and Market Weighton recorded by Smith do not allow a definite identification of the location of the land described in the following deeds (*PN YorksER*, pp. 23, 205, 229; *PN YorksWR*, v, 51). But the attestion of Gerard Salvain (R687), and the appearance of *Wighton* immediately after Thorpe le Street in the post-Dissolution accounts of the hospital's lands (*Dissolved Houses*, IV, 226) show the place is Market Weighton. Market Weighton was *terra regis* in 1086, and so remained in 1302–03 (*KI*, p. 261).

**R686.** Confirmation to the hospital by William son of Hervey of Weighton, of the grant in alms made by his father, of a toft and croft in Weighton between the dwelling of Robert the shoemaker and the dwelling of Robert son of Ulf, quit of service beyond the boon-work of one man at harvest time, for which service the hospital will have common of pasture and other easements belonging to such a tenement [1178 × 1198]

PRINTED: *EYC*, I, no. 443, where dated 1160 × 1170.

**[f. 232ʳ]** *Confirmatio Willelmi filii Heruei de tofto et crofto in Wighton'.*[1]
Omnibus hominibus presentibus et futuris ad quorum noticiam littere iste pervenerint, Willelmus filius Heruei[2] de Whictun salutem. Sciatis me concessisse et confirmasse presenti carta fratribus et infirmis hospitalis beati Petri Ebor' elemosinam quam dedit eis pater meus, scilicet toftum et croftum, quod iacet in Wictu(n) inter mansuram Roberti sutoris et mansuram Roberti filii Ulfi, libere et quiete ab omni servicio et exactione preter una(m) precaria(m) cum uno homine in autumpno. Et ipsi habebunt pro hoc servicio communem pasturam in campis et alia aisiamenta ad tantam tenuram pertinentia. Hiis testibus, Haimone precentore, Geroldo can(onico), Adam de Thornouer, Willelmo vicearch(i)d(iacano), Rogero de Bauvent, Herberto de Ostun, Willelmo filio eius, Ric(ardo) veteri, Hugone Totheman et multis aliis.

The date range is the period for Hamo as precentor (FN).

**R687.** Acknowledgement of receipt, with recital, by James of Weighton, clerk, of the deed of William, rector, and the brethren of the hospital, granting him the toft in Weighton which Richard son of Geoffrey formerly held of them, paying 14*d.* annually and 1*m.* as a portion of chattels on death [1235 × 1240 or 1245 × 1252]

*Terra in Wighton' dimissa ad firmam et pro portione in obitu i. marca.*
Sciant presentes et futuri quod ego Iacobus de Wihton' clericus recepi cartam hospitalis in hec verba: Omnibus cristi fidelibus ad quos presens scriptum pervenerit, Willelmus rector et fratres hospitalis sancti Petri Ebor' salutem. Noverit universitas vestra nos dedisse et presenti carta nostra confirmasse Iacobo de Wihton' clerico quoddam toftum cum pertinenciis suis in Wihton', illud videlicet toftum quod Ricardus filius Galfridi aliquando de nobis tenuit, tenendum et habendum dicto Iacobo et heredibus

---

[1]  See R676 for the pilcrow in blue ink separating the text and the rubric.
[2]  Possibly *Hernei*.

suis vel assignatis exceptis iudeis et viris religiosis aliis a nobis predictum toftum cum pertinenciis suis aisiamentis et libertatibus suis infra villam et extra libere integre et quiete iure hereditario, reddendo inde nobis annuatim pro omni servicio ad nos pertinente quatuordecim denarios, medietatem ad Pent' et medietatem ad festum sancti Martini in yeme. Predictus vero Iacobus et heredes sui vel assignati sui vel quicumque in predicta terra manserint vel dictam terram tenuerint pro portione catallorum ipsos in obitu contingente unam marcam argenti pauperibus domus nostre nomine testamenti fideliter persolvent, ita scilicet quod de residuo omnium catallorum ipsos contingentem licite et sine contradictione libere suum possent condere testamentum et per se et per suos executores ipsum plenius perficere. Hoc autem fideliter faciendum pro se et suis tactis sacrosanctis iuravit predictus Iacobus et affidavit. Nos autem predictum toftum cum pertinenciis suis eidem Iacobo et heredibus suis vel assignatis suis warantizabimus quamdiu donatores nostri illud nobis warantizaverint. In huius rei testimonium huic scripto sigillum nostrum apposuimus. Hiis testibus, domino Galfrido[3] Salvey', domino Roberto constabulario, Ricardo Veil', Thoma de Neubalde, Simone fratre suo, Hugone filio Willelmi, Roberto Frankeley', Henrico clerico, Waltero coco, Ricardo de Wytewell' et aliis. In cuius rei testimonium huic scripto sigillum meum apposui.

The date range is the widest period possible for William as rector. As Sir Geoffrey Salvain does not otherwise appear, it can be assumed that the first witness is a mistake for Gerard Salvain, who in 1254 held 3 ct. in Thorpe le Street, par. Market Weighton, of St Mary's Abbey (*EYC*, xii, 110). The second witness is doubtless Robert Constable III of Flamborough, who succeeded his father William between 1224 and 1243, occurs as a knight in 1246 and 1251, and died in 1272 × 1274 (*EYC*, xii, 147–48). Gerard Salvain, Robert le Veyll, and Godfrey Franklin were tenants in Market Weighton (*Wighton cum membris*) in 1302–3 (*KI*, p. 261), and may have been the representatives of the families of the first, third, and seventh witnesses respectively. The 4th witness presumably took his name from one of the places named Newbald lying between Market Weighton and Little Weighton.

**R688.** Final concord between Roger le Wauters and Mildonia his wife, claimants, and brother William master of the hospital, tenant, concerning a toft in Weighton, whereof there had been a plea before them in the same court. Roger and Mildonia recognised the toft to be the right of the master and brethren, and released it and quitclaimed for themselves and the heirs of Mildonia. The master gave 1*m*. 25 June 1246.

ORIGINAL: *a* PRO, CP/25/1/262/39, no. 89, not collated. COPY: *b* Rawl., f. 232ʳ. CALENDAR: *YF*, 1232–1246, p. 157, from *a*.

*Cirograph(um) in curia regis de tofto in W(ychton).*
Hec est finalis concordia facta in curia domini regis apud Ebor' in crastino sancti Iohannis baptiste anno regni regis Henrici filius regis Iohannis tricesimo coram Rogero de Thurkelby, Gilberto Preston', magistro Simone de Wauton' et Iohanne de Cobbeham iusticiariis itinerantibus et aliis domini regis fidelibus tunc ibidem presentibus inter Rogerum le Wauters et Mildon(iam) uxorem eius petentes et fratrem Willelmum magistrum hospitalis sancti Petri Ebor' tenentem de uno tofto cum

---

[3] sic, but see the note to the deed.

pertinenciis in Wychton', unde placitum fuit inter eos in eadem curia, scilicet quod predicti Rogerus et Mildon(ia) recogn(overunt) predictum toftum cum pertinenciis esse ius ipsius magistri et fratrum predicti hospitalis et illud remiser(un)t et quiet' clam(averunt) de se et heredibus ipsius Mildon(ie) predicto magistro et successoribus suis et predictis fratribus imperpetuum. Et pro hac recognitione remissione quiet(a) clam(ancia) fine et concordia idem magister dedit predictis Rogero et Mildon(ie) unam marcam argenti.

The remainder of f. 232$^r$ is blank. f. 232$^v$ is blank except for the well-known Latin palindrome *Roma tibi subito motibus ibit amor*, followed by a note *the contents of this bowke is xi$^{xx}$ and xii leaves*.

# SUPPLEMENTARY DOCUMENTS

## West Riding Deeds

Dodsworth's transcripts in MS Dods. 120b provide abstracts from many deeds copied to leaves of the West Riding division of the Rawlinson volume that are now missing. These transcripts are printed below, together with the texts of deeds from other sources belonging to vills in the West Riding. Also included here are brief notes on the hospital's holdings in places in the West Riding which had no section in the cartulary, like Bagley and Barnburgh. Section headings, if not in square brackets, are taken from the Contents List or from MS Dods. 120b.

### [Bagley]

There was no section for Bagley in the Rawlinson volume. King Stephen gave the hospital 5 bv. in Woolthwaite and 1 bv. in Bagley (both par. Tickhill) by a charter of 1135 × 1148 (C1 [*Regesta*, III, no. 994]). The papal confirmations for 1148 and 1157 include these gifts but the donor is not named. There is no mention of either place in the confirmation of 1173 (C178–C180 [*EYC*, I, nos 179, 186, 197]). In 1155 × 1170 Henry II confirmed 4 bv. in Woolthwaite and 1 bv. in Bagley 'of my gift' (C10 [*EYC*, I, no. 175]), and 1155 × 1173 he ordered the constable and bailiffs of Tickhill to allow the brethren of the hospital to hold their land in Woolthwaite and *Colsilanda* in Bagley in peace (C25 [Cott., f. 5ʳ]). No subsequent trace of the hospital's Bagley holding has been found.

### [Barnburgh]

In 1086 Barnburgh lay partly in the fee of Roger de Busli, and partly in that of William de Warenne. The papal confirmation of 1148 includes *in Barnaburc terra de qua pauperes habent iiii. solidos*. The confirmations of 1157 and 1173 include similar phrases, but do not identify the donor (C178–C180 [*EYC*, I, nos 179, 186, 197]). There was no section for Barnburgh in the Rawlinson volume, and nothing more is known of the hospital's holding.

### [Bramhope]

For Bramhope, see R6–R54.

**R701.** Grant at fee-farm by Thomas, rector of the hospital, to Marmaduke son of Marmaduke of Dishforth, of five tofts, 7 bv. and 14½ a. in Bramhope, for 2s. 6d. annually, and an obituary payment of ½m. [1263 × 1276, probably c. 1270–71]

COPY: MS Dods. 83, f. 7ʳ⁻ᵛ, from the original at Skipton Castle, copied by Dodsworth in 1646.

*Carta facta Marmeduco filio Marmaducis de Disceford.*

Universis cristi fidelibus ad quos presens scriptum pervenerit, Thomas rector et fratres hospitalis sancti Leonardi Ebor' salutem in domino sempiternam. Noveritis nos, cum consilio et assensu capituli nostri, concessisse dedisse et confirmasse Marmeduco filio Marmeduci de Disceford, quinque tofta cum septem bovatis terre et quatuordecim acris et dimidia in villa [et]¹ territorio de Bramhop: scilicet illam bovatam terre quam Adam Wauncy quondam de nobis tenuit, et unum toftum cum duabus bovatis terre iuxta toftum Willelmi Northiby que Radulfus Forestarius quondam tenuit, [et aliud toftum cum duabus bovatis terre que Helias prepositus quondam tenuit,]² <et tertium toftum quod iacet propinquius capitali messuagio nostro versus occidentem, cum illis duabus bovatis terre que Thomas Morolf quondam tenuit>, et quartum toftum iacens ex orientali parte propinquius tofto Ade de Karleton, et quintum toftum quod vocatur pars curtilagii cum quatuor buttis³ terre abbuttantibus super curtilagium et croftum dicti Marmaduci, et sex acras terre et dimidia(m) quas Willelmus Northiby et Robertus filius eius tenuerunt, quarum sex acre iacent in cultura que vocatur Le Ridding, iacens versus occidentalem partem vie, que ducit de Bramhop usque Pouel, inter terram dicti Marmaduci ex una parte et illam acram quam Ricardus prepositus tenuit ex altera, et dimidiam acram ex occidentale parte prati dicti Marmaduci in Murelethes et Ruggeknollerane sicut se extendit de Noutegate in longitudine, usque ad viam que ducit Dibbe versus Lathebote, et in latitudine⁴ versus occidentem de Ruggeknollerane, usque ad viam que ducit de Bramhop <usque> ad Pouel, et unam acram terre que iacet infra eandem Ruggeknol[f. 7ᵛ]lerane, et dimidiam acram quam Anabella uxor Roberti Vilayn quondam tenuit, scilicet que iacet iuxta prenominatam acram, et septem acras terre et dimidiam, quarum due acre et dimidia iacent in cultura que vocatur Pristekroune, unam acram terre que iacet ex utraque parte de Ruggeknollerane ad caput orientale, et quatuor acras que iacent iuxta boscum de Bramhope, in loco qui dicitur Langgeridding, tenend(a) et habend(a) de nobis et successoribus nostris dicto Marmaduco et heredibus suis et suis assignatis, exceptis viris religiosis aliis a nobis et capitalibus dominis feodi, libere quiete integre et honor-ifice et pacifice, cum omnibus pertinenciis libertatibus et aisiamentis, in pratis et pasturis, et tot animalia quot idem Marmaducus et heredes sui perquirere poterint, excepto bosco nostro, et dominicis nostris, reddendo inde annuatim nobis et succes-soribus nostris duos solidos et sex denarios duobus terminis anni, videlicet quindecim denarios ad Pentecosten, et quindecim denarios ad festum sancti Martini in hyeme, pro omni <seculari> servitio, sectis curiarum, exactione, et demand(a). Nos vero et successores <nostri> totum predictum tenementum cum omnibus pertinenciis suis supradictis, sepedicto Marmaduco et heredibus suis et suis assignatis ut predictum est, per predictum servitium contra omnes gentes warantizabimus adquietabimus et defendemus, quamdiu carte donator(um) nostri quas inde habemus, nobis predictas terras <et> tenementum warantizare adquietare poterunt et defendere. Et sciendum est quod dictus Marmaducus et heredes sui et sui assignati seu quicumque dictum tenementum cum pertinenciis tenuerint, vel in eo manserint, pro portione catallorum suorum in obitu suo ipsos contingente dimidiam marcam pauperibus domus nostre nomine testamenti relinquent. In cuius rei testimonium duo scripta unius tenoris

¹   Supplied.
²   The text *et aliud toftum . . . Helias prepositus quondam tenuit* is supplied from Marmaduke's deed to the hospital (R43). The insertion of this phrase, with the other suggested amendment, supplies the necessary five tofts and 7 bv.
³   MS: *bovatis*. This correction follows the text in R43.
⁴   MS: *et in latitudine* repeated.

in modum cyrographi sunt confecta, quorum unum residet penes nos, sigillo dicti Marmaduci signatum, et aliud penes dictum Marmaducum communi sigillo <nostro> munitum. Hiis testibus, domino Patricio de Westwyc, domino Symone Ward tunc rectore de Giselay, Radulfo de Arthington, Ricardo de Goldesburgh, Roberto [de] Pouell, Willelmo de Alwardlay, Adam de Tofhuse, Henrico Wigan, Roberto Vilayn, Radulfo <de> Tresck clerico et aliis.

The date range is the period for Thomas as rector. The reference to 'our capital messuage', which in another deed is the 'capital messuage of Thomas (son of Marmaduke of Dishforth)' (R43), implies a date after Thomas of Dishforth's gift of his manor to the hospital in c.1270–71 (R7). The majority of the property listed here was given by Thomas son of Marmaduke of Dishforth and Marmaduke son of Marmaduke of Dishforth by deeds which have different descriptions of the land, but almost identical witness lists to the present deed (R43, R44). All four deeds were probably given at about the same time, as part of a single transaction. The deed by which the hospital acquired the bovate held by Adam Wauncy has not been preserved.

# [Brotherton]

A rent in *Broderton* was noted in the account of 1542, following entries for Knottingley and Fairburn (*Dissolved Houses*, IV, 225). Nothing further is known of this holding, and there was no section for Brotherton in the Rawlinson volume. In c.1030 Brotherton was included in a list of the soke of the archbishop's manor of Sherburn (*EYC*, I, no. 7), and 1316 was jointly held by the archbishop of York and John Markenfield (*KI*, p. 345).

# [Copmanthorpe]

For Copmanthorpe, see R95–R102.

**R702.** Truncated inspeximus by Roger, the dean, and the chapter of St Peter's, York, of the deeds of Ralph de Fontibus, chaplain, and his assigns [1220 × c.1233 or 1258 × 1263]

ORIGINAL: WYAS, Leeds, Ingilby MS, WYL230/11, 19 cm. (wide) × 34 cm. The bottom of the document has been cut off, and the seal tag reinserted through a new pair of slits cut in the text. Seal, red wax, badly broken, fragment 25 mm. (wide) × 40 mm. remaining, a robed standing figure, hands clasped together over a stole with ends joined forming a v-shape, presumably for St Peter (cf. the chapter seals described in *BM Cat. Seals*, I, 382–83). No medieval endorsements.

Rogerus decanus et capitulum sancti Petri Ebor' omnibus cristi fidelibus salutem. Noveritis nos inspexisse cartas Radulfi capellani de Fontibus et assignatorum suorum in hec verba: [*texts of R703, R704, R102 with interlineation, and R705 follow*]

The loss of the attestation, if there was one, makes it difficult to determine whether the inspeximus belongs to Roger de Lisle, who was dean 1220–c.1233, or Roger of Holderness, alias of Skeffling, dean 1258–1263. The hand is suggestive of the earlier period, but is not conclusive. The full inspeximus form, with recital, was in use in York by the early thirteenth century. Archbishop Geoffrey issued such a document in 1191 × 1205 (*EEA*, xxvii, no. 3), and Simon de Apulia, the dean, did so in 1213 × 1214 (C359 [Cott., f. 69ʳ]).

**R703.** Bond by Hugh, rector, and the brethren of the hospital, to maintain a chaplain in their house at the altar of St Edmund in the church of St Leonard, to pray for the living and the dead, and to pay him his stipend of 20*s.* annually, and to provide 4*lb.* of wax yearly to light the altar, from the rent which Ralph de Fontibus chaplain gave to the hospital for the purpose. Ralph has also given, for the service of God and St Edmund at the said altar, a silver chalice, two silver phials, and vestment and ornaments for the altar [1214 × 1218]

COPY: Inspeximus R702.

Omnibus presentes litteras visuris vel audituris magister H[ugo] rector et fratres hospitalis sancti Petri Ebor' eternam in domino salutem. Noverit universitas vestra nos teneri ad exhibend(um) unum capellanum in domo nostra qui ad altare sancti Edmundi in ecclesia sancti Leonardi tam pro vivis quam pro defunctis in perpetuum celebrabit. Tenemur etiam ad solvendum eidem capellano stipendia sua, scilicet viginti solidos annuos, et ad inveniendum quatuor libras cere annuas ad luminare eiusdem altaris de redditu quam Radulfus de Fontibus capellanus caritative domui nostre dedit et ad predicta invenienda assignavit. Dedit autem dictus Radulfus ad serviendum deo et sancto Edmundo ad predictum altare calicem argenteum duas fialas argenteas librum vestimentum et ornamenta ad altare pertinentia. In huius autem rei robur et testimonium huic scripto sigillum nostrum apposuimus. Testibus, domino H[amone] thesaurario etc.

Hamo was still treasurer in August 1217, but was dean by 1 March 1218. Hugh succeeded Ralph as rector of the hospital between 1214 and September 1217.

**R704.** Grant by Hugh, rector, and the brethren of the hospital, to Ralph de Fontibus, chaplain, of the ½ ct. in Copmanthorpe which Thomas de Camera gave them at the request of the same Ralph, and which John Malebisse confirmed for 100*s.* paid by Ralph, to be held by Ralph according to the deeds of Thomas and John, paying the hospital ½*m.* annually, and a portion of chattels as an obituary payment, for a pittance on St Edmund's day to those in the infirmary [1214 × 1231]

COPY: Inspeximus R702.

Omnibus cristi fidelibus ad quos presens scriptum pervenerit magister Hugo rector hospitalis sancti Petri Ebor' et fratres eiusdem domus eternam in domino salutem. Noverit universitas vestra nos concessisse et presenti carta nostra confirmasse Radulfo de Fontibus capellano dimidiam carucatam terre in territorio de Copmantorp cum toftis et croftis ad illam terram pertinentibus et cum communi pastura eiusdem ville, illam scilicet dimidiam carucatam terre quam Thomas de Kamera ad instanciam et petitione predicti Radulfi capellani nobis dedit, et Iohannes Malebisse, pro centum solidis quos sepedictus Radulfus ei dedit, confirmavit, tenendam et habendam totam predictam terram cum omnibus pertinenciis suis et asiamentis et libertatibus infra villam et extra, secundum tenorem cartarum predictorum Thome et Iohannis Malebisse, prenominato Radulfo vel cui eam asignare voluerit, de nobis libere integre et quiete iure hereditario, reddendo inde nobis annuatim dimidiam marcam argenti pro omni servicio et exactione et proportione catallorum eis in obitu contingente, ad unam pitanciam faciendam in die sancti Eadmundi infirmis de infirmitorio pro anima predicti Radulfi et antecessorum et successorum suorum imperpetuum. In huius autem rei robur et testimonium huic scripto sigillum nostrum apposuimus. Hiis testibus, Iohanne Malebisse etc.

John Malebisse was dead in 1231.

**R705.** Grant by Isolda of Copmanthorpe, truncated [1214 × c.1235]

COPY: Inspeximus R702.

Omnibus presentes litteras visuris vel audituris, Ysoude de Copmantorp salutem. Noverit universitas vestra me in libera potestate mea constitutam ad instanciam et petitione domini mei Radulfi de Fontibus et aliorum amicorum meorum dedisse [remainder cut away]

## [Cridling Stubbs]

There was no section for Cridling Stubbs in the Rawlinson volume. The papal confirmations of 1157 and 1173 include 1 bv. and 42 a. in *Cridlinc* (C179–C180 [*EYC*, I, nos 186, 197]). In 1155 × 1173, Henry II ordered Henry de Lacy to allow the brethren of the hospital to hold in peace 42 a. in *Credelyng*, which Robert de Campeaux had given them before he was impleaded for the death of William Maltravers (C18 [*EYC*, III, no. 1455]). As Maltravers was killed immediately after the death of Henry I, and King Stephen pardoned those involved soon afterwards (*EYC*, III, 143–44; Richard of Hexham, *Historia*, III, 140), Henry II's charter indicates that the hospital gained its land in Cridling during the reign of Henry I, or very soon after his death. But as the hospital was prepared to fabricate evidence to improve its title to lands given during the reign of Stephen (R1n) this cannot be regarded as certain. In 1166 Cridling formed part of the 1 k.f. held by Ralph son of Nicholas [of Cridling] of Henry de Lacy. Ralph's son Adam of Cridling resigned the vill and other property to Roger de Lacy, constable of Chester, in 1193 × 1211 (*EYC*, III, 387). No subsequent trace of the hospital's holding in Cridling has been found.

## *Grimston in Elmett* [par. Kirkby Wharfe, WR]

The Contents List shows that ff. 52, 53 and 54, now missing, contained deeds belonging to Grimston 'in Elmet', which lies 2 m. south of Tadcaster. Dodsworth made abstracts from deeds on ff. 52–53. In 1086 Grimston was in the fee of Ilbert [de Lacy]. Like many places in the Lacy fee it is absent from the returns of 1284–85 (*KI*, p. 50n). The deeds copied by Dodsworth show that the hospital acquired 1 bv. in Grimston from William son of Henry of Grimston in c.1245 × c.1275 (R706–R707), and the service of the tenant of 2 bv. in Grimston from William son of John of Lotherton in c.1260 × c.1280 (R708). Apart from these deeds, no evidence for the hospital's interest in Grimston has been discovered.

**R706.** Gift to the hospital by William son of Henry of Grimston of 1 bv. in Grimston
[*c*.1245 × *c*.1275]

NOTED: MS Dods. 120b, f. 10ʳ, from Rawl., f. 52, now missing.

Willelmus filius Henrici de Grimeston dedit hospitali sancti Leonardi Ebor' 1 bovatam
terre in Grimston etc. Teste Philippo de Milford, Iohanne de eadem etc. fo. 52.

Philip and John of Milford head a list of jurors in an inquisition concerning an
accusation of murder procured by the householder (*husbandi*) of the grange of Lead
in 1249 (*YI*, I, 14). Philip of Milford was party to a fine concerning North Milford
in 1268 (*YF*, 1246–1272, p. 161). He attested a Hornington deed in *c*.1260 × *c*.1280
(R195), and with John of Milford and William of Grimston another, possibly at a
similar date (R197). Philip of Milford attested two Lead deeds, one with John of
Milford, at about the same time (R261–R262); Philip and John of Milford attested a
Saxton deed in 1263 × 1274 (R400).

**R707.** Confirmation of R706 by Thomas of Grimston, brother of William [*c*.1245 ×
            *c*.1275]
NOTED: MS Dods. 120b, f. 10ʳ, from Rawl., f. 52, now missing.

Tho(mas) de Grymston frater ipsius W(illelm)i confirm(avit) etc. ibidem.

Thomas son of Henry of Grimston attested a Saxton deed in 1263 × 1276 (R404).

**R708.** Grant to the hospital by William son of Jordan of Lotherton of the service
            of Alan son of Alan [son of Gilbert] of Grimston pertaining to 2 bv. which
            (Alan) holds of (William's) fee in Grimston [*c*.1260 × *c*.1280]

ABSTRACT: MS Dods. 120b, f. 10ʳ, from Rawl., f. 52, now missing.

Willelmus filius Iordani de Lutrington dedit et confirm(avit) hospitali sancti Leonardi
Ebor' servitium Alani filii Alani <{filii Gilberti}> de Grimeston de 2 bovatis terre
quas t(enet) de feodo suo in eadem villa. Testibus, Rogero de Saxton, Iohanne filio
Simonis de eadem, Iohanne de Milford, Iohanne de Saxton. fo. 52.

In 1269 Alan son of Alan of Grimston paid 5*m*. to Thomas of Ulleskelf and Modesty
his wife for a toft in Grimston (*YF*, 1246–1272, p. 175), and in 1284 he demised to
Roger of Saxton a messuage, mill, and 104 a. of land in Saxton and Barkston, for
the life of Roger (*YF*, 1272–1300, p. 70). Alan of Grimston was named in abutments
as a holder of lands in Saxton in *c*.1289 (R396). John son of Simon of Saxton made
quitclaims in 1263 × 1274 (R400) and *c*.1250 × 1269 (R402). The first witness was
probably the rector of Finghall, who with John of Milford, John of Saxton, Alan of
Grimston and others attested a deed of 1263 × 1276 (R405). John of Milford and
John of Saxton attested together in 1264–65 (R709).

**R709.** Dated attestation [28 October 1264 × 27 October 1265]

NOTED: MS Dods. 120b, f. 10ᵛ, from Rawl., f. 53, now missing.

Iohannes de Milford, Thoma de Grimeston, Iohannes de Saxton testes 49.H.3. fo. 53.

# [North Grimston, ER]

For North Grimston, see R499–R500.

**R710.** Gift to the hospital by Richard son of Sir Walter of Grimston of 1 bv. and a toft in [North] Grimston [1214 × 1245, dubious authenticity]

COPY: *d* Burton transcripts 5, f. 85ʳ, p. 161, B10 N24, abbreviated. ABSTRACT: *c* MS Dods. 120b, f. 10ᵛ (1st, 8th, 9th, 11th witnesses only) from Rawl., f. 52, now missing. NOTED: Drake, *Eboracum*, p. 335, via Torre's collections.

Universis etc. Ricardus filius domini Walteri de Grimestona salutem. Noverit etc. me dedisse etc. deo et beato Petro et beato Leonardo et pauperibus hospitalis Eboraci in puram etc. unam bovatam terram in Grimestona et unum toftum in eadem villa, tenend(a) et habend(a) libere etc. Hiis testibus, magistro Hugone rectore hospitalis, fratre Ada, fratre Ricardo, Stephano et Waltero, fratre Willelmo de Trent, Willelmo capellano de Kernetebi, Radulfo de Fribi, Thoma filio Galfridi de Grimestona, Roberto filio Willelmi de eadem villa, Alano Westibi de Diugilby, Roberto de Gin'ai de eadem villa, Willelmo filio suo etc.

The donor appears in connection with [North] Grimston (HN) and so this deed was misplaced in the West Riding division of the Rawlinson volume. This deed has several unusual features: the attestation of the master to a benefaction to the hospital is very uncommon; the repeated use of *fratre* is unusual at this period; and the expression *deo et beato Petro et beato Leonardo* is also uncommon. Some suspicion must therefore attach to it. The date range suggested is the period for rector Hugh.

## Hickleton

The Contents List gives f. 58, now missing, for Hickleton. The two deeds copied by Dodsworth were both from this folio. For the hospital's interest in Hickleton, and the Neufmarché family's holdings there, see HN: Cadeby.

**R711.** Gift to the hospital by John son of Henry [?] of Goldthorpe of a toft in Hickleton next to the land of Nicola, daughter of Randulf de Neufmarché [1219 × 1240]

NOTED: MS Dods. 120b, f. 10ᵛ, from Rawl., f. 58, now missing.

Iohannes filius Hernici⁵ de Goldthorp dedit hospitali sancti Leonardi Ebor' unum toftum cum pertinentiis in villa de Hikelton iuxta terram Nicholee filie Randulfi de Novomercato. Testibus, Radulfo de Novomercato, Anselino de Kateby, Ricardo de Schauceby, Elia de eadem villa, Willelmo de Bareville, Thoma de Lascy, Rogero de Lascy de Thirnesco etc. fo. 58.

The date range is limited by the period for Ralph de Neufmarché (FN).

⁵ sic.

**R712.** Confirmation of R711 by Ralph de Neufmarché [1219 × 1240]

NOTED: MS Dods. 120b, f. 10ᵛ, from Rawl., f. 58, now missing.

Radulfus de Novo Mercato de Hikelton confirmat donacionem predictam. Eysdem testibus, ibidem.

## *Harley*⁶ [in Wentworth, par. Wath on Dearne]

The Contents List states that f. 59 contained Harley deeds, and the single deed abstracted by Dodsworth is referenced to this folio. The witnesses support the identification of the place as Harley, near Wentworth, although it is not otherwise recorded as Herlay (*PN Yorks WR*, I, 121), and is not otherwise noticed amongst the possessions of the hospital.

**R713.** Quitclaim to the hospital by Henry son of Robert de Herlay, of all right and claim he had in 60 a. in Harley which he pleaded by writ of mort d'ancestor from Laurence son of John before the king's justices [October or November 1208 or later]

ABSTRACT: MS Dods. 120b, f. 11ʳ, from Rawl., f. 59, now missing.

Ego Henricus filius Roberti de Herlay <dedi et> confirm(avi) hospitali beati Petri Ebor' totum ius et clam(eum) quod habui in 60 acris terre in Herlay quas petii per breve de morte an(te)cessorum a Laurentio filio Iohannis coram Ada de Port, Simone de Pateshil', Godefrido de Insula et aliis sociis eorum tunc iusticiariis domini regis. Testibus, Willelmo filio Iohannis, Willelmo de Morthing, Nicholao de sancta Maria, Rogero de Swinton, Radulfo de Wath, Thoma Barbot, Willelmo Barbot. fo. 59.

Port, Pattishall and Lisle were amongst the justices in eyre in Yorkshire in October and November 1208 (*General Eyre*, p. 68).

## *Helleby* [Hellaby]

For Hellaby, which lay in the honour of Tickhill, see *SY*, I, 260. The Contents List gives f. 59 for Hellaby. A rent there, formerly belonging to the hospital, was noted in 1542 (*Dissolved Houses*, IV, 225). The hospital also had land in Bramley and Hooton Levitt nearby, but nothing more is known of the Hellaby holding.

## [Hoylandswain]

There was no section for Hoylandswain, a member of the Lacy fee, in the Rawlinson volume. In 1300 the master claimed against John Reyner of Hoylandswain 1 a. there as the right of the hospital (Baildon, *Monastic Notes*, II, 76). The account of 1542 included a rent in *Hullanswan* (*Dissolved Houses*, IV, 225). Nothing more is known of the hospital's holding.

---

⁶  MS Dods. 120b: *Herlay.*

## *Hutton=Lyvet* [Hooton Levitt]

The Contents List gives f. 60 for Hooton Levitt. The deeds copied by Dodsworth are referenced to this folio. In 1086 the count of Mortain held Hooton [Levitt], where there were 3 ct. 6 bv. Its subsequent tenure by Mauley indicates it passed to Fossard after Mortain's forfeiture. A mesne tenancy was held by Vescy (*KI*, pp. 7, 11; *SY*, 1, 264–65). A bovate in Hooton and another in Wickersley were included in the papal confirmations to the hospital of 1148, 1157 and 1173, but no further details are given (C178–C180 [*EYC*, 1, nos 179, 186, 197]). Wickersley, assessed at 4 ct., was held in 1086 by Roger de Busli, whose fee later became the honour of Tickhill. Richard son of Turgis, a co-founder of Roche Abbey, held land in both Wickersley and Hooton. It was Richard son of Turgis who gave the hospital its bovate in Hooton Levitt, and it is probable that the bovate in Wickersley was also his gift.[7] Richard's son Roger made two deeds to the hospital. Styling himself Roger son of Richard of Wickersley he confirmed the bovate in Hooton given by his father, which had belonged to his grandmother; and as Roger son of Richard of Hooton, he exchanged 8 a. for an assart (R714, R720). In 1194 × 1198 William de Livet, who was husband to Roger's daughter Constance, confirmed the land in Hooton given by his predecessors to the hospital, and in 1205 × 1229 Constance confirmed 2 bv. in Hooton given by her predecessors, and gave a further bovate in Wickersley and another in Hooton (R715, R716). Constance's descendants were the hospital's tenants in Hooton. Richard Livet of Hooton undertook not to sell the land he held of the hospital in 1277, and in 1288 × 1293 the master confirmed to Nicholas de Livet the 3 bv. in Hooton which had been given to Nicholas by Richard son of Richard Livet (R718, R719). The hospital's holdings in Hooton Levitt and Wickersley do not appear in the extents of the late thirteenth century, nor in the *Valor Ecclesiasticus*, but a rent in *Hutton* is recorded in the account of 1542 (*Dissolved Houses*, IV, 225).

The family of HOOTON [Levitt] or WICKERSLEY was descended from Richard son of Turgis, who was living in the reigns of Henry I and Stephen. The family held ½ k.f. in Wickersley of Neufmarché, who held of the honour of Tickhill, and 2 k.f. in Rotherham, Hooton Levitt, Pickburn and elsewhere of Vescy, who held of Fossard. Richard son of Turgis and Richard de Busli, another Tickhill tenant, were joint founders of the monastery of Roche. The two men issued similar deeds, with identical witnesses, to 'God and St Mary and the monks of Roche' in *c*.1147.[8] Richard son of Turgis gave the monks his land in *Etrichetorp*, and the right to fifty cartloads (presumably of brush or wood) each year from his wood of Wickersley. Busli's deed gives land close by, with rights of pasture. The deeds gave the abbot freedom to build the abbey by whichever part of the water[9] should seem best. Adam de Neufmarché,

---

7   The hospital's Wickersley deeds were copied at f. 134, now missing, but Dodsworth made no abstracts from them.

8   The date usually given for the abbey's foundation, 30 July 1147, is derived from a list of the early abbots which has the appearance of being drawn up at the end of the rule of Abbot Walter in *c*.1258, with some later additions (*MA*, v, 505, no. 14). This seems to be the only source for the date. The old edition of the *Monasticon* also cites *Annal. Cestr. in bibl. Cotton.*, and this reference was copied verbatim to the new edition (*MA1*, 1, 835; *MA*, v, 502n). But the printed edition of the Chester annals makes no mention of Roche, and the editor does not mention a Cotton manuscript (*Annales Cestriensis*, passim). There is no volume of 'Chester Annals' in the catalogue of the Cotton MSS. The list of witnesses to Richard son of Turgis' deed is truncated in *MA*. A fuller version, which corresponds exactly with that of Busli's deed, is given at MS Dods. 8, f. 271ᵛ; cf. MS Dods. 9, f.165ᵛ.

9   Maltby Dike, which formed the boundary between Maltby and Hooton.

WICKERSLEY, WILSIC, LIVET AND HOOTON

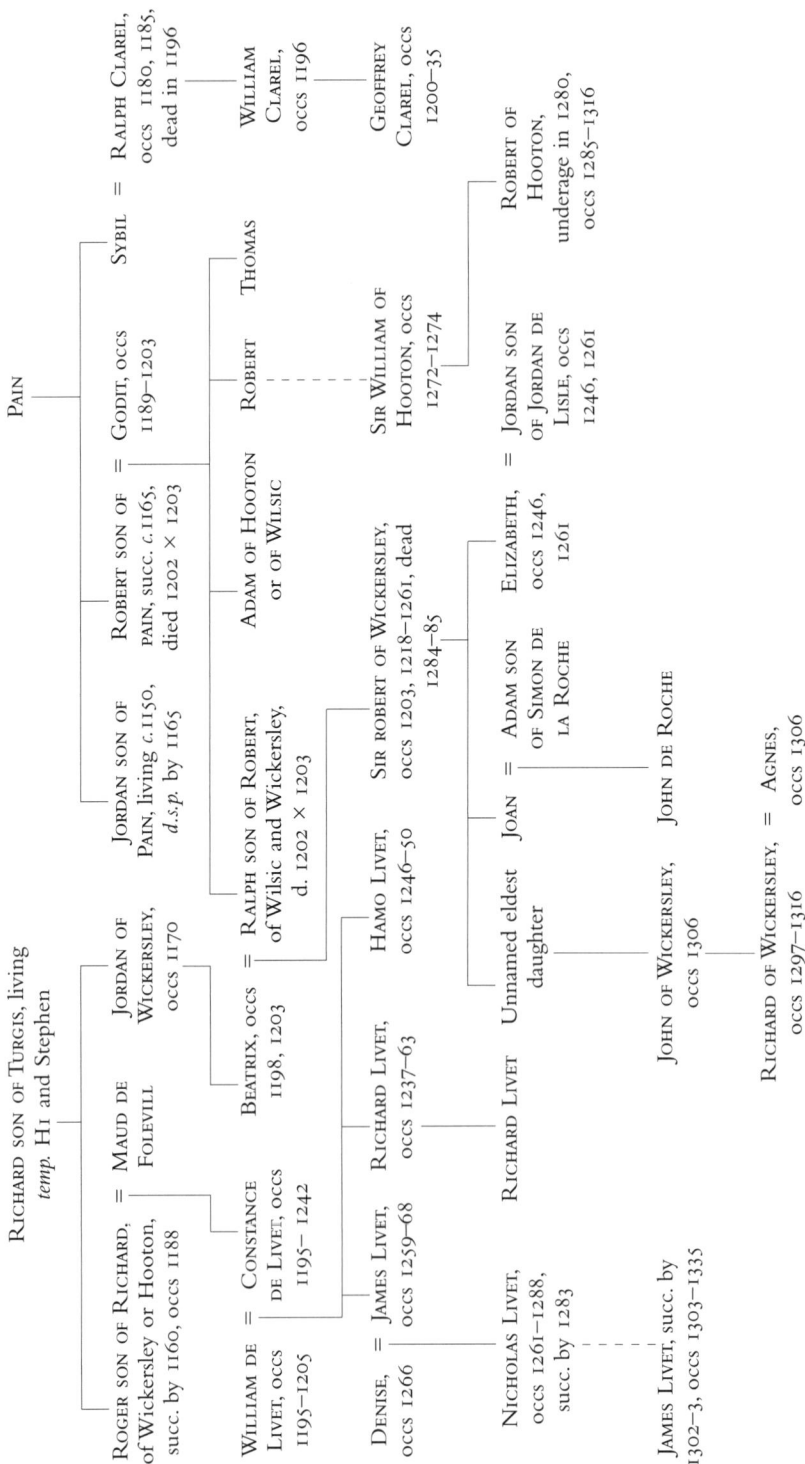

RICHARD SON OF TURGIS, living *temp.* H1 and Stephen

PAIN

ROGER SON OF RICHARD, of Wickersley or Hooton, succ. by 1160, occs 1188 = MAUD DE FOLEVILL

JORDAN OF WICKERSLEY, occs 1170

ROBERT SON OF PAIN, succ. *c.*1165, died 1202 × 1203 = GODIT, occs 1189–1203

JORDAN SON OF PAIN, living *c.*1150, *d.s.p.* by 1165

SYBIL = RALPH CLAREL, occs 1180, 1185, dead in 1196

WILLIAM CLAREL, occs 1196

GEOFFREY CLAREL, occs 1200–35

WILLIAM DE LIVET, occs 1195–1205 = CONSTANCE DE LIVET, occs 1195–1242

BEATRIX, occs 1198, 1203 = RALPH SON OF ROBERT, of Wilsic and Wickersley, d. 1202 × 1203

ADAM OF HOOTON or of WILSIC

ROBERT

THOMAS

SIR WILLIAM OF HOOTON, occs 1272–1274

ROBERT OF HOOTON, underage in 1280, occs 1285–1316

HAMO LIVET, occs 1246–50

RICHARD LIVET, occs 1237–63

SIR ROBERT OF WICKERSLEY, occs 1203, 1218–1261, dead 1284–85

ELIZABETH, occs 1246, 1261 = JORDAN SON of Jordan de Lisle, occs 1246, 1261

DENISE, occs 1266 = JAMES LIVET, occs 1259–68

RICHARD LIVET

Unnamed eldest daughter

JOAN = ADAM SON of Simon de la Roche

NICHOLAS LIVET, occs 1261–1288, succ. by 1283

RICHARD LIVET

JOHN OF WICKERSLEY, occs 1306

JOHN DE ROCHE

JAMES LIVET, succ. by 1302–3, occs 1303–1335

RICHARD OF WICKERSLEY, occs 1297–1316 = AGNES, occs 1306

of whom Richard son of Turgis held his land in Wickersley, was the first witness (*MA*, v, 502–3, nos 1–2). In 1186 Pope Urban III confirmed to Abbot Osmund 'by the gift of Richard de Busli and Richard of Wickersley the place in which your abbey is situated' (ibid., 505, no. 13).

Richard son of Turgis was succeeded by Roger son of Richard of Wickersley, who confirmed the gift to the hospital of 1 bv. in Hooton which his grandmother had held, and which his father had given previously (R720). As Roger son of Richard of Hooton he gave the hospital 8 a. in exchange for an assart (R714). Constance, daughter of Roger of Hooton, confirmed 2 bv. in Hooton given to the hospital by her ancestors (R715). Entries in the now lost cartulary of Worksop confirmed the descent from Richard to Roger to Constance, who was wife to William de Livet. Roger son of Richard of Wickersley granted the canons of Worksop his lordship of the church of Wickersley; Maud de Folevill, wife of Roger of Wickersley, confirmed her husband's grant. William de Livet, with the consent of Constance his wife, confirmed the grant of the advowson of the church of Wickersley which Roger of Wickersley, Constance's father, had made (MS Dods. 126, f. 148$^{r-v}$ [ex f. 57, cap. 1–5]).[10] In January 1161 the church of Wickersley (*Willeley*), with other property, was confirmed to Worksop by Pope Alexander III (*MA*, VI, 120, no. 7). 1160 would therefore seem to be the latest date for the succession of Roger.[11] In 1170 Roger of Wickersley and Jordan his brother owed 10*m.* for right in 2 k.f. which Roger de Tilly was holding of Henry de Lacy (*PR*, 16 Hen. II, p. 41). The entry was repeated in subsequent years, with the statement that [Tilly] 'did not have the right, nor a writ of right' appended in 1175 and 1176 (*PR*, 17–22 Hen. II, passim). Payment in full for 'right in 2 k.f. against Roger de Tilly' was made in 1176–77 (*PR*, 23 Hen. II, p. 70). In view of the dispute between Eustace de Vescy and Ralph de Tilly concerning 1 k.f. in Rotherham, mentioned in 1203 (*CRR*, 1203–1205, p. 74), and the lack of evidence for a significant Wickersley holding of Lacy, the 2 k.f. must be those held in the first half of the thirteenth century by Constance de Livet of Vescy, who held of Mauley; and were presumably included in the 7 k.f. held by William de Vescy of William Fossard in 1166 (*EYC*, II, no. 1003 and n). The interest of Henry de Lacy is difficult to explain, but is further evidenced by his confirmation to Roche of the grant of common pasture in Hooton made by Richard of Wickersley and Roger and Jordan his heirs (MS Dods. 117, f. 18$^r$).

Roger of Wickersley was a benefactor of Blyth Priory, to which he gave an *acrescot*[12] annually (*Ctl. Blyth*, no. 302). In 1188 Roger de Hotton owed ½*m.* in Yorkshire as he had not carried out what he pledged. The entry continued onto subsequent rolls and the money was never paid (*PR*, 34 Hen. II, p. 93; ibid., 6 Ric. I, p. 148). This suggests Roger died *c.*1188 or soon afterwards. He was certainly dead in 1200, when William Livet and Constance his wife (Roger's daughter) were plaintiffs in a case in the king's court. Further details on this case, and notes on the Livet family, are given below.

A subsidiary interest in Wickersley and Hooton Levitt was held by Roger of Wickersley's brother Jordan, and passed to Jordan's daughter Beatrix, wife to Ralph son of Robert son of Pain, who also occurs as Ralph of Wilsic and Ralph of

---

[10] Dodsworth's abstracts concerning Wickersley are copied from '*liber S.K.A.T.*', ff. 165–66 (MS Dods. 126, f. 109), apparently a volume of transcripts or abstracts from various sources by the Derbyshire antiquary Saint Loe Kniveton, then in the hands of Richard Gascoigne (*SC*, II, 941). Dodsworth's notes appear to be the source of the details given in Holland, *Worksop*, pp. 78–79, whence *SY*, I, 277.

[11] So Richard de Hoton, who was named in the account for Notts. and Derbs. in the pipe roll for 1176–77, paying an amercement for forest offences, cannot be Richard son of Turgis (*PR*, 22 Hen. II, p. 94; ibid., 23 Hen. II, p. 59).

[12] A rent or charge per acre.

Wickersley.[13] Ralph of Wickersley, son of Robert son of Pain, with the consent of Beatrix his wife, granted his right in Wickersley church to Worksop, and confirmed the grant of the advowson of the church made by [his wife's uncle] Roger son of Richard. Beatrix daughter of Jordan of Wickersley issued a separate confirmation (MS Dods. 126, f. 148ᵛ [ex f. 57, cap. 6, 8]). The gift of 1 bv. in Wickersley to Worksop Priory by Ralph of Wilsic (*Wilgesic*) and his wife Beatrix was noted in a confirmation charter of Edward II (*CalCh*, 1300–1326, p. 302; *MA*, vi, 120–22, no. 8). Matthew of Hathersage (*Hathersen*) brought a case against Ralph of Wilsic (*Wilesec*) for a plea of *bosc(i) abscisi* in 1194 (*RCuria*, i, 67). The plaintiff can be identified as Matthew of Hathersage, or of Withington, who was a son of William of Withington, and husband to Emma de Mesnil (Statham, 'Domesday Descendants', *DAJ*, pt 49, pp. 307–10). In 1198 Matthew son of William impleaded Ralph of Wickersley (*Wicherle*) and Beatrix his wife for wood and land of *Hailwinetorp*,[14] as the maritagium of Emma de Mesnil, Matthew's wife, wherof Matthew had been seised in time of peace in the reign of Henry [II]. Wager of battle was ordered between Hugh of Flockton, for Ralph and Beatrix, and Utting, for Matthew. The pledges for Hugh of Flockton were Ralph [of Wickersley], his lord, and Robert son of Pain (*CRR*, i, 40–41; ibid., 1213–1215, pp. 344–45; *MemR*, 10 John, p. 100). Ralph of Wickersley was apparently dead in 1203, when Robert of Wickersley for himself, and for Beatrix daughter of Jordan, and Constance wife of William Livet, put in a claim for 1 k.f. in Rotherham, whereof there was wager of battle between Eustace de Vescy and Ralph de Tilly (*CRR*, 1203–1205, p. 74).

It seems that Sir Robert of Wickersley, who was holding the Wickersley undertenancy of Livet in the mid-thirteenth century, was the son of Beatrix and Ralph of Wickersley. Robert of Wickersley's plea of 1203 can be reconciled with Sir Robert's apparent survival until 1261 if we suppose the plea was made in his name whilst he was underage. A period in wardship would also help explain Robert's subsequent absence from records until 1218. But the occurrence of Robin son of Ralph in 1218–19, and the confusion as to whether it was Ranulf or Robert of Wickersley who claimed disseisin by the men of Robert de Vipont in the same period, leaves some room for doubt (FN: Wilsic).

Robert son of Ralph of Wickersley was the leading witness to a deed of uncertain date made by Mabel, widow of Matthew of Tickhill, to Roche (Burton transcripts 3, f. 78ʳ, p. 129, B21 N20).[15] In Michaelmas term 1225 and Hilary term 1226 Robert of Wickersley failed to defend an action by Ragenild widow of Peter de Rodes for a third part of a mill in *Rodes*.[16] Ragenild was given seisin by default (*CRR*, 1225–1226, nos 1118, 1788). In 1230 Robert of Wickersley quitclaimed the advowson of the church of Wickersley to the prior of Worksop, and was received into the benefactions of the priory (*YF*, 1218–1231, pp. 130–31). Sir Robert of Wickersley attested in 1236 and 1245[/46] (*SY*, i, 247–48; *Ctl. Monkbretton*, p. 45). On several occasions in 1246 and 1251–52 he served as recognitor on a grand assize, or as one of four knights to choose twelve (*YF*, 1232–1246; ibid., 1246–1272, passim; *Three Yorks. Assize Rolls*, p. 60). Robert of Wickersley, knight, heads the list of jurors at an inquisition into certain lands held of the manor of Tickhill in 1252 (*YI*, i, 33). In 1261, Robert of Wickersley, who did not describe himself as *dominus* or *miles* but was doubtless the

---

[13]  Notes on Robert son of Pain, and the descent of the two half fees he held of the honour of Tickhill, are given below.

[14]  Unidentified. 'Ellenthorpe in Gisburn' is suggested in *CRR* and *MemR*, but seems unlikely.

[15]  The other witnesses were Nicholas de St-Paul, Henry son of Jordan of Todwick, Walter son of Besing of Woolthwaite.

[16]  Identified as Royds, Rotherham.

same person, confirmed to Roche the lands they had by gift and sale in Hooton Levitt by Jordan, son of Jordan de Lisle, and Elizabeth his wife (MS Dods. 152, f. 118[2]ʳ). Elizabeth was one of Sir Robert's daughters and coheirs.

In 1284–85 the heirs of Robert of Wickersley held ½ k.f. in Wickersley of Nicholas Livet, who held of [the manor of] Bentley,[17] of the honour of Tickhill (*KI*, p. 6). An inquisition of 1297 concerning the tenants of Blyth Priory in Billingley (2 m. north west of Bolton upon Dearne) gives details of Sir Robert's descendants. It states that Robert of Wickersley had held 15 bv. in Billingley, paying 11*s*. 8*d*. yearly. Robert died leaving three daughters. The eldest of these had a son John, and John a son Richard, who was then holding the tenancy with Oliver of Wickersley and Jordan de Lisle, who shared with him (doubtless representing Robert's two younger daughters) (*Ctl. Blyth*, p. 468, no. A81). The account is in accord with other evidence. Oliver of Wickersley and John of Wickersley were amongst the jurors in a Tickhill inquisition of 1282 (*YI*, I, 257). Adam, son of Simon de la Roche, and Joan, Adam's wife, daughter of Robert of Wickersley, gave 1 bv. in Hooton Levitt to Roche Abbey, which was confirmed by her father Sir Robert of Wickersley, knight (*Monasticon Eboracense*, p. 321; MS Dods. 8, f. 300ʳ). John, son and heir of Adam de Roche, and 'one of the heirs of Robert of Wickersley', gave all the land and annual rent he held in Wilsic by hereditary right after the death of Joan his mother, to Peter de Boseville ('Ctl. Nostell', no. 347 [ex f. 48ᵛ]). In 1306 John of Wickersley enfeoffed Richard his son and Agnes his wife, and the heirs of Richard, with all his lands and tenements in Wickersley, Hooton Levitt, *Byletsyke*,[18] Loversall and Billingley, with woods, meadows, homages, fealties, wards, marriages, rents, reliefs, escheats etc (*SY*, I, 277).[19]

The lords of Wickersley named in the *Nomina Villarum* of 1316 were Jordan de Lisle, Thomas of Wickersley, and Richard of Wickersley (*KI*, p. 365).[20] In 1326, Thomas de Boseville and Elizabeth his wife made a fine with Thomas of Wickersley and Denise his wife concerning 140 a. land and other property in Wickersley and other places (*YF*, 1314–1326, no. 667). In 1428 it was said that William Livet formerly held ½ k.f. in Wickersley, which John Frickley, Robert Wickersley, and the prioress of Kirklees were now holding separately, such that none held more than ¼ k.f. (*Feudal Aids*, VI, 278). Some details of later members of the Wickersley family are given by Hunter (*SY*, I, 277–78).

The marriage of Beatrix, daughter of Jordan of Wickersley, to Ralph son of Robert son of Pain [of WILSIC] is mentioned above. The earliest notice of the Wilsic family occurs during the archiepiscopate of Henry Murdac (1147–1153), when Jordan son of Pain gave the vill of Wilsic (*Wilgesic*), with pasture in Wellingley (between Wilsic and Stancil) to Roche Abbey (Burton transcripts I, f. 113ᵛ, p. 174, B23 N5, cited *Monasticon Eboracense*, p. 323; also at MS Dods. 8, f. 304ʳ). The deed is doubtful, as it is sealed 'with the seal of my brother Robert, because I have lost my seal'. It is unlikely that Robert can then have been far into his twenties, as he was still living in 1202. There is no further trace of a Roche interest in Wilsic, and it is likely the abbey's land there was exchanged for the land in Wellingley and Wadworth given subsequently. At an uncertain date William Chaworth and William son of Eudo of Wadworth, chief lords of Wadworth, released to Roche all claim in the lands of Sir Jordan son of Pain, lord

---

[17]  See HN: Wickersley for the mesne tenancy of Neufmarché, lords of the manor of Bentley.
[18]  Unidentified.
[19]  The inquisition of 1297 cited above shows that John had acquired his tenancy in Billingley before this feoffment.
[20]  The entry reads *Iordanus de Ilde, Thomas de Wykereslai et Ricardus de Dred* (i.e. *de eodem*), cf. *SY*, I, 277.

of Stancil, Wellingley and Wilsic, which Jordan had given to the abbey, by specified bounds which mention Wadworth, Wellingley, and Stancil (*SY*, I, 247, 249).[21] Jordan son of Pain apparently died without surviving issue, as the interest in Wilsic passed to Robert son of Pain. In 1165 William de Serton and Robert son of Pain owed relief for I k.f. of the honour of Tickhill; Robert son of Pain also owed relief for a further ½ k.f. held of Tickhill. The debt was paid over the ensuing two years (*PR*, II–13 Hen. II, passim). A confirmation by Urban III to Roche of 1186 includes 'by the gift of Robert son of Pain' Wellingley with appurtenances and all the land which the abbey had in Wadworth (*Wadburthe*) (*MA*, v, 505, no. 13). Robert's deed to Roche, or a copy of it, was seen by John Burton, who intended to print it in his appendix to the *Monasticon Eboracense* (*op. cit.*, p. 323 and n).[22] Robert's wife was Godit, who can be identified with Godida of Wilsic (*Willesich*), who in 1188–89 paid 2*m*. for recognition of the death of Jordan her brother, concerning 19 bv. of land against Hugh son of William (*PR*, I Ric. I, p. 84). In 1196, Hugh son of William of Brinsworth (*Brunesford*) attorned Robert or Henry, his sons, in a plea of land against Robert son of Pain and Goditha his wife (*Fines*, 10 Ric. I, p. 219; *MemR*, 10 John, pp. 74, 77).

Robert son of Pain, often with one or more of his sons, was a frequent witness to deeds. He attested at least three gifts to the hospital (R343, R344, R762). Robert son of Pain and Ralph his son attested Robert son of Gerbod's gift to Roche, which was also witnessed by Richard de Busli, William his brother, John de Busli, and Hugh his brother (Burton transcripts 3, f. 79ʳ, p. 131, B21 N63). Described similarly, father and son attested John de Busli's confirmation of his father Richard de Busli's gifts to Roche (*MA*, v, 503, no. 4; *YD*, VII, no. 453); a quitclaim made in the court of Tickhill to Hugh of Stainton (MS Dods. 8, f. 307ʳ); and two grants to Kirkstall of land in Bessacarr, one made after 1190[23] (*EYC*, II, nos 816, 822). A quitclaim to Kirkstead Abbey (Lincs.) in property in Handsworth was attested by Robert son of Pain and Ralph of Wilsic (*EYC*, III, no. 1276); and a deed of Nicholas de St-Paul was witnessed by William Livet, Robert son of Pain and Ralph of Wickersley (MS Dods. 152, f. 116ʳ). In or before 1194,[24] Robert son of Pain, with Ralph and Adam his sons, witnessed a deed of William son of Gerbod to Roche (Burton transcripts 3, f. 58ʳ, p. 89, B13 N22), and in 1202–03 Robert son of Pain, Ralph, Robert and Thomas his sons witnessed a deed of Nicholas de St-Paul (*EYC*, III, no. 1413). In Michaelmas term 1200 there was a plea between Geoffrey Clarel and Robert son of Pain concerning 6 bv. land in Tickhill, which Robert had claimed against William, father of Geoffrey. William said he had warranty thereof, and a deed of Jordan, eldest brother of Robert, by which Jordan had given the land to Ralph, father of William, in frank-marriage with Sybil, Jordan's sister. Robert claimed the deed was a forgery, produced six or seven years after the death of Jordan. The outcome of the case does not appear (*CRR*, I, 296). Robert son of Pain was named during the years 1201–07 as the holder of I k.f. of Tickhill, on which scutage was due (*PR*, 3–9 John, passim). But he was dead before Michaelmas 1203, when Godit *que fuit uxor Roberti f. Pagani* owed 2*m*. for common belonging to her in Aston (*Eston*) and in Aughton (*Acton*) (*PR*, 5 John, p. 213).

The attestations cited above indicate that Ralph was the eldest of Robert son of Pain's sons. Ralph appears to have died in 1202 × 1203, the same period as his father. Although the property Ralph held in Wickersley and Hooton Levitt by right of his

---

[21]  For the problems associated with this deed, see p. 161 n. 15.
[22]  Not found in Burton transcripts.
[23]  Attested by John of Birkin, who succeeded in or after that year (FN).
[24]  Also witnessed by Gerard of Styrrup, who was dead in that year (FN: Oldcotes).

wife Beatrix passed to their presumed son Robert of Wickersley, who held it in the mid-thirteenth century, it was apparently Ralph's brother Adam who succeeded to the two half fees held of Tickhill by Robert son of Pain, comprising holdings in Wilsic and elsewhere. The possibility that Adam was the eldest son of Robert son of Pain and an unknown first wife should not perhaps be ruled out, but it seems more likely that he had Wilsic by his father's gift. Adam was sometimes called 'of Wilsic', but often took the surname 'of Hooton', from Hooton Roberts, and this was the family name used by his heirs. Adam of Wilsic (*Wulvessic*) was holding 1 k.f. of Tickhill in 1208 × 1213 (*Bk of Fees*, p. 32; *Red Bk*, p. 593). Adam *de Wileshic* appears on a muster roll of 1213 (Vincent, 'Knights', p. 96). He can probably be identified with Adam de Hoton, who accounted in Yorkshire for ½m. for a concealment in 1202–03 (*PR*, 5 John, p. 218; ibid., 6 John, p. 203). In October 1217 a writ was issued in the king's name ordering the sheriff of York to deliver seisin of his lands to Adam de Hoton who had come to allegiance (*RClose*, 1, 331b). In 1218–19 there was an assize of novel disseisin to determine whether Geoffrey Cryol, Adam of Hooton, Adam de Medburn, Ralph and Andrew sons of Adam, and Thomas of Hooton, described as men of R[obert] de Vipont, had disseised Robert[25] of Wickersley of his free tenement in Tickhill. Vipont was at that time trying to establish his claim to the honour of Tickhill by right of his wife Idonea (*Yorkshire Eyre Rolls*, pp. xxii–xxv, 179). In December 1218, probably in settlement of the assize, Robert son of Ralph of Wickersley and Adam of Hooton made a fine as to 1 k.f. [held of the honour of Tickhill] in Tickhill, Stancil, Wadworth, Wilsic, Hooton [Roberts], Hesley[26] and *Marton*,[27] 1 ct. in Aston and Aughton,[28] 12 bv. in Stancil, 1 bv. in *Wirhal*,[29] and an assart in Stainton called *Painistubing*. They were the right of Adam, who granted to Robert all the vill of Wilsic, the bovate in Wirhal and the assart in Stainton, to hold to him and his heirs, of Adam and his heirs, doing the service of an eighth part of 1 k.f. for Wilsic, the forinsec service due on 1 bv. in Wirhal, and 12d. annually for *Painistubing* (*YF*, 1218–1231, pp. 10–11). Robin son of Ralph (*Robinus f. Radulfi*) owed 100s. for having a writ of right against Adam the parson of *Hocton*, concerning 1 k.f. in Hooton (*Hocton*), Wilsic (*Welesic*), Wadworth *et alibi* in 1218–19 (*PR*, 3 Hen. III, p. 195). It is tempting to imagine that the plaintiff and defendant were the same Robert and Adam, but this is far from certain. The first witness to a deed of Eudo son of Geoffrey of Wadworth to Roche, of the first half of the thirteenth century,[30] is Adam, *persona de Hotun*. Thomas of Wilsic (*Wikhesic, Wilskhesic*) also attests (Burton transcripts 3, f. 78ᵛ, p. 130; ibid. 5, f. 69ʳ, p. 129, B10 N12).[31]

That Adam was son of Robert son of Pain appears only from his attestations. It was probably after the deaths of Ralph of Wilsic and Robert son of Pain, and before June 1213,[32] that Adam son of Robert son of Pain, with Robert and Thomas his brothers, witnessed a deed of Nicholas de St-Paul, son of William (*EYC*, VI, no. 111). Adam son of Robert of Wilsic attested a gift of Hugh son of William of Stainton to the hospital in 1202 × 1209 (R433).

---

25  Stenton gives Ranulf rather than Robert. The name is rather faded in the original, but appears to be *Rob(ertu)m* (PRO, JUST 1/1040, m. 12d). *YF*, 1218–1231, p. 10n gives Robert.

26  Par. Harworth, Notts., near Stancil.

27  Identified by Parker as Martin [Hall] by Bawtry, known as Marton in earlier times (cf. *PN Yorks WR*, I, 48; *SY*, I, 75, 248).

28  Adjoining vills 6 m. south east of Rotherham.

29  Placed in Wadworth by Smith, but no other occurrence cited (*PN Yorks WR*, I, 62).

30  Witnessed by Peter son of William of Wadworth (FN).

31  Two copies. The second gives *Adam, priore de Hoton*, but this must be an error.

32  Also witnessed by Sir John de Busli, who was dead in that month (R433n).

It has not proved possible to establish the connection between Adam of Hooton and the men who held the fee later in the century. Hunter gives a pedigree, taken from 'the great pedigree of Wentworth compiled by William Gascoign for the first earl of Strafford in the reign of Charles I', which shows the interest passed through one Robert of Hooton, a younger brother of Adam of Hooton, to Robert's son Sir William of Hooton, and from William to his son Sir Robert of Hooton. Sir Robert of Hooton had issue William of Hooton and Lucy, who married Sir Henry of Tinsley. But Hunter notes that 'other accounts of this descent are given', and the details are not to be trusted (SY, I, 399). By 1272 the interest was in the hands of William of Hooton, who made presentations to the church of Hooton Roberts in that year and in 1274 (Fasti Parochiales, I, 147). The sale of the custody of the land and heir of William of Hooton (Hoton) to master John Clarel, by Constance de Béarn, widow of Henry of Almain, who then held the honour of Tickhill, was ratified by the king in 1280 (CalPat, 1272–1281, p. 377). It was this purchase which enabled Clarel to present master William of Orleans to the church of Hooton Roberts in 1280 (Reg. Wickwane, p. 32). The survey of 1284–85 states that Robert son of William of Hooton held ½ k.f. in Hooton Roberts of the honour of Tickhill. Henry of Tinsley (Tenneslowe) also held ½ k.f. there (KI, pp. 2–3, 9). In 1302–03 Robert of Hooton held 1 k.f. of Tickhill in Hooton Roberts, Stancil and Wilsic, and in 1316 was named as lord of Hooton Roberts (Hoton sub Haia) and Stancil (KI, pp. 233, 283, 365). In January 1314[/15] Robert of Hooton, lord of Stancil, confirmed the gifts of William de Boseville of land in Wilsic to the prior and convent of St Oswald, Nostell ('Ctl. Nostell', no. 335 [ex f. 47ʳ]). In an extent of the honour of Tickhill taken in the reign of Edward IV (1461–1483) it was said that in 1374–75 William Estefeld 'formerly held immediately of the honour' a knight's fee in Stancil, Wilsic, Wadworth, Tickhill, Marton 'and else-where' (SY, I, 248). A feodary of 1428 states that William Wentworth held 1 k.f. in Hooton Roberts, which [another] William of Wentworth had formerly held; and that Anota de Herthill formerly held 1 k.f. in Stancil, Wilsic, Wadworth, and Tickhill, which was then held separately by several tenants, none of whom held more than ¼ k.f. (Feudal Aids, VI, 279).

Several men with the surname Wilsic occur after Adam of Wilsic assigned the vill of Wilsic to Robert of Wickersley in 1218. It is not improbable that the Robert of Wilsic (Wilwersic), who in 1220 was a recognitor when Peter de Mauley [I] and Isabel his wife claimed land in Rossington (2 m. north east of Stancil), was the same Robert of Wickersley. He had essoined, and was removed. The following year Nicholas of Wilsic (Wuleswic) and Thomas of Wilsic (Wilessic) were to be removed from the recognitors in the same case, and replaced with men who were not entitled to essoin (CRR, 1220, p. 278; ibid., 1221–1222, p. 35). A series of thirteenth century deeds in the Nostell cartulary show that a William of Wilsic had sons Nicholas, probably the eldest, and William, a chaplain. Nicholas had a son John,[33] and almost certainly another, named William[34] ('Ctl. Nostell', nos 336–46 [ex ff. 47ᵛ–48ᵛ]). A grant

---

[33] Nicholas son of William of Wilsic sold his brother William a toft in Wilsic (no. 340). William of Wilsic, chaplain, gave the same toft to his nephew John, son of Nicholas of Wilsic, his brother (no. 341). John of Wilsic son of Nicholas son of William of Wilsic gave the same toft to Nostell, describing it as the toft his uncle (patrui) William had given him (no. 342). Subsequently Nicholas of Wilsic, son of William of Wilsic, confirmed the gift made by John his son to the priory (no. 339).

[34] This William, as William son of Nicholas of Wilsic, confirmed to the priory 4 a. in Wilsic adjoining land his father had given. Nicholas of Wilsic confirmed the gift of 4 a. made by William his son (nos 336–37). William of Wilsic son of Nicholas gave Nostell two parts of his toft in Wilsic, of which his father held the third part, with a hedge (sepes vivam) and other property. This too was confirmed by Nicholas of Wilsic as the gift of his son William (ibid., nos 343–44). Frost identifies this William as

of ½ bv. in Wilsic, of the gift of William son of Nicholas of Wilsic, is the last item in Edward I's general confirmation to Nostell made in 1280 (*CalCh*, 1257–1300, p. 235). But there is nothing to connect these men to either Adam of Hooton or Robert of Wickersley, and they may not have been related.

Clay gives several references for William de LIVET, who was a steward of Earl Hamelin in 1198 (*EYC*, VIII, 244–45). If he held land in his own right, his tenure has left no trace. He may perhaps have been a descendant of Robert (*Rtibertus*) de Livet, who witnessed a deed of William of Stainton to Roche with several tenants of the honour of Tickhill in *c.*1160 × 1194 (MS Dods. 152, f. 117ʳ).[35] William de Livet, with his son William, elsewhere called William de Livet *iunior*, attested deeds dated within *c.*1200 × *c.*1210 by Clay (*EYC*, VIII, nos 90, 121). Simon son of William de Livet witnessed a Roche deed in 1202–03 (*EYC*, III, no. 1413). Neither the younger William de Livet nor his father occurs after *c.*1212. It was almost certainly the younger William who was married to Constance, daughter of Roger son of Richard of Wickersley. The couple were married by 1195, when William de Livet and Constance his wife owed 100*s.* for right in 1 k.f. in Rotherham against Ralph de Tilly, Geoffrey de Saucusemare and Maud his wife (*PR*, 7 Ric. I, p. 92). In 1194 × 1198, William de Livet confirmed to the hospital the gifts in Hooton made by his predecessors (R716). In 1200 a case between Geoffrey de Saucusemare, Maud his wife, and Ralph de Tilly, tenants, and William Livet and Constance his wife plaintiffs, remained without day (*CRR*, I, 189). Constance, wife of William Livet, was party to a claim in 1203 concerning 1 k.f. in Rotherham whereof there was wager of battle between Eustace de Vescy and Ralph de Tilly (*CRR*, 1203–1205, p. 74).[36] William de Livet attested a quitclaim with Robert Waleys, sheriff of Yorkshire, in 1204 × 1209[37] (*YD*, IV, no. 508). In 1205 he was summoned as one of four knights to choose twelve for a grand assize concerning land in Scawsby, and was attached for default (*CRR*, 1203–1205, p. 285). This was presumably the younger William, who had the tenurial qualification for knighthood by right of his wife. Constance lived for many years after William's death, and there is no evidence that she remarried. In 1237, Constance de Livet attorned Richard de Livet in a plea against Maud de Saucusemare concerning ½ k.f. in Rotherham (*CloseR*, 1234–1237, p. 568). In 1242–43 she was said to hold 2 k.f. of Mauley in Pickburn and Hooton Levitt (*Bk of Fees*, p. 1099). At the inquisition after the death of Sir Peter de Mauley [II] in 1279 it was said that John de Vescy held 3½ k.f. in Rotherham, Pickburn, and Hooton Levitt, of which Constance Livet was 'wont to hold' 2 k.f. (*YI*, I, 200), though she must then have been dead for some years.

Three sons of William and Constance de Livet can be named. James de Livet was the eldest; his brothers were Richard and Hamo or Hamond.[38] The identity of William Scorh, son of William de Livet, who gave the land he held of the hospital to

the father of the Nicholas who confirmed the gift of his son John. As the witnesses to the deeds are not copied, this cannot be ruled out entirely. It is however unlikely, as it requires that two men named Nicholas of Wilsic confirmed the deeds of their sons, one being grandfather to the other. The deeds do not appear to be widely separated in time, and it is likely that they were issued by members of just two generations rather than the four proposed by Frost.

35 For this deed, and its date, see FN: Stainton. It is unlikely that the witness was the Robert de Livet who held 2 k.f. of Ferrers in 1135, and derived his name from Livet-en-Ouche in Eure (*ANF*, p. 55).

36 For these cases, see FN: Tilly.

37 The period during which Waleys was sheriff.

38 This is deduced from the references which follow. The rubrics of Dodsworth's copies of certain deeds provide a measure of supporting evidence: '*Carta Iacobi de Lyvet senior fratris Ricardi*'; '*Carta Hamonis de Lyvet tertius filius Constantie*' (MS Dods. 152, ff. 117ᵛ, 118[1]ᵛ).

his sister Erneburga in *c*.1200 × 1218, has not been ascertained (R717). He may have been illegitimate, or a son of a previous marriage of William de Livet I or II. James Livet and Richard Livet are the second and fourth witnesses respectively to a deed of June 1260 (MS Dods. 8, f. 299ᵛ); they attested a deed of Robert of Wickersley as second and fifth witnesses (Burton transcripts 1, f. 121ʳ, p. 189, B17 N30). James Livet and Richard his brother attested a deed of Walter, abbot of Roche in 1241 × 1259³⁹ (MS Dods. 8, f. 31ʳ); a deed of Alan, abbot of Roche in 1259⁴⁰ (MS Dods. 152, f. 117ᵛ); and a Catwick (ER) deed dated 1263 (Burton transcripts 1, f. 114ʳ, p. 175, B23 N13). In 1266 James de Livet and Denise his wife gave ½*m*. in Yorkshire for an assize (*RFine Excerpta*, II, 433). In September 1268 James de Livet, having lost his sight, had a grant from the king that he be quit of suit in person at county, hundred, wapentake and all other of the king's courts (*CalPat*, 1266–1272, p. 260). Constance, widow of William de Livet, in widowhood, gave her son Richard de Livet 2 bv. in North Hooton (*Northoton*),⁴¹ for his homage and service, and 2*s*. 6*d*. and a pair of gloves annually (MS Dods. 8, f. 305ʳ). On 9 March 1245[/46] Richard son of William Livet gave half the mill of North Hooton, with the mill-pond and the watercourse to the mill at Maltby as far as the mill-pond of the monks, which his mother Constance had granted him after the death of his father (Burton transcripts 2, f. 130ʳ, p. 224, B17 N40; cited *Monasticon Eboracense*, p. 321). Subsequently Constance de Livet gave to Roche Abbey the 2*d*. annual rent which her son Richard de Livet was accustomed to pay for half the mill of North Hooton (MS Dods. 8, f. 316ʳ⁻ᵛ). Hamo son of William de Livet gave Roche a toft and croft, and 1 bv. in Hooton Levitt (Burton transcripts 3, f. 79ʳ, p. 131, B5 N37); and in the presence of similar witnesses gave 1 bv. in Hooton Levitt and 5 r. abutting the land which his brother Richard had given (MS Dods. 152, f. 118[1]ᵛ). Hamond de Livet occurs in February 1249[/50], when two Jews, Manselin of Doncaster and Manselin of Brodsworth, released to Roche Abbey the lands they held of him in Hooton Levitt (*SY*, I, 265).⁴² Shortly before 18 May 1246,⁴³ Richard de Livet and Hamo his brother attested a deed of Jordan son of Jordan de Lisle and the younger Jordan's wife Elizabeth, which mentions a rent of 4*d*. to be paid annually to Constance de Livet and her heirs (MS Dods. 8, f. 292ʳ).

The next generation is shown by the attestation to a deed of Robert of Wickersley of 1261, which includes James de Livet, Richard his brother, and Nicholas son of James Livet (MS Dods. 152, f. 118[2]ʳ). Nicholas had succeeded by February 1283, when King Edward I inspected a deed of John de Vescy, son and heir of William de Vescy, confirming property in Rotherham to Rufford Abbey, but reserving the homage of Nicholas de Livet from the fees he held of the donor in Hooton 'by the abbey of Roche' (*CalCh*, 1257–1300, pp. 264–65). In 1284–85 Nicholas Livet

---

³⁹  The extreme dates for Abbot Walter (see the next note).

⁴⁰  This deed proves that Abbot Alan preceded Abbot Jordan, who occurs in 1263. In 1895 Baildon published a list of the abbots of Roche based on the list in *MA*, which follows a mid-thirteenth-century memorandum of the names of the abbots and the number of years they remained in office. Baildon added further documentary references and omitted parts of the medieval list when it was not in accordance with other evidence. Clay reconciled the list to dated occurrences by proposing that the period for Abbot Osmund, given in the list as thirty-nine years, should be amended to twenty-nine. *Heads* accepts Clay's list, which ends with Walter of Wadworth (*c*.1244–*c*.1258) but cites Baildon for the accession of Alan in 1268, and so gives a date ten years too late, placing him after Jordan (Baildon, *Monastic Notes*, I, 183; Clay, 'Early Abbots', pp. 37–39; *Heads*, II, 304; *MA*, v, 501, 505, no. 14).

⁴¹  North Hooton does not appear in *PN YorksWR*. It was almost certainly another name for Hooton Levitt, which is about a mile north of Slade Hooton.

⁴²  Indirectly from a transcript at MS Dods. 152, f. 118[1]ᵛ.

⁴³  The date of the corresponding fine (*YF*, 1232–1246, p. 139).

held 1 k.f. in Pickburn (elsewhere said to be ½ k.f.) and 1 k.f. in Hooton Levitt, of John de Vescy, of Mauley. He also had ½ k.f. in Wickersley, which was held of him by the heirs of Robert of Wickersley (*KI*, pp. 6, 7, 9, 11). Nicholas Livet of Hooton witnessed a deed in July 1288 (MS Dods. 8, f. 318ʳ). By 1302–03⁴⁴ Nicholas had been succeeded by James Livet, who held 1 k.f. (elsewhere said to be ½ k.f.) in Hooton Levitt and Pickburn of Mauley, and ½ k.f. in Wickersley of the honour of Tickhill (*KI*, pp. 231–32, 282–83). At an inquisition in Yorkshire following the death of Peter de Mauley [III] held in summer 1309, it was said that James Livet held 1 k.f. of him in Hooton Levitt, Pickburn and *Stane*,⁴⁵ 'rendering nothing' (*CalInqPM*, v, no. 199). James Livet and William Darell were named as lords of Pickburn and Brodsworth in 1316 (*KI*, p. 359). James Livet attested as lord of Hooton in 1335 (*YD*, x, no. 445). At the inquisition following the death of Earl John Warenne in 1347, it was said that James Livet (*Lynet*) lately held of the earl 1 ct. in a hamlet called Lupset in Stanley, for 43s. annually, which rent the earl had quitclaimed to Maud de Nerford, tenant of the land by Livet's enfeoffment (*CalInqPM*, ix, 53). Brief notes on some later members of the family were given by Hunter (*SY*, i, 265).

**R714.** Gift to the hospital by Roger son of Richard of Hooton of 8 a., of which 4 a. are on the east side of his culture at *Hertheshou*, and 4 a. are in another culture at *Witunehill*, also on the east side, in exchange for an assart called the Lady's Assart, as his father's deed and the donor's confirmation testify [*c.*1150 × *c.*1188]

COPY: MS Dods. 120b, f. 11ʳ, from Rawl., probably f. 60, now missing.

Sciant universi litteras has videntes sive audientes quod ego Rogerus filius Ricardi de Hotuna conc(essi) et ded(i) deo et beato Petro et pauperibus hospitalis sancti Petri Ebor' viii. acras terre assensu [heredum]⁴⁶ meorum, quarum viii. acrarum iiiiᵒʳ de cultura mea apud Hertheshou in parte orientali, et iiiiᵒʳ de alia cultura apud Witune-hill' similiter in orientali parte in escambium per sartam quod vocabatur sartum domine, in puram et perpetuam elemosinam, sicut scriptum patris mei et confirmatio mea testantur. Et si in aliquo modo excessi, sive minus dedi quam ibi habetur, prom-itto me in prefatis locis adimplend(um). Hiis testibus, Alano presbitero, Iohanne capel-lano, Ricardo diacono, Roberto clerico de Edlington, Druelin de Malteby, Rogero Restold', Ada' de Neuhall, Orm et Ailsi de Hotuna, Guil(lelm)o filio Eilsi, Osberto Puddins, Norman coco et multis aliis.

The date range is the donor's potential period of tenure (FN).

**R715.** Gift to the hospital by Constance daughter of Roger of Hooton of 2 bv. with a toft, being 1 bv. and a toft in Wickersley which Robert son of Peter held, and 1 bv. in Hooton which William son of Ailsi held. Also confirmation of another 2 bv. in Hooton which her predecessors gave [probably 1205 × 1229]

---

44 The exact date of James' succession is obscure. A note taken from a Wakefield court roll states that James 'de Heton', son and heir of Nicholas de Livet, gave £4 6s. for his relief for lands in Lupset, which his father held of the earl [Warrene], but Dodsworth was uncertain whether the date was August 14 Edw. I (1286) or 14 Edw. II (1320) (MS Dods. 117, f. 157ʳ, cited 'Dodsworth's Yorkshire Notes', *YAJ*, VII, 418). Neither can be correct. The entry does not appear in the printed volumes of the rolls.

45 Unidentified.

46 Deleted by Dodsworth.

COPY: MS Dods. 120b, f. 11ᵛ, from Rawl., f. 60, now missing.

Omnibus cristi fidelibus ad quos presens scriptum pervenerit Constancia filia Rogeri
de Hotun salutem. Noverit universitas vestra me caritatis intuitu conc(essisse)
d(edisse) et hac presenti carta mea confirm(asse) deo et pauperibus hospitalis sancti
Petri Ebor' duas bovatas terre cum 1 tofto, scilicet unam bovatam et unum toftum
in Wykerslay quod Robertus filius Petri tenuit, et unam bovatam in Hotun quam
Willelmus filius Ailsy tenuit, cum omnibus pertinenciis suis aisiamentis et libertatibus suis et cum communi pastura, tam in villa de Wykerslaya quam de Hotun infra
et extra in puram <et perpetuam> elemosinam. Et preterea conc(essi) et presenti
carta mea c(onfirmavi) predictis pauperibus alias duas bovatas terre in Hotun quas
antecessores mei eis caritative contulerunt, tenend(um) scilicet et habend(um) totum
predictum tenementum memoratis pauperibus libere integre et quiete sicut aliqua
elemosina liberius et melius teneri potest. Ego autem et heredes mei prenominatum
tenementum cum omnibus pertinenciis suis sepedictis pauperibus warantizabimus
adquiet(abimus) et defend(emus) in omnibus et contra omnes homines imperpetuum.
Hec autem omnia fideliter observanda tactis sacrosanctis iuravi affidavi, et in huius rei
robur et testimonium huic scripto sigillum meum apposui. Hiis testibus, [Radulfo][47]
de Normanville, Hugone de Langewehit, Radulfo Selueyn, Iordano de Morthing,
Thoma de Crigleston, Iohanne de Touetona, Reynero de Waumewell et multis aliis.
fo. 60.

It is unlikely that this deed was given before the death of Constance's husband
William de Livet in or after 1205 (FN). The witness Thomas of Crigglestone was dead
in 1226 × 1229, when Robert son of Adam of Crigglestone made a gift to Healaugh
for the soul of Thomas of Crigglestone his brother, by a deed attested by Rainer of
Wombwell (*EYC*, I, 511–12; *CalCh*, 1300–1326, p. 152).

**R716.** Confirmation to the hospital by William de Livet of all the lands in Hooton
which his predecessors gave, as their deeds testify [1194 × 1198]

COPY: MS Dods. 120b, f. 12ʳ, from Rawl., f. 60, now missing.

Omnibus hominibus cartam istam visuris vel audituris Willelmus de Livet salutem.
Noveritis me con(cessisse) deo et hospitali beati Petri Ebor' et magistro et fratribus
ibidem deo servientibus omnes illas terras in Hotun cum omnibus liberis pertinenciis
suis quas predec(essores) mei ded(erunt) eis in puram et perpetuam elemosinam sicut
eorum carte testantur. Et ut eas libere honorifice et quiete possideant sine impedimento et retenemento pro me et pro heredibus meis, sicut predicte carte testantur,
eas terras eis presenti carta mea confirmavi. Hiis testibus, S[imone] decano et capitulo
Ebor', Rogero de Batevent tunc vic(ecomite), Odard(o) celerario et conventu eiusdem
domus et multis aliis. fo. 60.

Simon was dean of York from 1194; Roger de Bavent was undersheriff from Easter
1194 to Michaelmas 1198.

---

[47] A blank space in the MS. A succession of men named Ralph de Normanville were lords of Thrybergh,
some 6 m. north west of Hooton Levitt, in the late twelfth and early thirteenth centuries (*EYC*, XI,
289–91).

**R717.**   Gift by William Scorh, son of William de Livet, to Erneburga his sister, of all
his land in Hooton which he held of the hospital, paying to the brethren 6s.
annually [c.1200 × 1218]

COPY: MS Dods. 120b, f. 12ʳ, abbreviated, from Rawl., f. 60, now missing.

Omnibus visuris vel audituris has litteras Willelmus Scorh[48] filius Willelmi de Liveth
salutem. Sciatis me dedisse etc. Erneburge sorori mee et heredibus suis totam terram
meam in Hoton' quam tenui de ministro hospitalis beati Petri Ebor', et reddendo
inde annuatim fratribus sex solidos. Testibus, Thoma de Horburi, Willelmo filio Ade,
Roberto de Sandall, Ada persona de Himl'wrt', Iohanne de Deusbury, Suano de
Bretton, Hugone filio eius, Willelmo filio Willelmi de Keteltorp, Ada filio Petri de
Wdethorp. fo. 60.

The first witness, Thomas of Horbury, succeeded his father Matthew of Horbury in
1188 × 1196, and was steward of Earl Warenne after William de Livet. He died not
later than 1218, and was succeeded by his son Ralph (*EYC*, VIII, 211–13, 245). Adam,
parson of Hemsworth, attested in 1223 × 1227[49] (*Ctl. Pontefract*, no. 95). Ralph de
Wennerville attested in c.1188 × 1202 as parson of Hemsworth (*EYC*, VIII, no. 136).
Thomas of Bretgate was presented to the rectory of Hemsworth in 1242 (*Fasti Parochiales*, I, 135). It is likely that the third and fifth witnesses were also clerks. Robert,
parson of Sandal, occurs c.1188 × 1202 (*EYC*, VIII, nos 136, 143, 167) and 1202 × 1218
(ibid., no. 172). John, parson of Dewsbury, was joint rector of Dewsbury in 1225 and
appears to have died in or before September 1230 (ibid., 209; Chadwick, 'Dewsbury
Church', p. 393; *Reg. Gray*, pp. 37, 41). Swain of [West] Bretton, who was succeeded
by his son Hugh, also occurs during the early thirteenth century (*Ctl. Byland*, nos
40–45; *EYC*, III, 408).

**R718.**   Grant at fee-farm by James de Ispania, master of the hospital, and the brethren,
to Nicholas de Livet, of a toft which the hospital had by the gift of the late
Richard Livet. Also confirmation of 3 bv. in the same place, which Richard
son of Richard Livet held of the hospital and gave to Nicholas and his heirs
by his deed, paying the hospital 12s. annually [1288 × 1293]

ABSTRACT: MS Dods 120b, f. 12ᵛ, from Rawl., f. 60, now missing.

Sciant presentes et futuri quod nos Iacobus de Ispania magister hospitalis sancti Leonardi Ebor' et fratres eiusdem loci dedimus etc. Nicholao de Livet quoddam toftum
quod habuimus de dono quondam Ricardi Livet. Preterea conc(essimus) eidem Nicholao 3 bovatas terre in eadem villa, quas Ricardus filius Ricardi Livet de nobis ten(ui)t,
et dicto Nicholao et heredibus suis per chartam suam dedit, tenend(a) etc., reddendo
annuatim nobis et successoribus 12s. argenti. Testibus, Olivero de Wikerley, Elia de
Burton, <Ricardo Luuecok>. fo. 60.

The date range is given by the extreme dates for James de Ispania as master.

---

48   Unclear, perhaps *Scoth* or *Scoch*.
49   Attested by John of Birkin, who was dead in 1227, and whilst Gilbert of Notton was steward of
     Pontefract (FNs).

**R719.** Undertaking by Richard Livet of Hooton that he and his heirs would not sell the tenements he holds of the hospital. 5 September 1277.

ABSTRACT: MS Dods. 120b, f. 12ᵛ , from Rawl., f. 60, now missing.

Ricardus Livet de Hoton spontanea voluntate sua tactis sacrosanctis iuravit quod nec ille nec heredes sui tenementa que tenet⁵⁰ de predicto hospitali venda(t) etc. Testibus, Thoma de Heseleby, <Ricardo filio Luuecok>. Dat' apud Doncaster 5 Sept. 1277. fo. 60.

**R720.** Confirmation to the hospital by Roger son of Richard of Wickersley of the gift of his father, being the bovate which Roger's grandmother had in Hooton, with common of pasture [*c.*1160 × *c.*1188]

ABSTRACT: MS Dods. 120b, f. 12ᵛ, from Rawl., f. 60, now missing.

Ego Rogerus filius Ricardi de Wicoresleia et heredes mei dedimus et conc(essimus) deo et sancto Petro et pauperibus hospitalis beati Petri Ebor' donacionem quam pater noster Ricardus eis prius dederat, scilicet totam illam bovatam terre quam ava mea habuit in Hotuna cum communi pastura etc. Testibus, Radulfo capellano, Henrico capellano, Iohanne clerico, Hugone de Wil', Rogero de Dalton, Holfe de Fossgate etc. fo. 60.

Roger of Wickersley succeeded his father between 1147 and 1160, and died *c.*1188 (FN). The chaplains Ralph and Henry were leading witnesses to deeds of *c.*1160 × *c.*1182 (R150, R152, R329).

## *Heck* [par. Snaith]

The Contents List gives f. 61 for Heck, but Dodsworth's abstracts are said to be from f. 62. The Contents List has Heslewood and Hornington on f. 62. Both folios are now missing. Heck does not appear in Domesday, but in 1316 it was a member of the Lacy fee (*KI*, p. 363). It is not mentioned in the papal confirmation to the hospital of 1148, but the confirmations of 1157 and 1173 include 1 bv. in *Hecca*. The donor is not named (C178–C180 [*EYC*, I, nos 179, 186, 197]). It is likely that this was the bovate given by Godwin, which was confirmed by his son William de Lisle before 1177 (R722). In later years Henry de Lisle and Amabel de Lisle each gave a toft to the hospital (R721, R724). Heck is not mentioned in the extents of the later thirteenth century, the *Valor Ecclesiasticus*, or the account of 1542.

The St Leonard's deeds, when considered with others in the Selby cartulary, allow the construction of a plausible descent of several generations of this branch of the LISLE family, which had interests in Pollington and Balne (both par. Snaith) as well as Heck. Godwin's gift to the hospital, probably made before 1157, which was confirmed by his son William de Lisle, has been mentioned above. Henry de Lisle, son of William de Lisle, gave to Jordan his brother, for his homage and service, ½ ct. in Pollington,

---

⁵⁰ MS: *teneo.*

including the service of Ilard of Heck (*EYC*, I, no. 496). Afterwards Jordan de Lisle gave the land to Selby, to be held of William son of Henry de Lisle, by a deed witnessed by John of Birkin (*Ctl. Selby*, no. 938). Amabel, sister and heir of Jordan de Lisle confirmed Jordan's gift to Selby (ibid., no. 939). Oliver de Vendouer confirmed the grant of his uncle (*avunculus*) Jordan de Lisle to Selby before 1227[51] (ibid., no. 941). Thus it appears that William de Lisle, son of Godwin, was father of Henry, Jordan, and Amabel de Lisle. Henry, the eldest son, who issued a deed in *c.*1210 × 1226 (M: Ramsholme [MS Dods. 120b, f. 76r]) was succeeded by his son William, who was succeeded in turn by his uncle Jordan and aunt Amabel. Later Amabel was succeeded by Oliver de Vendouer, probably her son-in-law.[52] Farrer pointed out that Holmes had confused this branch of the Lisle family with that of Brodsworth (*EYC*, I, 382; *Ctl. Pontefract*, p. 139). Farrer's statement that Amabel sister of Henry de Lisle confirmed the gifts of Godwin her grandfather, William her father, and Henry her brother (*EYC*, I, 381–82) is supposition based on the single line by which Dodsworth reported R723.

Ilard of HECK, who is mentioned in R724, gave land in Hensall to Osbert of Hensall, probably in the first quarter of the thirteenth century[53] (*EYC*, I, no. 498). He attested at Easter 1219 (*Ctl. Selby*, no. 765), and occurred several times with John of Birkin, implying *c.*1190 × 1227, and also with Adam de Bellewe, therefore after 1202 (*Ctl. Selby*, nos 336, 938, 953, 970; FN: Birkin, Bellewe). Richenda daughter of Ilard of Heck issued an acknowledgement, witnessed by John of Birkin, that she held 1 bv. in Pollington of Selby Abbey, which Jordan [previously] held of Jordan, her brother (ibid., no. 940). Ilard of Heck and John his son attested a deed of H[enry] de Vernoil, given probably in the first quarter of the thirteenth century[54] (MS Dods. 8, f. 161ʳ). John of Heck and Amice his wife were impleaded in 1218–19 by Alice widow of Adam of Preston for land in Preston, and in the same period John of Heck was suspected of the death of Idonea wife of Henry of Pocklington (*Yorkshire Eyre Rolls*, nos 132, 592). Ilard of Heck was dead in October 1226, when his widow Agnes claimed dower of a third part of 14 bv. in Heck against John of Heck (*YF*, 1218–1231, p. 67).

**R721.** Gift to the hospital by Henry de Lisle of a toft in Heck, which John the miller
held [*c.*1175 × *c.*1210]

COPIES: *d* MS Dods. 8, f. 191ᵛ; *c* MS Dods 120b, f. 13ʳ, from Rawl., f. 62, now missing, with the minor omission noted. CALENDAR: 'Dodsworth's Yorkshire Notes', *YAJ*, XI, 52, no witnesses, from *c* via Jennyns and Tillotson. NOTED: *EYC*, I, 381, from *YAJ*.

---

51  Attested by John of Birkin, who was dead in that year.
52  As Oliver's wife was named Mabel, she was probably a daughter of Amabel, the names being broadly equivalent. Oliver was probably of the family which had interests in Glentworth and Hackthorn, Lincs., who may have taken their name from Wendover in Bucks. (*Danelaw Docs*, pp. xxviii n, 25, 213; *Gilbertine Charters*, pp. xxviii, 84–86). Oliver de Vendouer was a knight on a grand assize in Lincolnshire in 1203, 1204, 1205 and 1220 (*CRR*, 1203–1205, pp. 26, 225, 309; ibid., 1219–1220, p. 369). There was a plea of land against him in Lincolnshire in 1208 (ibid., 1207–1209, p. 307). He made a fine in 1211 concerning land in Newton and Toft; and another in 1219 concerning land in Hackthorn (*Lincs. Fines*, I, 101, 151). Mabel, widow of Oliver de Vendouer, quitclaimed land in Hackthorn, probably in 1240 (*Reg. Antiquissimum*, IV, 67), and was summoned to respond to William de Vendouer concerning land in Brattleby (Lincs.) in 1242–43 (*CRR*, 1242–1243, no. 2236).
53  Attested by Alexander of Roall, Alexander his son, Roger of Roall, Simon of Roall, and Otes his son (FN).
54  Also attested by Alexander and Ralph of Roall (FN).

*Carta Henrici de Insula.*

Sciant tam presentes quam futuri quod ego Henricus de Insula dedi hospitali sancti Petri Eboraci in puram elemosinam, pro anima patris mei et antecessorum meorum, toftum unum[55] in Hecca, quod Iohannes molendinarius tenuit, liberum et quietum ab omni servitio. Hiis testibus, H(er)nulfo capellano, Widone cappellano, Ada diacono, Turgisio de abbatia Eboraci, W(illelm)o clerico de Sneheit,[56] Reginaldo preposito de Goldale et multis aliis. Et hoc sigillo meo confirmavi.[57]

It is difficult to assign secure limits of date to this deed, which has been dated with reference to the likely period for the donor. Turgis of the Abbey occurs in 1204, and may have been a descendant of the man of that name who had a grant of land in York in the time of Savaric, abbot of St Mary's between 1138 and 1161 (*EYC*, I, no. 271 and n). Adam the deacon may be the witness to an Eggborough deed of 1166 × *c*.1190 (R132).

**R722.** Confirmation to the hospital by William de Lisle of 1 bv. of land in Heck which his father Godwin had given in alms [*c*.1150 × 1177]

COPY: *d* MS Dods. 8, f. 192a^r, probably from the original deed. ABSTRACT: *c* MS Dods. 120b, f. 13^r, from Rawl., f. 62, now missing, possibly from a slightly different original. CALENDAR: 'Dodsworth's Yorkshire Notes', *YAJ*, XI, 52, no witnesses, from *c* via Jennyns and Tillotson. NOTED: *EYC*, I, 381, from *YAJ*.

*Carta Willelmi de Insula.*

Notum sit omnibus sancte matris ecclesie filiis tam presentibus quam futuris quod ego Will(elmus) de Insula et heredes mei concessimus et confirmavimus deo et sancto Petro et pauperibus hospitalis beati Petri Ebor' terram quam pater meus Godwinus eis prius dederat in puram et perpetuam elemosinam, videlicet unam bovatam terre in Hech, cum omnibus appenditiis suis in bosco et plano in aquis in pratis et pascuis et in omnibus q(ue) ad terram pertinent. Illam vero prefatam terram contra omnes homines warantizabimus solutam et quietam, liberam et immunem ab omni geldo et consuetudine et exactione et omni seculari servitio preter orationes pauperum. Et simus participes omnium bonorum et orationum que fiunt in illa sancta domo in vita et in morte. Isti sunt testes, Umfridus de Ruhala, Alexander de Ruh(ala),[58] <Herbertus de Hetheneshaia,> Ada de Pontef(racto), Tomas de Snait, Hugo de Insula, Robertus de Thirna, Arnulfus filius Dolfin, Alanus filius Osberti, Alfredus Peliparius, Iordanus de Pouelintun, Robertus filius Ingeram, Radulfo capellano, Roberto clerico de Scakeltorp, Gamello de Bugthorp, Gaufrido clerico.[59]

Godwin's gift, made in 1148 × 1156, was apparently not marked by a deed, so it is likely that this confirmation was issued after his death. Humphrey and Alexander of Roall witnessed together not later than 1177 (R130). Humphrey was dead in the latter year (FN).

---

[55]  *c*: *unum toftum.*
[56]  *d*: *Soneheit.*
[57]  *c* omits *Et hoc . . . confirmavi.*
[58]  *c* has the first two witnesses, followed by *Ada de Egburc*, who does not occur in *d*.
[59]  *sic*, with later witnesses in ablative.

**R723.** Confirmation of R722 by Amabel daughter of William de Lisle [*c.*1210 × *c.*1230]

NOTED: *c* MS Dods. 120b, f. 13ᵣ, from Rawl., f. 62, now missing. NOTED: 'Dodsworth's Yorkshire Notes', *YAJ*, XI, 52, from *c* via Jennyns and Tillotson; whence *EYC*, I, 381–82.

Amabil(ia) filia Willelmi de Insula confirm(avit) donacionem predictam.⁶⁰

**R724.** Gift to the hospital by Amabel daughter of William de Lisle of the toft between the toft of Ilard of Heck and the toft which John the miller held of Adam of Lund [*c.*1210 × *c.*1230]

COPY: MS Dods. 8, f. 192aᵛ.

*Carta Amabil(ie) filie W(illelm)i de Insula.*
Omnibus presentes literas visuris vel audituris Amabil(ia) filia Willelmi de Insula salutem. Noverit universitas vestra me caritatis et pietatis intuitu concessisse dedisse et hac presenti carta mea confirm(asse) deo et pauperibus hospitalis sancti Petri Ebor' illud toftum quod iacet inter toftum Ylard' de Hecka et toftum quod Iohannes molendinarius tenuit de Ada de Lund, tenend(um) et habend(um) predictis pauperibus cum omnibus pertinentiis infra villam et extra, in liberam puram et perpetuam elemosinam, sicut aliqua elemosina liberius et melius dari potest. Ego a(utem) et heredes mei predictam elemosinam meam warantizabimus, acquietabimus et defendemus predictis pauperibus in omnibus contra omnes homines imperpetuum. In cuius rei testimonium huic scripto sigillum meum apposui. Testibus, Roberto, Bernardo, Willelmo fratribus et capellanis, Godefrido de celler(io), Waltero et aliis fratribus hospitalis, Radulfo de Fontibus, Alexandro, Thoma, Ada capellanis, Ricardo Fossard, Ada de [ ]⁶¹ et multis aliis.

Robert, William, and Bernard, brothers and chaplains, and Richard Fossard attested a deed of *c.*1210 × 1217 (R390); and with the addition of Ralph de Fontibus, a deed of 1214 × *c.*1230 (R24). The three brother-chaplains, with Fontibus, attested a deed of *c.*1214 × *c.*1230 (R443), and with Walter, Fontibus, and Fossard, attested another with the same limits of date (R497). Individually the witnesses attested frequently in the period assigned.

## *Heselwood* [Hazlewood, near Tadcaster ?]

The Contents List gives f. 62 for *Heselwood*, but nothing more is known of the hospital's holdings there, and so the identification of the place remains uncertain.

---

⁶⁰ Dodsworth's writing is very hurried, possibly *donationes predictas* is intended.
⁶¹ Space left for surname.

# [Knottingley]

For Knottingley, see R209–R215.

**R725.** Gift by Paulinus, minister of the hospital, with the consent of the chapter, to the abbot and monks of Meaux, of a messuage in the hospital's land in Knottingley, 60 ft in width and in length from the river called *Frith* as far as the land of Robert de Lacy, next to the land which a certain widow holds of the hospital on the east side, under condition that no married or cohabiting man should live there to the shame of the donors or the injury of the brethren [1181 × c.1202, probably 1181 × 1193]

COPY: *d* Meaux cartulary, f. 156ʳ. NOTED: *e* Meaux register, f. 44ᵛ; *f* ibid., f. 50ʳ; *g* JRUL, MS Latin 219 (Meaux chronicle), f. 47; *h* BL, MS Egerton 1141 (Meaux chronicle), f. 35ᵛ. PRINTED: 'Ctl. Meaux', no. 397, imperfectly, where dated 1197 × 1202, from *d*. NOTED: *Chron. Meaux*, I, 322–23, from *g* and *h*;[62] 'Ctl. Meaux', p. 629, from *f*.

*Carta per quam Paulinus minister hospitalis sancti Petri Ebor' dedit mon(achis) de Melsa mansionem in Knottyngley.*
Universis cristi fidelibus litteras has videntibus sive audient(ibus) Paulinus hospitalis sancti Petri Ebor' humilis minister salutem. Universitati vestre notificetur me communi consilio et assensu capituli nostri concessisse et presenti carta nostra confirmasse deo et abbatie de M(elsa) et monachis ibidem deo servientibus mansionem quamdam in terra nostra in Cnottyngleia, latitudine sexaginta pedum et in longitudine quantum terra nostra extenditur ad flumine quod dicitur Frith usque ad terram Roberti de Laceio iuxta terram quam tenet vidua quedam de nobis ex parte orientali, ut predicti monachi prefatam terram habeant et possideant propriis usibus imperpetuum libere et quiete ab omni seculari servicio preter orationes devotas in Christo prefate domus sicut in carta domus commemorate continetur. Conditione vero tali predictis monachis terram prefatam concedimus ut nullus uxoratus neque mulierum cohabitatio ad nostrum dedecus aut gravamen fratrum nostrorum inhabitet. Hiis testibus, Reginaldo, Svano, Ricardo, presbiteris et fratribus, Osmundo, Dolfino[63] etc.

The date range given is that for Paulinus as master of the hospital. The witness list is truncated, as is normally the case in the Meaux cartulary. Orange's dating relies on the note concerning this deed in *Chron. Meaux* falling under the heading *Alexander abbas quartas*. However, it is probable that the Robert de Lacy mentioned was the lord of Pontefract, and that he was living when this deed was drawn up, indicating a date of 1193 or before. The deed has several unusual features. The restriction to single men does not appear elsewhere in the hospital's deeds, and is suggestive of a particular problem with respect to this location. There is no occurrence of the word *flumen* in the Rawlinson volume, where *aqua* is usual. The river or stream named *Frith* is not otherwise recorded.

---

[62] Abbas itaque ipse acquisivit in Knottyngle de hospitali sancti Petri Eboraci quandam mansionem, ut eam haberemus in proprios usus imperpetuum; ita quod nullus uxoratus aut mulierum cohabitatio, ad suum dedecus aut gravamen, eam inhabitaret. Sed qualiter ipsa mansio fuit alienata penitus ignoratur.
[63] MS: *Doffino.*

# [Leathley]

For Leathley, see R221–R253.

**R726.** Grant by Hugh of Leathley to Roger his son, for his homage and service, of
half his mills in Leathley, whether built or to be built, with all suit, which the
grantor would not alienate or diminish, for 1*d.* annually [1219 × 1237]

COPY: MS Dods. 8, f. 179ᵛ, probably from the original.

*Carta Hugonis de Lelai.*
Sciant omnes presentes et futuri quod ego Hugo de Lelai dedi concessi et hac mea
carta confirm(avi) Rogero filio meo pro homagio et servitio suo totam medietatem
omnium molendinorum meorum in Lelai, tam factorum quam faciendorum, cum
tota sequela eorum et cum omnibus pertinenciis integre et plenarie sine retenemento,
tenendam et habendam predicto Rogero et heredibus suis de me et heredibus meis in
feodo et hereditate libere quiete et honorifice imperpetuum, reddendo inde annuatim
michi et heredibus meis unum denarium ad natale domini, pro omnibus servitiis et
demandis, ita quod ego Hugo et heredes mei non alienabimus nec minuemus aliquid
de predicta sequela predictorum molendinorum imperpetuum. Et ego et heredes mei
totam predictam medietatem omnium predictorum molendinorum cum omnibus
pertinenciis warantizabimus et defendemus predicto Rogero et heredibus suis pro
predicto servitio contra omnes homines imperpetuum. Hiis testibus, Nicholao Warde,
Willelmo Vavasore, Ricardo de Mohaut, Willelmo clerico de Lindelai, Willelmo <de>
Plumton, Henrico de Westscoth', Willelmo de Castelai, Rogero de Hugebi, Thoma
<de> Hurteschi et multis aliis.

Whether the half of the mills granted here was the half which Roger held of the
hospital is uncertain (R225, R230). The first witness, Nicholas Ward, who held 1 k.f.
in Guiseley of the archbishop, appears to have succeeded his father William Ward in
1216 × 1217, and to have died in 1248 × 1252 (*Baildon*, I, 224–29). William Vavasour
succeeded his father Mauger probably in 1219 (FN). Richard de Mohaut was dead
in 1236[/37] (R221n).

**R727.** Gift to the hospital by Ellis and William of Leathley, sons of Jordan of Leathley,
of a waste toft in Leathley where their father used to live [*c.*1240 × *c.*1280]

NOTED: MS Dods. 95, f. 48ʳ, apparently from the original found in the rubble of
St Mary's Tower.

Elias de Lethelay et Willelmus de Letheley filii Iordani de Lethelay dederunt hospitalis
sancti Leonardi Ebor' unum vastum toftum in Letheley in quo Iordanus pater eorum
habitabat. Test(e) Iacobo de Monte Alto.

William son of Jordan of Leathley occurs in 1257 and was probably dead in 1280
(R226, R227).

# [Pudsey, par. Calverley]

For Pudsey, see R331–R342.

**R728.** Grant at fee-farm by master Hugh, rector, and the brethren of the hospital to William the clerk of Calverley, of 1 a. land in Wadelands, which they had by gift of Henry Scot of Pudsey, paying 12*d.* annually and 1*m.* as an obituary payment [*c.*1229 × 1245]

ORIGINAL: YAS, DD57/B.oo, at Woolley Hall in 1859 and *c.*1922, 16 cm. (wide) × 12 cm., bottom turn-up, slit for seal tag (present), seal gone in 1859. Medieval endorsement: *carta de hospitali de i. acra terre pro xii.d. redd'.* PRINTED: 'Charters of the thirteenth century, communicated by G. Wentworth esq. of Woolley Park, Wakefield,' *Journal of the British Archaeological Association*, XV (1859), 332–33, no. 2. CALENDAR: *YD*, III, no. 35, imperfect. FACSIMILE: Plate VII.

Omnibus cristi fidelibus ad quos presens scriptum pervenerit, magister Hugo rector et fratres hospitalis sancti Petri Ebor' salutem in domino. Noverit universitas vestra nos concessisse et presenti carta nostra confirmasse Willelmo clerico de Calverlay unam acram terre in Wadelandes quam habemus de dono Henrici Scotti de Pudekeseya, tenendam et habendam predicto Willelmo et assignatis suis preterquam iudeis et viris religiosis aliis a nobis cum omnibus pertinenciis suis aisiamentis et libertatibus suis infra villam et extra libere integre et quiete, reddendo inde nobis annuatim duodecim denarios, medietatem ad Pentecoste(n) et aliam medietatem ad festum sancti Martini in hieme. Predictus autem Willelmus et assignati sui vel quicunque in predicta terra manserint pro portione catallorum eos contingente in obitu suo unam marcam argenti pauperibus domus nostre persolvent. Nos autem predictam terram cum suis pertinenciis predicto Willelmo et assignatis suis warantizabimus quamdiu carte donatorum quas inde habemus nobis illam warantizare poterunt. In huius autem rei robur et testimonium huic scripto sigillum nostrum apposuimus. Hiis testibus, Ricardo de Tanga, Simone de Fersleya, Rog(ero) Alano,[64] Stephano de Ecclesclif', Roberto de Eccleshil', Ricardo de Tirsal', Fulcone de Ulvestthorp', Iordano filio Willelmi et multis aliis.

Henry Scot's gift of this land to the hospital was probably made in 1229 or later (R332). Margaret of Tyersal, daughter of the late William, clerk of Calverley, gave to master William de Wudehal 'what her father had held of the hospital of St Leonard, York' with other land in Wadelands and *Arnesrode* (*YD*, III, no. 36).

# [Reedness]

There is no trace of a section for Reedness deeds in the Rawlinson volume. Deeds belonging to Inklemoor nearby were copied to ff. 205–7 in the East Riding division, under the heading Morhamwick (R792–R799). In April 1295, commissioners were appointed on complaint by Walter de Langton, king's clerk and master of the hospital of St Leonard, that persons having lands near the bank of the Ouse between

---

[64] sic, in full.

the towns of Hook and Reedness did not repair the walls and dykes as they should. A few days later a similar commission was issued, covering a much longer stretch of the river from Cawood to Faxfleet (*CalPat*, 1292–1301, p. 160). The resulting inquisition is preserved at Lichfield RO, D30/12/108, but is not included in *CalInqMisc*.

**R729.** Gift to the hospital by Ralph, son of Reginald the serjeant, of *Scoter*, of 12 perches of moor, with land and appurtenances, in the moor of Reedness, and a toft, containing 2 perches, paying 18*d*. annually to Thomas son of Robert of Reedness and 6*d*. to his heirs [*c*.1214 × *c*.1230]

COPY: Burton transcripts 3, f. 118ʳ, p. 209, B18 N34.

Omnibus has litteras etc. Radulfus filius Reginaldi servientis de Scoter salutem. Noverit etc. dedisse deo et pauperibus hospitalis sancti Petri Ebor' duodecim pertic(atas) de mora cum fundo et terra et pertinenciis in latitudine in mora de Rednesse et in longitudine quantum mora se extendit a Fulesike ..⁶⁵ versus austrum, et unum toftum continens duas perticatas terre iacent(is) inter Kerdic et ripam Use, tenend(a) et habend(a) libere etc., reddendo inde annuatim pro omni servicio etc. decem et octo denarios Thome filio Roberti de Rednesse et heredibus suis sex denarios. Hanc elemosinam feci pro salute etc. et ut participes simus omnium beneficiorum que facienda sint in dicta domo dei in perpetuum. In huius autem rei etc. apposui. Hiis testibus, magistro Gulielmo de Gerunden, Henrico de Hedun capellano, magist(ris) T[homa] de Languat, I[ohanne] de Lada, Willelmo de Rednesse, Radulfo de⁶⁶ Gaitington, Roberto de Stowa, et aliis.

The date range is the period during which Thomas de Langwath attested as master.


# [Rufforth]

For Rufforth, see R368–R391. Five folios (ff. 105–9), containing deeds numbered 21–53, are missing from the Rufforth section of the Rawlinson volume.

**R730.** Confirmation to the hospital by Geoffrey of Bugthorpe and Ellen his wife of land in Rufforth [*c*.1210 × 1218]

NOTED: MS Dods. 120b, f. 22ʳ, from Rawl., f. 105, now missing, no. 22.

<Ego> Galfridus de Buggethorp et Elena {filia et heres Ful(c)onis de Rugheford c. 23} uxor mea confirm(avimus) terram in Rugheford hospitali sancti Petri Ebor'. Testibus, Hamone thesaurario ecclesie beati Petri Ebor', Roberto⁶⁷ Langwath, Roberto de Stow cleric(is) hospitalis. c. 22.⁶⁸ fo. 105.

Hamo was treasurer between 1197 and 1217 or 1218; Robert de Stowe attests after *c*.1210. Fulk of Rufforth died in 1214 × 1217, but this deed may have been issued

---

⁶⁵  sic in MS.
⁶⁶  *de* supplied.
⁶⁷  sic, presumably a mistake for Thomas.
⁶⁸  Apparently altered to c. 23, but as Dodsworth references c. 23 within this abstract, c. 22 is more likely.

during his lifetime. As the witnesses are included in those of Fulk's deed giving *Karte-gathe Hyrste* in Rufforth to the hospital (R386), the present deed may be a confirmation issued on the same occasion.

**R731.** Confirmation to the hospital by Ellen, daughter and heir of Fulk of Rufforth, of all the grants and gifts her father made, that is, all the land on the west side of the hospital's wood, *Kartegatehirst* by the bounds named in his deed, with everything according to the deed. Also confirmation of the advowson of Rufforth church, which her father left by his will, with his body. Also gift of the land with the wood called *Moshaghe*, and whatever right she has in the Foss stream. Also gift of part of the land in *Baregathes*. She has subjected herself to the jurisdiction of the dean and chapter of York, under penalty of 40*m.*, in the event of any dispute [1218 × 1220]

COPY: *b* C98 [Cott., f. 14ᵛ (old f. 12ᵛ)]. ABSTRACT: *c* MS Dods. 120b, f. 22ʳ, omitting last three witnesses, from Rawl., f. 106, no. 25, now missing.

*Elena⁶⁹ fil(ia) et her(es) Fulconis de Rughford' confirmat⁷⁰ omnes donationes patris sui, et preterea ded(it) Moshaghe et illam partem terre in Baregathes et confirmat⁷⁰ donacionem ecclesie de Rughford.*
Omnibus cristi fidelibus ad quos presens scriptum pervenerit, Elena filia et heres Fulconis de Rughford' salutem. Noveritis quod ego caritatis et pietatis intuitu et pro salute anime mee et animarum patris mei matris mee et omnium antecessorum et successorum meorum concessi et presenti carta mea confirmavi deo et pauperibus hospitalis sancti Petri Ebor' omnes concessiones et donationes quas Fulco pater meus eis caritatem⁷¹ dedit, videlicet totam terram ex occidentali parte bosci hospitalis quam eis dedit, et Kartegatehirst per terminos et metas in carta patris mei expressos cum omnibus secundum tenorem carte eiusdem illis concess(is). Confirmavi etiam eisdem pauperibus advocationem ecclesie de Rufford' quam eis pater meus cum corpore suo in testamento suo reliquit. Preterea sepedictis pauperibus concessi dedi et presenti carta mea confirmavi totam terram illam cum bosco quod appellatur Moshaghe q(ue) scilicet protenditur versus occidentem a supradicta terra quam pater meus illis prius dederat ultra Fossam usque ad metas et terminos positos inter Fossam et culturam que appellatur Bradele versus austrum. Vero protenditur eadem terra a cultura que appellatur Akumhag usque ad divisam de Haskeham secundum metas et terminos iuxta cursum Fosse positos, et quicquid iuris habui vel habere potui in sepedicta aqua. Et preterea concessi et dedi eisdem pauperibus illam partem terre in Barega-thes que protenditur a meta et termino iuxta pontem Fosse posito que protenditur versus occidentem usque ad metam et terminum ibi positum, continentem in latere aquilonali triginta et sex perticatas et in latitudine versus meridiem usque ad fossatum hospitalis continentem viginti et unam perticatas et dimidiam, tenenda scilicet et habenda omnia predicta cum omnibus pertinenciis suis et aisiamentis infra villam et extra in puram et perpetuam elemosinam liberam quietam et solutam ab omni seculari servicio et exactione sicut aliqua elemosina liberius et melius dari potest, ita quod ego et heredes mei totum predictum tenementum et omnia preenumerata sepe-dictis pauperibus in omnibus et contra omnes homines warantizabimus aquietabimus

---

⁶⁹ *b: Elene.*
⁷⁰ *b: confir'ᵗ.*
⁷¹ sic, probably for *caritative.*

et defendemus imperpetuum. Hec autem omnia pro me et heredibus meis affidavi et tactis sacrosanctis iuravi. Et sub pena quadraginta marcarum firmiter promisi, ita quod si aliqu(is), instinctu diaboli, quod deus avertat, per me vel per alium predictis pauperibus super aliqua prenumeratorum controversia movere presuma(t) vel contra fidem et iuramentum meum veniens concessiones et donationes patris mei et meas predictas in aliquo infringere attempte(t), iurisdictioni decani et capituli Ebor', appelatione remota omn(is) iuris auxilio renuncians, me subieci, ut ipsi me et heredes meos ad solutionem predictarum quadraginta marcarum nomine pene premissarum per excomunicationem vel quocumque alio modo voluerint me compellant et insuper maledictionem omnipotentis dei et genitricis eius Marie et beati Leonardi necnon et omnium sanctorum et infirmorum dicte domus dei incurram. In huius rei robur et testimonium huic scripto sigillum meum apposui. Testibus, H[amone] decano, magistro Waltero archidiacono de Hestrithing, Willelmo filio Ricardi, magistris Ricardo Cornub', Galfrido de Norwis, Iohanne Rom', Roberto de Wynton', Erardo, Bernardo et aliis canonicis Ebor', Radulpho de Fontibus, magistro Thoma de Languad', Ricardo Fossard', Henrico de Cava, Roberto de Stouhe et multis aliis.

For the date, indicated by the attestations of Hamo the dean, and master Walter the archdeacon, see R368n. There are other examples of explicit penalty clauses in deeds given by women during the early thirteenth century. A penalty of £40 was included in one of Ellen's deeds to Fountains made in 1214 × 1226 (*Ctl. Fountains*, pp. 770–71; FN: Rufforth). Emma, widow of Ralph son of Baldwin [of Bramhope] agreed to a penalty of 40*m.* if she initiated any subsequent dispute in a deed of 1214 × *c.*1230 (R24).

**R732.** Agreement between Fulk of Rufforth and master Ralph, rector of the hospital, for the maintenance of a chaplain celebrating daily at the altar of St Katherine for the souls of Fulk and his ancestors. Fulk gave the master lands in Rufforth by named bounds [1204 × 1217]

ABSTRACT: MS Dods. 120b, f. 23ʳ, from Rawl., f. 106, now missing.

Fulco de Rugheford convenit cum magistro Radulfo rectore hospitalis sancti Petri Ebor' pro habendo capellano singulis diebus ad altare sancti Katerine celebratur pro animabus dicti Fulconis et antecessorum. Et dedit predicto magistro terras in Rugheford per divisas. Test(e) H[amone] thesaur(ario) Ebor'. fo. 106.

It is unclear whether the altar of St Katherine was in the hospital or Rufforth church. Master Ralph indicates 1204 × 1217; Fulk died in 1214 × 1217 (FN).

**R733.** Gift and release to the hospital by Adam son of Alan of Knapton of all *Mikelmor*, so that the brethren may enclose it, and plough and sow as they wish [*c.*1200 × 1214]

COPY: Burton transcripts 2, f. 80ʳ, p. 126, B12 N56. NOTED: Drake, *Eboracum*, p. 336, via Torre's collections.

Sciant omnes presentes[72] et futuri quod ego Adam filius Alani de Knapetona dedi reddidi et concessi et hac presenti carta mea confirmavi deo et pauperibus hospi-

---

[72] *presentes* supplied.

talis beati Petri Ebor' totum Mikelmor cum omnibus liberis pertinenciis suis, ita quod bene licet fratribus predicti hospitalis circumfossare, includere, arare, seminare, et facere totum libitum suum de toto predicto Mikelmor cum omnibus liberis pertinenciis suis, sive ullo impedimento vel retenemento, scilicet habendum sibi in puram et perpetuam elemosinam, libere integre honorifice et quiete ab omni servicio, et ab omni exactione, sicut ulla elemosina liberius potest dari vel confirmari, ita quod ego et heredes mei warantizabimus defendemus adquietabimus et pacifice possidere faciemus predictis pauperibus totam predictam donationem et concessionem sine ullo retenemento et impedimento contra omnes homines ut simus participes omnium bonorum que fiunt et fient in predicta domo dei. Hiis testibus, Alano filio Elys', Willelmo de Stiveton, Roberto de Wivelestorp, Fulcone de Rucford, Willelmo de Popleton, Iohanne filio Widonis, Henrico Bustard, domino S[imone] decano et capitulo beati Petri Ebor', Thoma de Langwath, et multis aliis.

The hospital's meadow of Mikelmor is mentioned in a Rufforth deed of 1214 × 1230 (R369). The Knapton family held land in Bustardthorpe, Knapton (which adjoins Rufforth), Amotherby, and Swinton, par. Appleton-le-Street (*EYC*, VI, 147). The donor gave the hospital 1 ct. in Bustardthorpe by a deed with similar witnesses (R75). Simon de Apulia was dean of York between 1194 and 1214; Fulk of Rufforth died in 1214 × 1217; Robert de Wivelestorp died in 1214; Alan of Knapton, the donor's father, was living in 1197 and was probably dead in 1207. William de Stiveton succeeded his father Bertram in 1200 or later (FNs). The position of the dean and chapter in the witness list is unusual, but is perhaps idiosyncratic rather than suspicious.

For the sixth witness, John son of Guy, who also attests R735, see *EYC*, I, 435–36. He occurs in the early thirteenth century, sometimes with the surname *Hoton*, from Hutton Wandesley.

**R734.** Gift to the hospital, and to endow the church of All Saints in Rufforth, by Geoffrey of Rufforth and Elena his wife, of a messuage in Rufforth, and a culture in the field of Rufforth, being that which Robert son of Gamel formerly held of the donors in the new assart towards York [1235 × 1248]

COPY: MS Dods. 8, f. 150ʳ, presumably from the original.

*Carta Galfridi de Rufford et Elene uxoris eius.*
Omnibus cristi fidelibus ad quos presens scriptum pervenerit Galfridus de Rufford et Elena uxor eius salutem. Noverit universitas vestra nos caritatis intuitu et pro salute animarum nostrarum et animarum antecessorum et successorum nostrorum dedisse concessisse et presenti carta nostra confirm(asse) deo et pauperibus hospitalis sancti Petri Ebor' et ad ecclesiam omnium Sanctorum de Rufford dotandam unum messuagium cum pertinenciis suis in Rufford, continens in latitudine septem percatas et quinque pedes cum pertica viginti pedum et in latitudine triginta tres pedes, et iacent iuxta messuagium pertinens ad ecclesiam de Rufford ex parte australi. Et unam culturam in campo de Rufford, videlicet illam quam Rob(ertus) filius Gamelli aliquando de nobis tenuit que iacet in novo essarto versus Eboracum, tenendum et habendum predictis pauperibus in liberam puram et perpetuam elemosinam cum omnibus pertinenciis suis aysiamentis et libertatibus suis infra villam et extra, sicut aliqua elemosina liberius et meleius⁷³ teneri potest et haberi. Nos autem et

---

⁷³ sic.

heredes nostri predictum tenementum cum pertinenciis suis predictis pauperibus warantizabimus adquietabimus et defendemus in omnibus et contra omnes homines imperpetuum. In huius autem rei robur et testimonium huic scripto sigilla nostra apposuimus. Hiis testibus, Gilberto Candide Case episcopo, Willelmo persona de Helaw tunc decano de Aynsti, Petro de Knapeton et Thoma fratre suo, Iohanne de Merston, Ada clerico de Rufford, Iohanne talliatore et multis aliis.

The date range is limited by the election and consecration of Bishop Gilbert of Galloway in 1235, and the death of Geoffrey of Rufforth in 1246 × 1248 (FN). Lawton was unable to establish the patron saint of Rufforth church, but noted that Guy Wright, gent., of Rufforth, by his will of 1574 gave his soul to God, St Mary and All Saints, and his body to be buried in the church before the image of All Hallows (Lawton, *Collections*, p. 72).

**R735.** Gift by Fulk of Rufforth to William Cunin, for his life, for his homage and service and 1*lb.* of pepper annually, of 40 a. in Rufforth, situated between the boundary of Askham and the assart of William, Fulk's brother, with so much pasture as belongs to 2 bv. in Rufforth [*c.*1190 × 1207]

COPY: MS Dods. 8, f. 150$^{r-v}$, presumably from the original.

*Carta Fulconis de Ruhford.*
Sciant omnes presentes et futuri quod ego Fulco de Ruhford' dedi et concessi et hac presenti carta mea confirmavi Willelmo Kunin pro homagio et servitio suo quadraginta acras terre in territorio de Ruhford, scilicet inter divisam de Askham et essartam Willelmi fratris mei, tenendas sibi tota vita eiusdem Willelmi et habendas libere integre honorifice et quiete cum pastura et claustura et cum omnibus liberis pertinenciis suis, quantum pasture scilicet pertinet ad duas bovatas terre in Ruhford, ita quod prefatus Willelmus reddet inde michi et heredibus meis [f. 150$^v$] annuatim tantummodo unam libram piperis infra octavas apostolorum Petri et Pauli. Et ego predictus Fulco et heredes mei warantizabimus predicto Willelmo tota vita sua totum predictum tenementum cum omnibus liberis pertinenciis suis sine impedimento et retenemento contra omnes homines per predictum servitium. Hiis testibus, Nigello de Plumton', Rob' de Wivelestorp, Alano filio Helie de Katerton, Bertramo de Stiveton, Willelmo filio eius, Iohanne filio Widonis, Alano de Knapton', Ada et aliis filiis eius, Thurstino de Merston, Henrico persona de Hoton, Thoma de Langwath et multis aliis.

Fulk of Rufforth died in 1214 × 1217; Nigel de Plumpton died in 1212; Robert de Wivelestorp died in 1214; Alan of Knapton was probably dead in 1207; Bertram de Stiveton last occurs in 1200 (FNs). Thomas de Langwath attested from *c.*1190. William Cunin later released this land to Fulk of Rufforth, who gave it to the hospital (R388–R390).

**R736.** Confirmation to the hospital by Ellis parson of Rufforth of the gift which Fulk of Rufforth his brother gave, being the land in Rufforth lying next to the boundary of the hospital's wood [*c.*1210 × 1217]

COPY: MS Dods. 8, f. 150$^v$, presumably from the original.

*Carta Elye persone de Rughford.*
Omnibus presentes litteras visuris vel audituris Elyas persona de Rughford salutem.

Universitati vestre notum facio me ratam gratam et acceptam habere donacionem quam Fulco de Rughfort frater meus dedit pauperibus hospitalis sancti Petri Ebor', scilicet de terra illa in territorio de Rughfort cum suis pertinenciis que iacet iuxta metas bosci fratrum eiusdem hospitalis. In huius a(utem) rei robur et testimonium huic scripto sigillum meum apposui. Testibus, Roberto, Willelmo, Bernardo capellanis et fratribus hospitalis, Anketino, Godfrido, Waltero, Thoma cellerario et aliis fratribus hospitalis, Fulcone de Rughfort, Radulfo Nuuel, Alano de Knapeton', Thoma de sancto Salvatore, Petro, Rogero, Willelmo capellanis, Thoma de Langwath, Roberto de Stowe, Watero de Alredale, Malgero, Ricardo, et multis aliis.

For the date, see R390, which has very similar witnesses.

**R737.** Confirmation and quitclaim to the hospital by Ellen, daughter of Fulk of Rufforth, in widowhood, of all lands and possessions she and Geoffrey of Bugthorpe, formerly her husband, had given, namely the land with wood called *Molesawe*, the culture called *Bradele*, a culture called *le Hag*, a plot in *Scaleker*, a culture in the new assart which Robert son of Gamel formerly held, the culture called *Smalwyht*, the land called *Husbonde croft* in *Baregates*, a toft where the priest lives, a toft where Nigel lives with his 2 a. in *Smalwyt*. She also confirmed the land and pasture the hospital has by the gift of Fulk her father, being all *le Sumergang, Cunungriding, Acumgate Hyrst, Ca[rtegate] Hyrst, Hesylhyrst,* and the toft where Thomas Tod lives; also the land given by her uncle John in *Doleker* and *Zel* and *Linthweit* with the toft that belonged to the said John; also the advowson of the church of Rufforth with 2 bv. of land and the tofts and crofts belonging. She confirmed all the gifts made by Fulk, John, Geoffrey and herself, as the hospital held them on 17 May 1257.

COPY: MS Dods. 8, f. 151ʳ, from the original. Drawing of seal on tag, vesica, a raven close, facing dexter, SIGILL': ELIANORE: FILIE: FVE+.

*Carta Elene filie Fulconis de Ruford relicte Galfridi de Buggetorp.*
Omnibus cristi fidelibus hoc scriptum visuris vel audituris Elena filia Fulconis de Ruford eternam in domino salutem. Noverit universitas vestra me in mea viduitate et pro(p)ria potestate concessisse et hac carta mea confirm(asse) <ac> quietum clamasse deo et pauperibus hospitalis beati Leonardi Ebor' omnes terras et possessiones quas Galfridus de Buggetorp quondam vir meus et ego Elena concessimus et dedimus eisdem, videlicet totam illam terram cum bosco que appelatur Molesawe sicut includitur sepe et fossato, et totam illam culturam que dicitur Bradele sicut includitur inter divisas de Ascham et terram que fuit Galfridi filii mei in Morlflat, et una(m) cultura(m) que dicitur le Hag iacentem ex parte aquilonali de Mosehawe secundum metas ibidem factas, et unam placcam terre iacentem in Scaleker iuxta terram dicti hospitalis illam scilicet quam Ranulfus de Merston aliquando tenuit, et unam culturam in novo assarto quam Robertus filius Gamelli aliquando tenuit, et totam illam culturam que dicitur Smalwyht sicut includitur fossato, et totam illam terram que dicitur Husbonde croft iacentem in Baregates, et unum toftum longitudinis septem perticarum et quinque pedum in quo sacerdos manet, et unum toftum in quo Nigellus manet cum duabus acris terre quas <idem> tenet in Smalwyht. Et preterea confirmavi deo et eisdem pauperibus totam illam terram et pasturam quam habent ex concessione et donacione Fulconis patris mei, scilicet totum le Sumergang,

Cunungriding, Acumgate Hyrst, Ca---[74] hyrst, Hesylhyrst, secundum metas positas et sicut includuntur, et illud toftum in quo Thomas Tod manet, et totam illam terram quam habent ex concessione Iohannis avunculi mei in Doleker[75] et Zel[76] et Linthweit cum tofto quod fuit eiusdem Iohannis. Et pretered confirmavi eisdem pauperibus advocationem ecclesie de Rugford cum duabus bovatis terre, et cum toftis et croftis eidem ecclesie pertinentibus. In super concessi et confirmavi eisdem pauperibus omnes concessiones et donaciones eisdem a dicto Fulcone patre meo, Iohanne avunculo meo, Galfrido viro meo, et a me factas, de omnibus terris reddititibus possessionibus et quibuscumque tenementis sicut eas possederunt usque ad diem ascensionis domini anno gracie millesimi ducentesimi quinquagesimi septimi, habenda et tenenda omnia prescripta eisdem pauperibus et suis successoribus in lib(er)am puram et perpetuam elemosinam. Ego autem et heredes mei omnia prescripta eisdem pauperibus waran-tizabimus adquietabimus et defendemus in [f. 151ᵛ] omnibus et contra omnes homines in perpetuum. In huius autem rei robur et testimonium huic scripto sigillum meum apposui. Hiis testibus, domino Ricardo de Lutterington, domino Alano de Catherton, domino Thoma filio Willelmi de Merst(on), domino Iohanne de Reygate, Iohanne de Merston, Elya de Burel, Iohanne de Crancewyhc', Roberto le Frankeleyn de Acum, Olivero de eadem, Willelmo de Heshey, Gylone[77] de Ascham, Thoma fratre domini Petri de Knapeton, Ada de Ruford, Thoma de Bram, Michaele et multis aliis.

This may be the last occurrence of Sir Richard de Lutterington (Lotherton), who was one of twelve knights on a grand assize in January 1252 (*YF, 1246–1276*, p. 69n; see Wheater, *Sherburn and Cawood*, p. 127 for some notes on the family).

## [Sandbeck]

The papal confirmations of 1148, 1157 and 1173 include 'land of Sandbeck' (*Sandbec, Sambec, Sanbec*), but the donor is not named (C178–C180 [*EYC*, I, nos 179, 186, 197]). There is no evidence for a Sandbeck section anywhere in the cartulary. There are several habitations of that name in Yorkshire, but it is clear the hospital's interest lay in Sandbeck in Maltby, near Hooton Levitt. Sandbeck formed part of the 6½ k.f. held by Idonea de Vipont of the honour of Tickhill in the second quarter of the thirteenth century. She gave the manor of Sandbeck to Roche abbey in 1241 (*SY*, I, 272–73). The *Valor Ecclesiasticus* (1535) for Roche included a rent of 2s. *ballivio de Tikhill per annum hospitali sancti Leonardi Ebor' de terr(a) in Sandebek*. A rent in Sandbeck, listed amongst several in the southern part of the West Riding, was included in the account of 1542 (*Dissolved Houses*, IV, 225).

## [*Sandhala*]

The papal confirmation of 1148 includes 2 bv. in *Sandhala* (C178 [*EYC*, I, no. 179]). Long Sandall, in the Fossard fee, or possibly Kirk Sandall, a member of the honour of Warenne, seem the most likely places, as the entry appears between entries for lands in

---

[74] Illegible to Dodsworth, but probably *Kartegatehurst*, which was given by Fulk (R386, R731).
[75] Elsewhere *Scaleker* (R379).
[76] Elsewhere *Ekel*, *Ethzel* (R378–R379).
[77] sic.

Doncaster and lands in the neighbourhood of Tickhill. There was no Sandall section in the Rawlinson volume, and nothing further is known of the hospital's holding.

# [Saxton]

For Saxton, see R392–R407. Three folios (ff. 115–17), containing deeds numbered 17–38, have been removed from the Saxton section.

**R738.** Note stating that the mill [of Lead] was previously held by Hereward, by grant of the master of the hospital, and was thus called Hereward's mill.

NOTE: MS Dods. 120b, f. 16$^r$, from Rawl., f. 115$^v$, now missing, appended to an abstract of R257, contained in notes on the descendants of Ascelin de Day.

Hoc molendinum qui(dam) Herewardus p(rius) tenuit ex dimissione magistri hospitalis, a quo dictum erat molendinum Herewardi. Titulo de Saxton, fo. 115.b.

**R739.** Confirmation to the hospital by Pope Adrian [IV] of land in the fields of Saxton [1154 × 1159]

NOTED: MS Dods. 120b, f. 23$^r$, from Rawl., f. 117, now missing, no. 35, marginal note to an abstract of R392.

Adrianus papa confirm(avit) terram in campis de Saxton rectori[78] hosp(italis) imperpetuum. carta 35. fo. 117 Maidencastell.

The date range is given by the papacy of Adrian IV.

**R740.** Confirmation to the hospital by Roger son of Thomas Peitevin of the gifts in his fee in the territory of Saxton and Woodhouse made by his ancestors Roger Peitevin and Robert Peitevin. 27 June 1260.

COPY: MS Dods. 120b, f. 24$^r$, from Rawl., f. 115, now missing. CALENDAR: Wheater, *Sherburn and Cawood*, p. 137 [from MS Dods. 120b, via Jennyns and Tillotson, BL, Harley 795, f. 53]. NOTED: Baildon, 'Leathley', p. 36, from Harley 795.

Universis presens scriptum visuris vel audituris Rogerus filius Thome Pictaviensis salutem in domino. Noverit universitas vestra me confirmasse et ratificasse omnes donaciones quas Rogerus Pictaviensis et Robertus Pictaviensis antecessores mei dederunt et conc(esserunt) magistro et fratribus hospitalis sancti Leonardi Ebor' de omnibus terris quas habent de feodo meo in territorio de Saxtun et de Wodehuse. Teste, dominis Iohanne le Vavasor, Gilberto de Bernevale militibus, Willelmo rectore ecclesie de Rither, Rogero de Saxton. Dat' Ebor' 5 kal' iulii 1260. fo. 115.

**R741.** Grant to the hospital by William [recte Walter ?] son of Otes of Barkston of the tithes of his windmill next to Barkston in the fields of Saxton [1202 × 1214]

---

[78] MS unclear, apparently *rem'*.

MS Dods. 120b, f. 24ᵛ, from Rawl., f. 117, now missing. CALENDAR: Wheater, *Sherburn and Cawood*, p. 138 [from MS Dods. 120b via Jennyns and Tillotson].

Willelmus[79] filius Otonis de Barkeston dedit hospitali sancti Petri Ebor' decimas molendini mei ad ventum iuxta Barkeston in campis de Saxton. Testibus, S[imone] decano et capitulo Ebor', Rogero Pictaviensi, Rogero de Birkin, Hugone de Thouleston, Turstino et aliis fratribus eius, Roberto de Barkeston, Nicholao de Barkeston, Thoma de Langwath. fo. 117.

Simon de Apulia was dean between 1194 and 1214. Roger Peitevin succeeded his brother Robert in 1202 or afterwards. Roger and Robert were half-brothers to the grantor. Otes of Barkston was living in 1199; his son Walter was dead in 1218 (FN: Peitevin; *EYC*, VI, 111).

## [Stockeld, par. Spofforth]

For Stockeld, see R417–R427.

**R742.** Grant to the hospital by Maud de Percy, countess of Warwick, in widowhood, of common pasture for its beasts and the beasts of its men in Stockeld, in her 'hay' at the path from *Kirkeby* to *Holebec*, paying 12*d.* annually [1184 × 1204]

COPY: R743 (inspeximus, witnesses omitted). CALENDAR: *YD*, VI, no. 475.

Omnibus filiis sancte matris ecclesie Matild(is) de Perci comitissa de Warewic eternam in domino salutem. Noverit universitas vestra me caritatis intuitu pro salute anime mee et patris mei Willelmi de Perci et animabus omnium antecessorum et heredum nostrorum in viduali libertate mea dedisse et concessisse[80] et hac presenti carta mea confirmasse deo et hospitalis sancti Petri Ebor' in puram et perpetuam elemosinam communem pasturam omnibus bestiis suis et hominum suorum de Stokelde de haia mea quantum durat ipsa haya apud semitam que venit de Kirkeby et cadit in Holebec, et si ultra transeant sine custodia facta ne vexentur tam porcis quam aliis bestiis suis, ita quod prefatum hospitale persolvet inde mihi et heredibus meis annuatim duodecim denarios scilicet infra octabas sancti Martini. Hoc donum dedi eis tam libere honorifice et quiete sicut ulla elemosinam liberius dari potest ut ego et antecessores mei et heredes simus participes omnium orationum elemosinarum et aliorum beneficiorum qui fiunt vel facienda sunt in illa sancta domo dei. Et ego predicta Matildis et heredes mei warantizabimus prefatum donum predicto hospitali in perpetuum contra omnes homines in perpetuum. Hiis testibus etc.

The date is limited by the widowhood of Maud de Percy (*EYC*, XI, 5).

**R743.** Inspeximus by H[amo], dean, and the chapter of St Peter's York, of four Stockeld deeds in favour of the hospital [1217 × 1220]

---

[79] sic, probably a mistake for Walter. William son of Otes of Barkston does not otherwise occur.
[80] MS: *concessessisse*.

ORIGINAL: YAS, MD59/1/76/24, formerly MD59/21/Spofforth/1, 15–16 cm. (wide) × 39–40 cm., bottom turn-up, slit for seal tag, seal gone. No medieval endorsements. CALENDAR: *YD*, VI, no. 475.

Omnibus cristi fidelibus ad quos littere presentes pervenerint H[amo] decanus et capitulum sancti Petri Ebor' salutem. Noverit universitas vestra nos inspexisse cartas hospitalis sancti Petri Ebor' in hec verba: [*texts of R418, R420, R421, and R742 follow, in full, except witnesses omitted*]. In huius autem rei testimonium huic scriptum sigillum nostrum apposuimus. Valete.

The date range is the period for Hamo as dean.

**R744.**  Acknowledgement by Baldwin of Stockeld, as brother and heir of Richard of Stockeld, that he had received from the hospital the vill called Stockeld, and the land Richard his brother held in Deighton of the fee of William Trussebut. Richard held for ½*m.* annually; Baldwin would pay 10*s.* annually, and a third part of his chattels as an obituary payment [*c.*1214 × *c.*1230]

ORIGINAL: YAS, MD59/1/76/7, formerly MD59/1/Hospitals/15, 16 cm. (wide) × 9 cm., bottom turn-up, three slits for seal tag; seal, pink wax, round, 35 mm. diameter, a large bird walking to the dexter, + SIGILL . . . [NIG ?]ELLI, chipped. Medieval endorsement: *Baldewin' de Stockeld' de incremento veteris firme de Stockeld', scilicet de xl.d. et de tertia parte catallorum in obitu.* PRINTED: *EYC*, x, no. 45, where dated *c.*1208 × *c.*1225. CALENDAR: *YD*, IV, no. 489.

Omnibus presentes literas visuris vel audituris Baldewinus de Stockeld' salutem. Noveritis me tamquam fratrem et heredem Ricardi de Stockeld' suscepisse a magistro et fratribus hospitalis sancti Petri Ebor' totam villam que appellatur Stockeld' cum omnibus ad eandem villam pertinentibus infra villam et extra, et totam terram quam dictus frater meus tenuit in campis de Dichton' de feudo Willelmi Trussebot, quod quidem totum predictum tenementum sepedictus Ricardus frater meus de illis tenuit pro dimidia marca annua, tenendum scilicet et habendum totum predictum tenementum decetero mihi et heredibus meis libere integre et quiete de predictis magistro et fratribus in perpetuum, reddendo inde eis pro omni servicio ad illos pertinente decem solidos annuos, medietatem ad festum sancti Martini et medietatem ad Pentecost'. Et insuper ego et heredes mei terciam partem catallorum nos contingentem in obitu nostro pauperibus dicte domus caritative relinquimus. Hoc autem pro predicto tenemento accrementum veteris firme et catallorum portionem memoratis pauperibus de me et de heredibus meis in perpetuum concessi ut ego et heredes et antecessores et successores mei in fraternitatem dicte domus recipiamur et partem beneficiorum que in dicta domo dei fiunt vel in perpetuum facienda sunt consequamur. In huius autem rei robur et testimonium huic scripto sigillum meum apposui. Testibus, Anket(ino), Godefrido, Waltero hosp(italis), Iohanne, Rogero, Roberto, Ricardo, Stephano et aliis fratribus hospitalis, Radulfo de Fontibus, Willelmo fratre eius, Iohanne, capellanis, Roberto de Sgegness', magistro T[homa] de Langwath', Thoma fratre meo, Roberto de Stow', Rogero de Hunton', Waltero de Beningburg' et multis aliis.

Thomas de Langwath attested as master between *c.*1214 and *c.*1230. Richard of Stockeld was apparently dead in 1221 (FN), and it is unlikely this deed was issued many years afterwards.

**R745.** Notification by Baldwin of Stockeld that he is bound to the hospital to pay 20*s.* annually, and 8*s.* to the heirs of William Trussebut, for the vill of Stockeld, and the culture in the fee of William de Percy called *Crauwelflat*, and all the land which Nigel the grantor's father gave to the hospital in the fields of Deighton in the fee of William Trussebut; and also to pay a portion of chattels as an obituary payment [*c.*1214 × *c.*1230]

ORIGINAL: YAS, MD59/1/76/8, formerly MD59/1/Hospitals/16, 16 cm. (wide) × 8 cm., bottom turn-up, seal tag through three slits, seal gone. Medieval endorsement: *Baldewini de Stockeld' de xx.s. annuis hosp' solvendis et viii.s. annuatim solvendis heredibus Willelmi Trussebut pro toto tenemento suo.* PRINTED: *EYC*, X, no. 46, where dated 1208 × *c.*1225. CALENDAR: *YD*, IV, no. 490.

Sciant presentes et futuri quod ego Baldewinus de Stockeld et heredes mei tenemur dominis meis magistro et fratribus hospitalis sancti Petri Ebor' ad solutionem viginti solidorum annuorum, medietatis ad festum sancti Martini et medietatis ad Pentecost', et preterea ad solutionem octo solidorum annuorum pro eis faciendam ad eosdem terminos heredibus Willelmi Trussebut pro omni servicio ad predictos dominos meos pertinente de toto tenemento quod de illis teneo in feudo et hereditate, videlicet de tota villa de Stockeld' cum omnibus suis pertinentiis et de cultura de feudo Willelmi de Percy que appellatur Crauwelflat cum suis pertinentiis, et de tota terra quam Nigellus pater meus predicte domui dedit in campis de Dichton' que est de feudo Willelmi Trussebut. Et preterea ego et heredes mei in perpetuum porcionem catallorum in obitu nos contingentem predicte domus pauperibus pro animabus nostris et animabus antecessorum et successorum nostrorum fideliter relinquimus. Hec autem omnia predicta fideliter observanda pro me et pro heredibus meis tactis sacrosanctis iuravi affidavi et sigillo meo confirmavi. Test(ibus), Bernardo, Rogero, Iohanne, fratribus hospitalis capellanis, Radulfo de Fontibus, Radulfo de Gaitington', Willelmo de Notingh' capellanis secularibus, magistro Thoma de Langwath', Roberto de Stow', Waltero de Alredale, Waltero de Beningburg' et multis aliis.

In the same hand as R744, and of similar date.

**R746.** Receipt by Richard of Stockeld, knight, of 1*m.* lent by master Geoffrey of Aspall, to be repaid at the quindene of Easter 1285. Bristol, 24 December 1284.

ORIGINAL: YAS, MD59/1/76/11, formerly MD59/1/Hospitals/17, 15 cm. (wide) × 6 cm., 8 mm. tongue for seal, 4 mm. wrapping tie, ends cut, no trace of seal. Medieval endorsements: (?) *dnf'*; *Ric' de Stoch'.* CALENDAR: *YD*, IV, no. 493.

Omnibus cristi fidelibus ad quos presentes littere pervenerint Ricardus de Stockhild miles salutem in domino. Noveritis me recepisse de magistro Galfrido de Haspall' unam marcam argenti ex causa mutui de qua quidem marca me bene voco pacatum die confectionis presencium. Quam quidem marcam promitto per legitimam stipulationem solvere predicto magistro Galfrido vel suo certo nuncio a die pasche in quindecim dies anno regni regis Edwardi terciodecimo sine ulterior(i) dilacione. In cuius rei testimonium presenti scripto sigillum meum apposui. Dat' apud Bristall' in vigilia natalis domini anno regni domini regis Edwardi supradicto.

Aspall was master of the hospital from 1281 until 1287. The king was at Bristol when the receipt was given (*CalPat*, 1281–1292, p. 148).

**R747.** Surrender and quitclaim to his chief lords, the master and brethren of the hospital, by Richard of Stockeld knight of two tofts with 42½ a. arable land and a piece of meadow called *Horsheng*, of the grantor's demesne in Stockeld, without detriment to the rent of 28*s*. which the grantor paid annually for the manor. Licence of pasture and turbary, but no right of common in the grantor's park. If the hospital's animals were found in the park by the *wardfet*, then moderate amends were to be made, according to the view of honest and lawful men. The hospital was to be allowed sufficient fencing to renew that of their lands and tenements, the old fencing to be left to Richard. For the surrender the hospital released all claim to arrears of rent until 2 February 1298 [1298]

ORIGINAL: YAS, MD59/1/76/17, formerly MD59/1/Hospitals/22A, 26 cm. (wide) × 21 cm., stained, holed, bottom turn-up, slit for seal tag, seal gone. Medieval endorsement: *indentur' Ricardi de Stockeld de terra in Stockeld*. CALENDAR: *YD*, IV, no. 498.

Sciant presentes et futuri quod ego Ricardus de Stockeld miles concessi sursum reddidi et quiet' clamavi pro me et heredibus meis in perpetuum capitalibus dominis meis . . magistro hospitalis sancti Leonardi Ebor' et pauperibus eiusdem hospitalis ac etiam fratribus ibidem deo servientibus duo tofta que quondam Willelmus filius Hawisie et Annotus fil[ ][81] consueverunt una cum quatraginta duabus acris et dimid(ia) terre arabilis et una pecia prati que vocatur Horsheng' de dominicis meis in villa de Stockeld quarum quindecim acre et dimidia iacent in campo de Esckelriding' et quatuordecim acre in Le Morflat et decem acre et dimidii in Le Roberdriding' et due acre et dimidia in L[ ] iuxta Le Lideyhat et dicta pecia prati iacet iuxta Thwaytheng' ex parte australi, habend(a) et tenend(a) dictis magistro pauperibus ac fratribus predicti hospitalis ac eorum assignatis dicta tofta terram et pratum cum omnibus aisiamentis et communis ut in pratis pascuis pasturis turbariis et mariscis et cum omnibus aliis comoditatibus infra villa de Stockeld' et extra ad me pertinentibus libere quiete sine aliqua diminutione seu decremento viginti et octo solidorum annui redditus quos ego et successores mei tenemur solvere annuatim dicto hospitali pro manerio meo de Stockeld' prelibato, ita quod possint habere cuiuslibet generis animalia in predictis pasturis et communis ad libitam voluntatem suam et in turbaria predice ville fodere et asportare pro suo libito voluntatis sine admensuracione vel contradictione me[ ] autem magister pauperes et fratres et eorum assignati in parco meo nullam habebunt communam nec vendicare poterunt [ ] et cariando huic inde de terra ad terram. Et si contingat animalia dicti hospitali vel eorum assignatorum dicta tenementa [ ] libere sine aliqua lesione vel inpedimento vel dampni emendacione vel inparcamento mei vel heredum meorum benign' debent esse [ ] nisi forte per wardfet in dicto parco ad pascend' inveniantur et tunc iuxta visum proborum et legalium virorum secundum quantitatem debiti rationabile et moderata fieri debet emenda. Volo et concedo pro me et heredibus meis quod dicti magister pauperes ac fratres dicti hospitalis et eorum assignati habeant et percipiant in dicto parco meo rationabile competentem et sufficientem clausturam pro terris et tenementis superius nominatis, ita quod quocumque tempore predicta claustura renovata fuerit dicti magister pauperes et fratres et eorum assignati nichil inde poterunt assportare videlicet michi et heredibus meis inveterata claustura pl[ ] debet remanere salve quod clasura inveterata. Duo tofta memorata sine calumpnia mei vel heredum meorum cum contigerit ipsam renovari. Pro hac autem

---

[81]  There are several places where the text cannot be read.

[ ] clamatione dicti magister pauperes et fratres hospitalis antedicti michi remiserunt omnimoda debita et arreragia reddit(us) in quib[ ] usque ad festum purificationis virginis gloriose Marie anno regni regis Edwardi filii regis Henrici vicesimo
sexto, ita tamen quod [ ] ex nunc et in futurum teneamur solvere eisdem viginti et
octo solidis annuos superius nominatos pro manerio meo de Stockeld' antedicto. In
cuius rei testimonium parti huius scripti indentati penes hospitale remanenti sigillum
meum apposui et alteri[82] parti penes me residenti sigillum commune dicti hospitalis est
appensum. Hiis testibus, domino Willelmo de Ros de Ingmanthorp' seniore, domino
Willelmo filio eius militibus, domino Iohanne de Schardeborg' rectore ecclesie de
Spofforth', Thoma Gulias, Nicholao de Dichton', Mattheo de Stodfald', Hugone de
Bilton', Roberto de Ribbestan', Nigello de Wetherby et aliis.

**R748.** Notification by Richard of Stockeld, knight, that for default of the rent of 28s.
a year which he was bound to pay to the hospital for the manor of Stockeld,
the bailiffs of the hospital had made many distraints on his cattle, horses, oxen
and other livestock. He assigned four oxen, taken in distraint, to the hospital,
for one year's rent. York, 5 February 1298.

ORIGINAL: YAS, MD59/1/76/12, formerly MD59/1/Hospitals/20, 22 cm. (wide) ×
9 cm., bottom turn-up, slit for seal tag; seal fragments of light brown wax. No medieval endorsements. CALENDAR: *YD*, IV, no. 494.

Universis sancte matris ecclesie filiis presentes litteras inspecturis Ricardus de Stockeld'
miles salutem in omnium salvatore. Noverit universitas vestra quod cum pro detentione redditus viginti et octo solidorum annuorum quos capitalibus dominis meis
magistro pauperibus ac fratribus hospitalis sancti Leonardi Ebor' teneor solvere pro
manerio meo de Stockeld', per captionem et detentionem averiorum meorum ac
equorum boum et aliorum animalium frequenter rationabiles super me per ballivos
dicti hospitalis facere fuiessent districtiones. Demum in allocatione viginti et octo
solidorum pro firma unius anni debitorum quatuor boves pro quandam districtione
facta captos assignavi et sponte liberavi eisdem. De qua quidem assignatione et boum
liberatione bene me voco contentum ipsos que magistrum pauperes et fratres de dicta
captione et detentione boum quietos pro me et heredibus meis clamo imperpetuum.
In cuius rei testimonium presenti scripto sigillum meum apposui. Dat' apud Ebor'
die mercurii prox' post festum purificationis beate Marie anno regni regis Edwardi
filii regis Henrici vicesimo sexto.

**R749.** Conveyance to the hospital by Richard of Stockeld, knight, of a piece of his
meadow in Stockeld, called *Thwaiteng*, with free passage for carts and livestock throughout the year. The hospital would pay 100s. yearly. Richard had
received twenty years' rent beforehand, so the hospital was quit of the rent
for the next twenty years. 5 February 1298.

ORIGINAL: YAS, MD59/1/76/13, formerly MD59/1/Hospitals/18, 25 cm. (wide) ×
8 cm., bottom turn-up, slit for seal tag; seal, vessica, brown wax, 35 mm. (wide) ×
45 mm., a fleur-de-lis, S . RICARDI . D' . STO. . .D. Medieval endorsement: *Carta Ricardi
de Stockeld de una pecia prati in Stockeld*. CALENDAR: *YD*, IV, no. 495.

[82] sic.

Sciant presentes et futuri quod ego Ricardus de Stockeld' miles dedi concessi et hac presenti carta mea confirmavi magistro pauperibus hospitalis sancti Leonardi Ebor' ac fratribus eiusdem hospitalis ibidem deo servientibus unam peciam prati mei in villa de Stockeld' que vocatur Thwaiteng', habendam et tenendam eisdem magistro pauperibus ac fratribus eiusdem hospitalis predictam peciam prati cum libera via ad cariand(um) et fugand(um) carectas et animalia per totum annum cum omnibus aliis pertinenciis et aisiamentis ad dictum pratum pertinentibus libere quiete bene in pace et imperpetuum hereditarie, reddendo inde annuatim michi et heredibus meis vel meis assignatis centum solidos argenti tantum die sancti Michaelis pro omnibus secularibus serviciis et demandis. Et ego predictus Ricardus et heredes mei predictum pratum prefatis magistro pauperibus ac fratribus dicti hospitalis contra omnes gentes warentizabimus acquietabimus et in perpetuum defendemus. Et sciendum est quod ego dictus Ricardus recepi premanibus de predictis magistro pauperibus et fratribus dicti hospitalis totum redditum annuum predictorum centum solidorum de viginti annis. Ita quod quieti erunt de solutione dicti redditus per predictum terminum viginti annorum proximorum et plenarie completorum. In cuius rei testimonium huic carte sigillum meum apposui. Hiis testibus, domino Willelmo de Ros de Ingmanthorp iuniore milite, Thoma Guliaas, Nicholao de Dihton', Matheo de Stodfald', Hugone de Bilton', Roberto de Ribbestayn, Nigello de Wehebi et aliis. Dat' apud Ebor' die mercurii in festo sancte Agath' virginis anno regni regis Edwardi filii regis Henrici vicesimo sexto.

**R750.** Agreement between Richard of Stockeld, knight, and the hospital. Richard had enfeoffed the hospital with a piece of meadow in the vill of Stockeld called *Thwaitheng*, for 100s. annual rent which the hospital had paid for twenty years in advance, so was quit for twenty years from the date of the agreement. If the hospital kept the land beyond the term, it would pay yearly 100s. If the hospital surrendered the land to Richard at the end of the term, or at another time, he would have no further right in the rent. 14 February 1298.

ORIGINAL: YAS, MD59/1/76/16, formerly MD59/1/Hospitals/19, 25 cm. (wide) × 15 cm., bottom turn-up, slit for seal tag, seal gone. Medieval endorsement: *Stokelle*. NOTED: *YD*, IV, no. 495n.

Die sancti Valentini martir' anno regni regis Edwardi filii regis Henrici vicesimo sexto convenit inter dominum Ricardum de Stockeld militem ex parte una et magistrum et pauperes hospitalis sancti L[e]onardi Ebor' ac fratres ibidem deo servientes ex altera, videlicet quod cum dictus dominus Ricardus feofasset dictos magistrum pauperes et fratres de una pecia prati in villa de Stockeld' que vocatur Thwaitheng' pro centum solidis argenti dicto domino Ricardo heredibus suis et assignatis annuatim in festo sancti Michaelis solvend(is), quem redditum centum solidorum annuorum dicti magister pauperes et fratres dicti hospitalis pro predicto prato prefato domino Ricardo pro viginti annis premanibus solverunt, ita tamen quod de dicta solutione centum solidorum annuorum erunt quieti per predictos viginti annos proximos et plenarie completos post confectionem presentium. Et quod dictus Ricardus nec heredes sui vel assignati aliquem redditum pro predicto prato de prefatis magistro pauperibus ac fratribus dicti hospitalis ante finem predictorum viginti annorum nec pro predictis viginti annis exigere poterunt vel vendicare. Si vero dicti magister pauperes et fratres hospitalis antedicti ultra terminum viginti annorum detinuerint pratum memoratum tunc dicto domino Ricardo heredibus seu assignatis suis quolibet anno dabunt centum solidos prout carta super hos confecta plenius inde testatur. Et dictus dominus

Ricardus concessit pro se heredibus suis et assignatis quod si dicti magister pauperes et fratres dicti hospitalis in fine viginti annorum predictorum vel quoquo alio tempore dictum pratum reliquerint seu eidem domino Ricardo vel heredibus suis illud reddiderint quod ipse dominus Ricardus nec heredes sui nec aliquis nomine eorundem de predictis magistro pauperibus ac fratribus dicti hospitalis de predicto redditu centum solidorum de predicto prato ex tunc aliquid exigere poterunt vel vendicare. In cuius rei testimonium parti huius scripti ad modum cirographi confecti penes dictos magistrum pauperes et fratres remanenti dictus dominus Ricardus sigillum suum apposuit et alteri[83] parti penes eiusdem dominum Ricardum residenti sigillum commune dicti hospitalis est appensum. Hiis testibus, domino Willelmo de Ros de Ingemanthorp' iuniore milite, Thoma Gulias, Nicholao de Dighton', Matheo de Stodfald, Hugone de Bilton', Roberto de Ribbestayn', Nigello de Werherby et aliis. Dat' apud Ebor' die et anno supradictis.

**R751.** Number not used.

**R752.** Agreement (in the form of a tripartite indenture between the parties and William de Bemys) between the hospital and Sir Richard of Stockeld, knight, whereby Richard quitclaimed to the hospital a rent of 100s. annually from a piece of meadow called *Thweytengg* in the vill of Stockeld. The quitclaim was placed in the indifferent keeping of William de Beumys by consent of both parties. If Richard paid 60s. to William next Michaelmas, the quitclaim was to be returned to him. If not, the hospital would pay William 10m., for Richard, and William would give the quitclaim to the warden (*gardiano*) of the hospital; and because part of a certain indenture remains in the hands of Sir Richard concerning payment of the 100s. after a term of twenty years, it will be surrendered to the hospital or William and will be void. 23 February 1298.

ORIGINAL: YAS, MD59/1/76/15, formerly MD59/1/Hospitals/22, 32 cm (wide) × 11 cm., bottom turn-up, slits for two seal tags, seals gone. Medieval endorsement: *Indentura facta inter magistrum hospitalis sancti Leonardi et fratres huiusdem loci et dominum Ricardum Stokkeld' militem.* CALENDAR: YD, IV, no. 497, imperfect.

Anno regni regis Edwardi vicesimo sexto septimo kalend' marcii convenit inter magistrum hospitalis sancti Leonardi Ebor' et fratres eiusdem hospitalis ex una parte et dominum Ricardum de Stockeld' militem ex alia parte, quod predictus Ricardus remisit et quietumclamavit pro se et heredibus suis dictis magistro et fratribus centum solidos annuum redditus in quibus iidem sibi tenebantur annuatim pro quadam pecia prati que vocatur Thweytengg' in predicta villa de Stockild'. Et dictum scriptum quieteclamancie dicti redditus traditum fuit in equali manu Willelmo de Beumys ex utriusque partis assensu. Ita quod si dictus Ricardus vel heredes sui vel aliquis attornatus eorundem partem istius scripti indentati sigillo communi dicti hospitalis et sigillo dicti Willelmi signat(am) dicto Willelmo de Beumys ad festum sancti Michaelis proxim' post confectionem presentium solverint sexaginta solidos quod dictum scriptum quieteclamancie de predictis centum solidis dictis domino Ricardo vel heredibus suis aut attornato suo partem istius scripti deferenti retradatur sine contradictione vel calumpnia dictorum magistri et fratrum hospitalis memorati. Et si

[83] sic.

dictus Ricardus vel heredes sui vel attornatus suus predictos sexaginta solidos predicto Willelmo ad prenominatum festum sancti Michaelis non solverint, dicti magister et fratres solvant dicto Willelmo de Beumys decem marcas ad solvend(um) dicto Ricardo vel heredibus eiusdem Ricardi et reddet dictum scriptum quieteclam(ancie) de predictis centum solidis gardiano dicti hospitalis sine contradictione vel calumpnia dicti domini Ricardi heredum suorum aut alicuius nomine eorundem. Et quod pars cuiusdam scripti indentati penes dictum dominum Ricardum remanens de solutione predictorum centum solidorum annuatim pro predicto prato solvendorum predicto domino Ricardo et heredibus suis post terminum viginti annorum in eodem scripto contentorum gardiano dicti hospitalis vel Willelmo de Beumys retradatur et ex tunc pro nullo habeatur et viribus suis careat omnino. In cuius rei testimonium parti huius scripti penes dictum dominum Ricardum rem(anenti) sigillum commune dicti hospitalis una cum sigillo dicti Willelmi de Beumys est appensum, et alteri parti penes gardianum dicti hospitalis rem(anenti) sigilla dictorum domini Ricardi et Willelmi sunt appensa et tercie parti penes dictum Willelmum de Beumys rem(anenti) sigillum commune dicti hospitalis una cum sigillo dicti domini Ricardi est appensum. Hiis testibus, Ricardo Oysel', Thoma Guliaas, Iohanne Lunge Speye, Iohanne filio suo, Nicholao de Dihton', Matheo de Stodfald', Roberto Broun de Ribbestayn et aliis. Dat' apud Ebor' die et anno supradictis.

In view of Beumys' long association with the hospital[84] it is surprising to find him acting in a supposedly independent capacity.

**R753.** Surrender to his chief lords, the master and brethren of the hospital, by Ralph son of Richard of Stockeld, of 3 a. arable land in the field of Stockeld in *Guteringkeldflat*, between the land of the hospital and the land of the grantor [*c.*1298 × *c.*1301]

ORIGINAL: YAS, MD59/1/76/18, formerly MD59/1/Hospitals/23; 21 cm. (wide) × 11 cm., bottom turn-up, slit for missing seal tag. Medieval endorsements: (in the deed hand) *Carta Radulphi filii Ricardi de Stockeld de tribus acris terre in campo de eodem*; another very faded endorsement. CALENDAR: *YD*, IV, no. 499.

Sciant presentes et futuri quod ego Radulphus filius Ricardi de Stockeld concessi sursum reddidi et quietum clamavi pro me et heredibus meis imperpetuum capitalibus dominis meis magistro hospitalis sancti Leonardi Ebor' et pauperibus eiusdem hospitalis ac etiam fratribus ibidem deo servientibus tres acras terre arabilis in campo de Stockeld sicut iacent in Guteringkeldflat', videlicet inter terram dicti hospitalis ex una parte et terram meam ex parte altera, tenend(as) et habend(as) predictis magistro fratribus ac pauperibus eiusdem hospitalis in puram et perpetuam elemosinam cum omnibus suis pertinenciis aisiamentis et libertatibus suis infra villam et extra libere integre et quiete ab omni servicio et exactione, sicut aliqua elemosina liberius et melius teneri et haberi potest. Ego autem predictus Radulphus et heredes mei predictas tres acras terre cum omnibus suis pertinenciis sine aliquo retenemento prefatis magistro fratribus ac pauperibus warantizabimus acquietabimus et defendemus in omnibus et contra omnes gentes in perpetuum exept(a) comunia in parco meo. In cuius rei testimonium presenti carte sigillum meum apposui. Hiis testibus, domino Willelmo de Ros milite, domino Iohanne de Scartheborg' rectore ecclesie de Spofford', Thoma

---

[84] Beumys frequently attested the hospital's deeds. He occurs as the master's steward in *c.*1263 × *c.*1276 (R512), and was named amongst the employees of the hospital in 1295 (Benson, *St Leonard's*, p. 15).

Gillias, Nicholao de Dichton', Matheo de Stodfald', Hugone de Bilton', Nigello de Wetherby et aliis.

R747 and R749, issued *c.* 2 February 1298 and 5 February 1298, have very similar witness lists, but this deed may have been issued after the settlement made by Richard of Stockeld in October 1298 (FN).

**R754.** Surrender to his chief lords, the master and brethren of the hospital of St Leonard, York, by Ralph son of Richard de Stockild, of a messuage and 2 bv. land in Stockild, which Robert le Grayve formerly held of Richard the grantor's father in diverse places in the vill and territory of Stockild, paying a rose yearly at the feast of the nativity of St John the baptist for the first twenty years starting at Pentecost 1301 for all secular service, and afterwards £10 yearly at the feasts of St Martin and Pentecost by equal portions. Also grant of common pasture for ten oxen and two horses each year in the grantor's wood of Stockild called Le Parke. Right to cut underwood in the grantor's park sufficient for the messuage and to enclose the curtilage. The grantor would not have more than thirty oxen and horses in the said wood, saving to John de Scartheborg parson of the church of Spofforth common pasture for ten oxen and two horses. Licence for the hospital to impound animals beyond that number, saving strays (*eschapio*) in the wood to Ralph. Warranty. Alternate seals [1301]

ORIGINALS: *a1, a2* YAS, MD59/1/76/19–20 (indenture and counterpart), formerly MD59/1/Hospitals/24, no textual variations, both 22 cm. (wide) × 23 cm., bottom turn-up, slits for seal tag, *a1* retains seal, red wax, circular, impression 18 mm. diameter, a shield with three eagles displayed, s' RADULFI DE STOCHELD. *a1* endorsed (med.): *indentura Radulfi filii Ricardi de uno mesuagio et ii. bovatis terre in Stockeld*; *a2* endorsed (med.): *Stockeld*. CALENDAR: *YD*, IV, no. 500, imperfect.

Hiis testibus, domino Roberto de Plumton', domino Henrico de Hertlington', Rogero de Linton', Thoma Chaunberlayn de eadem, Roberto filio Ricardi de eadem, Nigello de Whetherby et Matheo de Braham et aliis.

**R755.** Indenture witnessing that whereas Ralph de Stokkyld had been bound to Gilbert de Houson, deceased, in £19 12*s.*, by recognizance made before the mayor of York and Robert de Sexdecim Vallibus, king's clerk, appointed for the recognizance of debts at York; the executors of Gilbert, as the debt had not been paid, took seisin of all lands and tenements which Ralph held in the vill of Stokkyld, according to the form of the king's statute, as more fully contained in the king's writ. At the request of Ralph, and so he might be more quickly freed from the debt, the executors sold the lands to the master and brethren of the hospital of St Leonard, York, to hold until the debt was satisfied according to the form of the statute and as extended by the king's writ. Afterwards the hospital and Ralph agreed that the hospital would hold the manor of Stokkyld, without any retention by Ralph, from 11 November 1301 [*a festo sancti Martini in hyeme anno regni regis E. xxix$^{mo}$*] for four years. The hospital would then surrender the statute made to Gilbert, and seisin of the manor, saving the lands which it held before in the manor. Alternate seals. No witnesses [November 1301]

ORIGINAL: YAS, MD59/1/76/42, formerly MD59/20/Stockeld/14, 20 cm. (wide) ×
17 cm., bottom turn-up, slit for seal tag; seal, oval, red wax, 18 mm. (wide) × 22 mm., a
shield, three eagles displayed, s' RADULFI D' S. . . . No medieval endorsements. CALENDAR:
YD, v, no. 423.

The extent mentioned in the deed is dated 5 November 1301 (R426).

**R756.** Agreement between the master and brethren of the hospital of St Leonard,
York, and Sir Thomas, son and heir of Sir Peter de Midelton, knight. There had
been discord between the parties concerning certain services and demands
made by the hospital on Sir Thomas for the manor of Stokeld, and it was
agreed as follows. Sir Thomas recognised he and his ancestors held of the
hospital as their chief lords, for 28s. paid annually at Pentecost and St Martin
in winter by equal portions, and agreed to pay 28s. for the terms of Pentecost
and St Martin last past for all arrears. The hospital released to Sir Thomas all
other arrears to the date of the agreement. The hospital granted that Thomas
and his heirs should hold the manor at the service of 28s., and also all other
lands and tenements of the hospital in the vill of Stokhild, namely two tofts,
2 bv., 45½ a. land, 10 a. 1 r. meadow; and also all lands and tenements of
the hospital in Midelton in Whervedale, namely three messuages, seven tofts,
6 bv. 22 a. land, 4 a. meadow, 19 a. waste, and an assart called Arnald Riddyng,
for a term of twenty-four years from the date of the agreement, paying 7m. at
the terms of Pentecost and St Martin in winter, that is 28s. for the said manor
and then 65s. 4d. additional to make up the 7m. If Thomas died within the
term, an obituary payment of 40s. as the portion of chattels would be made.
Right of entry to distrain if the rent or obituary payment were in arrear for a
month. Warranty. Alternate seals. In the hospital's chapter, York, 14 November
1358. No witnesses.

ORIGINAL: YAS, MD59/1/76/23, formerly MD59/1/Hospitals/27; 34 cm. (wide) ×
17 cm., slot for seal tag; seal dark brown wax, circular, diameter 23 mm., a shield,
fretty a canton (Middleton), within a decorated border, legend indistinct. Medieval
endorsement: *Stokeld et Middelton.* CALENDAR: YD, IV, no. 504.

Dat' apud Ebor' in capitulo predicti hospitalis quartodecimo die mensis novembris
anno domini millesimo trescentesimo quinquagessimo octavo et regni regis Edwardi
tertii post conquestum Anglie tricesimo secundo.

## *Shipton*[85] [Skipton]

The appearance of the following deed in the West Riding rather than the Craven
division of the cartulary shows that *Schiptune* was not correctly identified by the
cartularist. The heading of f. 126 was *Shipton*. There is no indication of a Skipton
section in the Missing volume. A rent in Skipton was noticed in 1542 (*Dissolved
Houses*, IV, 225), and an appurtenance in Skipton belonging to the manor of Nappa,
formerly held by the hospital, was mentioned when Nappa was sold by the Crown
in 1544 (*LPFD*, XIX (1), no. 80.23), but there is no further evidence for the hospital's

[85] MS Dods. 120b: *Skypton.*

holding. The location of the property given by William, nephew of the king, is not described in Dodsworth's abstract, and may have been assumed from the place-date.

**R757.** Gift to the hospital by William, nephew of the king, of a messuage with the toft belonging to it [1135 × 1154, probably 1151 × 1154]

COPY: MS Dods. 120b, f. 27ᵛ, from Rawl., f. 126, now missing.

Willelmus nepos regis omnibus probis hominibus totius terre sue francis et anglis clericis et laicis salutem. Sciatis me dedisse et imperpetuum concessisse in puram et perpetuam elemosinam unam mansuram cum tofto pertin(enti) solutam et quietam ab omnibus servitiis hospitali de Ebor', pro remissione peccatorum meorum et uxoris mee et antecessorum meorum. Test', Ada' fil' Sueni et Adelis de Rumeli et Willelmo Flandrensi et Galtero de Vianes, Eduard' dispensator et Druilloni magistri et Galteri clerici,[86] qui hanc cartam conscripsit et multis aliis. Et hoc in burgo de Schiptune. Valete. fo. 126.

William 'nephew of the king', was son of Duncan II, king of Scotland in 1094, and nephew to Duncan's half brothers Alexander I (reigned 1107–1124) and David I (reigned 1124–1153). The second witness was Alice de Rumilly, William's wife, through whom he acquired the honour of Skipton. They were married probably in 1135 × 1138, and William died probably 1152 × 1154. Clay doubted whether William could have taken part in transactions concerning the honour of Skipton between 1138 and 1151, and indeed it is possible that he acquired the honour only after the death of his mother-in-law Cecily de Rumilly, who may have been living as late as 1151. According to John of Hexham, William was confirmed in the honour of Skipton by King David in 1151, and destroyed a small castle set up by his enemies (*EYC*, VII, 10–11, 58–59).

## *Towton* [par. Saxton]

According to the Contents List, Towton deeds were copied on ff. 127–28. For Towton, which was held of Lacy by Peitevin, and which passed to the Stopham family with other Peitevin property in the second half of the thirteenth century, see FN: Peitevin of Altofts; Wheater, *Sherburn and Cawood*, pp. 149–53. Towton is not mentioned in the extents and rentals of the later thirteenth century, the *Valor Ecclesiasticus*, nor the account of 1542, presumably because the property acquired by these deeds was subsumed into the grange of Lead.

**R758.** Confirmation by Roger Peitevin to God, and the mother church of Saxton, and the master and brethren of the hospital, of the homage and service of William son of John of Towton and his heirs, from all land, meadow and tenements with the capital messuage, and whatever rights may come to the grantor and his heirs from William and his heirs, in the vill of Towton [1263 × 1274]

COPY: MS Dods. 120b, f. 28ʳ, from Rawl., f. 127, now missing.

---

[86] Witness names sic, in genitive and ablative, probably reflecting a genitive witness list in the original.

Sciant presentes et futuri quod ego Rogerus <le> Paytevyn dedi c(oncessi) et hac presenti carta mea con(firmavi) deo et matrici ecclesie de Saxton magistro et fratribus sancti Leonardi Ebor' homagium et servitium Willelmi filii Iohannis de Toueton et heredum suorum de tota terra et prato et cum omnibus terris et ten(ementis) cum capitali messuagio et quidquid michi vel heredibus meis iure hereditario predictis Willelmo et heredibus suis de predicta terra et prato accidere poterit sine aliquo retenemento in villa de Touetona. Testibus, Iohanne le Vavasur, Radulfo de Norman-vill', Rogero de Ryvill', Thoma de Barkeston etc. fo. 127.

This deed is associated with the gift made in R759, and so must have been made in or after 1263. As it is not a quitclaim, it is probable that the date is before 1274, when Roger Peitevin was in prison and was 'former lord' (FN). In 1279 William son of John of Towton called John of Towton to warrant a messuage and 1 ct., less 1½ bv., of land in Cocksford [in Lead], and in 1285 made a fine whereby he sold a messuage, 104 a. land, 3 a. of meadow, and 4s. rents in Cocksford and Hazlewood to William Vavasour and Nicola his wife (YF, 1272–1300, pp. 21, 75). Ralph son of John of Towton, rector of Sproatley, and his brother William occur in several deeds in the Nostell cartulary, of similar date to the present deed, concerning land in Oglethorpe ('Ctl. Nostell', nos 1177–83).

**R759.** Gift by William son of John of Towton, to God and Blessed Mary and the chapel of St James of Towton, of lands in Towton, being 1 bv. with the principal messuage and 8 a. demesne with other plots, towards the sustenance of a chaplain celebrating daily for the soul of Ralph, the donor's brother [1263 × 1276]

ABSTRACT: MS Dods. 120b, f. 28ʳ, from Rawl., f. 128, now missing.

*De sustentatione unius capellani[87] in capella de Toueton.*
Willelmus filius Iohannis de Toueton dedit deo et beate Marie et capelle sancti Iacobi de Toueton ad sustentacionem unius capellani qui ibidem diatim celebrabit imper-petuum pro anima Radulfi fratris sui etc. omnes terras subscriptas in territorio de Toueton, videlicet unam bovatam terre cum <principali>[88] messuagio in Thoueton et 8 acras terre de dominico cum diversis aliis parcellis. Testibus, Thoma tunc magistro hospitalis sancti Leonardi, Iohanne le Vavasur, Willelmo filio eius, Willelmo filio Willelmi[89] de Rye, Iohanne filio Iohannis de Lede, Thoma de Grimeston, Thoma de Barkeston, Willelmo de Wodehuse', Ricardo de Malesouer de Kokesford. fo. 128.

The date range is indicated by the attestation of Thomas, master of the hospital. The deed shows that there was a chapel at Towton almost two hundred years before the battle of 1461. Richard III's ill-fated project to build a memorial chapel at Towton is well documented. Three quarters of a century after the battle Leland noted 'Towton village is a mile from Saxton, where is a great chapel begun by Richard III, but not finished. Sir John Multon's father laid the first stone of it.' Elsewhere Leland mentions 'a chapel or hermitage upon Towton field in token of prayer and memory of men slain there' (Leland, *Itinerary*, I, 43; ibid., IV, 77). A warrant to the receiver of Pontefract

[87] MS: *cappli'*.
[88] *capitale* corrected to *principali*.
[89] MS: *Willelmo*.

to pay £40 towards the chapel dates probably from October 1484 (*Cat. Harleian*, I, 263, no. 344). In 1486 an indulgence of forty days, for two years, was issued to assist the building of a chapel in the midst of fields where many killed in the battle were buried. In 1502 the indulgence was renewed to support the 'newly built' chapel (Raine, *Fabric Rolls*, pp. 241–42). The original chapel was presumably a dependency of Saxton church, which belonged to the hospital.

## *Trunfleet* [Trumfleet, near Thorpe in Balne]

For Trumfleet, see *SY*, I, 207–08. The Contents List's reference to f. 129, now missing, is apparently the only notice of the hospital's holdings in Trumfleet.

## *Touleston* [Toulston, par. Newton Kyme]

According to the Contents List, Toulston deeds were copied at f. 129, now missing. The following deed provides the only known evidence for the hospital's interest there. In 1086 the Arches fee included slightly less than 11 ct. in Newton [Kyme], Toulston, and Oglethorpe, and a further 3 ct. in Toulston were soke of the Fossard manor of Bramham. 1 ct. in Toulston which had belonged to William Malet was within the boundary of Ilbert [de Lacy's] land. In the early twelfth century Fulk [the steward] gave 2 ct. of the Arches fee in Toulston to Whitby Abbey (*EYC*, I, nos 529–32). Peter of Toulston gave a rent of 3s. in Toulston, and [his brother] Thomas son of Robert of Toulston gave a toft in Toulston to Pontefract Priory in the later part of the twelfth century. Farrer printed Peter's deed in his section on the Fossard fee; but assigned Thomas' deed to the Lacy fee, on the grounds that it was witnessed by three of Lacy's knights (*EYC*, II, no. 1040; ibid., III, 1612). Nevertheless it is possible that Peter of Toulston held of Arches in Toulston (FN: Toulston). The inquisition following the death of William de Kyme [whose ancestors had succeeded to the steward's fee][90] in 1260 establised that William of Elkington (Lincs.)[91] held 1½ ct. in Toulston, Thomas of Catterton held 1 ct. and Healaugh Priory held ½ ct. of William of Catterton (*YI*, I, 86). In 1284–85 Philip de Kyme had 2½ ct. in Toulston, where 14 ct. made a fee. The lords of the vill in 1316 were Simon de Kyme and the prior of [Healaugh] Park (*KI*, pp. 50, 345). William son of Alan of Catterton had sold Healaugh 6 bv. in Toulston, apparently of the Kyme fee, noting in his deed that 6 bv. were reckoned as 1 ct. in the vill (*EYC*, I, no. 533; *Ctl. Healaugh*, pp. 42, 45).[92]

**R760.** Gift to the hospital by Hugh son of Peter of Toulston of 1½ bv. with a toft and croft in Toulston [1192 × 1226]

ABSTRACT: MS Dods. 120b, f. 28ʳ, from Rawl., f. 129, now missing.

Hugo filius Petri de Touleston dedit hospitali beati Petri Ebor' unam bovatam terre

90  FN: Catterton.
91  Where the Kyme family had interests (*EYC*, XI, 89–91).
92  For the suggested date of *c.*1225 × 1254 see FN: Catterton.

et dimidiam cum tofto et crofto in Touleston etc., ut[93] ego et heredes mei simus participes omnium beneficiorum que fiunt vel facienda sunt in predicta sancta domo dei. fo. 129.

The date range is the period for Hugh of Toulston (FN).

## Thorp in Balne

For Thorpe in Balne, which was held by Otes de Tilly, and subsequently by the Neufmarché family, of Vavasour, see *SY*, I, 217–19; *EYC*, VIII, 145n; *CalInqPM*, x, no. 25. The Contents List gives f. 130, now missing, for Thorpe in Balne, but nothing is known of the hospital's holdings there.

## Tadcaster

The Contents List gives f. 130, now missing, for Tadcaster, which was in the Percy fee. Nothing is known of the hospital's holdings.

## Tykehill' [Tickhill, WR and Notts.]

According to the Contents List, Tickhill deeds were copied on f. 131, now missing. For Tickhill, the *caput* of the honour of Tickhill, held in 1086 by Roger de Busli, and Stainton 3 m. to the west, which was a member of the honour, see *SY*, I, 220–247, 255–60; *Ctl. Blyth*, pp. cxv–cxl. Little is known of the hospital's holdings in Tickhill. King Stephen granted the tithes of toll and of the mill of Tickhill to the hospital (C1 [*Regesta*, III, no. 994]). A dwelling in Tickhill was confirmed to the hospital by Adrian IV in 1157 (C179 [*EYC*, I, no. 186]), but does not appear in the confirmations of 1148 or 1173. It is not clear that the gift of Hugh de Drincourt, probably made *c.*1154, contained property in Tickhill (R761). Walter Clarel's gift of a toft with buildings in Tickhill (R762) was probably made after the confirmation of 1157. Tickhill does not appear in the extents of the later thirteenth century, the *Valor Ecclesiasticus*, or the account of 1542.

Walter CLAREL was a member of a prominent Tickhill family, but his relationship to the first witness to his gift, Ralph Clarel, is not known. Ralph's son John, another witness, does not otherwise occur. Ralph Clarel, who also attested Hugh de Drincourt's gift to the hospital (R761), was named as a serjeant of Tickhill castle in 1180, and in 1185 was summoned by Gilbert de Arches to warrant his land, of which he had been discharged in the court at Tickhill (*PR*, 26 Hen. II, p. 76; ibid., 31 Hen. II, p. 75). Ralph Clarel and William his son witnessed a Wadworth deed of the later twelfth century (*EYC*, II, no. 1011). It is likely that Ralph was dead in 1196, when William Clarel and Geoffrey son of Edric assessed the account for renovations at Tickhill castle (*ChancR*, 8 Ric. I, p. 274). William had probably inherited his father's role as serjeant of the castle, and his tenure of the office shows he was not amongst

---

93  MS: *et.*

the Tickhill tenants who had joined the rebellion of the count of Mortain. William Clarel attested deeds of William Barbot and John de Busli to the Hospitallers in *c*.1190 × 1200[94] (MS Dods. 8, f. 212ʳ).

Three generations of the Clarel family are shown by the plea between Geoffrey Clarel and Robert son of Pain [of Wilsic] in 1200, concerning 6 bv. in Tickhill. The plea referred to a previous case in the court of Tickhill, in which Robert son of Pain had sued William, father of Geoffrey Clarel, for the land. In that case, it was said, William had claimed his father Ralph had the land from Jordan, Robert's older brother, in marriage with Sybil sister of Jordan (FN: Wilsic; *CRR*, I, 296). In 1204 Geoffrey Clarel owed ½*m*. in Yorkshire for a writ concerning 5 bv. in *Rutepel* (*PR*, 6 John, p. 189), and in 1218–19 there was an assize of mort d'ancestor to determine whether William Clarel, father of Geoffrey Clarel, had been seised in demesne as of fee of 40 a. land and 4½ a. meadow in Tickhill on the day he died. It was stated that the land was in the fee of Gilbert de Arches, who had been disseised by King Richard because he was in rebellion at the castle of Tickhill with the count of Mortain. The king gave the land to the bailiff of Tickhill, who gave it to William Clarel. But afterwards Gilbert de Arches made his peace with the king, and his lands were restored, and his heirs granted the land to two tenants. After the hearing Geoffrey quitclaimed a moiety of the lands to one of the tenants, Thorald son of Wulfoth, for 2½*m*., but there is no record of an agreement with the other tenant, who had taken the cross and was in the land of Jerusalem (*Yorkshire Eyre Rolls*, nos 15, 36; *YF*, 1218–1231, p. 22). Geoffrey Clarel of Tickhill was a pledge for ½*m*. for Adam de Deneby in 1218–19 (*Yorkshire Eyre Rolls*, no. 473). Described similarly he sold a toft in Lindrick (in Tickhill) to Ailwin son of Robert of Tickhill at an uncertain date, by a deed witnessed by John Clarel, clerk (A2A: DD/FJ/1/282/7).[95] He attested a deed made to Alice, countess of Eu, in 1219 × 1229[96] (MS Dods. 8, f.316ᵛ). Geoffrey Clarel attorned William Clarel against Andrew de Wydrington and Alice his wife, tenants, concerning 1 ct. land in Misson (Notts.) in 1235 (*CloseR*, 1234–1237, p. 176).[97]

Proof of the next step in the descent is elusive. John Clarel, son of Geoffrey Clarel of Tickhill, purchased a plot of 1 a. in Tickhill by a deed attested by Thorald son of Wulfat, one of the tenants named in the action of 1218–19 (A2A: DD/FJ/1/282/8). It is clear that William Clarel, brother to master John Clarel, the diplomat and pluralist, was holding the fee in the mid-thirteenth century. William and John may have been Geoffrey's sons, or were perhaps of the subsequent generation. Geoffrey appears to have had seisin of his lands in 1200, but he may have been of full age only just before that. Arrangements for the marriage of William were not made until *c*.1243 or later, and John was still living in 1293, having gained his first benefice in 1245–46.

William Clarel appears to have succeeded by 1240–41, when it was claimed he had wrongly entered a plea in the ecclesiastical rather than the king's court (*CRR*, 1237–1242, nos 1283, 1289, 1368). In 1242–43 he was involved in a dispute with Archbishop Gray concerning the service he owed for a free tenement in Misson, which was due to the archbishop as ward of the heir of Roger of Mattersey (*CRR*, 1237–1242,

---

94 Attested by Adam, Jordan and Nicholas de Ste-Marie, and Ralph of Wickersley and others. William Clarel was dead in 1200.

95 NottsA, Foljambe of Osberton papers.

96 After Alice had succeeded to the honour of Tickhill (*CP*, v, 163–64), and before Reginald had been succeeded as abbot of Roche.

97 A further indication of the Clarel interest in Misson is shown by the quitclaim in the advowson of the church of Misson issued by John Clarel, which was included in a general confirmation to Mattersey Priory (Notts.) in 1323 (*CalCh*, 1300–1326, p. 455).

## CLAREL, QUATREMARS AND MAUREWARD

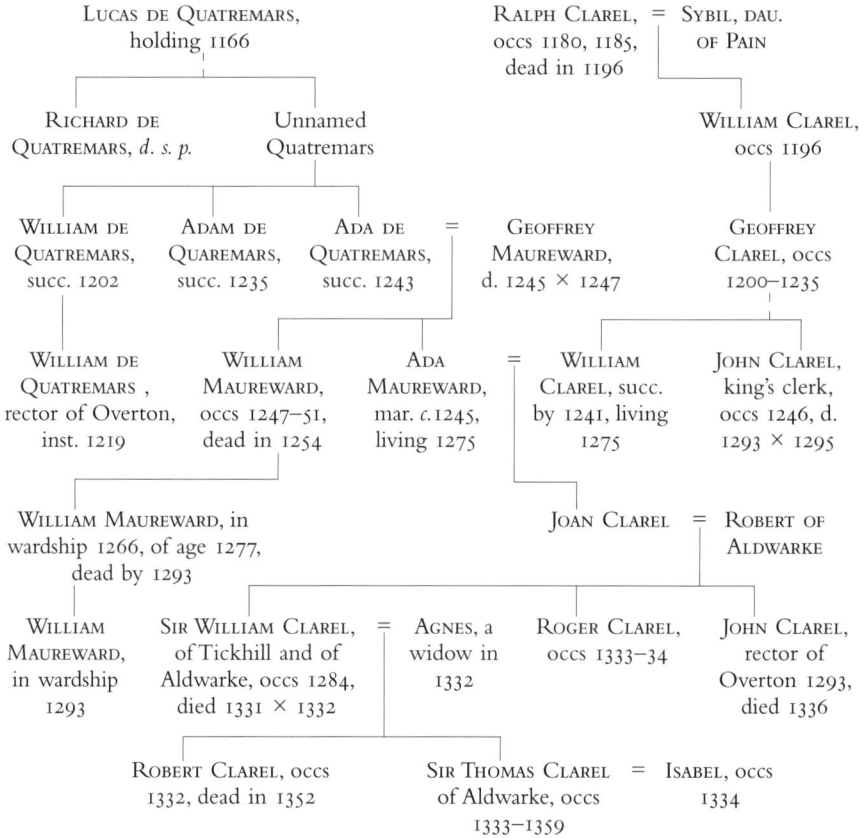

LUCAS DE QUATREMARS,
holding 1166

RALPH CLAREL, = SYBIL, DAU.
occs 1180, 1185,     OF PAIN
dead in 1196

RICHARD DE          Unnamed
QUATREMARS, d. s. p.   Quatremars

WILLIAM CLAREL,
occs 1196

WILLIAM DE    ADAM DE     ADA DE     =   GEOFFREY        GEOFFREY
QUATREMARS,   QUAREMARS,  QUATREMARS,     MAUREWARD,      CLAREL, occs
succ. 1202    succ. 1235  succ. 1243      d. 1245 × 1247  1200–1235

WILLIAM DE     WILLIAM     ADA      =   WILLIAM       JOHN CLAREL,
QUATREMARS ,   MAUREWARD,  MAUREWARD,   CLAREL, succ.  king's clerk,
rector of Overton,  occs 1247–51,  mar. c.1245,  by 1241, living  occs 1246, d.
inst. 1219     dead in 1254  living 1275  1275       1293 × 1295

WILLIAM MAUREWARD, in                    JOAN CLAREL  =  ROBERT OF
wardship 1266, of age 1277,                              ALDWARKE
dead by 1293

WILLIAM      SIR WILLIAM CLAREL,  =  AGNES, a   ROGER CLAREL,  JOHN CLAREL,
MAUREWARD,   of Tickhill and of      widow in   occs 1333–34   rector of
in wardship  Aldwarke, occs 1284,    1332                      Overton 1293,
1293         died 1331 × 1332                                  died 1336

ROBERT CLAREL, occs      SIR THOMAS CLAREL  =  ISABEL, occs
1332, dead in 1352       of Aldwarke, occs       1334
                         1333–1359

no. 2039; ibid., 1242–1243, no. 1405). William was called to warrant 1½ a. in Tickhill
in 1251 (*YF*, 1246–1272, p. 51). In December 1256 the sheriff of Leicestershire was
ordered to give him respite from knighthood until the Michaelmas following, at the
instance of John Mansel (*CloseR*, 1256–1259, p. 112).

William's wife was Ada, daughter of Geoffrey Maureward and Ada de Quatremars.
William Maureward confirmed to William Clarel, in frankmarriage with his sister
Ada, all the lands and wood which Maureward's parents Geoffrey Maureward and
Ada had previously given. The place is not named (A2A: DD/FJ/4/32/1). Geoffrey
and Ada's grant, which does not survive, was probably made in *c.*1243 × 1247,[98] and
the confirmation by William in 1245 × 1254.[99] It seems the marriage settlement also
made provision for William's brother John, as he was presented to his first benefice,
Cole Orton (*Overton*)[100] in Leicestershire, by Geoffrey Maureward in 1245–46 (see
below).

[98] After the death of Adam de Quatremars, brother of Ada, and before the death of Geoffrey Maureward
(FN).
[99] During William son of Geoffrey Maureward's tenure (FN).
[100] For Overton Quatremars, which with Overton Saucey comprised the parish of Cole Orton, or
Coleorton, see Nichols, *Leicestershire*, III, 733★. It is sometimes confused with Cold Overton, a parish

The heir of William Clarel was his daughter, Joan. It was probably on her marriage that William assigned all his lands and tenements in Chellaston in Derbyshire (*Chelardeston*) to Robert of Aldwarke and Joan [his wife], daughter of the grantor, for their lives, with remainder to their male heirs (A2A: DD/FJ/1/63/3). By another deed, known only from a later copy, William assigned to master John Clarel his brother all his lands in Tickhill, *Lyncepoll*, *Heselay* and *Marlhouer*, for the life of John, with remainder to Joan, William's daughter. John was to pay William 15*m.* annually (A2A: DD/FJ/1/282/4–5). William Clarel and Ada his wife were living in 1275–76, when they arraigned an assize of novel disseisin against William Maureward and another concerning a tenement in Overton Quatremars (*Rep. Dep. Keeper*, XLV (1885), App. II, p. 272).

William Clarel, son of Robert of Aldwarke, to whom William son of Jordan of Tickhill granted the manor of Westfold (in Tickhill),[101] was doubtless Joan's son (A2A: DD/FJ/1/282/2). He occurs as William Clarel of Tickhill, son of Robert of Aldwarke, when he exchanged land in *Otherton*[102] for land in Tickhill (A2A: DD/FJ/1/282/15). William Clarel of Aldwarke must have been of age in 1284, when [his great uncle] master John Clarel gave him a messuage, 1 ct. land, 20 a. meadow, and 100*s.* rent in Tickhill. William was to pay John £10 yearly during his life (*YF*, 1272–1300, pp. 68, 72). Gilbert son of William del Hill of Dalton gave land in Dalton to William Clarel of Aldwarke in 1302 (A2A: DD/FJ/1/209/2). William was apparently heir to his father as well as his mother, as he inherited substantial holdings in Aldwarke. Sir William Clarel of Aldwarke, knight, occurs in 1312 (A2A: DD/FJ/7/80/2). In 1319 William Clarel and his wife Agnes enfeoffed Adam of Rotherham, chaplain, with the manors of Penistone and Newton on Derwent and property in Wadworth, which the chaplain regranted them for life, with remainder to Thomas Clarel, their son (A2A: DD/FJ/4/32/2). In March 1328 the sheriff of York was ordered to appoint a new coroner in place of William Clarel, who was incapacitated by infirmity (*CalCl*, 1327–1330, p. 265). In 1331 William Clarel, knight, assigned rents in Great and Little Dalton and other places, and a watermill in Aldwarke to Thomas his son (A2A: DD/FJ/4/32/3), and in March 1332 Agnes, widow of Sir William Clarel, granted half the manor of Adwick [upon Dearne] to her son Thomas, with remainder to John Stainton and his wife Joan. Thomas promptly regranted the property to his mother for life (A2A: DD/FJ/4/32/4–7).

William Clarel was apparently succeeded by his son Robert. In October 1332 two grants were made to Robert Clarel, son and heir of William Clarel, knight (A2A: DD/FJ/1/194/40–41). In 1352 the king confirmed a grant of Queen Philippa to her damsel Margery de Sutton of all lands late of Robert Clarel, deceased, in the queen's honour of Tickhill and in *La Folde* and Adwick, which were in her hands by reason of a forfeiture and trespass done by Robert. In 1354 a similar confirmation was made, for the same lands, with the addition of Swinton, which were in the queen's hands as Robert had died without heir of himself, and his kinsman John son of John of Stokesley was outlawed for felony (*CalPat*, 1350–1354, p. 329; ibid., 1354–1358, p. 53). But matters seem to have been arranged so that Robert's brother Thomas inherited the family interests, and members of the Clarel family held substantial property in Tickhill, Aldwarke, and Adwick in the fifteenth century.

In 1333–34 Thomas Clarel, son of Sir William Clarel, knight, confirmed to Roger

---

on the other side of the county, for which see ibid., II, 137. Cole Orton is described in these notes as Overton or Overton Quatremars, following the individual documentary references.

101   *PN Yorks WR*, I, 54; *YD*, X, no. 448.
102   Cole Orton ?

Clarel his uncle 1 bv. in Kilnhurst which Sir William had given to Roger (MS Dods. 139, f. 73ᵛ). In 1334–35 John de Paldene and his wife Alice granted Thomas son of Sir William Clarel, and his wife Isabel, certain tenements in Adwick (A2A: DD/ FJ/1/194/43–44). Thomas Clarel is described as 'of Aldwarke' in 1333 and frequently thereafter (A2A: DD/FJ/7/36/6), and occurs as a knight in 1347, 1349, 1350 (with Isabel his wife), 1356 and 1359 (A2A: DD/FJ/1/232/10; DD/FJ/7/43/1; DD/FJ/1/194/33; DD/FJ/1/194/13; DD/FJ/8/7/2).¹⁰³

Hunter gives several references for the succeeding generations of the Clarel family (*SY*, II, 52–53, 334), and many of their deeds may be found amongst the Foljambe papers at Nottinghamshire Archives. Nathaniel Johnston compiled a history of the Clarels, and the FitzWilliams and Foljambes, who were their successors in Aldwarke, which he dated January 1705, stating it to be his last work (A2A: DD/FJ/10/10/1–3; cf. HMC 5, *6th report* (1877), p. 460).

Master John Clarel, mentioned above, was a prominent pluralist and diplomat.¹⁰⁴ He was presented as subdeacon to his first benefice of Cole Orton (*Overton*) by Geoffrey Maureward (father-in-law of his brother William) in 1245–46 (*Rot. Grosseteste*, p. 427). In January 1251, John Mansel, provost of Beverley, was allowed to grant a dispensation to his clerk John 'called Clarel' to add another benefice with cure of souls in the province of Canterbury to his rectory of Overton (*CalPapalL*, 1198–1304, p. 265). John is first given the title *magister* in a cancelled entry in the close rolls, at the instance of J[ohn] Mansel, in 1251 (*CloseR*, 1247–1251, p. 486). Clarel continued his association with Mansel, and occurs as his clerk in 1257 (*CalCh*, 1257–1300, p. 8). On the death of Archbishop Gray in 1255 the king, describing Clarel as his clerk, appointed him and another to the custody of the province of York, and in the same year rewarded him with the prebend of Norwell in Southwell minster (*CalPat*, 1247–1258, pp. 409, 421). He is named frequently in the White Book of Southwell ('Ctl. Southwell', passim). Amongst other commissions, he served King Henry III as deputy to John Mansel on his diplomatic mission to Castile in 1253–54, he was emissary to Rome in 1258–59 (*CalPat*, 1247–1258, pp. 230, 321, 643; ibid., 1258–1266, p. 51; *CloseR*, 1251–1253, p. 476) and emissary to France in 1272 (*CalPat*, 1266–1272, p. 662).¹⁰⁵ Papal letters of 1262 and 1283 describe him as a papal chaplain (*CalPapalL*, 1198–1304, pp. 376, 467). He continued in royal service after the accession of Edward I, going to Rome on the king's affairs in 1282 (*CalPat*, 1281–1292, p. 26).¹⁰⁶ Clarel's possession of the royal free chapel of Tickhill is apparent from the papal mandate issued in 1286 for him or his proctor to appear before the pope concerning certain churches and chapels held to the use of the dean and chapter of Rouen (*CalPapalL*, 1198–1304, pp. 488–89).¹⁰⁷ He and 'master Bertrand' occur as 'stewards of the honour and castle of Tickhill' in a deed of uncertain date (*YD*, x, no. 442). Clarel was again sent abroad by the king in 1287, and was probably absent from the kingdom in January 1292, when he was believed dead and Tickhill chapel was granted to Boniface de Saluzzo. The grant was

---

¹⁰³   See Young, 'Religious Houses', p. 73 for brief notes on some later members of the Clarel family and the friary at Tickhill.

¹⁰⁴   Brief accounts of his career are given in Boulay Hill, 'Rectors of East Bridgford', pp. 76–77; *Reg. Romeyn*, I, 282–83n.

¹⁰⁵   In this last commission he is described, almost certainly mistakenly, as a canon of York, rather than Southwell. This is the only such reference to him and it is unlikely Clarel ever held a York canonry. For background to these diplomatic missions, and Clarel's role in them, see Powicke, *Henry III*, pp. 232–33, 386–90, 587–88, and for John Mansel, see *ODNB*.

¹⁰⁶   For the business at hand, see *CalPapalL*, 1198–1304, p. 467.

¹⁰⁷   For Rouen's possession of Tickhill chapel, and other churches in the honour of Tickhill, see *YMF*, II, 148–49.

revoked when it was discovered Clarel was still living (*CalPat*, 1281–1292, pp. 278, 470). On 2 April 1293, as prebendary of Norwell, he requested a case be determined by two others ('Ctl. Southwell', no. 197 [ex p. 120]). In 1295 he was dead, when Tickhill was again granted to Saluzzo (*CalPat*, 1292–1301, p. 135). In 1301 John de Stokwell, executor of the will of master John Clarel, formerly prebendary of Norwell, appointed a proctor in the case pending with the chapter of Southwell concerning the repair of the chancel of the prebendary church of Norwell ('Ctl. Southwell', no. 364 [ex p. 228]).

In 1265 × c.1274,[108] describing himself as a papal chaplain, John Clarel founded the Austin friary of Tickhill, by giving to the brothers heremite of St Augustine his manor of Tickhill, for the souls of himself, his family, and John Mansel, formerly treasurer of York, on the condition that six brothers were always to reside there (A2A: DD/FJ/1/282/1). Master John Clarel's grant of a messuage in Tickhill to Walter, prior of the order of St Augustine of Tickhill, was confirmed by a fine of November 1276 (*YF*, 1272–1300, p. 12). A licence was issued in the same year for the Austin friars of Tickhill to enclose a way outside the town on the north of their church between their place and the land of William Clarel (*CalPat*, 1272–1281, p. 164). The house of Austin Friars at Tickhill stood just west of Tickhill, close to a building known as Clarel Hall (*SY*, I, 244), doubtless the Tickhill residence of the family in the thirteenth century.[109]

Master J[ohn] Clarel 'the younger' (*minor*) occurs in 1292 (*Reg. Romeyn*, II, 107–08 and n). He was presented to Overton Quatremars in May 1293 as a clerk in minor orders, on the resignation of John Clarel the elder, and was ordained subdeacon at about that time. He was given licence to receive the diaconate and priesthood from any Catholic bishop, within two months of his ordination, as he was to travel to Rome on business. He was thus ordained to the diaconate by the bishop of Bologna in December 1293, and ordained to the priesthood in Bologna the following March (*Reg. Sutton*, VII, 38–39, 52–53; ibid., VIII, 53). It has been suggested he was an illegitimate son of John Clarel the elder, but it seems more probable that he was a great nephew,[110] and that he can be identified with John Clarel, son of Robert of Aldwarke, who issued a deed concerning Somerby (Leics.) at Overton Quatremars in 1299 (A2A: DD/FJ/1/149/1). It was this younger master John Clarel who was prebendary of Pipa Minor in Lichfield in 1319, and who exchanged the rectory of Cole Orton[111] for the archdeaconry of Stafford in 1323. In 1329 he was granted licence to alienate in mortmain land in Overton Quatremars to establish a chantry in the church there, for his soul and those of his ancestors (*CalPat*, 1327–1330, p. 412). He held the archdeaconry of Stafford until his death in 1336.

The marriage of William Clarel to Ada MAUREWARD, daughter of Geoffrey Maureward and the heiress Ada de QUATREMARS, which took place in c.1243 × 1247, has been mentioned above. Lucas de Quatremars held 12 ct. in the Leicestershire vills

---

[108]  After the death of John Mansel as treasurer in 1265. In 1274 one friar of the house was ordained deacon, and three friars ordained priest (*VCH Yorks*, III, 280–81, which gives a brief history of the friary).

[109]  For the remains of the Austin priory and Clarel hall as they were in 1817, see Euphrastus, 'Tickhill', pp. 323–24, 487. The buildings were noticed by Leland c.1544 (Leland, *Itinerary*, I, 36).

[110]  That master John Clarel had children is shown by the quitclaim made in 1298 by Jordan de Lisle of Great Houghton (*Haluton*), co. York, and Alice his wife, grand-daughter and one of the heirs of master John Clarel, late rector, to Robert, rector of Hemingford Abbots (co. Huntingdon), of all right in a messuage and land in Hemingford. Clarel had been instituted rector of Hemingford Abbots in 1253 (*VCH Hunts*, II, 307 and n).

[111]  Cold Overton according to Emden, *Oxford*, p. 437, s.n. Clerole; and *FEA 1300–1541*, X (Coventry and Lichfield), 19.

of Cole Orton (*Overton*) and Goadby Marwood (*Godesby*) of Geoffrey Ridel[112] in 1166 (*Red Bk*, p. 330). In 1202 William de Quatremars paid 20*m*. relief for £10 land in Shorne (*Sornes*), Kent, which had belonged to his uncle Richard de Quatremars, whose heir he was. It was probably the same William de Quatremars who paid 20*m*. for the king's grace in 1216, when orders were sent to the sheriffs of Leicester, Norfolk, Nottingham, Dorset and Kent to restore his lands (*RFine*, pp. 185, 585). William de Quatremars, knight, presented his son W[illiam] to Overton rectory, who was granted dispensation *eo quod puer et iuvenis erat*. He was instituted in 1219 (*Rot. Welles*, I, 11, 155). The older William was succeeded by his brother Adam de Quatremars in 1235, who paid a relief for his land in Kent. In 1243, Adam was dead, and Geoffrey Maureward, husband of Ada, sister and heir of Adam Quatremars, paid a relief for Adam's land in Cobham and Shorne (*RFine Excerpta*, I, 273, 402). Before 1247, when the deed was inspected and confirmed, Geoffrey Maureward (*Mauregard*) quitclaimed the rent of £10 in Cobham and Shorne paid to him and his wife Ada by Sir John of Cobham, which John had previously held of Adam Quatremars, brother of Ada (*CalCh*, 1226–1257, pp. 322–23).

As has been noted, Geoffrey Maureward presented John Clarel to Overton in 1245–46. Geoffrey seems to have died soon afterwards, for a jury in April 1254 found that William Maureward had demised the manor of Overton Quatremars to William de la Ferté for a six year term, which had expired at Michaelmas 1253 (Wrottesley, 'Plea Rolls Hen. III', pp. 130–31). William Maureward was living in 1251–52, when he made a presentation to Goadby [Marwood] (*Rot. Grosseteste*, p. 440), but was dead in April 1254, the jury stating that he had been 'languishing in distant parts . . . until he died'. In 1266 the land of William son of William *Mauregard* was in the wardship of *dom*. J. Clarel (*Rot. Gravesend*, p. 146). William Maureward was of age in 1277, when he presented master John Clarel, subdeacon, to Overton, and was living in 1278, when he presented to Goadby [Marwood] (ibid., pp. 160, 164). In 1293 William son of William Maureward was in ward to Sir Ralph Basset, who held the superior interest in Overton (*Reg. Sutton*, VIII, 53).

**R761.** Gift to the hospital by Hugh de Drincourt, his wife, and William his son and heir, of all the land which Walter the mason of Tickhill held, and all the land which William and Basing hold, with a certain woodland pasture in Stainton [*c*.1145 × 1165, probably *c*.1154]

COPY: MS Dods. 120, f. 28ᵛ, from Rawl., f. 131, now missing.

Notum sit omnibus etc. quod ego Hugo de Dreincurt et sponsa mea et Willelmus filius meus et heres meus et nostri heredes concedimus imperpetuum et <in elemosinam> damus fratribus et pauperibus hospitalis sancti Petri Ebor' et sancti Leonardi Ebor' totam illam terram quam tenuit Walterus cementarius de Ticheil in bosco et in terra arabili, et totam illam terram quam Willelmus et Basing' tenent <plenarie> in bosco et in terra arabili, liberam et quietam et cum quodam virgulto in Stainton. Hii sunt testes, Willelmus de Clerefait, Rogerus de Funtenai, Willelmus de Cressi, Radulfus Clarel, Walterus cementarius, Alanus de Folifate. Acta in curia hospitalis sancti Leonardi apud Ebor'. fo. 131.

Although this deed was included in the Tickhill section, it is not clear from Dodsworth's abstract that any of the land lay in Tickhill, and so it is not entirely

---

[112]   For Ridel, and other members of the Basset family, see Sanders, *English Baronies*, pp. 49–50.

safe to assume that the deed can be dated by the papal confirmation of a *mansum* in Tickhill to the hospital in 1157. The confirmation does not mention Stainton (C179 [*EYC*, I, no. 186]). Hugh de Drincourt was dead in 1165 (FN: Stainton); William de Clairfait, who held the castle of Tickhill in 1141, was dead in 1166 (FN). The reference to St Leonard is suggestive of a date close to the dedication of the church of the hospital to St Leonard in 1154 (C194 [*EYC*, I, no. 185]). The land in Stainton previously held by William and Besing was confirmed to the hospital by Hugh de Drincourt's grandson Hugh, son of William of Stainton, in 1202 × 1209 (R433).

**R762.** Gift to the hospital by Walter Clarel of a toft in Tickhill with the buildings on it [*c.*1160 × 1181]

COPY: *d* MS Dods. 8, f. 266ʳ. ABSTRACTS: *c* MS Dods. 120b, f. 28ᵛ, omits Thomas of Tickhill, Giffard, Richard the chaplain, and the last three witnesses, from Rawl., f. 131, now missing; *e* Burton transcripts 6, f. 69ʳ, p. 129, corrupt, from notes by Nathaniel Johnston from an unidentified Dodsworth MS (not *c*, as Tickhill and Giffard are given as witnesses).

*Carta Walteri Clarel.*
Notum sit archiepiscopo Eboraci totique capitulo sancti Petri et omnibus sancte matris ecclesie filiis tam presentibus quam futuris quod ego Gualterus Clarel[113] et heredes mei concessimus et dedimus deo et sancto Petro et pauperibus hospitalis sancti Petri Eboraci unum toftum in Tichehil et hedeficia que sunt superposita, cum omnibus appenticiis suis in puram et perpetuam elemosinam liberam solutam et quietam et immunem ab omnibus geldis et auxiliis et consuetudinibus et exactionibus et ab omni humano servitio que ad nos pertinent preter orationes pauperum. Hanc prefatam elemosinam dedimus et presenti carta confirmavimus pro salute animarum nostrarum et pro animabus omnium antecessorum nostrorum ut simus part(ic)ipes omnium beneficiorum et orationum que fiunt vel facienda sunt in illa sancta domo dei tam in vita quam in morte. Hiis testibus, Radulfo Clarel, Iohanne eius filio . . .[114] Thoma de Tichehil, Franceis Giffard, Pagano presbitero de Donecast', Radulfo eius filio, Ricardo capell(ano), Roberto de Scalcebi, Radulfo de Insula, Roberto filio Pagani, Iurdano de Reinesuil, Roberto clerico de Edlint', Roalto filio Waldig, Rad' . . .[114]

Few hospital deeds are addressed to the archbishop, and none can be shown to date to the archiepiscopate of Geoffrey or his successors.[115] The attestation of Pain priest of Doncaster suggests a date during the archiepiscopate of Roger rather than Geoffrey (FN: Doncaster rectors). It is reasonably certain therefore that this deed was issued before the death of Archbishop Roger in 1181. As the first witness Ralph Clarel was married to a sister of Jordan son of Pain [of Wilsic] it is improbable that he could have attested with a son before *c.*1160.

---

[113]  *c: Darel*, with *Clarell* inserted immediately above in a different hand.
[114]  sic in *d*.
[115]  For the contrasting example of Byland, benefactions to which were frequently addressed to the archbishop, see *Mowbray Charters*, pp. lxix–lxx; *Ctl. Byland*, pp. xlvii–xlviii.

## Wickersley

The Contents List gives f. 134, now missing, for Wickersley, a member of the honour of Tickhill. In 1284–85 the heirs of Robert of Wickersley held Wickersley of Nicholas Livet for ½ k.f. Nicholas held in turn of [the manor of] Bentley, of the honour of Tickhill (*KI*, p. 6; *SY*, I, 276–77). The 4 k.f. held in 1208 × 1213 by Adam de Neuf-marché of the honour of Tickhill are described as 'the manor of Bentley with the members' in an extent dating from the reign of Edward IV. The render to the lord of the manor included 20s. from the heirs of William Livet for ½ k.f. in Wickersley (*SY*, I, 324; *Bk of Fees*, p. 32). For what is known of the hospital's holdings in Wickersley, see HN: Hooton Levitt.

## Wath [Wath-upon-Dearne]

According to the Contents List, Wath and Wickersley deeds occupied f. 134. In 1086 Roger de Busli held 6 ct. in Wath; Wulfsige, a thane of the king, held over 7 ct. in Wath, West Melton, Wentworth, and *Eldeberge*. In 1284–85 the manor was held by William Fleming for 2 k.f. of the honour of Skipton (*KI*, p. 1). The deeds which follow show that the hospital was given 1 bv. in Wath by William le Fleming before 1166 (R763), and received two small gifts of land in the early thirteenth century (R764, R765). Wath does not occur in the papal and regal confirmations to the hospital, nor in the extents of the later thirteenth century. Land in Wath, late belonging to the hospital, was sold with much other property to Richard Andrewis and William Romsden of Longley, Yorks, in 1543 (*LPFD*, 1543, XVIII (1), 527).

The FLEMING family and its holding of the honour of Skipton have been discussed in detail by Clay (*EYC*, VII, 193–202). William le Fleming gave the hospital 1 bv. in [West] Melton in *c.*1140 × 1148 (R306). His son Reiner le Fleming [II], who held the fee in 1166, accounted for an amercement at Michaelmas 1205, and was dead in 1218–19 when the prioress of Kirklees complained that William le Fleming had not adhered to the deed of his father Reiner (*EYC*, VII, 196–97). Before 1207, Reiner le Fleming attested with his sons Adam, William, Walter and Thomas (*EYC*, VII, no. 108; *Ctl. Bolton*, no. 42). The order of witnesses gives the impression that Adam was Rein-er's eldest son, but if so he presumably died before his father, as there is no evidence he inherited.[116] Reiner le Fleming attested another deed with his sons William, Walter, Thomas and Reiner (*Ctl. Bolton*, AII 30). Reiner's son and heir William died in 1228 × 1235, when he was succeeded by his brother John (*EYC*, VII, 197–98).

**R763.** Gift to the hospital by William Fleming, son of Reiner, of 1 bv. in Wath which belonged to Suelmar [*c.*1140 × 1166]

COPY: MS Dods. 120b, f. 29ʳ, from Rawl., f. 134, now missing.

Notum sit omnibus sancte matris ecclesie filiis tam presentibus quam futuris quod ego Willelmus Flandrigena, Reneri filius, dedi et c(oncessi) et hac presenti carta mea

---

[116]   However, another deed is witnessed by Reiner Fleming, and William, Adam and Thomas his sons (*Ctl. Monk Bretton*, p. 188). Adam son of Reiner le Fleming, who made an agreement with the prior of Bolton in 1243, was tentatively identified by Clay as the son of Reiner II. This led Clay to the conclu-sion that Adam son of Reiner II could not have been the eldest son (*EYC*, VII, 197, and no. 134a). But it is more probable that the Adam of 1243 was a son of Reiner II's younger son Reiner.

confirm(avi) deo et sancto hospitali sancti Petri Ebor' in perpetuam elemosinam unam bovatam terre in Wath que fuit Suelmari sine retenemento alicuius rei, liberam et quietam ab omni seculari servitio et consuetudine in silvis in campis in pratis in aquis et in omnibus locis cum thol et theam et infagethef' pro anima patris mei et matris mei et Renerio filio meo et pro sponsa et pro animabus omnium heredum et successorum meorum. Et precor omnes heredes meos ut hanc elemosinam manute- neant et conservent. Huius donacionis testes sunt Suenus decanus de Wath, Godricus filius Ketelb(er)ti, Lasinc Tacun. fo. 134.

By a deed of probable date *c.*1140 × 1148, William Fleming assigned the hospital 1 bv. in West Melton (*Midilton*), near Wath, and 12*d.* annually from the mill of Agemund, for the alms which his father had given (R306). Presumably the 1 bv. given by the present deed was additional to the 1 bv. in West Melton. William Fleming, son of Reiner, was dead in 1166, when his son Reiner, named in this deed, held the fee (*EYC*, VII, 196). The leading witness, Swain dean of Wath, was probably the same man as Swain clerk of Wath, who attested Fleming's gift in West Melton. Godric son of Ketelbert, who occurs in 1130 when he owed 4*m.* for an amercement in Yorkshire, was the ancestor of the FitzWilliams of Emley and Sprotbrough (*EYC*, III, no. 1690n; *PR*, 31 Hen. I, p. 33; *Baildon*, I, 345).

**R764.** Gift to the hospital by Robert son of Richard son of Ulkel of Wath of 2 a. in the field of Wath [1205 × *c.*1230]

ABSTRACT: MS Dods. 120b, f. 29ʳ, from Rawl., f. 134, now missing.

Omnibus sancte matris ecclesie filiis Robertus filius Ricardi filii Ulkelli de Wad' salutem. Noveritis me etc. dedisse hospitali sancti Petri Ebor' duas acras terre in campo de Wad. Test(ibus), Willelmo Flandri, Reinero, Willelmo[117] fratribus suis, Roberto de Ecclefelde, Rogero de Suinish,[118] Radulfo de Wad, Iohanne, Willelmo filiis eius, Waltero, Godfrido, Willelmo fratribus hospitalis Ebor' etc. fo. 134.

Richard son of Ulkel of Wath, father of the grantor, gave 1 a. in Wath to Monk Bretton by a deed witnessed by Reiner le Fleming (*Ctl. Monk Bretton*, p. 196). The present deed was probably issued after William le Fleming succeeded his father Reiner in 1205 × 1219, and certainly before William's death in 1228 × 1235 (FN). Godfrey, brother of the hospital, attested within *c.*1200 × *c.*1230. Ralph of Wath and Juliana his wife were named in a fine of 1202 concerning land in Cadeby (*PF John*, p. 24). Roger of Swineshead witnessed deeds of Walter le Fleming in *c.*1170 × 1184 and 1171 × 1181, and attested with Ralph of Wath in the 'late twelfth or early thirteenth century' (*EYC*, VII, nos 87, 111, 133).

**R765.** Gift to the hospital by Robert son of Richard of Wath of all that land in Well Croft [*c.*1200 × *c.*1220]

ABSTRACT: MS Dods. 120b, f. 29ʳ, from Rawl., f. 134, now missing.

---

[117]   sic, possibly for Walter, though it was not unknown for two brothers to have the same Christian name. Reiner and William Fleming, parsons, attest a deed of William Fleming, knight, given in 1205 × 1235 (*Ctl. Fountains*, p. 140).

[118]   Probably for Swineshead.

Robertus filius Ricardi de Wath ded(it) hospitali sancti Petri Ebor' totam illam terram in Wellecroft etc. Testibus, Girardo, Waltero, Godfrido, Willelmo et aliis fratribus hospitalis Ebor'. fo. 134.

Godfrey attested between *c.*1200 and *c.*1230; Girard had ceased to attest by the time Thomas de Langwath gained the title of master. Well Croft Moor is named in the Wath tithe award of 1843 (*PN Yorks WR*, I, 119).

## [*Wodall*]

A rent in *Wodall* is noted amongst West Riding rents in the account of 1542 (*Dissolved Houses*, IV, 225), but it is difficult to identify which of several places with similar names is intended. It is possible there was a section for *Wodall* in the Rawlinson volume, as the gathering comprising the end of the West Riding division and the start of the East Riding division had been lost by the time the Contents List was written and Dodsworth made his abstracts.

## [Worsbrough]

As with *Wodall*, we cannot be certain whether there was a section for Worsbrough in the Rawlinson volume or not. The papal confirmations of 1148, 1157 and 1173 include 1 bv. in Worsbrough (*Wircasburc, Wyrcaburc, Wirkeburg*), but do not name the donor (C178–C180 [*EYC*, I, nos 179, 186, 197]). Nothing more is known of the hospital's holdings in Worsbrough, which was a member of the Lacy fee.

# East Riding Deeds

Dodsworth's transcripts in MS Dods. 120b provide abstracts from many deeds copied to leaves of the East Riding division of the Rawlinson volume that are now missing. These transcripts are printed below, together with the texts of deeds from other sources belonging to vills in the East Riding. Also included here are brief notes on the hospital's holdings in places in the East Riding which had no section in the cartulary, like Catfoss and Etton. Section headings, when not in square brackets, are taken from the Contents List, from MS Dods. 120b, or in the case of Aughton immediately below, from elsewhere in the cartulary.

## *Aghton'* [Aughton]

The Aughton section of the Rawlinson volume is known only from the note referring to it under the heading *Guthmundham* (Rawl., f. 165[r]). It was in the gathering which had been lost by the time Dodsworth made his abstracts and the Contents List was written. For the postulation that Emma Hay, or a close relation, was the hospital's benefactor in Aughton, see HN: Goodmanham.

## [Brandesburton]

For Brandesburton, held by the St-Quintin family of the Aumale fee of Holderness, see *VCH Yorks ER*, VII, 245–54. On 24 March 1371 the hospital had licence to acquire in mortmain from William Tiddeswell, parson of the church of St George in Fishergate, York, Walter Nafferton, parson of the church of St Margaret in Walmgate, York, John Braweby, Thomas Kirkeby, Ralph Tiddeswell and Hugh Catalle, chaplains, two messuages and 7½ bv. land in Brandesburton and Seaton, and the reversion of a messuage and 1 bv. land in Brandesburton which master William Melton, late parson of the church of Brandesburton, held for life of 'brother John Burton', to the yearly value of 10s., to hold in satisfaction of 1m. of the £10 land and rent which the hospital had licence to acquire (*CalPat*, 1370–1374, p. 67). The property had previously been conveyed to the same trustees[1] by Beatrix, daughter and heir of Robert Brandesburton or Burton, and sister of another Robert Burton. On 14 October 1369 she appointed Hugh Myton, clerk of the hospital of St Leonard, as her attorney to deliver seisin to the six trustees (BL, Addit. Chs 5754–55). As Brandesburton is not mentioned in the *Valor Ecclesiasticus* or the post-Dissolution accounts, it is likely that this estate had been disposed of by 1535. Brandesburton does not otherwise feature in the muniments of the hospital, and in view of the late date of the hospital's acquisition of this land it seems unlikely that the Rawlinson volume contained a section for Brandesburton deeds.

---

[1]   The rector of St George is called William Kettlewell in both these deeds.

# [Catfoss]

Catfoss, in Holderness, is not mentioned in the Contents List or Dodsworth's abstracts, so it is unlikely the Rawlinson volume included a Catfoss section. The vill was held by the Fauconberg family of the earl of Aumale. A bovate in Catfoss was included in the papal confirmations of 1148, 1157 and 1173, but the donor is not named (C178–C180 [*EYC*, I, nos 179, 186, 197]). No subsequent notice of the hospital's land in Catfoss has been found.

# [Etton]

The East Riding section of the account of 1542 includes a rent in Etton (*Dissolved Houses*, IV, 226). The hospital held land in Lockington, 2 m. to the north east of Etton, but nothing more is known of the holding, and there was no section for Etton in the Rawlinson volume.

# [Filey]

A messuage with a mill in Filey (*Fifle*, *Fifley*, *Fiflei*) was included in the papal confirmations of 1148, 1157 and 1173, but the donor was not named (C178–C180 [*EYC*, I, nos 179, 186, 197]). There was no section for Filey in the Rawlinson volume, and nothing more is known of this holding. Filey was in the Gant fee, and the mill was presumably given by Walter de Gant, who died in 1139, or his son Gilbert de Gant, who was underage in 1141, gained the earldom of Lincoln in *c.*1147–48, and died in 1156 (*EYC*, II, 432–33; *CP*, VII, 672–73). This was not the only mill in Filey, for in '*c.*1125 × 1130' Walter de Gant granted to Bridlington Priory the church of Filey *cum molendino uno* and other property (*EYC*, II, no. 1135).

# *Hoothom* [Hotham]

The Contents List cites f. 188 for Hotham, which is now missing. The two deeds abstracted by Dodsworth were from this folio. For Hotham, see *VCH Yorks ER*, IV, 115–123. Nigel Fossard had land in Hotham in 1086. The Hotham family held 2 k.f. of Fossard, and afterwards of Mauley, in the later twelfth and thirteenth centuries, which included land in Hotham. The deeds which follow show that the hospital acquired a toft and a croft in Hotham early in the thirteenth century (R766). The hospital let the property at fee-farm to Robert son of Hugh de Trehus (R767); Robert's son Alan subsequently granted at least part of the holding to Robert son of Ranulf of Broomfleet (R768). Apart from these deeds, there is no trace of Hotham in the hospital's muniments. The toft and croft, and other land in Hotham held by the hospital, appear to have been subsumed into the manor of Broomfleet. At the Dissolution the hospital held 20 a. in Hotham appurtenant to the manor of Broomfleet. An extent of the manor of Broomfleet from the later sixteenth century includes a messuage with 6½ a. freehold land, and a messuage with 13 a. in Hotham (*VCH Yorks ER*, IV, 118, citing PRO, SC 6/HenVIII/4601, m. 8d; *YD*, II, no. 128).

Philip Saltmarshe published his extensive history of the HOTHAM family in 1914. He made the plausible suggestion that Durand son of William, who held 2 k.f. of old feoffment of William Fossard in 1166 (*EYC*, II, no. 1003), was the ancestor of the family,[2] but the evidence used by Dodsworth to connect Durand with subsequent generations eluded him (Saltmarshe, *Hothams*, pp. 25–26; MS Dods. 79, f. 69ᵛ). Durand of Hotham (*Hodum*) owed 1m. in the wapentake of Harthill in 1166 (*PR*, 12 Hen. II, p. 48). He was a witness to a gift by William Fossard [I] to St Mary [of Merton, Surrey] made in c.1154 × 1164[3] (*EYC*, II, no. 1118) and a confirmation made by William Fossard [II] to Watton in 1164 × c.1183[4] (*EYC*, II, no. 1116).

Durand of Hotham was succeeded by his son Robert. Apparently in or before 1171[5] Robert of Hotham and Walram his brother attested William Fossard's gift of 1 bv. in Lockington to Roger of Lockington (*EYC*, II, no. 1121). Robert of Hotham witnessed a confirmation of Jordan son of Geoffrey *Britonil* [of Bugthorpe] before Easter 1192[6] (Burton transcripts 1, f. 141ʳ, p. 229, B12 N67).[7] He married a sister of master Roger Arundel,[8] whose name, according to pleadings of 1291, was Agnes (Saltmarshe, *Hothams*, pp. 26–27, citing De Banco, Hil., 19 Edw. I, no. 90, mm. 70, 107; *EYC*, XI, 198, citing PRO, CP 40/88, m. 149). Robert was presumably dead when Thomas of Hotham witnessed the agreement between William son of Peter [of Goodmanham] and Thomas Hay made in 1197 × 1211[9] (*EYC*, II, no. 1130). A quitclaim copied on f. 275 of the lost cartulary of Ormsby proves that Thomas was a grandson of Durand. By this deed Thomas of Hotham son of Robert son of Durand renounced all right in Michael son of Thurstan of Bursea to the nuns of Ormsby (MS Dods. 135, f. 143ʳ). In September 1213 Thomas de Holm' (sic, but doubtless a mistake for Hotham) fined for 500m. and five palfreys for having the land which had belonged to master Roger Arundel, his uncle (*RFine*, p. 491). Thomas son of

2   Both Farrer and Clay placed Durand son of William as a member of the Butterwick family, but he is difficult to fit into that descent (FN: Butterwick).

3   Confirmed by Archbishop Roger before he became legate (*EYC*, II, no. 1119).

4   Of similar date to an associated confirmation of William de Vescy (*EYC*, II, no. 1115), who was dead in 1183 (*CP*, XII (2), 274–75), witnessed by Roger, prior of Malton, who succeeded in or after 1164. The period for Roger is not clearly indicated in *Heads*. According to *The Book of St Gilbert*, written during Roger's lifetime, he had been a canon of Sempringham, and became head of Malton, before becoming *de facto* head of the order of Sempringham during Gilbert's old age. Roger was confirmed in the position on Gilbert's death in 1189 (*St Gilbert*, pp. 68–69, 86–87, 130–33). In 1946 C.R. Cheney pointed out that Prior Roger was named in the address clauses of a number of associated privileges for houses of the Gilbertine order made in 1178, giving the impression that a man of that name was simultaneously prior of Malton, Alvingham, and Chicksands. Cheney reasonably concluded that the man addressed was Roger, now effectively head of the order. Cheney used the term 'prior superior' to describe Roger's position, as he had authority over the priors of the individual houses. He further reasoned that a papal privilege for Malton dated 1169, addressed to 'Gilbert prior of the church of St Mary the virgin of Malton', was probably addressed to the head of the order, and should not be taken as evidence for a prior of Malton named Gilbert (Cheney, 'Papal Privileges', pp. 45–52). Foreville and Keir suggested that Gilbert's resignation fell in the period 1176 × 1178, but there is no firm evidence for the *terminus a quo* (*St Gilbert*, pp. xxiii n, 344), and it is quite possible that Roger remained as prior of Malton after becoming 'prior superior' to all the Gilbertine houses. Robert occurs as prior of Malton in 1164. Roger was prior in 1174, when master Gilbert of Sempringham, Roger prior of Malton, Hugh prior of Sixhills (*Sixle*), Thomas prior of Ormsby and Geoffrey prior of Alvingham attested an agreement (Alvingham cartulary, f. 130ᵛ). Roger is unlikely to have been described as prior of Malton in a witness clause after the death of Gilbert in 1189.

5   Witnessed by William Aguillun and William his son. The older William Aguillun was dead in 1171 (FN).

6   Witnessed by Amfrey de Chauncy, who died about that time (FN).

7   Calendared *Ctl. Byland*, no. 1161.

8   For master Roger Arundel and his coheirs see *EYC*, XI, 198–200.

9   For the date, see FN: Hay.

Robert of Hotham gave a toft and croft in Hotham to the hospital in *c.*1214 × 1223 (R766). He was in rebellion in the reign of John, but had come to allegiance by December 1217 (*RClose*, I, 376).[10] Thomas of Hotham was living in 1219, when he surrendered land in Belaugh [in Lockington] to Peter de Maulay and Isabel his wife, and possibly in 1220, when he was called to warrant land in Lockington but failed to appear (*CRR*, 1219–1220, pp. 35, 302; ibid., 1220, pp. 34, 150). He was dead in Michaelmas term 1223, when Margaret, or Margery, his widow, made many claims for dower. Thomas' son and heir Robert was a minor and in ward to Simon Hales in 1224 (ibid., 1223–1224, nos 770, 892, 1365, 1701, 2379, 2903). Robert was probably of age in 1228, when he made a claim against the abbot of Thornton and the prior of Watton concerning a tenement in Cranswick (*PatentR*, 1225–1232, p. 208), and was certainly of age in 1230, when he granted to Richard de Percy his interest in the mills of Scorborough. John de Beauver of Holme [on Spalding Moor] had previously granted to Robert of Hotham, son and heir of Sir Thomas of Hotham, all his part in the mills of Scorborough, doubtless part of the divided inheritance of Roger Arundel (*Ctl. Percy*, pp. 65, 116; *EYC*, XI, 199–200). In 1234 Robert of Hotham and Isabel his wife granted 2 bv. and two messuages in East Lutton to Roger son of Thomas of Thirkleby, for 14*m.* (*YF*, 1232–1246, p. 20). Robert of Hotham held 2 k.f. of Mauley in 1242–43, described as comprising land in Hotham, Cranswick, Seaton [Ross], and Easthorpe [par. Londsborough] (*Bk of Fees*, p. 1098). He died between 1250 and 1251, when his widow Alice, apparently his second wife, defended her right against Peter de Mauley. Alice, widow of Robert of Hotham, claimed dower in land in Beswick, Hotham, Cranswick and Hutton in 1252. The pleadings note that John, son and heir of Robert, was underage and in the wardship of Peter de Mauley, with certain of his lands in ward to John de Eyncourt, and Henry de Percy (Saltmarshe, *Hothams*, p. 30, citing Coram Rege, Easter, 36 Hen. III and Mich., 37 Hen. III).

Thomas of Hotham and Walter of Hotham, who witnessed an agreement between Marmaduke of Thwing and William Constable in 1227, have not been identified (*YD*, I, no. 273). They were perhaps younger brothers of Robert, attesting as minors. Robert enfeoffed his younger brother Thomas with 9 bv. and 70 a. in Cranswick in 1250. Thomas, brother of Robert of Hotham, was called to warrant by the prior of Watton when Robert's widow claimed dower in 1252 (Saltmarshe, *Hothams*, p. 30, citing Coram Rege, Mich., 35 Hen. III and Mich., 37 Hen. III). Thomas son of Thomas of Hotham gave Meaux Abbey property in Hutton and Cranswick, for which the monks paid 8*m.* to Jews, apparently in 1249 × 1269. In the same period John of Hotham confirmed all that the monks held in his fee (*Chron. Meaux*, II, 116). In 1253 Thomas of Hotham acknowledged receipt of 13*m.* from Robert, prior of Warter, for two plots of turbary with the foredales in the marsh of Cranswick (Warter cartulary, f. 78[r–v]). Thomas was dead in 1260, when Alice widow of Thomas of Hotham claimed against the abbot of Meaux her dower of a third part of two messuages and 28 a. land in Cranswick. The abbot called to warrant Geoffrey, son and heir of Thomas, who was in ward to John of Hotham (Baildon, *Monastic Notes*, I, 132). Geoffrey was the ancestor of the Hothams of Cranswick and Laxton. Saltmarshe suggests he came of age not many years before 1280, and lived until 1320 × 1322, though his son and heir Richard was holding on his own account in 1302 (Saltmarshe, *Hothams*, pp. 193–96).

We return now to the senior line of the family, known in later years as Hotham

---

[10]  This entry was doubtless the source for Saltmarshe's statement that Thomas of Hotham was sheriff of York in 1218 (Saltmarshe, *Hothams*, p. 28).

## HOTHAM OF SCORBOROUGH AND OF CRANSWICK

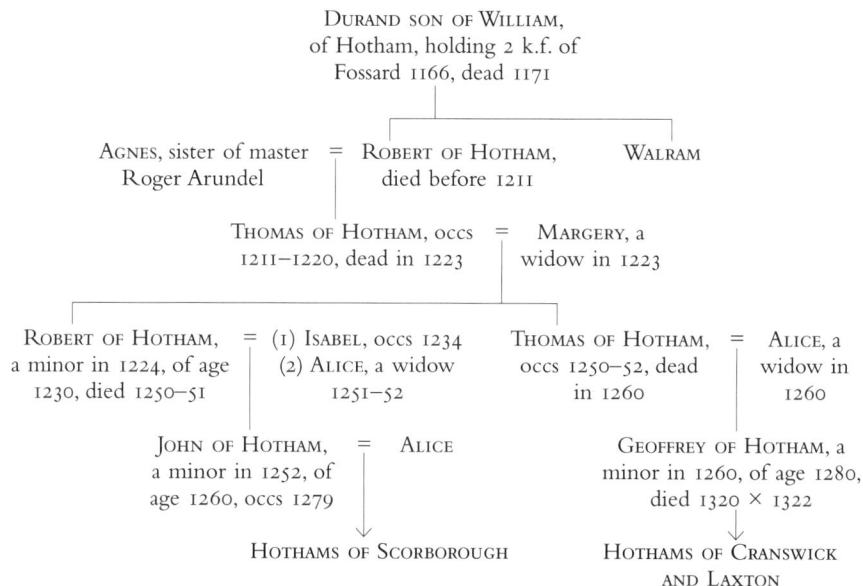

DURAND SON OF WILLIAM,
of Hotham, holding 2 k.f. of
Fossard 1166, dead 1171

AGNES, sister of master  =  ROBERT OF HOTHAM,         WALRAM
Roger Arundel                  died before 1211

THOMAS OF HOTHAM, occs  =  MARGERY, a
1211–1220, dead in 1223       widow in 1223

ROBERT OF HOTHAM,   = (1) ISABEL, occs 1234     THOMAS OF HOTHAM,  =  ALICE, a
a minor in 1224, of age  (2) ALICE, a widow       occs 1250–52, dead      widow in
1230, died 1250–51           1251–52                     in 1260                1260

JOHN OF HOTHAM,    =    ALICE           GEOFFREY OF HOTHAM, a
a minor in 1252, of                           minor in 1260, of age 1280,
age 1260, occs 1279                           died 1320 × 1322

HOTHAMS OF SCORBOROUGH          HOTHAMS OF CRANSWICK
                                                              AND LAXTON

of Scorborough. John, the son and heir of Robert of Hotham, was of age in 1260, when Geoffrey of Hotham was in his wardship. In 1275 John of Hotham and Alice his wife purchased a messuage and 1 bv. land in Hutton and Cranswick for 30m. (*YF*, 1272–1300, pp. 4–5), and in 1279–81, John, son of Robert of Hotham claimed services and other dues from Joan, widow of William of Upsall, which he claimed her grandmother, another Joan, had rendered to his father Robert in the time of Henry III for the manor of Sneaton (*Ctl. Gisborough*, 1, 274n, citing 'Yorkshire Assize Rolls 8 and 9 Edw. I, N.I., 9-1, fo. 69'). On the death of Peter de Mauley II in 1279 John of Hotham was found to hold 2 k.f. in Hotham, Easthorpe, and Cranswick (*YI*, 1, 196). John of Hotham had a grant of free warren in his demesne lands in Hotham, Scorborough and Bursea in 1290 (*CalCh*, 1257–1300, p. 366). For details of his successors, who were without exception named John Hotham until the end of the fifteenth century, see Saltmarshe, *Hothams*, passim.

**R766.** Gift to the hospital by Thomas son of Robert of Hotham of the toft with croft in Hotham, between the toft the hospital had before and the land of the canons of Watton [*c.*1214 × 1223]

ORIGINAL: *a* BL, Stowe Ch. 452, 14 cm. (wide) × 11 cm., bottom turn-up 25 mm., three slits for seal tag, each through both layers of parchment, with the two lowermost slits forming a narrow strip of 1.5 mm. width, rather than the usual arrangement of a slit in the bottom crease of the turn-up; remains of seal, brick red, round, 30 mm. diameter, design and legend indecipherable. Medieval endorsements: *Thom' fil' Roberti de i. tofto cum crofto in Hodhum*; *Hotham*. ABSTRACTS: *c* MS Dods. 120b, f. 37ᵛ, first six witnesses and Stowe only, from Rawl., f. 188, now missing; *d* MS Dods. 108, f. 80ᵛ, first seven witnesses only, drawing of outline of seal on tag, round, 'on horseback', from the original *ex bundello hosp. sancti Petri et sancti Leonardi Ebor'*, doubtless formerly in

St Mary's Tower. CALENDAR: *Cat. Stowe*, I, 779, from *a*. FACSIMILE: Saltmarshe, *Hothams*, pp. 28–29.

Omnibus presentes literas visuris vel audituris Thomas filius Roberti de Hodhum salutem. Noverit universitas vestra me caritatis et pietatis intuitu et pro salute anime mee et animarum antecess[orum][11] et successorum meorum concessisse dedisse et presenti carta mea confirmasse deo et pau[peri]bus hospitalis sancti Petri Ebor' illud toftum cum crofto quod iacet in predicta villa de Hodhum [inter] toftum quod ipsi prius habuerunt ibidem, et terram canonicorum de Watton'; tenendum scilicet et habendum predictis pauperibus in puram et perpetuam elemosinam liberam quietam et solutam ab omni seculari servicio et exactione sicut aliqua elemosina liberius et melius dari potest. Ego autem [et] heredes mei predictum toftum cum suis perti-nentiis et libertatibus et liberis consuetudinibus predictis pauperibus in perpetuum warantizabimus aquietabimus et defendemus in omnibus et contra omnes homines. In huius autem rei robur et testimonium huic scripto sigillum meum apposui. Testibus, Willelmo de Daiuill', Petro de Saunton', Thoma de Faxflet, Alano de Flaguill', Rogero Hay, Petro filio Petri, Dionis(io) de Ellerker, Thoma Braba'c', Iohanne Todhe, Roberto de Stow', Willelmo f(ilio) Osberti et Aluredo de Bru(n)g(ar)fl(eta) et multis aliis.

This deed was probably given shortly before master Hugh's grant of the same land (R767). Thomas of Hotham was dead in 1223 (FN); Alan de Flamville was dead in 1232 (*EYF*, p. 32). Thomas Hay appears to have resigned his interest in North Cave to his son Roger Hay between *c*.1210 and 1225 (FN).

**R767.** Grant at fee-farm by master H[ugh] and the brethren of the hospital to Robert son of Hugh de Trehus of a toft with a croft in Hotham, specified as in R766, paying 16*d*. annually, and a portion of chattels as an obituary payment [1214 × *c*.1223]

ORIGINAL: *a* BL, Stowe Ch. 451, 17 cm. (wide) × 8 cm., bottom turn-up, slit for seal tag, seal gone. Medieval endorsements: *Dimissio terre eiusd'*; Hotham. ABSTRACT: *c* MS Dods. 108, f. 80ᵛ, no witnesses, from the original deed in the St Leonard's bundle, presumably formerly in St Mary's Tower. CALENDAR: *Cat. Stowe*, I, 779, from *a*.

Omnibus presentes literas visuris vel audituris magister H[ugo] rector et fratres hospital(is) sancti Petri Ebor' salutem. Noverit universitas vestra nos concessisse et presenti carta nostra confirmasse Roberto filio Hugonis de Trehus unum toftum cum crofto in Hodhum, illud scilicet quod iacet inter toft(um) quod nos prius habuimus et terram canonicorum de Watton' in predicta villa, tenendum scilicet et habendum predicto Roberto et heredibus suis cum omnibus suis pertinenciis de nobis libere integre et quiete iure hereditario, reddendo inde nobis annuatim pro omni servicio ad nos pertinente sexdecim denarios, videlicet octo denarios ad festum sancti Martini et octo denarios ad Pentecost'. Predictus autem Robertus et heredes eius vel quicumque in predicta terra manserit portionem catallorum eos contingentem in obitu suo domui nostre fideliter relinquent. Hoc autem pro se et pro suis heredibus tactis sacrosanctis iuravit predictus Robertus et affidavit. In huius autem rei robur et testimonium huic scripto sigillum nostrum aposuimus. Testibus, Bernardo, Iohanne, Rogero fratribus hospitalis et capellanis, Radulfo de Fontibus, Fulcone, Rogero, Iohanne, Radulfo

---

[11] Left-hand side of the deed damaged by damp.

capellanis secularibus, Anketino, Godefrido, Waltero, Swano, Ricardo, Stephano, Willelmo et aliis fratribus laicis, Ricardo Fossard', Roberto de Stow', Waltero de Beningburg' et multis aliis.

This deed was probably given shortly after R766. Hugh became rector in 1214 × 1217. For *Threhous*, which lay between Hotham and North Cave, see *VCH Yorks ER*, IV, 118 and n.

**R768.** Grant and quitclaim by Alan de Trehus, son of Robert de Trehus, to Robert son of Ranulf of Broomfleet, of a toft in Hotham which the hospital had granted to Alan's father Robert [1232 × 1260]

ABSTRACTS: *c* MS Dods. 120b, f. 37ᵛ, from Rawl., f. 188, now missing; *d* MS Dods. 108, f. 80ʳ, 1st witness only, from the original deed in the St Leonard's bundle, presumably formerly in St Mary's Tower.

Omnibus hoc scriptum visuris vel audituris Alanus de Thehus[12] filius Roberti de Threhus salutem. Noveritis me conc(essisse)[13] et quiet' cl(amasse) de me et heredibus meis imperpetuum Roberto filio Ranulfi de Bromflete,[14] heredibus et assignatis, unum toftum et(c.)[15] in Hothum, illud scilicet toftum quod magister et fratres hospitalis sancti Petri Ebor' dederunt et conc(esserunt) Roberto patri meo, tenendum et habendum dicto Roberto et heredibus et assignatis suis libere quiete bene et in pace cum omnibus pertinenciis, ita videlicet quod ego Alanus et heredes mei numquam in eodem tofto aliquod ius vel clam(eum) possimus vendicare. In cuius rei testimonium presenti scripto sigillum meum apposui. Hiis [testibus] Elya de Flamvill', Petro filio Petri, Iohanne filio Simonis, Iohanne Thothe, Stephano Talun, Roberto filio David, W[illelm]o Thothe, Thoma de Hothom et aliis. fo. 188.

Ellis de Flamville succeeded Alan de Flamville after 1232, in which year Alan was dead and his heir under age (*EYF*, p. 32). The *terminus ad quem* depends on the identification of the last witness as Thomas son of Thomas of Hotham, which cannot be regarded as entirely certain.

## *Helmesley* [Upper Helmsley, NR]

[Upper] Helmsley deeds were entered on f. 191, now missing, and f. 220ᵛ. For the deeds copied on f. 220ᵛ, and a note on Upper Helmsley, see R638–R641.

**R769.** Notification by Nigel d'Aubigny, addressed to Th[omas] archbishop of York and the grantor's brother William, that he had surrendered to God and St Peter and the church of York, for the sustenance of the poor brethren near that church, 2 ct. land in Helmsley which he had taken from them. And to William son of Warin, to whom he had given the land, he gives in exchange 4 ct. in Thornton, with all the men there [1109 × 1114]

---

[12]  *d: Threhus.*
[13]  *d: dedisse.*
[14]  *d: Brungerflet.*
[15]  *d: cum pertinenciis.*

COPY:YML, Reg. Mag. Album, III, f. 29ʳ, new f. 231ʳ. PRINTED: Raine, *Historians*, III, no. 38, where dated *c*.1130; *Mowbray Charters*, no. 7, where dated 1109 × 1114.

*Carta Nigelli de Albeni de ii. carucatis terre in Hameseie.*
Th[ome] Ebor' archiepiscopo et vicecomiti et omnibus baronibus comitatus Ebor' et Willelmo fratri suo et omnibus amicis et omnibus suis francis et anglis Nigellus de Albeni salutem et amicitiam. Sciat dilectio vestra amici karissimi quod ego pro dilectione dei et redemptione anime mee reddidi et dedi deo et sancto Petro et ecclesie Ebor' et victui pauperum fratrum qui ecclesie illi adiacent ii. caracatas terre in Hameseie quas ego eis abstuleram. Et Willelmo filio Warini cui eas dederam dono Thornetun in excambio videlicet quatuor carucatas terre cum omnibus hominibus qui in eis sunt. Mando igitur tibi et precor Willelme frater meus ut sicut deum et animam diligis nullo modo hanc meam donationem violare presumas sed firmiter tenere studeas. T(estibus) Th[ome] archiepiscopo, et R[anulfo] Dunelm' episcopo, et Math(ilde) coniuge mea, et Guidone cap(ellano) et Roberto de Mainill' et Hugone de Ra(m)pan et Henrico de Monte Forti.

In view of its early date, it is unlikely that this deed was ever in the hospital's archive, or entered in the cartulary. It is one of a series by which Nigel d'Aubigny, gravely ill, repenting his *peccata maxima*, and preparing for death, returned lands which he had taken from St Peter's in York, its hospital, Durham cathedral, Serlo the monk, St Mary's in York and lay tenants (*Mowbray Charters*, nos 2–10). In a deed addressed to Henry I, he notifies the king that he had restored several estates to *Eboracensi ecclesie*, and to *hospitio pauperum fratrum eiusdem ecclesie ii. carrucatas terre in Hameseie* (ibid., no. 2). Appointing his brother William as his heir, he requested him to superintend the restorations (ibid., no. 3).

The witnesses to the present deed include Maud, Nigel's first wife, who was divorced from her previous husband in 1107, and was repudiated by Nigel before June 1118, when he married his second wife Gundreda (*CP*, IX, 368–69). It is likely therefore that the archbishop to whom the deed is addressed, and who attests, was Thomas, rather than his successor Thurstan. Thurstan, though elected and enthroned as archbishop soon after the death of Archbishop Thomas in 1114, was not consecrated until 1119, and was out of the country for much of the intervening period.[16]

Greenway was uncertain of the location of Thornton, given in compensation to William son of Warin, suggesting Thornton Bridge (NR). Roger de Mowbray also held in Thornton-on-the-Hill (par. Coxwold) and Thornton Dale (*Mowbray Charters*, p. 264).

**R770.** Gift to St Peter and [St] Leonard, York, by Ralph son of Wimund and Peter his brother, of the *mansio* of the priest in Helmsley, with the toft, bounded by a ditch, with half of the road which goes from the vill to the church, towards [Sand] Hutton, which the donors knew to be grant-in-alms in the time of their father and Robert their brother. The other part of the road was in the donors' fee [*c*.1150 × 1177, probably towards the end of the period]

ABSTRACT: MS Dods. 120b, f. 38ʳ, from Rawl., f. 191, now missing.

---

[16]  In addition, the abbreviation *Th'* rather than *T'* favours Thomas over Thurstan, but only slight weight can be attached to this as the deed is not an archiepiscopal act, nor an original (Clay, 'A Worcester Charter', pp. 134–35).

Radulfus filius Wimundi et Petrus frater eius dederunt sancto Petro et Leonardo Ebor' in puram elemosinam mansionem presbiteri in Hemelssi cum tofto sicut cinctum est certo fossato et extra cum medietate vie que vadit de villa ad ecclesiam versus Hotona', quod scimus tempore patris nostri et tempore Roberti fratris nostri elemosinam fuisse. Altera pars enim vie[17] est de feodo nostro. Test' Robertus decanus, Simon' canonico Ebor', Willelmo de Bridehala.[18] fo. 191.

As the survey of 1086 shows that Nigel Fossard held 4 ct. in [Upper] Helmsley, it is probable that the donor is the Ralph son of Wimund who held 1 k.f. of Fossard in 1166. Ralph son of Wimund held land in Lockington and Etton, but his interest in Upper Helmsley is otherwise unknown (FN). Sand Hutton (*Hoton* in 1086) is 1 m. to the north of Upper Helmsley. Peter son of Wimund attested in '*c*.1154 × *c*.1172', 'late Henry II' and '*c*.1160 × 1175' (*EYC*, XI, nos 159, 209, 218). Simon the canon was in all probability Simon de Sigillo, as there is no evidence for any other canon of York called Simon during the second half of the twelfth century. Simon, canon of York, occurs as a witness to an act of William, bishop of Durham, in 1143 × 1152[19] (*EYC*, II, no. 957); and in 1143 × 1154[20] Simon de Sigillo, canon of York, attested a deed of Robert, dean of York (ibid., I, no. 450). Simon de Sigillo was referred to as the former holder of Langtoft prebend in 1164 × 1177[21] (*EYC*, I, nos 161, 282–84). There is no evidence he was living after 1177. Robert the dean, Simon the canon, and William de Briddesh(ala) are amongst the witnesses to a gift to the hospital made most probably in 1173 × 1177 (C92 [*EYC*, III, no. 1562]). This may indicate the approximate date of the present deed.

**R771.** Grant at fee-farm by Hugh, rector of the hospital, and the brethren to William son of Roger Gernun, of the 2 ct. in Helmsley which the said Roger and Maud his wife held of the brethren, paying 24*s*. annually, and a portion of chattels as an obituary payment [1214 × *c*.1220]

ABSTRACT: MS Dods. 120b, f. 38ʳ, from Rawl., f. 191, now missing; see R772, which preserves a better text of parts of the deed.

Hugo rector hospitalis beati Petri Ebor' et fratres ipsius domus dederunt et conc(esserunt) Willelmo filio Rogeri Gernun illas duas carucatas terre in Hemeleseia quas dictus Rogerus et Matildis uxor eius de nobis tenuerunt, reddendo annuatim 24s. Et in obitu omnium hominum manentium in predicta terra habebimus port(ion)em catallorum que ipsos morientes contigerit. Test(e) Thoma de Langwath'. fo. 191.

Hugh became rector in 1214 or later. Thomas de Langwath is usually called master after *c*.1220.

---

[17] MS: *via*.
[18] Witnesses in both nominative and ablative.
[19] The period for William as bishop.
[20] The earliest date for Robert as dean, and the latest for the witness Hugh the treasurer.
[21] Whilst Archbishop Roger was legate, and before the deaths of Geoffrey, provost of Beverley, and master Robert [Magnus]. The attestation of Nicholas *de capella domini archiepiscopi*, with his colleague Peter, to nos 282–85 suggests a date late in the period. The presence of Jeremy as canon, rather than archdeacon, and of John, archdeacon of Nottingham, is not good evidence for an earlier date (see Carpenter, 'York Dignitaries', passim).

**R772.** Acknowledgement of receipt, with recital, by William son of Roger Gernun of Helmsley, of the hospital's grant R771 [1214 × c.1220]

ABSTRACT: MS Dods. 108, f. 80ʳ, from the original in the St Leonard's bundle, presumably formerly in St Mary's Tower.

Sciant presentes et futuri quod ego Willelmus filius Rogeri Gernun de Hemeleseya recepi cartam hospitalis sancti Petri Ebor' in hec verba: Sciant presentes et futuri quod ego magister Hugo rector hospitalis sancti Petri Ebor' et fratres ipsius domus concessimus et presenti carta nostra confirmavimus Willelmo filio Rogeri Gernun illas duas carucatas terre in Hemeleseya quas dictus Rogerus et Matildis uxor eius de nobis tenuerunt, tenendas scilicet et habendas de nobis in feudo et hereditate predictis Willelmo et heredibus suis etc., reddendo nobis annuatim viginti quatuor solidos etc.

## *Weaverthorp*²² [Everthorpe, par. North Cave]

The Contents List cites f. 192 for *Weaverthorp*, but it is clear from the position of the entry between the East Riding vills with initial 'H' and those with initial 'K', and from Dodsworth's abstracts, that Everthorpe, sometimes spelt *Iverthorpe* in early documents, was the place meant. Perhaps there were also Weaverthorpe deeds on f. 192, but there is no evidence for a hospital holding there. For Everthorpe, where 4 ct. were held by Thomas Hay of the Fossard fee in 1200, see *VCH Yorks ER*, IV, 25–26 and FN: Hay. By the following early-thirteenth-century deeds the hospital received 4½ a. in Everthorpe. In 1385 the master sued William Greg of Ellerker for cutting his grass at Everthorpe, and taking grass and hay to the value of 40s. (Baildon, *Monastic Notes*, II, 81). The account of 1542 includes a rent in Everthorpe (*Dissolved Houses*, IV, 226).

**R773.** Gift to the hospital by Thomas Hay of 2½ a. in Everthorpe [c.1210 × c.1220]

ABSTRACT: MS Dods. 120b, f. 38ʳ, from Rawl., f. 192, now missing.

Thomas Hay dedit hospitali sancti Petri Ebor' duas acras et dimidiam terre in Uverthorp iuxta Southcave. Testibus, Roberto de Stow, Thoma de Langwath, clericis hospitalis. fo. 192

The date range depends on the earliest date for Robert de Stowe and the latest for Thomas de Langwath, who is usually called master after c.1220. Thomas Hay died in 1226 × 1227, but appears to have resigned his interest in Everthorpe and North Cave to his son Roger by 1225 at the latest (FN).

**R774.** Gift to the hospital's brethren at Broomfleet, by Agnes daughter of Reginald Syre of Everthorpe, of 2 a. meadow in Everthorpe, which lie between the meadow of Sir Roger Hay and the meadow of William son of Hacon of North Cave [1226 × 1245]

ABSTRACT: MS Dods. 120b, f. 38ʳ, from Rawl., f. 192, now missing.

[Ego]²³ Agnes filia R<a>inaldi Syre de Yverthorp dedi <fratribus> hospitalis sancti

---

²² MS Dods. 120b: *Iverthorp al' Uverethorp.*
²³ Supplied.

Petri Ebor' <apud Brungarflet corporantibus> duas acras prati in territorio de Uverthorp que iacent inter pratum domini Rogeri Hai et pratum Willelmi filii Hacon de
Norcava. Testibus, domino Rogero Hay, domino Willelmo de Dayvilla, Rogero filio
eius etc. fo. 192.

The appearance of Roger Hay as *dominus* suggests a date after 1226 (FN). The deed
was issued before rector Hugh's grant of the same land (R775).

**R775.** Grant by Hugh, rector of the hospital, to Walter, chaplain, son of Peter Pugil
    of North Cave, of the property described in R774 [1226 × 1245]

NOTED: MS Dods. 120b, f. 38ʳ, in margin, from Rawl., f. 192, now missing.

Hugo rector hospitalis dedit hec Walt(er)io capellano filio Petri Pugil de Nor<th>cava.
fo. 192.

The date is between the grant to the hospital (R774) and the death of rector Hugh.


## *Karnetby* [Carnaby]

According to the Contents List, the Carnaby deeds were copied to the Rawlinson
volume on ff. 195–96, now missing. 13 ct. in Carnaby were in the hands of the king
in 1086, and passed to the Percy fee before the middle of the twelfth century (*EYC*,
XI, no. 101n). In 1284–85 Carnaby was assessed 12 ct. (*KI*, p. 59). At least two thirds
of the vill were held of Percy by the descendants of Picot, who held of William de
Percy in Bolton-upon-Dearne and Sutton upon Derwent in 1086, which family
took the surname Percy and frequently attested deeds with the additional description 'of Carnaby'. Clay has given a full account of the family (*EYC*, XI, 104–12). At
his death in 1267 Peter de Percy [of Carnaby] held, with other property, 8 ct. in
Carnaby. Carnaby does not appear in the papal confirmations to the hospital until
1204, when 1 ct. there was included in the bull of Innocent III (C182 [*Letters Innoc.
III*, no. 562]). This was presumably the 1 ct. given by Robert de Percy in 1157 × 1175,
later confirmed by his son and grandson (R776–R777, R779). In 1218–19 Robert
de Percy was found to have disseised the master of his free tenement in Carnaby,
carrying off his crop in time of peace (*Yorkshire Eyre Rolls*, no. 1114). The matter did
not rest there, for in 1221 Robert de Percy owed ½m. for a writ of attaint in his case
concerning common of pasture in Carnaby against the master of the hospital (*PR*,
5 Hen. III, p. 136), but agreement had apparently been reached by 1225 (R779). The
hospital's grange of Carnaby was granted protection by a bull of Pope Honorius in
1216 × 1227 (C228 [Cott., f. 50ʳ]). Carnaby is not mentioned in the extents of the
later thirteenth century. John son of Walter de Uppiby of Carnaby called the master
to warrant a toft and 8 bv. in Carnaby in 1317 (Baildon, *Monastic Notes*, II, 77). In
1429 the hospital held 10 bv. in Carnaby of Percy (*VCH Yorks ER*, II, 127). Carnaby
is not listed in the *Valor Ecclesiasticus*, but the account of 1542 includes a rent there
(*Dissolved Houses*, IV, 226), and the former possessions of the hospital in 1557 included
a manor house in Carnaby with 16 bv. A capital messuage and lands, and another
messuage, three cottages and lands in the tenure of Roger Cowton in Carnaby, late
of the hospital of St Leonard, were amongst the property sold to James Lambarte of
Well, co. York, gentleman, and George Cotton of London in 1557 (*CalPat*, 1557–1558,
p. 273). For the subsequent history of the hospital's estate, see *VCH Yorks ER*, II, 127.

**R776.** Gift to the hospital by Robert de Percy of 1 ct. land in Carnaby with so much toft as belongs to it [and a toft with vivary],[24] with part of the donor's culture in *Buckeldedaila*, just as the donor perambulated with master Swain and placed boundary markers with his own hand, for the health of his soul and that of his lord William [de Percy] [1157 × 1175]

COPIES: *d* MS Dods. 8, f. 139[r]; *e* Burton transcripts 6, f. 83[r], p. 157, B8 N5, slightly abbreviated, seventeen witnesses only, from an original 'penes M[armaduke] F[othergill] et F[rancis] D[rake]';[25] *f* Burton transcripts 1, f. 178[v], p. 304, B20 N45, from a slightly different original. ABSTRACT: *c* MS Dods. 120b, f. 38[v], ten witnesses only, from Rawl., f. 195, now missing. NOTED: MS Dods. 127, f. 10[v], from the same, via Richard Gascoigne's 'liber C', f. 12. NOTED: Drake, *Eboracum*, p. 335, via Torre's collections.

*Carta Roberti de Perceio.*[26]
Notum sit omnibus cristi fidelibus presentibus et futuris quod ego Robertus de Perceio et heredes mei concessimus et dedimus deo et pauperibus hospitalis sancti Petri unam carucatam terre in Carendebi[27] cum tanto tofto quantum ad ipsam carucatam pertinet, et toftum Ucca, [et unum toftum cum ipso vivario sicut mete sui[][28] posite ubi fratres hospitalis edificare debent][29] et ad illam carucatam [terre][30] addidi unam partem culture mee in Bickeldedaila[31] iuxta viam, et ex altera parte vie de altera cultura, sicut perambulavi cum magistro Suano et multis aliis et cruces posui in metis manu propria in puram et perpetuam elemosinam liberam et solutam et quietam ab omni geldo et consuetudine et auxilio et ab omni humano servicio, cum communi pastura eiusdem ville in campo et marisco, et in omnibus pertinentiis pro salute anime mee et omnium antecessorum meorum et pro domino meo Willelmo et heredibus eius, et pro[32] uxore mea et heredibus meis. Dedi etiam totam curtem meam deo et sancto Leonardo pro qua curte ego et heredes mei dabimus eidem hospitali singulis annis unam libram piperis. Hanc autem elemosinam eis dedimus ut participes simus omnium bonorum que fiunt vel facienda sunt in illa sancta domo in vita et in morte. Cuius[33] rei testes sunt Robertus decanus, Simon canon(icus), Radulfus capell(anus), Robertus cap(ellanus), Robertus Wal',[34] Uctredus cap(ellani),[35] Radulfus de Perceio, Paulinus filius episcopi, Robertus filius Stephani, Rogerus de Ruddestain, Waltero Darches, Hugo de Munbi, Willelmus filius eius, Willelmus de Besingbi, Malgerus frater eius, Uctredus, Willelmus filius eius,[36] Willelmus Caperun, Dodin frater eius, Robertus de Clara, Ada clericus, Rogerus prefectus, Hugo, Robertus filius Gamel[37] et ceteri omnes, Pichotus[38] filius meus, Ricardus Malerba, Osmundus, Ernaldus parmentarius.

[24] One copy only.
[25] For this collection of deeds, see Carpenter, 'Torre Charters', pp. 11–12.
[26] Rubric from *d*.
[27] *f: Kerendebi*.
[28] An overtight binding hides the end of this word.
[29] *f* only.
[30] *f* only.
[31] *f, c: Buckeldedaila*.
[32] *f* omits *pro*.
[33] *f: Huius* for *Cuius*.
[34] *f: Walter*.
[35] *f: capellani*.
[36] *f: eius filius*.
[37] *f* has *Hugo filius Gamelli* for *Hugo, Robertus filius Gamel*.
[38] *f: Pichoch filius mei*.

The donor, described as Robert son of Picot, held 3 k.f. of Percy in 1166, which lay in Bolton Percy, Carnaby, Nesfield, and Sutton upon Derwent. He had been succeeded by his son William in 1175 (*EYC*, XI, 104–7). William [de Percy II], mentioned as the donor's lord, died in 1169 × 1175 (ibid., p. 4). As Robert of the hospital had apparently been succeeded by master Swain the earliest date is 1157. For the witness Paulinus, son of Ralph Nuuel, bishop of the Orkneys, see Carpenter, 'Paulinus', pp. 12–13. He was of full age in 1133 × 1141, occurs in 1160, and was dead in 1184.

**R777.** Confirmation to the hospital by William son and heir of Robert de Percy of the grant in alms, as in R776, which his father had given before [*c.*1160 × 1177]

COPY: *d* Burton transcripts 3, f. 92$^{r-v}$, pp. 157–58, B16 N40, abbreviated. NOTED: *c* MS Dods. 120b, f. 38$^v$, 1st, 2nd, 3rd, 6th and 7th witnesses only, from Rawl., f. 195, now missing. NOTED: Drake, *Eboracum*, p. 336, via Torre's collections.

Notum sit omnibus etc. quod ego Willelmus filius Roberti de Perceio et heres concessi et dedi etc. pauperibus <hospitalis> sancti Petri Ebor' [92/158$^v$] illam elemosinam quam pater meus eis prius dederat, videlicet unam carrucatam terre in Kerendeby, tantum toftum$^{39}$ quantum ad ipsam carrucatam pertinet, et toftum Ucca, et unum toftum cum ipso vivario sicut mete sunt posite etc. et illas partes culture in Buck-eldedail ex utraque parte vie, in puram etc. liberam etc. ab omni geldo etc. humano servicio cum communi pastura eiusdem ville in campo et marisco etc. pro salute anime etc. Concessi etiam et dedi sicut pater meus concessit deo et sancto Leonardo totam curtem meam. Hanc autem donationem feci ut ego et uxor mea et heredes mei simus participes omnium bonorum que fiunt vel facienda sunt in illa sancta domo in vita et in morte. Huius rei sunt testes, Robertus Pict', Reinerus Flamm', Willelmus clericus de Wath, Henricus de Perceio, Picot filius Hugonis, Helias de Wlvel, Martinus Mala-herba, Willelmus filius Willelmi.

William son of Robert de Percy succeeded his father in 1166 × 1175, and died in 1209 × 1213 (*EYC*, XI, 107–8). The suggested date range rests on the identification of the first witness as Robert Peitevin of Altofts, who died in 1166 × 1177 (FN). The description of the grantor as 'son and heir' and the nominative witness clause are also suggestive of a date early in William's career. The second witness was probably Reiner the Fleming (*Flandrigena*), who with three others held a third part of 1 k.f. of Percy in 1166 (*EYC*, XI, 283).

**R778.** Final concord between Hugh, rector, and the brethren of the hospital and Sir Robert de Percy concerning land in Carnaby. October 1219 × October 1220.

ABSTRACT: *c* MS Dods. 120b, f. 38$^v$, from Rawl., probably f. 195. Not calendared in *YF*, 1218–1231.

Finis de premissis 4.H.3. inter Hugonem rectorem et fratres hospitalis sancti Petri Ebor' et dominum Robertum de Percy.

---

$^{39}$ MS: *tanto tofto.*

**R779.** Confirmation to the hospital by Robert son of William de Percy of the gift made by his grandfather Robert of 1 ct. in Carnaby, and particularly common in the whole of the marsh; also confirmation of the houses they have in Ryecroft and in the south of *Bukeldedaile* [1219 × 1225]

COPY: *d* Burton transcripts 3, f. 93ʳ, p. 159, B21 N55, abbreviated. NOTED: *c* MS Dods. 120b, f. 38ᵛ, in Percy pedigree, first two and last four witnesses only, from Rawl., f. 195, now missing.

Omnibus presentibus litteras etc. Robertus filius Willelmi de Percy salutem. Noveritis me ratam et gratam habere donationem Roberti avi mei de una carucata terre cum pertinenciis quam deo et pauperibus hospitalis sancti Petri Ebor' caritative dedit in territorio de Kerneteby, maxime autem communam per totum mariscum pro salutem anime etc. Domus autem quas habent in Ryecroft et in australi de Bukeldedaile, libere etc. concessi. In huius autem rei etc. apposui. Testibus, magistris Rogero decano, Galfrido precentore, Willelmo thesaurario, Waltero archidiacono de Estriding, Iohanne Romano, Willelmo de Lanum, Mauricio, canonicis, magistris Nicholao, Roberto de Holebech, Petro succentore et aliis capellanis Ebor' ecclesie, Roberto de Schegness, Radulfo Nuuel, Willelmo Fairfax, Roberto de Stow etc.

This confirmation presumably represents a resolution of the disputes between Robert de Percy and the hospital. Roger de Lisle became dean in 1219 or 1220, and Robert de Percy was dead in 1229 (*EYC*, XI, 106, 108). William of Laneham was archdeacon of Durham by 1224, and John Romeyn was subdean of York by 1228, but the absence of these titles is not an entirely secure indication of date. Peter the succentor was the predecessor of Richard, who was holding the office in 1219 × 1225 (R449; *YMF*, no. 30).

**R780.** Gift to the hospital by Robert son of William de Percy of 7 a. land and meadow in Carnaby, being those which Thomas the fisherman formerly held, which lie outside the enclosure of the hospital towards the south. Also a plot to extend their courtyard next to the road which goes from Carnaby to Auburn,[40] and as much common pasture as belongs to the hospital's tenement in Carnaby, with entry and exit within the donor's enclosure called *Flaskedaile*, and *Hunkelholm*, when they carry away their corn and hay [1224 × 1229]

COPY: *d* MS Dods. 7, f. 18ʳ, outline pencil drawing of a tag and seal, round, a shield, no further detail. NOTED: *c* MS Dods. 120b, f. 38ᵛ, with list of witnesses, excluding first and last, in Percy pedigree, from Rawl., f. 195, now missing.

*Carta Roberti filii Willelmi de Percy.*
Omnibus cristi fidelibus ad quos presens scriptum pervenerit, Robertus filius Willelmi de Percy salutem. Noverit universitas vestra me caritatis et pietatis intuitu dedisse et concessisse et hac presenti carta mea confirm(asse) deo et pauperibus hospitalis sancti Petri Ebor' septem acras terre et prati in Kernetby, scilicet illas quas Thomas Piscator aliquando tenuit, que iacent extra clausum dicti hospitalis propinquiores versus austrum. Et pretera dedi eis quamdam terram ad curiam suam augmentandum que extendit se a porta eorum usque ad capud australe curie eorum, iuxta viam

[40]   A depopulated village in Carnaby township (*PN YorksER*, p. 87).

que tendit de Kerneteby versus Aleburne. Et preterea dedi eis communem pasturam quantum pertinet ad tenementum eorum in eadem villa sine occasione, cum libero introitu et exitu infra clausum meum, quod appellatur Flaskedaile, et Hunkelholm, cum bladum et fenum inde asportato fuerit, tenendum scilicet et habendum totum predictum tenementum et predictam communiam cum omnibus pertinenciis suis predictis pauperibus in puram et perpetuam elemosinam libere integre et quiete ab omni <servicio et> exactione sicut aliqua elemosina liberius et melius teneri potest et haberi. Ego autem et heredes mei omnia predicta memoratis pauperibus warantizabimus et adquietabimus et defendemus in omnibus et contra omnes homines imperpetuum. In huius autem rei robur et testimonium huic scripto sigillum meum apposui. Hiis testibus, Ricardo abbate de Seleby, domino Ricardo de Percy, Eustachio de Ludeham <tunc> vic(ecomite) Ebor', Nicholao Basset, Willelmo Darel, Gilberto de Atona, Iohanne de Atona, Ricardo Gramayre, Nicholao de Hewich, Marmaduc Darel, Iohanne de Toueton, Galfrido de Rughford, Roberto de Bowelton et multis aliis.

Eustace of Lowdham was undersheriff from Michaelmas 1224 until May 1229. Richard was abbot of Selby throughout this period. The second witness was presumably the son of Agnes de Percy and Jocelin de Louvain, who was dead in 1244. The sixth witness was Gilbert of Ayton, in Pickering Lythe wapentake, who died early in 1235, when his son and heir William was underage (*RFine Excerpta*, I, 276, 281). For him and his family, later the Lords Aton, see *Baronage*, II, 98–99; *EYC*, II, no. 996; *CP*, I, 324–26.

## *Kexby* [par. Catton]

Little is known of the early tenure of Kexby, which is not mentioned in Domesday, but was doubtless included in the extensive soke of the manor of Catton (*VCH Yorks*, II, 219). Some details of the later tenants of the manor are given at *VCH Yorks ER*, III, 159–61. The Contents List gives f. 197 (now missing) for Kexby, and Dodsworth's abstracts are referenced to this folio. The hospital's possessions there were apparently restricted to the 2 a. noticed in Dodsworth's abstracts, and are not mentioned elsewhere.

It has not been possible to determine the ancestors of Alexander BURDUN, to whom he refers in his deed of confirmation to the hospital of 2 a. in Kexby made in *c.*1210 × *c.*1230 (R781), but it is likely he was the successor to, and possibly the son of, William Burdun, who was holding land in Grimston (in Gilling) in 1197 × 1214.[41] In view of the Percy tenancies held by later members of the family, it is not improbable that William Burdun, who attested deeds of William de Percy [II] in 1164 × 1175 and of Agnes de Percy in 1180 × 1204 (*EYC*, XI, nos 23, 27, 76; C522 [*EYC*, I, no. 231]), was the same man or at least of the same family. The coincidence of names suggests that William and Alexander Burdun, who held land in Sancton in the late twelfth and early thirteenth centuries, were the same men, but no proof is available. William Burdun gave land in *Alderges*, near Sancton, to Watton Priory in 1200 (*EYC*, XII, 22n, 82). Alexander son of William of Sancton quitclaimed to Watton a rent of 8s. from a carucate in Sancton, which Alexander Burdun used to hold of the grantor, with the

---

41 See below.

homage of the same Alexander Burdun, in 1217 × 1220[42] (Burton transcripts 2, f. 129ʳ, p. 222, B25 N7). Alexander Burdun gave Watton the service of Robert son of Walter of Skegness from a carucate of land in Sancton (MS Dods. 7, f. 354ᵛ).

Alexander Burdun was a recognitor in an assize of mort d'ancestor concerning a tenement in Wheldrake in 1218 (*Yorkshire Eyre Rolls*, no. 351), but again there is no proof that this was the ancestor of the Burduns of Kexby, and the relationship between Alexander Burdun and Thomas son of Robert Burdun, who confirmed the 2 a. in Kexby and 7 a. in Wilberfoss in 1267 × 1286 (R782) remains unclear. Robert Burdun, who attested a Wilberfoss Priory deed concerning land in Catton in 1239 × 1244[43] (MS Dods. 7, f. 352ʳ), was named as the tenant of lands amounting to 11 bv. in Wilberfoss, holding of Alan of Catterton, who held of William de Kyme, in 1260 (*CalInqPM*, I, 131). In a mid-thirteenth century Percy feodary Robert Burdun was said to hold 3 ct. in [Hund-] Burton[44] and 1 ct. in Catton (*Ctl. Percy*, p. 474). Robert was doubtless dead in 1276, when Thomas Burdun and Alexander Burdun attested a deed of Robert de Percy, lord of Bolton [Percy] in Ainsty, after the *milites* (*CalCl*, 1279–1288, p. 49). In 1267 × 1278,[45] Thomas Burdun of Kexby witnessed a deed of the prior and convent of Warter, also after the *milites* (*CalCh*, 1257–1300, p. 207); and in 1267 × 1286 Thomas son of Robert Burdun of Kexby confirmed to the hospital land in Kexby and Wilberfoss (R782). Some doubt is introduced into the apparently straightforward succession from Robert Burdun to his son Thomas by a deed of Roger Burdun, inspected in 1360 on the petition of Thomas Ughtred. By this deed, apparently dating from 1242 × 1253,[46] Roger Burdun of Kexby granted to Thomas Burdun of Kexby and Isabel his wife all his lands, to wit the manor of Kexby, and lands in Wilberfoss, Upper Catton, Hundburton, Stamford Bridge, and Elstob in the bishopric of Durham, the manor of Grimston (in Gilling, NR), and 6s. 11d. rent in Wiganthorpe (par. Terrington, NR), to hold to them and the heirs of their bodies, rendering to the grantor for his life 100m. annually, with remainder to William, brother of the said Thomas and the heirs of his body, with reversion to the right heirs of the grantor (*CalPat*, 1358–1361, p. 488). This is perhaps most plausibly explained as a simple error of transcription by which Robert Burdun became Roger Burdun, though the apparent date is rather early in the career of Thomas Burdun for such a feoffment.

In 1261 × 1290[47] Brian son of Alan gave lands in Fimber to Sir Thomas Burdun of Kexby, which the donor's grandfather Brian son of Alan had given to William de Neville of Muston in marriage with Isabel his daughter (MS Dods. 9, f. 86ᵛ, citing MS Dods. 156, f. 92a;[48] *EYC*, I, no. 632; ibid., II, 465).[49] Sir Thomas Burdun held 1 ct. in Kexby of R[obert] de Percy [of Bolton Percy], of the heirs of H[enry] de Percy, who

---

42   Whilst Hamo was dean of York.
43   Given with the consent of Richard de Percy, who was dead in 1244 (*CP*, x, 452), and attested by Sir Robert Chauncy, who had livery of his lands in 1239 and died in 1246 (*EYC*, II, 177).
44   For the identification of Burton as Hundburton, or Burton Fields, in Stamford Bridge East, see *VCH Yorks ER*, III, 151.
45   Witnessed by Sir Robert de Ros, who succeeded probably in 1264 (*CP*, xi, 94–95), Sir Robert de Percy [of Bolton Percy], who succeeded in 1267 (*EYC*, xi, 110), and inspected in 1278.
46   The witnesses were Sirs Picot Lascelles, Robert de Stuteville, Henry de Deyville, William Malebisse, Roger Lascelles, Roger de Hoton, Alan son of Brian, Robert his brother. Sir Picot Lascelles was dead in 1253 (*CP*, vii, 445). Sir Alan son of Brian of Bedale succeeded his father after July 1242, and was dead in 1267 (*CP*, v, 393).
47   Brian son of Alan of Bedale succeeded his father in 1261 or later, and died in 1306 (*EYC*, v, 204; *CP*, v, 393–94). Thomas Burdun was in possession of land in Fimber in 1290.
48   Abstracts from St Mary JR.
49   For the estate in Fimber, see *VCH Yorks ER*, viii, 69.

## BURDUN AND UGHTRED

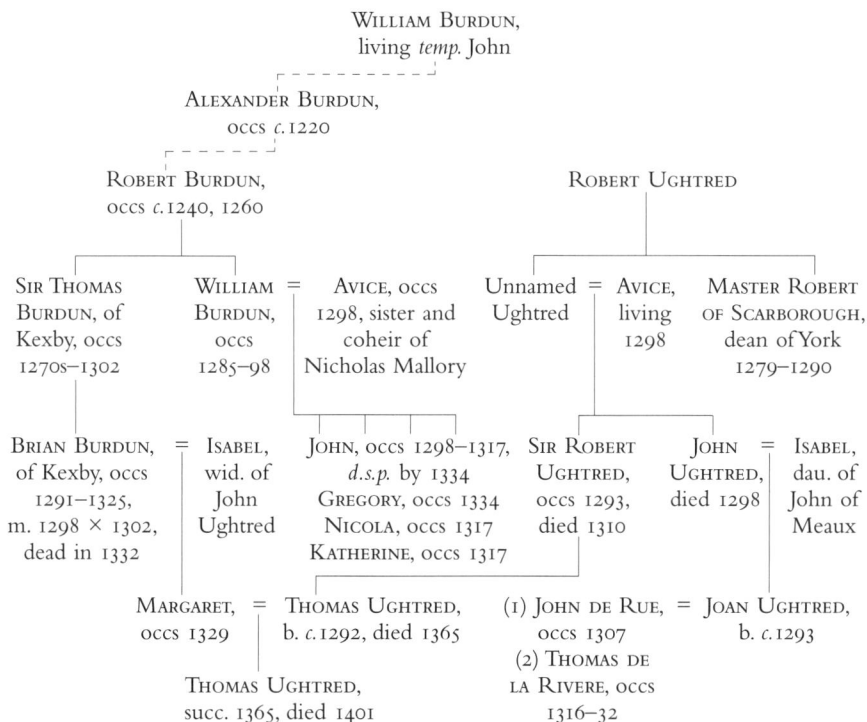

WILLIAM BURDUN,
living *temp.* John

ALEXANDER BURDUN,
occs *c.*1220

ROBERT BURDUN,                          ROBERT UGHTRED
occs *c.*1240, 1260

| SIR THOMAS BURDUN, of Kexby, occs 1270s–1302 | WILLIAM BURDUN, occs 1285–98 | = | AVICE, occs 1298, sister and coheir of Nicholas Mallory | Unnamed Ughtred | = | AVICE, living 1298 | MASTER ROBERT OF SCARBOROUGH, dean of York 1279–1290 |

| BRIAN BURDUN, of Kexby, occs 1291–1325, m. 1298 × 1302, dead in 1332 | = ISABEL, wid. of John Ughtred | JOHN, occs 1298–1317, *d.s.p.* by 1334 GREGORY, occs 1334 NICOLA, occs 1317 KATHERINE, occs 1317 | SIR ROBERT UGHTRED, occs 1293, died 1310 | JOHN UGHTRED, died 1298 | = ISABEL, dau. of John of Meaux |

MARGARET, = THOMAS UGHTRED,
occs 1329      b. *c.*1292, died 1365

THOMAS UGHTRED,
succ. 1365, died 1401

(1) JOHN DE RUE, = JOAN UGHTRED,
occs 1307            b. *c.*1293
(2) THOMAS DE
LA RIVERE, occs
1316–32

held in chief, in the survey of 1284–85. In the same survey Thomas was said to hold
1 ct. in Stamford Bridge or Catton, 3 ct. in [Hund-] Burton, and 20 bv. in Wilberfoss,
of which the church was endowed with 3 bv. His relationship to Alexander Burdun,
whose widow Custancia held 2 bv. in Wilberfoss in dower, and Let[it]ia and Alice
Burdun, who each held 2 bv. there, is not apparent. The land in all these places was
held of the heirs of Percy, who held of the earl of Chester, who held in chief (*KI*,
pp. 61, 86–87). In 1290 Thomas Burdun and his heirs had a grant of free warren in
his demesne lands of Kexby, Catton, [Hund-] Burton, Wilberfoss, Fimber and the
town of Stamford Bridge (*CalCh*, 1257–1300, p. 341). Sir Thomas Burdun, holding
land worth £40 in Ouse and Derwent wapentake, was in January 1300 summoned
to perform military service against the Scots, and again in the following year. There
was another summons in August 1314, but Thomas was then either dead or retired
(*Parl. Writs*, I, 332b, 356, 506; ibid., II (2), 429; II (3), 614). Sir Thomas Burdun, Brian
Burdun and Avice Burdun head the list of inhabitants of Kexby in 1301 (*Lay Subsidy
1301*, p. 104). In 1302–03 Thomas Burdun held 3 ct. 6 bv. in Catton with its soke.
[His son] Brian Burdun was then holding 2 bv. in [Bishop] Wilton and 1 ct. 5 bv. in
Gowthorpe, of the archbishop (*KI*, pp. 254–55, 258). Brian had acquired his interest
in these places by his marriage before February 1302 to Isabel, daughter of John of
Meaux, the widow of John Ughtred who had died in 1298 (*CalFine*, 1272–1307,
p. 449; *CalInqPM*, III, 356; and see below). Brian Burdun first occurs in 1291, when
he was granted protection whilst staying in Scotland with Brian son of Alan (*CalPat*,
1281–1292, p. 468). William de Ros of Helmsley complained that Brian Burdun and

others broke his park at Storthwaite (now Storwood, par. Thornton, ER) in 1298 (*CalPat*, 1292–1301, p. 381). Brian had succeeded his father by January 1313, when as Brian, son of Thomas Burdun, lord of Kexby, he issued a deed to Wilberfoss Priory confirming all their lands in his fee in Wilberfoss and elsewhere (MS Dods. 7, f. 359ᵛ). In 1315, after the death of Henry de Percy, Brian Burdun was said to hold a sixth of a fee in Hundburton, comprising 4 ct. where 23 ct. made a fee, and 1 ct. in Kexby, where 12 ct. made a fee (*CalInqPM*, v, 319). The order for dower for Henry de Percy's widow Eleanor included ¼ k.f. held by Brian Burdun in Hundburton and Kexby (*CalCl*, 1313–1318, p. 149). Brian Burdun was named as the lord of Gowthorpe, Kexby, and joint lord of Hundburton in 1316 (*KI*, pp. 310, 319). His name was returned in a list of knights in Yorkshire in response to a writ of May 1324 (*Parl. Writs*, II (2), 646; ibid., II (3), 614). As Sir Brian Burdun, knight, he witnessed a Catton deed in 1325–26 (*Ctl. Percy*, p. 173). He was dead in 1332, when a fine was made between Thomas Ughtred and Margaret his wife, plaintiffs, and John de Rouclyf and Richard Bernard, defendants, by which the manor of Kexby, with certain exceptions, was to be held to Thomas and Margaret and the heirs of their bodies, subject to the life estate of one third which Isabel, widow of Brian Burdun, held in dower, with remainder to the right heirs of Margaret (*YF*, 1327–1347, p. 58). There can be little doubt that Margaret was Brian Burdun's heir, and that Thomas Ughtred acquired the manor of Kexby and other Burdun estates through his marriage to her.

The interests of 'Roger' Burdun in Grimston and Wiganthorpe which are apparent in the deed examined in 1360 allow the identification of further members of the family. Geoffrey of Etton granted land in Grimston, in the fee of William Burdun, to the dean and chapter of York in 1197 × 1214[50] (Bilson, 'Gilling Castle', p. 110, citing MS Dods. 125, f. 87ᵛ). It is likely that William Burdun was the progenitor of Alexander Burdun, who issued the confirmation to the hospital in *c.*1210 × *c.*1230. Avice, wife of a later William Burdun, was one of the four sisters and coheirs of Nicholas, son of Sir Anketin Mallory, who died shortly before 19 September 1275, holding land in Mowthorpe, Terrington, Wiganthorpe, Huntington and Clifford (*YI*, I, 161). It seems probable that this William was the brother of Thomas Burdun mentioned in the deed of 'Roger' Burdun. William Burdun was holding 2½ ct. in Grimston in 1284–85 (*KI*, p. 120); and in 1298, William Burdun and Avice his wife quitclaimed to John Burdun (probably their son) all right in two messuages, eight tofts, 18 bv. 14 a. land, 20 a. meadow, 60 a. wood, and 6*s.* 11*d.* rent in Mowthorpe, Wiganthorpe and Clifford in exchange for John's grant to them of the manor of Grimston and 6*s.* 11*d.* rent in Wiganthorpe, to be held for their lives with reversion to John (*YF*, 1272–1300, p. 123). John Burdun, and representatives of the other coheirs of Mallory, were holding in Clifford, near Bramham, in 1302–3 (*KI*, pp. 214, 284). In 1317, John son of Sir William Burdun, knight, of Grimston in Ryedale, mentioning his sisters Nicola and Katherine, quitclaimed to Sir Anketin Salvain, knight, and Isolda his wife, all right in certain yearly rents in Mowthorpe, Terrington, and Wiganthorpe (*YD*, I, no. 338). John was dead in 1334 when Gregory, brother and heir of John Burdun, sued the prior of Malton for waste in a tenement in Grimston in Rydale that John had demised to the priory in 1307 for a thirty year term (Malton cartulary, f. 104/101ʳ, citing De Banco, rot. lxxxii).[51] In 1336 Gregory son of William Burdun sold the manor of Grimston to Sir John Moryn, knight, for 100*m.* (*YF*, 1327–1347, p. 98). Details of the subsequent tenants of the manor of Grimston are given at *VCH Yorks NR*, I, 482.

---

[50] Attested by S[imon] dean and H[amo] treasurer.
[51] Cited imperfectly *VCH Yorks NR*, I, 482.

The marriage of Brian Burdun to Isabel, widow of John UGHTRED, in 1298 × 1302, and the marriage of Brian Burdun's heir Margaret to Thomas Ughtred, have been mentioned above. John Ughtred was a younger brother of Sir Robert Ughtred, father of Thomas. The men were members of the family of master Robert [Ughtred] of Scarborough, who was dean of York between 1279 and 1290, and died before 10 March 1291 (*YMF*, I, 8–10). The inquisition following the death of John Ughtred, who died shortly before 24 September 1298, found that John held tenements in Scarborough by the bequest of his uncle master Robert of Scarborough. These tenements John bequeathed on his deathbed to Avice his mother for her life, saving the dower of Isabel his wife. John's grandfather Robert Ughtred is named in connection with the tenements. John's other holdings included land in Owstwick, held of the king as of the honour of Aumale; the grange of Octon held of Meaux Abbey for life; the manor of Gowthorpe which he held with his wife Isabel of the archbishop of York by gift of John of Meaux, father of Isabel; and land in Youlthorpe, [Bishop] Wilton, and Full Sutton. John's heir was his daughter Joan, described variously as 'five and more', 'five', and 'four and a half' years old (*CalInqPM*, III, no. 471; *CalCl*, 1296–1302, pp. 226–28). Joan was married by 1307 when an order was made to cause John de Rue and Joan his wife, daughter and heiress of John Ughtred, to have seisin of the late John's lands, as Joan had proved her age and the king had taken John de Rue's fealty for all the lands which Joan's father held in chief at his death (*CalCl*, 1302–1307, p. 495). It seems that John de Rue did not survive for long, and that Joan remarried Thomas de la Rivere. The lords of Owstwick *cum membris* in 1316 were listed as the abbot of Meaux, William de la Twyer, Amandus de Ruda and Thomas de la Rivere (*KI*, p. 304).[52] In 1326 Thomas de la Rivere of Brandsby, knight, and Joan his wife made a fine concerning lands in Owstwick in Holderness and Bishop Wilton, held partly by Brian Burdun and Isabel his wife [widow of John Ughtred] as Isabel's dower in Joan's inheritance (*YF*, 1327–1347, p. 7). Thomas de la Rivere, lord of Brandsby, knight, and Joan his wife were benefactors of the hospital, to which they gave a rent of 5s. in Scarborough in 1332–33 (M: Scarborough [MS Dods. 120b, f. 97ᵛ]).[53]

As has been noted, John Ughtred was the younger brother of Sir Robert Ughtred. In 1293, Robert Ughtred, knight, and John his brother, executors of the will of master Robert of Scarborough, were absolved from their sentence of excommunication (*Reg. Romeyn*, I, 37).[54] Their father's name is not known. Robert Ughtred died shortly before 24 May 1310, when his heir was his son Thomas, then aged eighteen (*CalInqPM*, V, no. 204).[55] The first notice of Thomas Ughtred's marriage to Margaret, the Burdun heir, comes in 1329, when Thomas Ughtred, Margaret his wife, and Thomas their son made a fine concerning Yearsley, near Coxwold (*YF*, 1327–1347, p. 20). The fine of 1332 noted above provides reasonable evidence that Margaret was the heiress of Brian Burdun, but it has not been possible to confirm that she was Brian's daughter, as is commonly stated. In 1334 Thomas Ughtred had licence to empark his woods of Kexby, Moor Monkton, and Scagglethorpe; and in 1342 he had licence to crenellate his dwelling places of Moor Monkton and Kexby. He died in 1365, when he was succeeded by his son Thomas, mentioned above (*CalPat*,

---

52  For the sale of the Rivere land in Owstwick in 1326 and 1328, and its subsequent tenure, see *VCH Yorks ER*, VII, 87.
53  For further references to the de la Rivere family, see FN.
54  See also MS Dods. 7, f. 213ᵛ, for a receipt given by Robert Ughtred, executor of the will of *dom*. John Ughtred, his brother, dated 20 July 1301.
55  For Robert Ughtred's wife Isabel, the daughter of Richard de Stiveton, see FN: Stiveton of Steeton in Ainsty.

1334–1338, p. 36; ibid., 1340–1343, p. 388; *CP*, XII (2), 160–61). This Thomas Ughtred left £10 in his will of 1398 for a memorial in Catton church, which was to include images of his mother and father and the arms of Ughtred and Burdun (*Test. Ebor.*, I, 243). The arms of Ughtred were quartered with the arms of Burdun by the descendants of Thomas and Margaret and were so displayed on the seal of Sir Robert Ughtred in 1520, and in the armorial window at Aughton hall recorded by Robert Glover in 1584 (*YD*, II, 162n; Ellis, 'Askes of Aughton', pp. 43, 45, 49). For further details of Sir Thomas Ughtred, first Lord Ughtred (*c.*1292–1365), and his family, see *ONDB*; *CP*, XII (2), 158–66; Crouch and Pearson, *Medieval Scarborough*, pp. 43–45. Dodsworth's pedigree of Burdun and Ughtred is at MS Dods. 2, ff. 32$^r$–33$^r$.

**R781.** Confirmation to the hospital by Alexander Burdun of 2 a. meadow in Kexby, which his predecessors gave a long time before [*c.*1210 × *c.*1230]

ABSTRACT: MS Dods. 120b, f. 39$^r$, from Rawl., f. 197, now missing.

Alexander Burdun dedit hospitali beati Petri Ebor' duas acras prati in territorio de Kexby, quas an(te)cessores sui multis temporibus transactis in elemosinam dederunt. Test(e) Roberto de Stowa etc. fo. 197.

The date range is the period for Robert de Stowe.

**R782.** Confirmation to the hospital by Thomas son of Robert Burdun of Kexby of 2 a. meadow in Kexby, being those which the brethren have by the gift of his predecessors, and gift of 7 a. in Wilberfoss, and a toft in the same vill near the exit of the vill towards Thornton [1267 × 1286]

ABSTRACT: MS Dods. 120b, f. 39$^r$, from Rawl., f. 197, now missing.

Thomas filius Roberti Burdun de Kexeby dedit predicto hospitali duas acras prati in territorio de Kexby, illas videlicet quas idem fratres habent de dono antecessorum suorum, et 7 acras terre in Wilberfosse et unum toftum in eadem villa iuxta exitum ville versus Thorneton. Testibus, <dominis Roberto de Percy et> Thoma de Huck militibus, Ricardo de Mureres, Waltero filio Walteri de Hemelesseya, Alexandro Burdun, Henrico Gernun etc. fo. 197.

Robert de Percy III of Bolton Percy succeeded his father Peter in 1267 (*EYC*, XI, 106); Thomas of Hook succeeded his father John between 1252 and 1260, and died shortly before 6 July 1286 (FN).

**R783.** Note stating that the hospital's 2 a. in Kexby are now in the tenure of William Cloubek, and they lie in length from the Derwent and from the chapel of St Olaf or Eligius, from the east, as far as *le Conygarth* of Lady Ughtred to the west [probably *c.*1410 × 1422]

COPY: MS Dods. 120b, f. 39$^r$, from Rawl., f. 197, now missing.

Sunt ibidem due acre prati hospitalis predicti modo in tenura Willelmi Cloubek, et iacent in longitudine a Derwent et a capella sancti Olavi seu Elegii ab orienti usque le Conygarth domine de Ughtred ad occidentem etc. fo. 197.

It is probable that this information was contained in a marginal note, and hence later than, or contemporary with, the compilation of the cartulary. For similar examples see HN: Skelton and R357. Lady Ughtred was probably Idonea, second wife to Thomas, second Lord Ughtred. She was widowed in 1401 and lived until 1419 × 1422 (*VCH Yorks ER*, III, 159–60; *CP*, XII (2), 161–62). The chapel in Kexby is mentioned in Thomas Ughtred's will of 1398 (*Test. Ebor.*, I, 244).

## *Litton* [par. Arncliffe, WR]

The Litton deeds, which should have been copied in the Craven division in the Missing volume, were instead copied to f. 200 of the East Riding division of the Rawlinson volume, now missing, perhaps indicating confusion with Lutton. For Litton, see *EYC*, XI, 312. There were 6 ct. in Litton, a berewick of Roger of Poitou's manor of Giggleswick, in 1086. The land passed to the Percy fee. The papal confirmations of 1148, 1157 and 1173 include 2 bv. in Litton, but the donor, William de Percy II, is not named (C178–C180 [*EYC*, I, nos 179, 186, 197], R784). It was presumably this 2 bv. which was granted by master P[aulinus] to Thomas son of Gamel of Litton in 1181 × *c*.1202 (R785). Agnes de Percy, a daughter of William de Percy II, gave the hospital a further 1 bv. in Litton (R786). This was presumably the 'land of *Lictona*' confirmed by the pope in 1183 (C166 [*EYC*, I, no. 199]). Before August 1239, Richard de Percy gave the vill of Litton, with the valley called Littondale, except the lands held by Sallay and the land which Thomas of Litton held of St Leonard's, to Fountains Abbey (*Ctl. Fountains*, pp. 449–51). The survey of 1284–85 lists only 2 bv. held by the hospital of the heirs of Percy. The hospital's tenant was then Agnes de Bressenay or Gressenay (*KI*, p. 19). Litton is not mentioned in the hospital's extents of the later thirteenth century, the *Valor Ecclesiasticus*, or the account of 1542.

**R784.** Grant to the hospital by William de Percy [II] of licence to mill at his mills of Stamford Bridge, free from multure. Also 2 bv. in Litton of his own gift, with common pasture, and confirmation of all gifts in his fee, as witnessed by the deeds of the donors [1164 × 1175]

COPIES: *d* PRO, C53/80, Charter Roll, 22 Edw. I, m. 9 (royal inspeximus and confirmation of 16 June 1294); *b* Rawl., 8ᵛ (transcript included in a report of the king's court at Spofforth, 1407 [R54]). ABSTRACT: *c* MS Dods. 120b, f. 39ᵛ, 5 witnesses only, from Rawl., f. 200, now missing. PRINTED: *MA1*, II, 394–95, abbreviated, six witnesses omitted, from *d*; *MA*, VI, 612, from *MA1*; *EYC*, XI, no. 26, from *d*, where dated 1164 × 1175. CALENDAR: *CalCh*, 1257–1300, p. 441, no. 15, from *d*.

Omnibus filiis sancte matris ecclesie videntibus et audientibus has litteras Willelmus de Percy salutem. Sciatis me concessisse et dedisse et presenti carta mea confirmasse deo et pauperibus hospitalis beati Petri Ebor' libertatem molendi annonam suam absque multura ad molendina mea de Ponte Belli et duas bovatas terre de propria donatione mea in Littun' cum communi pastura eiusdem ville, in puram et perpetuam elemosinam liberam et quietam ab omni seculari servicio preter preces in domino, pro salute anime mee et Sibille sponse mee et animabus omnium antecessorum meorum. Preterea concessi et hac carta confirmavi predictis pauperibus in puram et perpetuam elemosinam omnes donationes de feodo meo sicut carte donatorum inde testantur. Hiis testibus, Alano canonico Ebor', Nicholao capellano, Galfrido clerico, Iohanne

Lard(enario), Baldwyno filio Radulfi, Marmaduco de Arel, Rogero filio Radulfi,
Iohanne de Percy, Galtero de Bentu' senescallo, Willelmo filio Ernaldi, Radulfo de
Hallai et Goselano fratre suo, Orm filio Godefridi et Willelmo fratre suo.

For Stamford Bridge deeds see R642–R647. William de Percy II married his second
wife Sybil, named in this deed, in 1164 × 1166, and was dead in 1175 (*EYC*, XI, 3–4).
William had issued an earlier deed confirming the hospital's use of the mills at Stamford Bridge (R643). The papal confirmations of 1148 and 1157 show that the land in
Litton was also given well before the present deed was issued.

**R785.** Grant at fee-farm by P[aulinus], minister of the hospital, with consent of the
brethren, to Thomas son of Gamel of Litton, of 2 bv. land with a toft and croft
in Litton, which Thomas' father formerly held, paying 2s. annually and 5s. as
an obituary payment [1181 × c.1202]

COPY: YML, MS Add. 271, formerly MS Hailstone QQ 44, p. 19, nineteenth-century
transcript by J.R. Walbran, source not stated.

P[aulinus] humilis minister hospitalis Ebor' omnibus hominibus presentibus et futuris
ad quorum precentiam litere iste pervenerint salutem in domino sempiternam. Sciatis
me commune assensu omnium fratrum nostrorum concessisse et hac presenti [carta][56]
confirmasse Thome filio Gameli de Littun et heredibus suis vel suis assignatis duas
bovatas terre cum omnibus pertinenciis suis et aysiamentis cum uno tofto et crofto
in villa et in campo de Littun' que pater eius quondam tenuit de nobis et successoribus nostris libere quiete integre bene et in pace, reddendo inde annuatim nobis
et successoribus nostris duos solidos ad duos anni terminos videlicet mediatatem ad
Pentecost' et aliam mediatatem ad festum sancti Martini in hyeme et infirmis domus
nostri quinque solidos ad obitum s[uum] pro omni servicio ...[57] exactione ... Et nos
et succesores nostri predictas [duas][58] bovatas terre cum tofto et crofto et omnibus
pertinenciis suis predicto Thome et heredibus suis vel suis assignatis ut predictum
est pro predicto annuo servicio contra omnes gentes warantizabimus adquietabimus
et defendemus inperpetuum. In cuius rei testimonium sigillum nostrum commune
apposuimus. Hiis testibus, Thurstano domino archiepiscopo Ebor',[59] Reginaldo sacerdote, Swano sacerdote, fratre Ranulffo sacerdote, fratre Dolfino, fratre Siwath, fratre
Willelmo Lelchi,[60] Adam decano de Arnclive, Ulfo et Roberto de Littun, Willelmo
filio Ormi, Iohanne fratre eius, Iohanne de Ernclife, Willelmo de Cratham et aliis
pluribus.

There are several deeds of Thomas son of Gamel of Litton, and William his son,
at *Ctl. Fountains*, pp. 444–47. The date range for the present deed is the period for
Paulinus as rector. Adam succeeded Ralph as rural dean of Craven in the period 1176
× 1184, but the date of his death is unknown (*Fasti Parochiales*, IV, 5–6). The name of
the first witness is corrupt, as Archbishop Thurstan had been dead for many years by
the time this deed was issued. The attestation of an archbishop would in any case be
out of place in a deed of this type and date. Archbishop Roger had a steward named

---

[56]  A blank space.
[57]  sic here and elsewhere.
[58]  MS: . . .
[59]  sic.
[60]  sic, probably for *Balchi*.

Thurstan, but he occurs about twenty years before the earliest date for the present deed (*EEA*, xx, no. 23). The name of at least one other witness is corrupt, but the list does not otherwise invite suspicion.

Robert son of Ralph, with Gamel of Litton, held 1 ct. of Percy in 1175, which was assigned to the share of Jocelin of Louvain in the division of the barony (*EYC*, xi, no. 89). Robert of Linton, chamberlain of the countess of Warwick, gave ½ ct. in Litton to Thomas son of Gamel of Litton before 1204 (*EYC*, xi, no. 241).

**R786.** Gift to the hospital by Agnes de Percy of 1 bv. in Litton which Adam clerk of Arncliffe held, for the soul of Jocelin her husband. Also a toft in Gargrave containing 2 a. [1179 × 1204, probably 1179 × 1183]

ABSTRACT: MS Dods. 120b, f. 39ᵛ, from Rawl., f. 200, now missing. NOTED: *EYC*, xi, 82.

Agnes de Percy de una bovata terre in Litton hospitali sancti Petri Ebor' quam Adam clericus de Arnecliva ten(ui)t, pro anima Iocelini mariti sui <et 1 toftum in Gargrave contin(ens) 2 acras terre>. Testes Ricardus de Perci, Theobald de Dalton qui tunc fuit dapifer, Willelmo de Kilton, Willelmo de Perci, Willelmo de Dalton, Griffinus Walensis, Eustachio Burdon, Marmaduc Darel etc.⁶¹ fo. 200.

This deed was issued after the death of Agnes de Percy's husband Jocelin de Louvain, which occurred in the year ending at Michaelmas 1180. Agnes de Percy died between 1201 and 1204 (*EYC*, xi, 6; *CP*, x, 447–48). The 'land of Gargrave' given by Agnes de Percy was included in the papal confirmation of 1183, as was the 'land of Litton' (C166 [*EYC*, i, no. 199]). There is no trace of a Gargrave section in the Missing volume, and there seems to be no other record of the hospital's holdings there.

## *Lutton* [Luttons Ambo, par. Weaverthorpe]

The Contents List places Lutton at f. 200 of the Rawlinson volume, but Dodsworth cites f. 201. Both folios are now missing. In 1086 8 ct. in Lutton were soke of the archbishop's manor of Weaverthorpe. Archbishop Thomas granted Weaverthorpe and 'the two Luttons', with other property, to Herbert the chamberlain in 1108 × 1114 (*EYC*, i, no. 25). The following deed provides the only evidence for the hospital's tenure in Lutton. It is likely that the donor was a relation of Ralph de Turp, whose benefaction of a spring called Woodkeld in Dale (now Dale Town, par. Hawnby, NR) to Byland Abbey was confirmed by William Ingram, who appears to have inherited Ralph's interests in Dale. In 1218 Robert Ingram (son of William) sought to have his lands in Dale and Lutton replevied to him (*EYC*, iii, 449–50). By 1284–85 Dale was held by William de Coleville, who was son of Philip de Coleville and the heir of John Ingram; East Lutton was also in the hands of William de Coleville (*KI*, pp. 73, 98). Details of the subsequent tenure of East and West Lutton are given in *VCH Yorks ER*, viii, 157–60.

**R787.** Gift to the hospital by William de Turp of Lutton of 1 bv. in the fields of Lutton [*c.*1173 × 1185]

---

⁶¹ Witnesses in both nominative and ablative.

ABSTRACT: MS Dods. 120b, f. 39$^v$, from Rawl., f. 201, now missing.

Willelmus de Turp de Lutton dedit hospitali sancti Petri Ebor' unam bovatam terre in campis de Lutton etc., ut simus participes omnium beneficiorum etc. in vita et morte. Testes Gaufrido de Stuttevilla, Willelmo Salvain, Adam Luuel, Thoma filio Ragenild, Rogerus Pictaviensis, Thomas Pictaviensis. fo. 201.

The suggested date range depends on the identification of Roger and Thomas Peit-evin as the lords of Altofts and Headingley respectively (FN). Thomas son of Ragenild held land in York in 1178 × 1181[62] (*EYC*, I, no. 280).

## *Lokington* [Lockington]

Farrer gives details of the feudal tenure of Lockington, which in 1086 was held by Nigel Fossard and the church of St John of Beverley. In 1243 Peter de Percy had a tenancy in Lockington, held of Mauley; and in 1279 William Daniel had ¼ k.f. in Lockington and *Wynthorp*,[63] held of Mauley (*EYC*, II, 414–15; *YI*, I, 196; *CalInqPM*, II, 171). The Contents List gives ff. 202–203, now missing, for Lockington, and Dodsworth's abstracts are referenced to f. 202. Arnold of Lockington, chaplain, gave a toft and 13 a. land to the hospital in 1218 × 1243 (R788, R790). This land was granted to Thomas son of James of Lockington by the hospital (R789). The hospital received a further toft and 8 a. by gift of Walter de Matham in *c.*1230 × 1243 (R791). In 1280, the hospital had 22*m.* rent in *Parva Wald', Burtun, Lokyngton', Brunne et Hugate* (R901). A rent in Lockington is mentioned in the post-Dissolution accounts (*Dissolved Houses*, IV, 226).

It is likely that the hospital's benefactor Arnald of LOCKINGTON, chaplain, can be identified with Ernald son of James of Lockington, whose service from a toft and 1 bv. in Lockington was granted to Meaux by Geoffrey de Argenters, with his body, apparently in 1235 × 1249. Geoffrey also gave an annual rent of 4*d.* and ½*lb.* incense, doubtless the rent reserved in Arnald's gift to St Leonard's. In the same period Meaux granted 1 bv. in Lockington to Thomas son of James of Lockington for 12*s.* annually (*Chron. Meaux*, II, 53; R790).

Walter de MATHAM, who gave the hospital a toft and 8 a. in Lockington (R791), occurs as attorney for Thomas of Hotham in 1214 (*CRR*, 1213–1215, p. 248), for the prior of Watton in 1223–25, for Margery, widow of Thomas of Hotham, in 1223–24, and for Roger Aguillun in 1228 (*CRR*, 1223–1224, nos 345, 892, 2173, 2379; *YF*, 1218–1231, pp. 59n, 115n). His father was Thurstan de Matham, who occurs in 1218–19 as a pledge for Thomas son of Kade (*Yorkshire Eyre Rolls*, no. 114), paid ½*m.* at Easter 1222 for not prosecuting a plea (*Receipt Rolls*, 4–6 Hen. III, p. 108), and in the early thirteenth century made grants of 9 bv. and 13 bv. in Reighton to Walter son of Warin of Reighton and Gilbert Beusyre of Reighton respectively (*YD*, IX, nos 355, 356). John de Matham and Walter son of Thurstan de Matham his brother attested in 1218 × 1243 (R788). Walter de Matham attested a North Dalton deed assigned to 1190 × 1220 by Farrer (*EYC*, I, no. 590). According to the chronicle of Meaux, in

---

[62]  After Hamo became precentor and before the death of Archbishop Roger.
[63]  Thorpe, in Lockington, occurs as *Wymundthorp* and *Wynthorp* in the thirteenth century (*PN YorksER*, p. 162).

1210 × 1220 John de Matham gave the abbey half a capital message in *Newtona iuxta Gerthomiam*,[64] and ½ ct. there, and released a rent of 40*d*. from 2 bv. in Molescroft given by Ralph Savage (*Chron. Meaux*, I, 229, 372). In 1235 × 1249 Michael, abbot of Meaux, granted the property in Newton which had belonged to John de Matham to Robert son of Thomas *Iunioris* of Etton. The witnesses included John and Walter de Matham (*YD*, III, no. 239). The chronicle of Meaux assigns Walter de Matham's grant to the abbey of 2*s*. rent from a windmill in Lockington to the same period (*Chron. Meaux*, II, 53). Walter son of Thurstan de Matham's confirmation of Ralph Savage's gift to Meaux of 2 bv. in Molescroft, which Ralph had held of Walter's father ('Ctl. Meaux', no. 351), was doubtless of similar date. Walter de Matham, by a deed witnessed by John de Matham, gave all his meadow at *Aswartholm*, in Scorborough, with his body, to Watton Priory (Burton transcripts 2, f. 49ʳ, p. 69, B12 N62, cited *Monasticon Eboracense*, p. 416). He also confirmed to Watton ½ bv. in Kilnwick, with pasture for 160 or 180 sheep, which he had from Thomas of Hotham, and which had been given to Watton by Walter's tenant Daniel of Kilnwick (*YD*, VI, nos 323–24). Walter also had interests in Sledmere, issuing quitclaims to Kirkham in 6 a. there which Geoffrey de Colton had given the canons, and in a rent of 2*d*. from 2 a. in Sledmere. Robert son of Thomas de Colton confirmed 2 bv. in Sledmere to Walter, which the grantor's brother Geoffrey had given (Kirkham cartulary, ff. 36ʳ–37ʳ). Walter was dead by 1251,[65] the latest date for Robert of Hotham's deed giving to the hospital of St Giles of Beverley, in exchange for their land in Bursea, a meadow in Scorborough which Walter de Matham formerly held of him, saving the third part of Agnes, widow of Walter (Warter cartulary, f. 95ᵛ).

Sir Roger AGUILLUN, who attests three of the Lockington deeds, is omitted from Farrer's account of the family (*EYC*, II, 382–83, 388), but it is clear that he held in Kirby Grindalythe in the 1220s and 1230s. Several members of the Aguillun family were named in the mid-twelfth century. William Fossard's notification of the gift he and his father had made to the hospital of 2 bv. in Huntington, probably made before 1159, has Walter Aguillun as first witness (M: Huntington [*EYC*, II, no. 1060]). Walter Aguillun was the first lay witness to William Fossard's gift to Watton of 1154 × 1162 (*EYC*, II, no. 1095). William Aguillun was witness to a gift by Walter of Huggate and Alice his wife to Watton made in 1154–55 or soon afterwards[66] (*EYC*, I, no. 158). William Aguillun, Thurstan Aguillun and Geoffrey Aguillun attested a deed of Agnes Fossard in 1143 × 1158[67] (*EYC*, II, no. 1037), and a gift by Robert son of William of Birdsall, dated to 1160 × 1180 by Farrer, but presumably issued before Michaelmas 1171[68] (*EYC*, II, no. 1035). Agnes, wife of William Aguillun, with the consent of her husband, gave to Watton Priory the service from 3 ct. land in Kilnwick, which was her marriage portion. The deed was witnessed by Thurstan Aguillun and Geoffrey his brother (*YD*, VI, no. 297). The impression gained is that William, Thurstan and Geoffrey were brothers but of this there is no proof. W[alter ?] Aguillun, with Thurstan his brother, issued a confirmation of a deed of William Aguillun to Kirkham; Thurstan Aguillun issued a confirmation to Kirkham of the land in Woodhouse given by William Aguillun and Agnes his wife (Kirkham cartulary, f. 23ᵛ).

---

[64]  Lost, near Cherry Burton (*PN YorksER*, p. 191).
[65]  When Robert of Hotham was dead (FN).
[66]  Attested by Archbishop Roger and Osbert the archdeacon, who do not seem to have remained in the archbishop's company for long after his consecration (FN: Pontefract Stewards).
[67]  While Robert de Gant was dean of York.
[68]  When William Aguillun I was dead.

## AGUILLUN OF KIRBY GRINDALYTHE

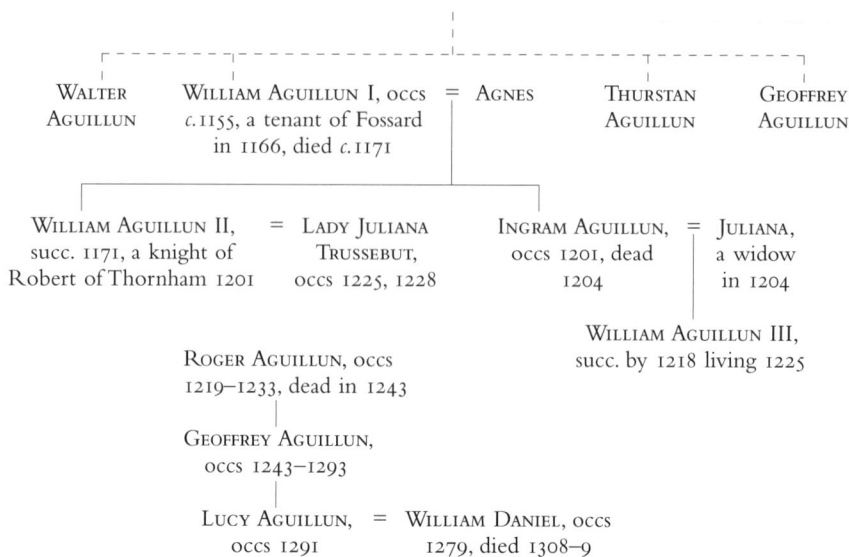

| WALTER AGUILLUN | WILLIAM AGUILLUN I, occs c.1155, a tenant of Fossard in 1166, died c.1171 | = AGNES | THURSTAN AGUILLUN | GEOFFREY AGUILLUN |
|---|---|---|---|---|

| WILLIAM AGUILLUN II, succ. 1171, a knight of Robert of Thornham 1201 | = LADY JULIANA TRUSSEBUT, occs 1225, 1228 | INGRAM AGUILLUN, occs 1201, dead 1204 | = JULIANA, a widow in 1204 |
|---|---|---|---|

WILLIAM AGUILLUN III,
succ. by 1218 living 1225

ROGER AGUILLUN, occs
1219–1233, dead in 1243

GEOFFREY AGUILLUN,
occs 1243–1293

LUCY AGUILLUN,    =    WILLIAM DANIEL, occs
occs 1291            1279, died 1308–9

William Aguillun held ½ k.f. of Fossard in 1166 (*EYC*, II, no. 1003).[69] Entries in the cartularies of Kirkham and Malton, noted below, indicate that this William was the husband of Agnes, and that William Aguillun, who in 1171 owed 5*m*. for his relief for 1 k.f. in Kirby [Grindalythe] (*PR*, 17 Hen. II, p. 73)[70] was his son and successor. Agnes survived her husband for many years as is shown by her gift of a croft to Ellerton Priory,[71] founded in 1199 or later, for the soul of her former husband William Aguillun and for her son William Aguillun (MS Dods. 95, f. 65ʳ). A large number of deeds issued by members of the family are noted in the Kirkham cartulary, but no witnesses are given, and the abstracts are usually very brief. From this source we learn that William Aguillun gave 2 bv. in Sutton *iuxta Malton* to William Basset in exchange for the release of the service he owed Basset for ½ ct. in Wharram. Basset gave the land in Sutton to Kirkham and his gift was confirmed by William Aguillun and Agnes his wife. William son and heir of William Aguillun issued a confirmation of the deed of his mother and father (Kirkham cartulary, f. 19ʳ⁻ᵛ). William Aguillun and Agnes his

---

[69] Farrer's statement that William was 'apparently son of Picot' should be treated with caution. The hypothesis appears to rest on the assumptions that Thurstan son of Picot was a brother of William Aguillun I and that Roger son of Thurstan son of Picot was the same person as Roger Aguillun (*EYC*, II, 382–83). But there is nothing to identify Thurstan Aguillun with Thurstan son of Picot, who made many gifts of land in Kirby Grindalythe to Kirkham. Roger son of Thurstan Picot was also a benefactor of Kirkham, and as Roger of Kirby confirmed land given by his father Thurstan (Kirkham cartulary, f. 40ʳ). Roger son of Thurstan witnessed a deed of William Aguillun [II] given in 1194 × 1198, so had presumably succeeded by then (Burton transcripts 3, f. 121ᵛ, p. 216, B13 N14, dating from the shrievalty of the witness Roger de Bavent). Roger Aguillun and Roger son of Thurstan attested together in 1226 (MS Dods. 7, f. 198ᵛ), and Roger of Kirby witnessed a deed of Alan Boniface in 1233 (Burton transcripts 3, f. 27ʳ, p. 319, B7 N5).

[70] The fine was due to the king, rather than Fossard, as the Fossard fee was then in the king's hands (*EYC*, II, 328).

[71] *canonicis de Ellreton qui sunt de ordine de Sempingham.*

wife also gave land in Woodhouse to Kirkham, which gift was confirmed by William Aguillun, doubtless the same son (Kirkham cartulary, f. 23$^{r-v}$).

The Aguillun deeds in the Malton cartulary are copied much more fully, but the witnesses are omitted. William Aguillun, doubtless again the husband of Agnes, gave the canons of Malton land and common of pasture in Mowthorpe, for which they received him *in specialem fratrem* in all the houses of the Gilbertine order, agreeing to make him a canon when he should wish, and if he died as a layman to receive his body and do for him as they would for a canon. The grange of Mowthorpe was confirmed to the canons by the pope in 1178 (*EYC*, II, no. 1084 and n). William Aguillun son of William Aguillun confirmed his father's gift in very similar terms (Malton cartulary, f. 190/186$^v$). Ingram Aguillun quitclaimed to his brother and lord William Aguillun [the younger] 6 bv. he held of him in Sutton *iuxta Malton*, which William then gave to Malton for a annual rent of 17$d$. William gave Ingram 6 bv. in Kirby Grindalythe in exchange (ibid., f. 64/62$^r$). William Aguillun also gave 1 bv. and a toft in Rillington to Malton, which was confirmed, with other property, by William de Forz, earl of Aumale, after 1190[72] (ibid., f. 173/169$^v$). In 1191 it was stated in the pipe roll that William Aguillun owed £20 as a fine concerning the debts of Aaron the Jew, in Yorkshire (*PR*, 3&4 Ric. I, p. 22). No payment was made against the debt until 1197–98. Payments continued sporadically well into the reign of Henry III, the debtor always being described simply as William Aguillun (*PR*, passim).

In 1194 × 1198[73] William Aguillun gave 3 bv. in Kirby [Grindalythe] to Kirkham, by a deed witnessed by Ingram Aguillun and Amaury Aguillun (Burton transcripts 3, f. 121$^v$, p. 216, B13 N14). In 1201 the king ordered that William son of Peter [of Goodmanham] and William Aguillun, knights of Robert of Thornham, the king's steward, were not to be summoned whilst they were in Robert's service, whether in England or abroad (*RChart*, p. 101). In the same year Ingram Aguillun witnessed a deed of William de Sumerville (MS Dods. 8, ff. 57$^v$–58$^r$). No evidence has been found to show that William Aguillun II was succeeded by his brother Ingram, and it is more probable the fee passed directly to Ingram's son William Aguillun III. Three deeds issued by Ingram Aguillun were noted in the Kirkham cartulary (Kirkham cartulary, ff. 41$^v$–42$^r$). These were a surrender of a toft in Kirby Grindalythe to William Aguillun [his brother], which he held of the same William (*EYC*, II, no. 1081); a gift of 2 bv. in the same place to Kirkham, which was confirmed by his brother William (*EYC*, II, no. 1080; Burton transcripts 2, f. 111$^r$, p. 186, B24 N78); and a gift of a toft in Kirby to Kirkham. Ingram Aguillun son of William Aguillun issued a confirmation to Malton of whatever the canons had by the gift of his brother William and his father, but this was apparently before William II's death, as it was made *pro salute mea et fratris mei* (Malton cartulary, f. 195/191$^r$). Ingram was dead in February 1204, when Juliana his widow claimed right in dower in a croft in Kirby Grindalythe against Walter of Sowerby (*PF John*, p. 84).[74] As it is uncertain whether Ingram Aguillun succeeded his brother, it is difficult to determine whether William Aguillun, to whom Nicholas son of Hugh and Cecilia his wife, formerly wife of Amaury Aguillun, released their

---

72 The earliest date for William de Forz as earl of Aumale (*CP*, I, 353). Farrer was in error when he stated the confirmation to belong to William le Gros (*EYC*, I, 491).

73 Witnessed by Roger de Bavent, sheriff of York.

74 Farrer says that Ingram 'married Juliana, relict of Gerard de Collum', and that Gerard of Thirkleby who held *temp*. Henry III 'seems to have been the son of Juliana, daughter of Gerald, by her husband Gerard de Kirkby, also known as Gerard de Collum' (*EYC*, II, 382–83), but the evidence for both statements is obscure. Cowlam is some 4 m. south east of Kirby Grindalythe. Whether Juliana can be identified with 'Lady Juliana, wife of Ingram' whose fee included 2 bv. in Gowthorpe (ER) is uncertain (*Ctl. Fountains*, p. 317).

claim in dower in Wharram in September 1206 (*PF John*, p. 105), was William II or his nephew William III. By 1218 the latter had succeeded to the fee.

William son of Ingram confirmed to Malton everything they had by gift of his grandfather William Aguillun, his uncle William *filii eius*, and Ingram Aguillun his father. He gave the canons on his own account 3 bv. in Mowthorpe, one of which was held in dower by Lady Juliana, widow of William Aguillun his uncle (Malton cartulary, f. 195/191ʳ). He made several further deeds in favour of Malton, including a confirmation dated 1218 of pasture sufficient for 600 sheep in the territory of Mowthorpe, which the canons had from William Aguillun the elder, William Aguillun his uncle, and himself (ibid., f. 195/191ᵛ). It is difficult to explain the interest of Peter son of Herbert, shown by his confirmation of the gifts in his fee in Mowthorpe made by William Aguillun the elder and William his son, and of 7 bv. given by William Aguillun son of Ingram Aguillun (ibid., f. 196/192ʳ).

Before September 1206[75] Thomas Boniface quitclaimed to his lord Robert de Ros a culture of land in Kirby [Grindalythe] which William Aguillun had claimed from him, so that William would hold it of Robert de Ros by hereditary right for 12*d.* annually (*EYC*, x, no. 103). By a deed issued in or before 1213,[76] witnessed by Roger Aguillun and Walter Aguillun, William Aguillun, without further description, gave the culture to Juliana his wife, noting that Thomas Boniface had quitclaimed it to him and that he held it by hereditary right of Robert de Ros for 12*d.* annually (ibid., no. 104). After 1225 Juliana Trussebut, formerly wife of William Aguillun, gave the land to Kirkham Priory, noting that she had been given the land by her husband (ibid., no. 29). Both Farrer and Clay believed that these deeds belonged to William Aguillun III and his widow, but this is doubtful. As has been noted above, the widow of William Aguillun II was named Juliana. William III describes himself as son of Ingram in all other deeds which have been ascribed to him. The period possible for the deeds allows both William II and William III, though no other deed of William III can be placed as early as the gift to Juliana. Juliana Trussebut occurs as *uxor* (probably widow) of William Aguillun in her confirmation and quitclaim to Kirkham of the wood of Woodhouse, 2 bv. in Kirby which Ingram Aguillun gave, and 2 bv. in Sutton *iuxta* Malton which William Basset gave (Kirkham cartulary, f. 23ᵛ). It seems unlikely that the widow of William Aguillun III would have confirmed these gifts, which were made during the time of William Aguillun I and his son William II.

In 1218 Walter of Sowerby called William Aguillun to warrant ½ ct. in Kirby Grindalythe, which Walter had been given by William Aguillun, uncle of the said William. Final concords were made in January 1219 settling the matter (*Yorkshire Eyre Rolls*, no. 360; *YF*, 1218–1231, p. 14). A further gift was made by William Aguillun son of Ingram Aguillun to Walter of Sowerby of ½ ct. land in Mowthorpe of the Fossard fee. Walter subsequently gave the land to Kirkham Priory, by a gift confirmed by William son of Ingram Aguillun (*EYC*, II, nos 1085–86 and n). On 19 February 1219 Hugh of Langthwaite paid William Aguillun 3*m.* for right in 1 bv. in Loversall, except the capital messuage, which was to remain to William (*YF*, 1218–1231, p. 25). At about the same time the burning by malefactors of William's house, probably in Loversall, and the slaying by William of Adam de Moncelles with a sword 'as they were playing' in Robert de Percy's house was reported to the visiting justices (*Yorkshire Eyre Rolls*, nos 494, 819). William Aguillun, son of Ingram Aguillun, gave to the Hospitallers all his demesne with the capital messuage in Loversall (MS Dods. 8, f. 310ʳ). William son

---

[75]  When the witness Aumary Aguillun was dead and his widow was claiming dower (*PF John*, p. 105).
[76]  The first witness, William de Percy [of Bolton Percy] was dead in that year.

of Ingram Aguillun gave Roger Caluum of Cathwaite[77] to Ellerton Priory before 1225.[78] The deed survives, with a portion of the seal which depicts a shield with a cross, or perhaps a sword, point downwards (BL, Addit. Ch. 20553).[79] It was presumably the same William Aguillun who in 1225 was said to outlawed *pro malo retto*, when his land in Loversall was given to John de Bithun for a year and a day. He was mentioned again in 1227, still an outlaw (*RClose*, II, 55, 188).

This is the last that is heard of William Aguillun. His relationship to Roger Aguillun, who in 1218–19 was a pledge for Thomas of Hotham (*Hoth*), has not been established. During the same eyre Robert of Watton failed to follow up his plea of novel disseisin against Roger Aguillun concerning a tenement in Beswick, which is about 1 m. from Lockington (*Yorkshire Eyre Rolls*, nos 67, 69). Roger occurs as a recognitor in 1220 and 1224, showing he was then of knightly status (*CRR*, 1220, p. 255; ibid., 1223–1224, no. 2479). Not described as a knight, he was the second witness to a Kirby Grindalythe deed dated 1226, the first being Gerard Salvain (MS Dods. 7, f. 198ᵛ). In Hilary term 1228 Gerard of Thirkleby sued Roger Aguillun and Juliana Trussebut in a plea of land, and the following Easter term Gerard and Roger came to an agreement concerning 9¼ bv. in Kirby [Grindalythe]. Roger Aguillun attorned Walter de Matham to take his chirograph. By the fine recording their agreement, made on 9 April 1228, Gerard of Thirkleby quitclaimed to Roger Aguillun half a carucate and two parts of a carucate of land in Kirby Grindalythe in return for 28*m*. Gerard's case against Juliana Trussebut continued. In 1228 the land he claimed was ordered to be taken into the king's hand, and seisin given to him, after she did not appear in court. It was noted that she was poor (*CRR*, 1227–1230, nos 465, 515, 1007; *YF*, 1218–1231, p. 115). Sir Roger Aguillun attested a Kilnwick deed in 1229 or later[80] (*YD*, VI, no. 325), and served as a knight on a grand assize in 1231 (*YF*, 1218–1231, pp. 149n, 154n). He last occurs in 1233, when he witnessed a deed of Alan Boniface of Kirby (Burton transcripts 3, f. 27ʳ, p. 27, B7 N5).

Roger Aguillun was dead in 1243, when Geoffrey Aguillun [his son] and Roger of Thirkleby held 1 k.f. in Kirby Grindalythe of Mauley (*Bk of Fees*, p. 1099). In 1247, Geoffrey Aguillun had exemption for life from all suit of ridings, hundreds, views of frank pledge and counties, and from being put on assizes, juries or recognitions; and in 1261, Robert of Thwing and Geoffrey Aguillun, his co-parcener, and their heirs, had a grant of free warren in all their demesne lands of Akenberg,[81] Beswick and Kirby Grindalythe, in co. York (*CalPat*, 1232–1247, p. 509; *CalCh*, 1257–1300, p. 37). Geoffrey produced these charters in quo warranto proceedings of 1293–94 (*YQW*, p. 208). In 1265 Geoffrey Aguillun confirmed to Marmaduke son of Robert of Thwing the gift made by Roger Aguillun his father to Marmaduke of Thwing, grandfather of the younger Marmaduke, of estovers in turbary in the marsh of Beswick (BL, MS Harley 1985, f. 96/287ʳ).[82] Geoffrey was involved in a dispute with the prior of Kirkham and others concerning the extent of pasture in Kirby Grindalythe in 1276 (MS Dods. 7, f. 207ʳ). In 1279 Geoffrey held a fifth part of a fee in Beswick, and ½ k.f. in Kilnwick, of Mauley (*YI*, I, 196–97). He was holding 2 ct. in Beswick of Mauley in 1284–85,

---

77  In Sutton on Derwent.
78  Witnessed by William son of Peter [of Goodmanham, the founder of Ellerton] who was dead in that year (FN).
79  Seen by Dodsworth, MS Dods. 152, f. 122ʳ.
80  Attested by Roger, prior of Watton, whose predecessor occurs in 1229.
81  Akenberg has been identified as the place later known as Barf Hill, in Lockington (*PN YorksER*, p. 161; *EYC*, x, pp. xvii–xviii, 124).
82  Abstract of a deed in the possession of John Lumley, baron of Lumley, co. Durham, in 1578.

but was not then noticed as a tenant in Kirby Grindalythe (*KI*, pp. 73, 83).[83] Geoffrey Aguillun was regularly appointed to hold inquisitions and was a justice of gaol delivery in Yorkshire during the 1270s and 1280s (*CalPat, CalCh, YI*, passim). He attested as steward of the York chapter in *c.*1270 × 1272 or 1278 × 1279[84] (BL, MS Cotton Claudius B. iii, f. 42/40[r]). He was summoned to the parliament at Shrewsbury in 1283 (*Parl. Writs*, I, 424).

Geoffrey's heir was his daughter Lucy, wife of William Daniel. William Daniel held ¼ k.f. of Mauley in Lockington and *Wynthorp* in 1279 (*YI*, I, 196), and was recorded as a tenant in Beswick in 1302–3 (*KI*, p. 259). In 1291 a fine was made between William Daniel and Lucy his wife, plaintiffs, and Geoffrey Aguillun, defendant, concerning tenements in Beswick which were acknowledged to be Lucy's right. A further fine concerning different property in Beswick was made between the same parties in 1293. Again the properties were acknowledged to be Lucy's right, and Geoffrey was to hold of William and Lucy, and Lucy's heirs, for his life at a yearly rent of 1*d.*, with reversion to William and Lucy and Lucy's heirs (*YF*, 1272–1300, pp. 94–95, 98). In 1304 a jury found that Roger Aguillun had died seised of 3 ct. in Beswick, of the Mauley fee, which was inherited by his son Geoffrey. Geoffrey gave the land by fine to William Daniel and Lucy his wife, daughter and heir of Geoffrey (MS Dods. 152, f. 25[v]).[85] It is likely that Geoffrey died not long after 1293, as he was over seventy in that year, and the references in 1300 to his gift of a rent of 20*s.* to Watton (*CalPat*, 1292–1300, p. 540) and his tenancy of an unspecified amount of land in Beswick in 1302–3 (*KI*, p. 259) ought not to be relied on as proof he was then still living. His name heads the list of those buried at the Franciscan friary at Beverley. Margery Aguillun, who appears later in the same list, was perhaps his wife (Young, 'Religious Houses', p. 129).

In 1308 licence was granted to William Daniel, knight, worn out with illness and old age, to have an oratory for three years in his manor of Beswick (*Reg. Greenfield*, III, 133). William was dead the following year, when Lucy, widow of William Daniel, gave a confirmation at Beswick to Robert Daniel her son (*Glover's Visitation*, p. 125).[86] Robert Daniel was lord of Beswick in 1316 (*KI*, p. 307), and was recorded as the tenant of Gerard Salvain in the same place in 1323 (*CalInqPM*, VI, no. 458). No Daniel interest in Kirby Grindalythe can be discerned.

**R788.** Gift to the hospital by Arnald of Lockington, chaplain, of a toft and 13 a. land with all his meadow in Lockington, with a piece of land, which he had by gift of Nigel Franceys [1218 × 1243]

ABSTRACT: MS Dods. 120b, f. 39[v], from Rawl., f. 202, now missing.

Arnaldus de Lokinton capellanus ded(it) hospitali sancti Petri Ebor' <unum toftum et> 13 acras terre cum toto prato suo in Lokinton <cum particula terre> q(ue) habuit ex dono Nigelli Franceis. Testibus, dominis Marmaduco de Tweng, Iohanne de Aton, Rogero de[87] Agelun militibus, Iohanne de Matam, Waltero filio Turstani de Maton fratre suo. fo. 202.

---

[83]  In 1316 John of Thirkleby and Gilbert Haunsard were named as the lords of Thirkleby and Kirby [Grindalythe] (*KI*, p. 315).

[84]  With Walter de Stokes, mayor of York (ML).

[85]  Indirectly from a *coram rege* roll, Hil. 32 Edw. I, 'rot. 1, f. 114'.

[86]  In his pedigree of Daniel of Beswick Glover made Lucy 'daughter and heir of . . . Aslakleby, outlived her husband, 30 Ed. II'.

[87]  sic.

The date range is the period for Roger Aguillun (FN). Marmaduke of Thwing, John of Ayton, and Walter de Matham attest together in 1227 (MS Dods. 8, f. 155ᵛ). Sir Marmaduke of Thwing I last occurs in 1234, but the date of his death is unknown (*CP*, XII (1), 736).

**R789.** Grant by Hugh, rector of the hospital, to Thomas son of James of Lockington, of the property described in R788 [1214 × 1245]

NOTED: MS Dods. 120b, f. 39ᵛ, in margin, from Rawl., f. 202, now missing.

Hugo rector hospitalis conc(essit) has 13 acras etc. Thome filio Iacobi de Lokinton et heredibus. Ibidem. Teste Stephano de Aldeford.

The date range is the period for Hugh as rector.

**R790.** Gift to the hospital by Arnald of Lockington, chaplain, with his body, of a toft in Lockington formerly held by James of Lockington, chaplain, and 13 a. and 1 r., with all the donor's meadow, paying the church of St Mary of Lockington ½*lb.* incense and the heirs of Geoffrey son of Fulk de Argentar 4*d.* annually [1218 × 1243]

COPY: (in two parts) Burton transcripts 2, ff. 170ʳ, 171ᵛ, pp. 304, 307, B25 N68.

Sciant omnes presentes et futuri quod ego Arnaldus de Lokington capellanus caritatis intuitu et pro salute anime mee et animarum antecessorum et successorum meorum cum corpore meo dedi concessi et hac presenti carta mea [f. 171ᵛ(p. 307)] confirmavi deo et pauperibus hospitalis sancti Petri Ebor' unum toftum in Lokintona et tresdecim acras terre et unam rodam cum toto prato meo in Scleythaker et Brunholm et Whyteholm in eadem villa, videlicet illud toftum quod Iacobus de Lokinton capellanus quondam tenuit, et illas duas acras et dimidiam que iacent in Brinighou, et unam acram in Gosehou et unam rodam in Heselhou, et unam acram et unam rodam in Mikeldail versus meridiem, et dimidiam acram in Swartmolde versus orientem, et unam acram et unam rodam in Becfurlanges, et unam acram et unam rodam in Langelandes versus occidentem, et duas acras et unam rodam in Lushou ex utraque parte, et tres rodas in Daltondale versus australem, et unam rodam Elbut de Fulmardsic, et duas acras in P-ngkeldedaile,⁸⁸ tenendum et habendum totum predictum tenementum cum omnibus pertinenciis suis aisiamentis et libertatibus suis infra villam et extra in liberam et perpetuam elemosinam predictis pauperibus, reddendo inde annuatim pro omni servicio et exactione ecclesie beate Marie de Lokintona dimidiam libram incensi, die assumptionis beate Marie, et heredibus vel assignatis Galfridi filii Fulconis de Argentar quatuor denarios tantum modo die beati Laurentii. Ego autem et heredes mei totum predictum tenementum cum omnibus pertinenciis suis predictis pauperibus per predictum servicium warantizabimus adquietabimus et defendemus in omnibus et contra omnes homines in perpetuum. Hiis testibus, domino Marmaduc(o) de Tweng, Iohanne de Atona, Rogero Agelun⁸⁹ militibus, Willelmo de Wimmethorp, Galfrido nepote decani, Iohanne de Matam, Willelmo nepote decani, Willelmo de Coupland, Thoma le Sumenur, Rogero fratre suo, Iacobo filio Aungeri et multis aliis.

---

⁸⁸ sic.
⁸⁹ MS: *Agelim.*

For the date range, see R788. Thomas le Sumenur occurs in 1226, when he quitclaimed 2 bv. in Lockington to Peter de Maulay and Isabel his wife for 5*m*. (*YF*, 1218–
1231, p. 87). In 1251 Thomas le Sumenur quitclaimed 2 bv. in Lockington to Roger
le Sumenur, possibly his brother who attests this deed, for 2*m*. (*YF*, 1246–1272, p. 43).

**R791.** Gift to the hospital by Walter de Matham of a toft and 8 a. in Lockington,
being the toft which Walter Chaplin formerly held of the donor, and 8 a.
from the 2 bv. which Thomas le Sumenur formerly held, which 8 a. Arnald
the chaplain formerly held of the convent of Swine [*c.*1230 × 1243]

COPY: *c* Burton transcripts 1, f. 170ʳ, p. 287, B12 N2. NOTED: *b* MS Dods. 120b, f. 39ᵛ,
first five witnesses only, from Rawl., f. 202, now missing. NOTED: Drake, *Eboracum*,
p. 336, via Torre's collections.

Omnibus cristi fidelibus ad quos presens scriptum pervenerit Walterus de Mathum
salutem. Noverit universitas vestra me caritatis intuitu et pro salute anime mee et
animarum antecessorum et successorum meorum dedisse concessisse et presenti
carta mea confirmasse deo et pauperibus hospitalis sancti Petri Ebor' unum toftum
in Lokintona et octo acras terre in territorio eiusdem ville, scilicet illud toftum
quod Walterus Chapeleyn aliquando de me tenuit et illas octo acras terre in territorio eiusdem ville sup--tas⁹⁰ ex illis duabus bovatis terre quas Thomas le Sumenur
aliquando tenuit, quas octo acras Arnaldus capellanus aliquando tenuit de conventu
de Swina, tenend(a) et habend(a) predictis pauperibus in liberam puram et perpetuam
elemosinam cum communa pasture pertinente ad tantum tenementum in eadem
villa et cum omnibus pertinenciis suis aisiamentis et libertatibus <suis> infra villam
et extra libere et quiete ab omni servicio et exactione seculari sicut aliqua elemosina
liberius vel melius teneri et haberi potest. Ego autem et heredes mei predictum
toftum et predictas octo acras terre cum communa pasture et cum omnibus pertinenciis suis warantizabimus adquietabimus et defendemus in omnibus et contra homines
omnes in perpetuum, ut ego et heredes mei simus participes in omnibus beneficiis
que fiunt vel facienda fuerint in predicto hospitali in perpetuum. In cuius rei robur
et testimonium huic scripto sigillum meum apposui. Hiis testibus, Galfrido de Rughford, Rogero Agwilun militibus,⁹¹ Roberto de Bugethorp, Iordano filio Galfrido de
Rughford, Iohanne de Touetona, Thoma de Killingwick, Willelmo ad Fontem, Iacobo
cementario et multis aliis.

The witness Geoffrey of Rufforth, also known as Geoffrey of Bugthorpe, who held
land in Lockington, died in 1246 × 1248. As Geoffrey's wife Helen survived until at
least 1258, it seems unlikely that their son Jordan would have been of age to attest
much before 1230. Roger Aguillun was dead in 1243 (FNs). The witness Robert of
Bugthorpe was probably brother to Geoffrey of Rufforth: Roger Aguillun, Geoffrey
of Bugthorpe, Robert his brother are amongst the witnesses to a grant by Agnes
Engaine daughter of Walter Engaine (*YD*, VI, no. 308).

---

⁹⁰ *c:* sic.
⁹¹ *c: militibus* omitted.

## *Morhamwicke* [Inklemoor, or Inkle Moors, par. Thorne, WR]

The Contents List shows that Inklemoor deeds were copied to ff. 205–7, now missing, under the heading *Morhamwicke*. Dodsworth makes reference to each of these folios. Inklemoor, Swinefleet, and Hook are not mentioned in Domesday or the survey of 1284–85, but appear to have been soke of the manor of Snaith. Henry de Lacy, earl of Lincoln (in possession 1268–1311),[92] confirmed a gift to Drax of land in the moor and marsh in Inklemoor 'in our manor and soke of Snaith, next to the vill of Swinefleet' (Drax cartulary, f. 66ᵛ, p. 133). A map of the area was produced *c.*1450 to illustrate a dispute between St Mary's Abbey, York, and the Duchy of Lancaster concerning turbaries and pasture in Inklemoor and Thorne Moor (PRO, MPC 1/56). A consider-able number of monastic houses held narrow strips of turbary in Inklemoor similar to those granted to the hospital by the deeds in this section of the cartulary. Their length has been estimated at about four miles (Thirsk, *Rural England*, p. 177). The hospital first acquired turbary in Inklemoor during the reign of John, when Roger son of Anketin of Hook gave two pieces of the moor, each at a rent of ½m. yearly, by two separate deeds possibly given on the same occasion (R792, R793). Roger's son John confirmed these gifts by two further deeds (R794, R795). In the 1260s Thomas son of John of Hook confirmed the previous gifts (R797), and added a further plot called *Le Strand*, for ½m. yearly (R796). In September 1269 he confirmed the grant in Inklemoor made to the hospital by Guy of Appleton (R798), and issued a further general confirmation (R799). Guy of Appleton had given the land in October 1266 in exchange for land in Appleton [Roebuck], which the hospital had by gift of Robert of Skegness (M: Appleton [St Mary JR, f. 377/386ʳ)]). In 1270 the master of the hospital, Thomas of Geddington, impleaded several people who had come to Morhamwick and carried away his corn there to the value of 40s. (Baildon, *Monastic Notes*, I, 246). In the 1280 extent the hospital's holdings in Morhamwick were given as 5 a. with 'a certain great turbary' (R901). The detailed extent of 1287 shows 13½ a. of profitable land, worth 4s., with a pasture and a turbary called Inklemoor which produced seventy-two boatloads of turf annually, worth 5s. a load, as well as forty quarters of salt. The whole was worth £22 3s. (R903). In 1371 the master sued three men for not mending the banks of the Ouse at Morhamwick, in consequence of which the master's meadows and pastures were flooded (Baildon, *Monastic Notes*, II, 80). Neither Morhamwick nor Inklemoor is mentioned in the *Valor Ecclesiasticus* or the account of 1542, but they were doubtless represented by the entries for Goole. The *Valor Ecclesiasticus* includes 106s. 8d. rent in *Goyll* (R905), and the 1542 account refers to the manor of Broomfleet with *Gowle*, which included a rent in *Gowle in Mershland* (*Dissolved Houses*, IV, 224). There was no section for Goole itself in the Rawlinson volume, and, apart from these entries, no evidence that the hospital held property there has been found.

As indicated, four generations of the Hook family are apparent in the hospital's deeds. Anketin, or Aschetill, of Hook made benefactions to a variety of religious houses. His gift of 26 perches of turbary in Inklemoor to Nostell was included in Edward I's general confirmation (*CalCh*, 1257–1300, p. 234).[93] By a deed made with the consent

---

92  *CP*, VII, 681–86.

93  It is probable that Anketin's deed was copied into the Nostell cartulary on p. 282, now missing, under the heading *Turbaria*. Hook deeds followed on pp. 283–84, also now missing, and doubtless included other gifts made by the family ('Ctl. Nostell', no. 1).

of Avicia his wife and Roger his son and heir, Anketin gave Drax Priory land in his
moor of Inklemoor for turbary (Burton transcripts 1, f. 54ᵛ, p. 56, B14 N39; Drax
cartulary, f. 66ᵛ, p. 133). His gift of moorland adjoining the land of Nostell, with
common of pasture in Morham and Swinefleet, was confirmed to Drax by his son
Roger (MS Dods. 8, f. 210ʳ). Roger also confirmed Anketin's gift to Selby Abbey of
moorland in Hook, with the *heremitagium* in the land of Hook, with land to make
a road to the river (*Ctl. Selby*, no. 873). To Thornton Abbey Anketin gave turbary in
Inklemoor with a toft in Swinefleet which was confirmed with other benefactions
by King Richard in 1190 (*EYC*, III, no. 1312). In 1189 or later[94] he gave a turbary in
Inklemoor at Swinefleet to the nuns of Nun Coton, with right of carriage by the
causeway from the moor to the water (*EYC*, I, no. 493). At about the same time[95]
Anketin gave an adjoining turbary, with a messuage next to his wood, with Anketin
(*Aschetill*) his son, to Newhouse Abbey (Lincs.). Anketin's seal, attached to his deed
recording this gift, is described as 'In armour: hauberk of mail, cap-like helmet, sword,
shield. Horse galloping, +SIGILLVM.ASCTIN DE HVC.' (*EYC*, I, no. 492; *BM Cat. Seals*, II,
no. 6122). To the abbey of Louth Park Anketin gave a turbary in his moor of Hook,
on the west side of Morham Flet, and a corner of land next to Morham Flet to
stack its turf (*CalCh*, 1300–1326, p. 253). His other gifts included part of the moor
between Swinefleet and Morham to [the chronicler] Roger, parson of Howden (*Cat.
Anc. Deeds*, III, B.3962); a toft in Swinefleet and a strip of moor in Hook to Simon
de Kyme (MS Dods. 8, f. 166ʳ); and land in Inklemoor to John of Crigglestone
[in marriage] with Anketin's unnamed daughter (R793). In 1198 Robert, abbot of
St Mary's, York, claimed 4 ct. of land in Hook from Anketill of Hook, who defended
his right (*MemR*, 10 John, p. 106). Anketin attested several deeds belonging to places in
the North Riding, including Amotherby (par. Appleton-le-Street, where a descendant
of Anketin had an interest in 1316), Little Danby (in Danby Wiske), and Baxby (par.
Husthwaite), dated 1182 × 1184, '*c*.1160 × 1175', and '*ante* 1190' respectively (*EYC*, V,
no. 354, ibid., VI, no. 25; M: Baxby [*EYF*, p. 110]). These attestations indicate that the
Hook interests in the parish of Appleton-le-Street apparent in the early fourteenth
century had been held since at least the late twelfth century.

Anketin had been succeeded by his son Roger by November 1208, when Savaric
of Hook quitclaimed to Roger son of Anketill 20 a. of land in Hook, whereof there
had been a recognition of mort d'ancestor (*PF John*, p. 132). In 1202 × 1214,[96] for
the health of the soul of his father, Roger son of Asketill of Hook gave to Pontefract
Priory moorland in Hook, with land to make a roadway to the Ouse (*Ctl. Pontefract*,
no. 451). Roger made gifts of turbary in Inklemoor to the hospital of St Peter by two
separate deeds, probably made on the same occasion in *c*.1200 × 1214 (R792, R793).
Roger's wife was Margaret, daughter of John of Criggleston, who as his widow gave
land in Barton[97] to Ormsby Priory (MS Dods. 135, f. 154), to which she also gave
½ bv. in Hook which she held by the gift of Richard son of Lambert. Ormsby Priory
let at farm 7 bv. of arable land in Barton to Margaret of Hook, daughter of John of

---

94  The gift was made *pro salute anime mee et pro anima Henrici regis*.
95  This gift was 10 perches, so possibly a different and later gift than the 5 perches in *Michelmore* at
    Swinefleet confirmed by Richard I in October 1189 (*CalCh*, 1300–1326, p. 387).
96  Attested by Richard abbot of Selby, whose successor was appointed in 1214, Adam de Bellewe, who
    was under age in 1202, Robert Waleys, who died in or before 1219, and John of Birkin, who died in
    1227 (FNs).
97  Presumably Barton-upon-Humber (Lincs.), where Ormsby held rents of £1 10s. at the Dissolution
    (*MA*, VI, 964).

Crigglestone, in 1229 (MS Dods, 135, f. 139ʳ),[98] which provides the latest date for the death of Roger of Hook.

John son of Roger son of Asketil of Hook made a gift to Pontefract in almost identical terms to his father's gift mentioned above, omitting the word *dedi*, and with different witnesses (*Ctl. Pontefract*, no. 450). As John son of Roger [of] Hook he confirmed to the nunnery of St Clement, York, 6 perches of moor in Inklemoor of the gift of William de Percy [of Carnaby] and Robert his son, which moor John's father Roger had given to William (Burton transcripts 1, f. 45ʳ, p. 37, B12 N59). John of Hook, son of Roger of Hook, gave 6 perches of land in Hook to Ormsby in 1244 × 1251[99] (*Gilbertine Charters*, p. 67). He was amongst those attending the court of St Mary, York, in 1245 (MS Dods. 7, f. 161ᵛ), and was chosen to appear on grand assizes in 1251 and early in 1252 (*YF*, 1246–1272, pp. 23n, 69n). Thomas, John's eldest son, was of age by 1251, when Ormsby granted him the 6 perches of moor which Sir John his father had given them, in exchange for 5*m.* and 4 perches of moor in Swinefleet (MS Dods. 135, f. 139ᵛ).

In 1260, the executors of Walter Kirkham, bishop of Durham, noted his debt of £100 to Thomas of Hook, which suggests that Thomas had succeeded his father John of Hook by that date. In 1261 Walter's successor as bishop, Robert Stichill, undertook to repay the debt (*EEA*, xxix, nos 96, 163). Sir Thomas attested at least five acta issued by Stichill and his successor, Robert of Holy Island, between 1261 and 1283 (ibid., nos 185, 196, 201, 210, 250). During the time of Abbot W[illiam], as Thomas of Hook, knight, he gave to Selby Abbey a piece of land in Hook, in exchange for a toft there which the monks had by gift of his father John (*Ctl. Selby*, no. 871; *Cat. Anc. Deeds*, iii, B.3996). Like his father, Thomas was a benefactor of Ormsby (*Gilbertine Charters*, p. 64). In 1269 Thomas was substituted for William de Rye, who was seriously ill, on a commission to assess the twentieth in Yorkshire, and in the following year was exempted from being put on assizes, juries, or recognitions, or being made sheriff, against his will (*CalPat*, 1266–1272, pp. 399, 457). On 6 July 1286 Archbishop Romeyn ordered the sequestration of the goods of Sir Thomas of Hook, deceased (*Reg. Romeyn*, i, 19), and on 7 August following he issued a bond to William, lord of Hook, for repayment of a loan of £200 (ibid., ii, 155).

William of Hook held several offices in Yorkshire during the years 1303–14 (Moor, *Knights*, s.n. Houk), including the shrievalty from 1304 to 1307. In 1309, with Alice his wife, he made a fine with John son of William of Hook, presumably a younger son, concerning a messuage and 2 ct. in Hook (*YF*, 1300–1314, p. 74).[100] Records of a debt of 18*m.* owed to him indicate that William was 'recently deceased' at the end of 1311 (PRO, C 241/80/120), but this is apparently a mistake, as he continued to be appointed to commissions until September 1314 (*CalPat*, 1307–1313, passim; ibid., 1313–1317, p. 234 and passim). His successor was Thomas [II] of Hook, who in 1316 was named as lord of Cotness and joint lord of Swinton (par. Appleton-le-Street, NR) (*KI*, pp. 316, 321). The latter interest he held before the death of his father, as in 1309 he and others held common of pasture in Swinton, Amotherby, Appleton[-le-Street] and Newsham (*CalPat*, 1307–1313, p. 172). He was a commissioner for walls and ditches in 1322 (*CalPat*, 1321–1324, p. 256). Thomas of Hook and Joan his wife occur in 1328, when they made a fine concerning seven messuages, 103 a. and 7½ bv.

---

98    Abstracts from Ormsby cartulary, Davis, no. 730, 'untraced'.
99    Before the corresponding grant to John's son Thomas made in 1251 noted below; and whilst the witness Thomas of Warthill was abbot of St Mary's, York.
100   Margaret de Alta Ripa, wife of Sir William of *Honk*, who was bequeathed a gold ring in the 1312 will of William Vavasour, is difficult to place (*Northern Wills*, i, 16).

land and other property in Hook (*YF*, 1327–1347, p. 14). In 1327 Thomas was allowed 22½*m*. for keeping Margaret, daughter of Hugh Despenser the younger, in his house with a nurse and a great household, for more than three years (*CalCl*, 1327–1330, p. 47). A fine made in 1337–38 shows that Thomas was then dead, and his widow remarried to Robert Constable [IV], and suggests that his estate had passed to three coheirs. By this fine a third part of the manor of Hook was conveyed by Thomas de la Rivere knight, to John de la Rivere [probably his son][101] and Isabel his wife, subject to the estate in a third of the third part, which was held by Alice widow of William of Hook in dower, and subject also to the estate in a third of two-thirds of the third part, which Joan wife of Robert the Constable of Flamborough held in dower, and her life estate in two-thirds of two-thirds of the third part of the manor (*YF*, 1327–1347, p. 125; *EYC*, xii, 150).

**R792.**  Gift to the hospital by Roger son of Anketin of Hook of part of his moor in Inklemoor, adjoining on the south that part of the moor which the monks of Louth Park hold of the donor's fee, for ½*m*. annually [*c.*1200 × 1214]

COPY: PRO, C 53/80, Charter Roll, 22 Edw. I, m. 6, no. 16 (royal inspeximus dated 16 June 1294). CALENDAR: *CalCh*, 1257–1300, p. 446, no. 2.

Omnibus sancte matris ecclesie filiis Rogerus filius Anketini de Huuc salutem. Noveritis me dedisse et concessisse et hac presenti carta mea confirmasse deo et pauperibus hospitalis beati Petri Ebor' pro salute anime mee et antecessorum et successorum meorum quandam partem more mee in Inkelmore cum tota terra eiusdem partis more que infra continetur proximam versus solem illi parti more quam monachi de Parco de Luue tenent de feodo meo, scilicet in longitudine quantum-cumque ipsa mora protentitur versus Usiam ex una parte sine diminutione et versus Bratchmere et versus Cruul ex alia parte et in latitudine ubique viginti perticarum et preterea octo pedum ita quod perticata mensuretur decem et octo pedum, ac scilicet quod amota turba facient de terra residua libitum suum ad profectum ipsius domus. Et preterea ab ipsa mora usque ad cursum aque Usie tres perticatas in latitudine ad liberum ingressum et egressum eorum ubicumque voluerint ex directo predicte more sue ad negocia sua peragenda et communem pasturam quantum pertinet ad tantum tenementum, scilicet tenendum et habendum totum predictum tenementum cum omnibus liberis pertinentiis suis predictis pauperibus in perpetuum honorifice quiete integre libere ab omni servicio et ab omni consuetudine et ab omni exac-tione, reddendo inde michi et heredibus meis annuatim in perpetuum tantummodo dimidiam marcam argenti, medietatem ad Pentecosten et medietatem ad festum sancti Martini. Et ego predictus Rogerus et heredes mei warantizabimus et adquietabimus predictam donationem et concessionem predictis pauperibus in perpetuum contra omnes homines pro predicto servicio. Hiis testibus, S. decano et capitulo beati Petri Ebor', Girardo, Godefrido, Waltero et aliis fratribus ipsius hospitalis, Willelmo, Petro, Lamberto et aliis capellanis predicti hospitalis, Thoma de Langwath, Willelmo de Notingh', Rogero de Derby et aliis clericis predicti hospitalis, Ingulfo, Ricardo fratre eius, Rogero Troueluue, Malgero marescaldo et aliis servientibus predicti hospitalis, Iohanne de Criglest', Iacob de Houeden, Iohanne de Warewyc, Gileberto de Huuc, Petro de Byrland', Adam fratre eius, Bernardo de Morh', Ricardo filio Lamberti, Matheo de Skelton', Waltero pistore et multis aliis.

---

[101]  See *VCH Yorks NR*, ii, 104–5 for the the de la Rivere family.

The date range is given by the attestions of S[imon de Apulia] the dean, brother Godfrey, and Mauger the marshall. The witness Gilbert of Hook was possibly the man, known also as Gilbert son of Pain, who was alleged in 1218–19 to have been killed by William of Crigglestone in a burglary ten years previously, but found by the court to have been living after this time (*Yorkshire Eyre Rolls*, no. 570; *RClose*, I, 378b).

**R793.** Gift to the hospital by Roger son of Anketin of Hook of part of his moor of Inklemoor next to the part which Anketin his father gave to John of Crigglestone with Roger's sister for ½m. annually [*c*.1200 × 1214]

COPIES: *c* MS Dods. 8, f. 116ʳ⁻ᵛ, probably from the original deed formerly in St Mary's Tower, York; *d* PRO, C 53/80, Charter Roll, 22 Edw. I, m. 6, no. 16 (royal inspeximus dated 16 June 1294); differences as noted, with further minor variations of spelling. NOTED: *b* MS Dods. 120b, f. 40ʳ, four witnesses named,[102] from Rawl., f. 205, now missing, rubric *De turbario de Inkelmore*. CALENDAR: *CalCh*, 1257–1300, pp. 446–47, no. 3 (imperfect), from *d*. NOTED: 'Dodsworth's Yorkshire Notes', *YAJ*, XI, 67, indirectly from *b*.

*Carta Rogeri filii Anketini de Hunc, al' Huc.*
Omnibus sancte matris ecclesie filiis Rogerus filius Anketini de Huuc salutem. Noveritis me dedisse et concessisse et hac presenti carta mea confirmasse deo et pauperibus hospitalis sancti Petri Ebor', pro salute anime mee et antecessorum et successorum meorum, quandam partem more mee in Inkelmore, cum tota terra eiusdem partis more, que infra continetur, proximam illi parti more quam Anketinus pater meus dedit Iohanni de Crigleston cum sorore mea, scilicet in longitudine quantumcumque ipsa mora protenditur versus Vsiam ex una parte sine diminutione, et versus Bratchemere et versus Cruul ex alia parte et in latitudine ubique viginti perticarum, et preterea septem pedes ex una parte ad fossatam faciendam, et similiter ex alia parte septem pedes ad aliam fossatam faciendam, ita quod perticata mensuretur decem et octo pedum sic scilicet quod, amota turba, facient de terra residua, libitum suum ad profectum ipsius domus, et preterea ab ipsa mora usque ad cursum aque Usie, duas perticatas in latitudine ad liberum ingressum et egressum eorum, ubicumque voluerint, ex directo predicte more sue, ad negotia sua peragenda, et communem pasturam quantum pertinet ad tantum tenementum, scilicet tenendum et habendum totum predictum tenementum cum omnibus liberis pertinentiis suis predictis pauperibus imperpetuum, honorifice quiete integre et libere ab omni servitio et ab omni consuetudine et ab omni exactione, reddendo inde michi et heredibus meis annuatim inperpetuum tantum modo dimidiam marcam argenti, medietatem ad Pent' et medietatem ad festum sancti Martini. Et ego predictus Rogerus et heredes mei warantizabimus et adquietabimus predictam donationem et concessionem predictis pauperibus imperpetuum contra omnes homines pro predicto servitio. Hiis testibus, S[imone][103] decano et capitulo sancti Petri Ebor', Gerardo,[104] Herberto, Anketino et aliis fratribus ipsius hospitalis, Willelmo, Waltero, Petro, et aliis capellanis, Thoma de Languad' et aliis clericis predicti hospitalis, Ingouf, Ricardo fratre eius, Rogero Truwelove, Bernardo et aliis servientis eiusdem domus, Iohanne de

---

[102]  *Test(ibus), S. decano et capitulo sancti Petri Ebor', Thoma de Languad', Iohanne de Crigleston, Willelmo filio Thome de Revill'* etc.
[103]  *c: Simon'.*
[104]  *d: Girardo.*

Crigleston, Willelmo filio Thome de Keuill', [105] Iohanne de Warewic [f. 116ᵛ], Gileberto de Huuc, Petro de Byrland', Adam fratre eius, Bernardo de Morham, Ricardo filio Lamberti, Matheo de Skelton et multis aliis.

See R792, which has similar witnesses, for the suggested date.

**R794.** Confirmation to the hospital by John, son of Roger of Hook, of a part of the moor in Inklemoor, next to the part which Anketil his grandfather gave to John of Crigglestone with his daughter, of width 20 perches and 14 ft; and another part of the moor adjoining to the south that part of the moor which the monks of Louth Park hold of the grantor's fee, of width 20 perches and 8 ft, according to the deeds of Roger the grantor's father [1219 × 1246]

COPY: MS Dods. 8, f. 116ᵛ, probably from the original deed formerly in St Mary's Tower, York.

*Carta Iohannis filii Rogeri de Huc.*
Sciant omnes presentes et futuri quod ego Iohannes filius Rogeri de Huc concessi et <presenti> hac carta mea confirm(avi) deo et pauperibus hospitalis sancti Petri Ebor' quandam partem more in Inkelmore, que iacet proxima illi parti more quam Anketinus avus meus dedit Iohanni de Crigelistona cum filia sua, habentem in latitudine ubique viginti perticatas et quatuorde(ci)m pedes, et preterea aliam partem more in Inkelmore, que est proxima versus solem illi parti more quam monachi de Parco de Luwe tenent de feodo meo, habente ubique in latitudine viginti perticatas et octo pedes, utaque autem pars more protenditur in longitudine quantumcumque mora de Inkelmore protenditur versus Usam ex una parte et versus Brademare et versus Cruul ex alia parte sine[106] diminutione. Et habebunt predicti pauperes hospitalis duas perticatas[107] in latitudine in directo pratis more iamdicto iuxta moram Iohannis de Criglestona ubicumque voluerint et tres perticatas in latitudine in directo alterius more iuxta moram monachorum predictorum ubicumque voluerint ad liberum ingressum et regressum eorum versus incursum aque de Use ad negotia sua peraganda. Perticata autem erit decem et octo pedum. Habebunt etiam communem pasturam quantum pertinet ad tantum tenementum. Tenebunt autem et habebunt predicti pauperes totum predictum tenementum et totam terram eiusdem tenementi q(ue) infra continetur, cum omnibus liberis pertinenciis suis imperpetuum et honorifice libere integre et quiete ab omni servitio et consuetudine et exactione secundum tenorem cartarum Rogeri patris mei, quas de eodem tenemento habent, et secundum concessionem eiusdem Rogeri. Sic videlicet quod, amota turba, facient de terra residua ad libitum suam, ad profectum domus hospitalis. Predicti autem pauperes reddent inde annuatim michi et heredibus meis imperpetuum tantum modo unam marcam argenti medietatem ad Pentec' et medietatem ad festum sancti Martini. Et ego predictus Iohannes et heredes mei warantizabimus et adquietabimus totum predictum tenementum cum omnibus prenominatis predictis pauperibus in perpetuum contra omnes homines pro predicto servitio. In huius autem rei robur et testimonium huic scripto sigillum meum apposui. Hiis testibus, Roberto de Schegnes, Thoma de Paulington, Willelmo

---

[105] b: *Revill'*; d: *Kenill'*.
[106] MS: *in* for *sine*.
[107] MS: *particulas*.

de Crigleston, Iohanne de Useflet, Ada fratre suo, Thome filio Rumfari de Houeden, Roberto Angers, Theobaldo de Thollerton et multis aliis.

The first witness was Robert of Skegness, doubtless attesting in his capacity as steward of St Mary's Abbey. The abbey had substantial interests in the area. Skegness' predecessor, Thomas of Wilton, occurs in 1219 (St Mary A1, f. 212ᵛ). Skegness first attested as steward on 24 November 1220 (ibid., f. 123ʳ), and last so occurs in 1239 × 1244[108] (ibid., f. 237ᵛ). He gave all his land in Bilbrough to St Mary's, where he wished his body to be buried, by an undated deed (St Mary JR, f. 368ᵛ). Skegness' successor, G[ilbert] de Kirketon, attested as steward on 11 May 1246 (St Mary A1, f. 213ʳ). The period for Skegness as steward is compatible with the period for John of Hook.

**R795.** Gift [confirmation] to the hospital by John son of Roger of Hook of part of the moor of Inklemoor, next to the part which Anketin his grandfather gave to John of Crigglestone with his daughter, and also another part of the moor adjoining on the south the part of the moor which the monks of Louth Park hold of the donor's fee, specified as in R794 [c.1235 × 1260]

COPY: c PRO, C 53/80, Charter Roll, 22 Edw. I, m. 6, no. 16 (royal inspeximus dated 16 June 1294). NOTED: b MS Dods. 120b, f. 40ʳ, briefly cited in Hook pedigree, 1st, 5th and 7th witnesses only, where dated circa 23.H.3., from Rawl., f. 206, now missing. CALENDAR: CalCh, 1257–1300, p. 447, no. 4, from c.

Sciant omnes presentes et futuri quod ego Iohannes filius Rogeri de Huuc caritatis et pietatis intuitu et pro salute anime mee et animarum antecessorum et successorum meorum dedi concessi et presenti carta mea confirmavi deo et pauperibus hospitalis sancti Petri Ebor' quandam partem more in Inkelmore que iacet proxima illi parti more quam Anketinus avus meus dedit Iohanni de Crigleston' cum filia sua, habentem in latitudine ubique viginti perticatas et quatuordecim pedes. Et preterea aliam partem more in Inkelmore que est proxima versus solem illi parti more quam monachi de Parco de Luwe tenent de feodo meo ubique in latitudine viginti perticatas et octo pedes. Utraque autem pars more protenditur in longitudine quocumque mora de Inkelmore protenditur versus Usam ex una parte et versus Brademor et versus Crul ex alia parte sine diminutione. Et habebunt predicti pauperes hospitalis duas perticatas in latitudine in directo partis more iamdicte iuxta moram Iohannis de Crigleston' ubicumque voluerint et tres perticatas in latitudine in directo alterius more iuxta moram monachorum predictorum ubicumque voluerint, ad liberum ingressum et egressum eorum usque in cursum aque Use ad negotia sua peragenda. Pertica autem erit decem et octo pedum. Habebunt autem communem pasturam quantum pertinet ad tantum tenementum. Tenebunt et habebunt predicti pauperes totum predictum tenementum et totam terram eidem tenemento que infra continetur cum omnibus liberis pertinentiis suis imperpetuum, ita videlicet quod, amota turba, facient de terra residua ad libitum suum ad profectum domus hospitalis libere integre et quiete in liberam puram et perpetuam elemosinam sicut aliqua elemosina liberius et melius dari potest et haberi, ut ego et heredes mei simus participes omnium bonorum que fient in predicta domo dei. Ego autem et heredes mei totum predictum tenementum cum suis pertinentiis predictis pauperibus warantizabimus adquietabimus et defendemus in omnibus et contra omnes homines imperpetuum. In huius autem rei robur

---

[108] Whilst W[illiam] was abbot.

et testimonium huic scripto sigillum meum apposui. Hiis testibus, domino Iohanne
de Useflet, Willelmo Wacelin militibus, Thoma de Redness', Willelmo de Redness',
Roberto filio Angor', Yone de Bauill', Roberto Bailloll', Ricardo Charite et multis
aliis.

As three of the witnesses attested a deed of 1269 (R799), it is likely that the present
deed was given late in the tenure of John of Hook, which ended in 1251 × 1260 (FN).
The witness Eudo de Bavill gave land in Hook to Nigel son of William of Pollington
by a deed attested by Sirs Thomas of Pollington, John of Ousefleet, and John of Hook
(*Cat. Anc. Deeds*, III, B.3997).

**R796.** Gift to the hospital by Thomas son of John of Hook, knight, of the plot of land
in Morhamwick called *Le Sand*, paying ½m. annually, with licence to impound
any animals straying onto it [possibly 28 October 1265 × 27 October 1266]

COPY: PRO, C 53/80, Charter Roll, 22 Edw. I, m. 6, no. 16 (royal inspeximus dated
16 June 1294). CALENDAR: *CalCh*, 1257–1300, p. 447, no. 5.

Omnibus cristi fidelibus ad quos presens scriptum pervenerit Thomas filius Iohannis
de Huk' miles salutem in domino sempiternam. Noverit universitas vestra me concessisse dedisse et presenti carta mea confirmasse pro salute anime mee et animarum
antecessorum et successorum meorum in liberam et perpetuam elemosinam deo et
pauperibus hospitalis sancti Leonardi Ebor' totam illam placeam terre in Moramwyk'
que vocatur le Sand sicut iacet in longitudine inter gottam monachorum de Pontefracto et gottam hospitalis sancti Leonardi et in latitudine inter aquam de Usa et
regiam stratam eiusdem ville sine aliquo retenemento, cum fossato illo quod quidem
dictus Thomas et tenentes sui facere consueverunt, habendam et tenendam dictam
placeam terre cum omnibus pertinentiis suis et aisiamentis deo et pauperibus dicti
hospitalis et eorum successoribus adeo libere quiete integre et pacifice sicuti eam
aliquando melius tenui et liberius vel tenere potui, ita scilicet quod si aliqua animalia
mea propria et heredum meorum seu tenentium nostrorum dictam placeam aliquo
tempore intrent, volo et concedo quod sine aliquo contradictione mei vel heredum
meorum aut aliquorum aliorum capiantur et imparcentur et illi quorum animalia
fuerint ibidem inventa solvent dictos pauperibus vel eorum attornato apud grangiam
suam de Moramwyk' commoranti pro quolibet animali per se unum denar' quale-
cumque fuerit animal et quocienscumque ibidem captum fuerit nomine eschapii seu
quocumque alio modo et tunc sine fraude et ulteriori detentione statim deliberentur.
Reddendo inde annuatim mihi et heredibus meis dimidiam marcam argentum tantum
ad duos terminos anni scilicet medietatem ad Pentecosten et aliam medietatem ad
festum sancti Martini in yeme pro omnibus secularis serviciis et exactionibus. Et
sciendum est quod dictum hospitale sustentabit dictum fossatum imperpetuum ita
quod nec animalia mea vel heredum meorum seu aliquorum aliorum herbagium
dicti fossati de wardo facto nisi tantum ea fugando depascere valeant et si ibidem
inventa fuerint depascendo in wardo facto licebit attornato dicti hospitalis sine
alicuius contradictione ei imparcare. Et ego Thomas et heredes mei totam dictam
placeam terre [et][109] fossatum predictum cum pertinentiis et omnibus aliis aisiamentis
sicut predictum est deo et dictis pauperibus et eorum successoribus contra omnes
gentes warantizabimus et pro predicto annuo redditu acquietabimus et defendemus

---

[109] Supplied.

imperpetuum. In cuius rei testimonium tam sigillum meum proprium quam sigillum commune dicti hospitalis presenti scripto in modum cirographi confecto alternatim sunt appensa. Hiis testibus, dominis Waltero de Useflet, Iohanne de Kayvill' militibus, Thoma de Redenes, Willelmo filio Roberti de eadem, Thoma de Holmer manente in Huk', Iohanne Sharp, Ricardo de eodem, Waltero filio Galfridi de Redenes, Iohanne le Grant de Useflet et aliis.

The suggested date is taken from R797, apparently dated 50 Hen. III, which has similar witnesses and was possibly given on the same occasion.

**R797.** Thomas son of John of Hook knight confirms R795 [28 October 1265 × 27 October 1266]

NOTED: MS Dods. 120b, f. 40ʳ, in Hook pedigree, from Rawl., f. 206, now missing.

Thomas filius Iohannis de Huk miles confirm(avit) donationem predictam 50.H.3., testibus domino Waltero de Useflete, Iohanne de Kayvile militibus, Thoma de Redenes. fo. 206.[110]

**R798.** Confirmation and quitclaim to the hospital by Thomas son of John of Hook, knight, of all right in the land and moor in Inklemoor which Guy of Appleton [Roebuck] formerly held of the grantor and gave to the hospital. 4 September 1269.

COPY: c MS Dods. 8, f.117ʳ, probably from the original deed formerly in St Mary's Tower, York; d PRO, C 53/80, Charter Roll, 22 Edw. I, m. 6, no. 16 (royal inspeximus dated 16 June 1294); differences as noted with further minor variations of spelling. CALENDAR: CalCh, 1257–1300, p. 448, no. 7.

*Carta Thome filii Iohannis de Huk militis.*
Omnibus cristi fidelibus ad quos presens scriptum pervenerit, Thomas filius Iohannis de Huk' miles eternam in domino salutem. Noverit universitas vestra me concessisse et presenti carta mea confirmasse ac omnino quietum clamasse pro me et [pro][111] heredibus meis in perpetuum, pro salute anime mee et [animarum][112] antecessorum et successorum meorum deo et pauperibus hospitalis sancti Leonardi Ebor' totum ius et clamium quod habui vel aliquo modo habere potui in tota illa terra et mora cum fundo in Inkelmore quam Wido de Apelton aliquando de me tenuit, et dictis pauperibus in liberam et perpetuam elemosinam dedit, tenend(as) et habend(as) sibi et successoribus suis in liberam [puram][112] et perpetuam elemosinam, ita videlicet quod nec ego Thomas nec heredes mei nec aliquis pro nobis vel ex parte nostra aliquod ius clamium seu calumpniam in tota predicta terra et mora cum fundo de cetero ponere poterimus et exigere. Et ut mea concessio et quieta clamatio perpetuum robur obtineat, presens scriptum sigilli mei impressione coroboravi. Dat' apud Huk die sancti Cuthberti episcopi in mense septembris anno domini M°CC°Lx° nono. Hiis testibus, domino Waltero de Useflet, domino Iohanne de Kayvill', Ric(ardo) de Vescy, Thoma de Metham, Eluardo de Salsomarisco, Willelmo de Beaumes et aliis.

---

[110] MS: fo. 106.
[111] d: omitted.
[112] c: omitted.

**R799.** Confirmation to the hospital by Thomas son of John of Hook, knight, of the gifts and grants of his father in Inklemoor, specified as in R795, with further gifts. 4 September 1269.

COPY: *c* PRO, C 53/80, Charter Roll, 22 Edw. I, m. 6, no. 16 (royal inspeximus dated 16 June 1294). NOTED: *b* MS Dods. 120b, f. 40$^r$, in Hook pedigree, first eight witnesses only, from Rawl., f. 207, now missing. CALENDAR: *CalCh*, 1257–1300, pp. 447–48, no. 6, from *c*.

Sciant presentes et futuri quod ego Thom' filius Iohannis de Huk' miles concessi et hac presenti carta mea confirmavi pro salute anime mee et animarum antecessorum et successorum meorum deo et pauperibus hospitalis sancti Leonardi Ebor' omnes concessiones et donationes quas Iohannes pater meus quondam fecit deo et predictis pauperibus in Inkelmore videlicet quandam partem more in Inkelemore que iacet proxima illi parti more quam Anketinus abavus meus quondam dedit Iohanni de Crigleston' cum filia sua habentem in latitudine ubique viginti perticatas et quatuor-decim pedes. Et in super aliam partem more in eadem que est proxima versus solem illi parti more quam monachi de Parco de Luthe tenent de feodo meo ubique in latitudine viginti perticatas et octo pedes. Utraque autem pars more protenditur in longitudine quantumcumque predicta mora protenditur versus Usam ex una parte et versus Brademere et versus Crul ex alia parte sine diminutione. Et habebunt dicti pauperes hospitalis duas perticatas in latitudine in directo partis more iamdicte iuxta moram Iohannis de Crigleston' ubicumque voluerint et tres perticatas in latitudine in directo alterius more iuxta moram monachorum predictorum ubicumque voluerint ad liberum ingressum eorum usque in cursum aque Use ad negotia sua peragenda. Pertica autem erit octo decim pedum. Et in super totam illam partem more cum fundo in Inkelmore sine ullo retenemento vel diminutione que iacet inter moram predicti hospitalis et moram que quondam fuit Heruio Carp et protenditur in longi-tudine ab aqua que vocatur Usa quantum mora de Inkelmore protenditur versus Brademere et Crul. Et in augmentatione more predicte dedi eisdem pauperibus decem perticatas more cum fundo iacentis inter moram sepedicto hospitalis et moram abbatis et conventus de Thorneton'. Preterea concessi dedi et hac presenti carta mea confirmavi deo et predictis pauperibus totam illam moram cum fundo q(ue) ad me vel ad heredes meos pertinere posset iacentem in longitudine et latitudine sine aliquo retenemento vel diminutione inter La Husemoram dicti hospitalis et moram quam Wydo de Apelton' quondam de me tenuit cuius capud boriale versus capitale mesua-gium dicti hospitalis incipit ad quandam divisam que distat a cursa aque Use fere per quatuor quarentenas et est ibi valde strictum et ex inde in latum crescendo extendit se in longitudine quantumcumque mora de Inkelmore protenditur versus Brademere et versus Crul salva tamen cuilibet parcenar(io) dicte more portione sua secundum quod quilibet eorum habuit die confectionis carte presentis sicut carte quas inde habent testantur, tenenda et habenda omnia supradicta ten(ementa) cum fundo et aliis pertinentiis suis sepedictis pauperibus et eorum successoribus libere quiete pacifice et integre, in liberam puram et perpetuam elemosinam sicut aliqua elemosina melius et liberius dari potest vel haberi sine aliquo seculari servicio consuetudine secta curie et demanda, ita videlicet quod amota turba dicte more faciant predicti pauperes de terra residua pro libitio suo ad profectum sepedicto hospitalis. Et habebunt dicti pauperes communam pasturam quantum pertinet ad tantum tenementum. Ego vero Thomas et heredes mei omnia supradicta ten(ementa) cum fundo communi pastura et cum omnibus aliis pertinentiis suis deo et sepedictis pauperibus et eorum successoribus contra omnes gentes warantizabimus acquietabimus et imperpetuum defendemus. Et simus participes omnium bonorum que fiunt vel fient in illa sancta domo dei tam in vita quam in morte. In cuius rei robur et testimonium presentem cartam sigilli mei impressione corroboravi. Hiis testibus, dominis Waltero de Useflet, Iohanne de Kayvill', Roberto de Thorni militibus, Ricardo de Vescy, Thoma de Metham, Thoma de Rednesse, Roberto de Bailloll', Waltero de Haukesworthe, Thoma de Holm', Iohanne Sparc, Ricardo Charite et aliis. Dat' apud Huk' die translationis sancti Cuthberti episcopi in mense septembris anno regni regis Henrici filii regis Iohannis quinquagesimo tertio.

## Middleton
## [Middleton-on-the-Wolds]

According to the Contents List, Middleton deeds were copied on ff. 209–10 of the East Riding division of the cartulary, but Dodsworth referenced ff. 208–09 when he drew up his three rough charts of the descendants of Serlo of Middleton. He made no substantial abstracts of Middleton deeds (MS Dods. 120b, ff. 40ᵛ, 46ʳ, 105ʳ). Farrer has given notes on the feudal tenure of Middleton-on-the-Wolds (*EYC*, II, no. 1099n). Apart from these deeds, no trace of the hospital's tenure in Middleton-on-the-Wolds has been found. There were many men who took the surname of Middleton from that place. It is not easy to distinguish between the generations, and so it has not been possible to give satisfactory limits of date to these deeds.

**R800.** Gift to the hospital by Serlo of Middleton, with the consent of Margaret his wife, of two tofts and 3 a. land in Middleton with common of pasture [probably *c.*1160 × *c.*1190]

ORIGINAL: *a* YAS, MD59/1/50/1, formerly MD59/1/Hospitals/1, 16 cm. (wide) × 7 cm., badly damaged and faded, top-left-hand corner separated, a sizeable piece missing from the left-hand side of the document, bottom turn-up, slit for missing seal tag. Medieval endorsements: [ ]*elton* [ ] *et tribus acris in Middelton'*; *ii.*; *script'*. NOTED: *c1* MS Dods. 120b, f. 40ᵛ, in Middleton pedigree, from Rawl., 1st, 2nd, 8th, 7th witnesses; *c2* ibid., f. 46ʳ, similar note in pedigree, from Rawl., 'fo. 209.a. et b.' now missing, 1st, 2nd, 7th, 8th, 9th, 10th witnesses; *c3* ibid., f. 105ʳ, similar, from 'fo. 209', no witnesses. CALENDAR: *YD*, IV, no. 347, from *a*, imperfect.

Notum sit omnibus videntibus et audientibus litteras has quod ego Serlo de Midelton assensu et consensu uxoris mee Margarete et heredum meorum concessi et dedi deo et sancto Petro et pauperibus hospital(is) beati Petri Ebor' duas toftas in Mideltun et tres acras terre in campis de Mideltune cum communi pastura eiusdem ville in puram et perpetuam elemosinam [ ] liberam ab omnibus geldis et consuetudinibus et exactionibus et auxiliis ab omni seculari servicio [ ] pro animabus omnium parentum et antecessorum [ ] bonorum et orationum que fiunt in illa sancta domo dei tam in vita quam in morte [ ] warentizabimus eis contra omnes homines. Cuius rei isti sunt testes, Thomas Tuschet, Reiner [de Midleton],[113] [G]amellus dispensator, Radulfus filius Malgeri, Guido fratre eius, Guill(elmus) miles, Symon Tuschet, Thomas [filius Rei]n(er)i,[114] Guill(elmus) Tuschet, Alexander filius Yuonis, Osebertus, Karolus,

---

[113] *a* has a hole in the MS sufficient for the surname, which is supplied from *c2*.
[114] Supplied from *c2*.

Girardus clericus, Alexander miles, Ada[ ], Iohannes capellan(us) et multi alii, Thom(as)
filius Serl(onis), Thom(as) filius Will(elmi), Alexand(er) frater Serl(onis).

The gift was confirmed by Thomas, son of the donor (R801). Thomas son of Serlo
of Middleton made a grant to Ralph son of Thurstan of Lund of land in Kilnwick
in 1189 or before[115] (*YD*, VI, no. 293). Thomas Tuschet occurs in 1169 (FN).

**R801.** Confirmation of R800 by Thomas son of Serlo [probably *c.*1160 × *c.*1190]

NOTED: *c1* MS Dods. 120b, f. 40ᵛ, brief note in pedigree, from Rawl., f. 208, now
missing; *c2* ibid., f. 105ʳ, similar, same source.

Thomas filius Serlonis confirm' cum patre, eisdem testibus. fo. 208.

**R802.** Note stating that Geoffrey, brother of Serlo of Middleton, was received into
the hospital [probably later twelfth century]

NOTE: *c1* MS Dods. 120b, f. 40ᵛ; *c2* name only, f. 46ʳ; *c3* similar to *c1*, ibid., f. 105ʳ, from
Rawl.

Gaufridus frater suscep' in hospitali.

**R803.** Gift to the hospital by Thomas son of Robert of Middleton of 2 a. ½ r. in
Middleton [possibly *c.*1200 × *c.*1230]

ORIGINAL: YAS, MD59/1/50/2, formerly MD59/1/Hospitals/2, 14 cm. (wide) ×
11 cm., bottom turn-up, slit for seal tag; seal oval, brick-red wax, SIGILL'. TOME. FIL'.
ROB', design indistinct, 38 mm. (wide) × 45 mm. Medieval endorsements: *Thom' fil'*
*Roberti de ii. acris terre et dimidia roda in Midelton'*; *vi.*; *script'*. CALENDAR: *YD*, IV, no. 349.

Sciant omnes presentes et futuri quod ego Thom' filius Roberti de Middelton' caritatis intuitu dedi concessi et hac presenti carta confirmavi deo et pauperibus hospitalis
sancti Petri Eboraci duas acras terre et dimidiam rodam in campis de Middelton',
scilicet unam acram et dimidiam ad Horni(n)g toftes que iacent inter terram Willelmi
de Ros et terram Elie de Beleby, et dimidiam acram et dimidiam rodam de illa
parte terre mee ad Foxpittes que est propinquior soli, tenendas et habendas predictis
pauperibus in puram et perpetuam elemosinam cum omnibus pertinentiis suis libere
integre et quiete ab omni servicio et exactione sicut aliqua elemosina liberius et
melius teneri et haberi potest. Ego autem et heredes mee predictum tenementum
cum pertinentiis suis warantizabimus adquietabimus et defendemus in omnibus et
contra omnes homines imperpetuum. In huius autem rei robur et testimonium huic
scripto sigillum meum apposui. Hiis testibus, Willelmo filio Thom', Amfrido filio
Gileberti, Iacobo fratre suo, Rogero filio Serlonis, Galfrido Gre(u)t, Willelmo filio
Gameli, Thom'[116] clerico, Galfrido Fossard', Thom' de Wimu(n)torp, Hugone apos-
toyse et multis aliis.

---

[115]   Witnessed by Reiner [of Waxham], steward of Ranulf de Glanville, then sheriff.
[116]   The form of the last character or characters is different from the other occurrences of *Thom'*, but no
satisfactory alternative reading can be suggested.

Some clues to the date are provided by the witnesses and others. The Ros family of Helmsley had interests in Middleton-on-the-Wolds (*EYC*, x, no. 92), but as William de Ros appears here without description he cannot be securely identified as Sir William de Ros who succeeded his father Robert de Ros II in 1225–26 (*CP*, xi, 93). Not many years removed from 1200,[117] Alan son of Alexander of Middleton made a deed concerning land in Middleton, witnessed by William son of Reiner of Middleton, Gilbert son of Amfrey, Amfrey his son, William son of Thomas, William son of Gamel and others (*EYC*, ii, no. 1104). In 1218–19 Peter Tuschet of Middleton [on-the-Wolds] impleaded William son of Thomas of Middleton for wounding him. Peter subsequently died and William son of Gamel of Middleton pledged ½m. for William son of Thomas (*Yorkshire Eyre Rolls*, no. 850).

**R804.** Gift to the hospital by Thomas son of Serlo of Middleton of a toft in Middleton near the land of William son of the priest [probably late twelfth century]

ORIGINAL: *a* YAS, MD59/1/50/3, formerly MD59/1/Hospitals/3, 15 cm. (wide) × 7 cm., bottom turn-up, three slits for seal tag, seal gone. Medieval endorsements: *Thom' f' Serlonis de i. tofto in Midelton'*; *iii.*; *script'*. NOTED: *c* MS Dods. 120b, f. 46ʳ, in pedigree, from Rawl., 3rd, 4th, 7th witnesses only. CALENDAR: *YD*, iv, no. 350, from *a*.

Universis cristi fidelibus ad quo notitiam littere iste pervenerint Tomas filius Serlonis de Midelton salutem. Universiti vestre notificetur me dedisse et presenti carta confirmasse deo et beato Petro et pauperibus hospitalis sancti Petri Ebor' unum toftum in Mideltun in parte occidentali propinquius terre Willelmi filius sacerdotis. Hoc feci pro salute anime mee et patris et matris mee et omnium antecessorum meorum ut simus participes omnium orationum beneficiorum q(ue) fiunt in illa domo dei die et nocte. His testibus, Roberto filio Gaufridi, Tom' filio Willelmi, Willelmo filio R(e)in(er)i,[118] Amfrido fratre suo, et Roberto filio Amfridi, Roberto filio Malgeri, Alexandro filio Iuonis, Simone Tuschet', Tom' filio Petri et pluribus aliis.

**R805.** Quitclaim by Denise, daughter of Thomas of Middleton, clerk [probably early thirteenth century]

NOTED: *c1* MS Dods. 120b, f. 40ᵛ, note in pedigree; *c2* ibid., f. 46ʳ, similar, no witnesses; *c3*, ibid., f. 105ʳ, similar, no witnesses; all from Rawl., 'fo. 209', now missing.

Dionisia filia Thome de Midelton clerici relax(avit).[119] Teste, Roberto de Kave, Radulfo de Halton. fo. 209.

The attestation of Robert of Cave suggests Middleton-on-the-Wolds rather than Middleton Tyas.

**R806.** Agreement between the master and brethren of the hospital of St Leonard, York, of the one part, and Richard son of Thomas de Baynton of Middleton, Margaret his wife,[120] and Thomas their son of the other part, whereby the master

---

[117] Farrer gives the date range '1190 × 1210', which is broadly compatible with the three canons of Beverley who attest.
[118] Unclear.
[119] *c2, c3* end.
[120] *uxorem eiusdem Thome* on first appearance, later *iidem Ricardus et Margareta uxor eius.*

and brethren have sold and demised at farm to the said Richard, Margaret and
Thomas and whichever of them lives longest, a messuage with a croft in the
vill of Middelton, being the messuage and croft which Richard and Margaret
already held at will, to hold the toft and croft with all appurtenances besides
(*preter*) a windmill built there, to Richard, Margaret and Thomas of the said
brethren for the life of the longest lived, paying the master and brethren 5s.
annually at two yearly terms, that is at St Martin in winter and at Pentecost,
and doing suit at the court of the hospital, as other tenants are bound to
do, and each one paying the portion of goods and chattels at death just as
other tenants have been accustomed to pay. Richard's seal is attached to this
indented part remaining in the hands of the master and brethren. 5 June 1316.
No witnesses.

ORIGINAL: YAS, MD59/1/50/4, formerly MD59/1/Hospitals/7, 23 cm. (wide) ×
13 cm., top indented, bottom turn-up, slit for seal tag; seal round, black wax, a piece
remaining 20 mm. × 20 mm., an axe, legend possibly . . . WALTER . . . Medieval
endorsements: *Middelton super Wald'*; *x.*; *script'*. CALENDAR: *YD*, IV, no. 352.

. . . in vigilia sancte Trinitatis anno regni regis Edwardi filii regis Edwardi nono . . .

The medieval endorsement *Middelton super Wald'* appears trustworthy. Thomas of
Bainton was holding 1 bv. of the Ros fee in Middleton [-on-the-Wolds] in 1302–3
(*KI*, p. 256). Bainton is 2 m. north east of Middleton-on-the-Wolds.

# [Middleton Tyas, NR]

There is no evidence that there was a section for Middleton Tyas in the North Riding
volume of the cartulary. The hospital's holdings there may have been restricted to
the property granted by the deed misplaced in the Middleton-on-the-Wolds deeds
in the East Riding division of the Rawlinson volume (R807). For the early history
and tenure of Middleton Tyas, see *VCH Yorks NR*, I, 192; *EYC*, IV, 142–44. Clay has
given notes on the family of Richard of Middleton and its holdings of the honour
of Richmond in Middleton Tyas and Kneeton. Richard of Middleton, who occurs
in 1208, was the son of Thomas son of William of Middleton. In 1210–11 Richard
sold his land in Middleton and Kneeton to Gilbert [FitzReinfrid] son of Roger son
of Reinfrid, to hold for the forinsec service for 3½ ct. Gilbert gave 100m. to enable
Richard to discharge a debt to the king for certain debts to Jews (*EYC*, IV, 142–44;
ibid., V, 177; *PR*, 13 John, p. 49).

**R807.** Gift to the hospital by Richard son of Thomas of Middleton of a toft in
Middleton between the toft of Alan Briton and the donor's demesne messuage,
and 3 a. land on the west side of Kirk Beck [1204 × 1215, probably 1204 ×
1211]

ORIGINAL: *a* YAS, MD59/1/51/1, formerly MD59/1/Hospitals/1A, 17 cm. (wide) ×
9 cm., bottom turn-up, three slits for seal tag; seal oval, brick-red wax, edges and
design partly gone, 28 mm. (wide) × 35 mm. remaining, . . . RICARDI DE MIDEL. . . ,
two axes, with long vertical shafts. Medieval endorsements: *Ric' fil' Thom' de Mideltun'
de pluribus particulis*; *vii.*; *script'*. NOTED: *c1* MS Dods. 120b, f. 40ᵛ, in Middleton pedigree,

1st, 3rd and 4th witnesses, from Rawl., 'fo. 209', now missing; *c2* ibid., f. 46ʳ, similar note in pedigree, first four witnesses only, from 'fo. 209.b.'; *c3* ibid., f. 105ʳ, similar, 1st, 3rd, 4th, 5th witnesses, from 'fo. 209'. CALENDAR: *YD*, IV, no. 348, from *a*.

Omnibus has litteras visuris vel audituris Ricardus filius Thome de Middilton' salutem. Noverit universitas vestra me pro salute anime mee et antecessorum et successorum meorum dedisse concessisse et hac presenti carta mea confirmasse deo et pauperibus hospitalis beati Petri Eborac' in puram et perpetuam elemosinam unum toftum in villa de Middilton' quod iacet inter toftum Alani Brittonis et meum d(o)m(ini)cu(m) mesuagium et tres acras terre in territorio eiusdem ville continuas ex occidentali parte de Kirkebec, tenendas et habendas predictas terras cum omnibus liberis perti-nenciis suis infra villam et extra libere integre honorifice et quiete sicut ulla elemosina liberius ac melius potest teneri et haberi, ut ego et heredes mei et antecessores et successores mei simus participes omnium bonorum que fiunt vel fient in prefata domo dei in perpetuum. Hanc autem donationem et concessionem ego et heredes mei predictis pauperibus warantizabimus adquietabimius et defendemus contra omnes homines. Et ad hoc tenendum pro me et pro heredibus meis tactis sacrosanctis iuravi et sigillo meo confirmavi. Hiis testibus, Henrico filio Heruei, Philippo filio Iohannis, Radulfo de Muleton', Nicholao de Stapelton', Conano de Sedberghe, Alexandro de Aloent, Willelmo Ruffo, David de Cuton', Willelmo filio Gilleberti, Thoma filio Hugonis, fratre Roberto capellano, Thoma celerario, Girardo, Godefrido, Waltero et aliis fratribus predicti hospitalis, Willelmo de Gerundun, Petro, Lamberto et aliis capellanis suis, Willelmo de Notingh', Gregorio, Reginaldo clericis, Malgero mares-caldo, Ingulfo, Ricardo, Waltero servientibus et multis aliis.

As rector Ralph's grant of the same land (R808) includes all the lay witnesses to the present deed the two deeds must have been issued on the same occasion, and prob-ably before Richard of Middleton's grant of his interests in Middleton Tyas to Gilbert FitzReinfrid in 1210–11. Henry son of Hervey, who was living in 1212, was dead on 9 January 1216 when an order was issued to restore his lands to Ranulf son of Henry (*EYC*, v, 319). The grantor gave land in Oulston to the hospital on the same occasion (M: Oulston [Burton transcripts 1, f. 171ʳ, p. 289, B23 N56]).

**R808.** Grant at fee-farm by master R[alph], rector, and the brethren of the hospital, to Alexander son of Ralph of Middleton, of the property described in R807, paying 2*s.* annually and a portion of chattels as an obituary payment [1204 × 1215, probably 1204 × 1211]

ORIGINAL: *a* YAS, MD59/1/51/2, formerly MD59/1/Hospitals/6, 15 cm. (wide) × 6 cm., bottom turn-up, three slits for seal tag, seal gone. No medieval endorsements. CALENDAR: *YD*, IV, no. 351, from *a*. FACSIMILE: Plate VI

Omnibus presentes literas visuris vel audituris magister R. rector et fratres hospitalis beati Petri Ebor' salutem. Noveritis nos concessisse et hac carta nostra confirmasse Alexandro filio Radulfi de Middelton' unum toftum in eadem villa quod iacet inter toftum Alani Britonis et dominicum mesuagium domini Ricardi filii Thome et tres acras terre in territorio eiusdem ville continuas ex occidentali parte de Kirkebec cum suis pertinentiis in villa et extra villam, tenenda de nobis in feodo et hereditate illi et heredibus suis libere et quiete, reddendo inde annuatim nobis pro omni servicio duos solidos videlicet duodecim denarios ad Pentecost' et duodecim denarios ad festum sancti Martini in yeme. Predictus autem Alexand(er) et heredes eius vel quicumque in predicta terra manserint relinquent nobis in obitu suo portionem catallorum eos contingentem. Hoc autem tactis sacrosanctis prenominatis Alexander iuravit. Testibus, Henrico filio Heruei, Philippo filio Iohannis, Rad(ulfo) de Muleton', Nicholao de Stapelton', Conano de Sedberge, Alexandro de Aloent, Willelmo Ruffo, David de Cuton', Willelmo filio Gileberti, Thoma filio Hugonis et multis aliis.

The same witnesses and date as R807, but in a different hand.

## Malton [NR]

According to the Contents List, Malton deeds were copied on f. 211, now missing. It is curious that Malton has been assigned to the East Riding section. Apart from a rent in Malton noted in the post-Dissolution accounts for the hospital, which is also assigned to the East Riding (*Dissolved Houses*, IV, 226) there is no other evidence for the hospital's holding in Malton.

## [North Cave]

For North Cave, see R598–R622.

**R809.** 'Grant by Paulinus, minister of the hospital of St Peter, York, with the consent of the brethren, to Osbert de Brungareflet, of half their mill of Cave, at 4s. yearly rent, payable at Whit Sunday and Martinmas. Witnesses, Ranulph the priest and brother Geoffrey, Osem', Dolfin, Siwat, Ralph, Girard, Teobald, Thomas, Swain, Robert, Roger, Henry and the other brethren, master William and Thomas, brothers of master P., Geoffrey, Thomas, John, Robert, Roger, chaplains, Rainer, William, Peter, Gilbert, Robert, Walter, clerks' [*c.* 1184 × *c.* 1191]

ORIGINAL: Broughton Hall MSS, Misc. A, not currently available for examination.
CALENDAR: *YD*, I, no. 129.

Ten of the twelve brothers and four of the five chaplains who attest witnessed another deed of P[aulinus] which can be dated with reasonable confidence to 1184 × 1191 (C828 [*EYC*, I, no. 221]).

## [North Dalton]

The papal confirmation of 1148 includes 4 bv. in *Daltuna* (C178 [*EYC*, I, no. 179]), but this is undoubtedly Dalton near Topcliffe (NR) where Alan de Percy gave 2 bv. and confirmed a further 2 bv. in the 1130s (M: Dalton [*EYC*, XI, no. 6]). There was no section for North Dalton in the Rawlinson volume, and the following deed provides the only evidence for the hospital's holdings there. The hospital may have disposed of its 4 bv. to Watton, which held the rectory and a grange at Dalton worth £26 13s. 4d. at the Dissolution (*MA*, VI, 957); or to Meaux, which had more than 300 a. in North Dalton ('Ctl. Meaux', no. 359n, citing Meaux register, f. 228).

**R810.** Gift to the hospital by Ernis, son of Ace the moneyer of York, with confirmation by his eldest son and heir Robert, of 2 bv. from the donor's 4 bv. in North Dalton, being those nearest the land of the canons of Watton on the east side, with the donor's capital messuage and two tofts and crofts in the same vill [1217 × 1220]

COPY: Burton transcripts 1, f. 177ʳ, p. 301, B8 N22. NOTED: Drake, *Eboracum*, p. 335, via Torre's collections.

Omnibus presentes litteras visuris aut audituris Ernesius filius Acci monetarii de Ebor' salutem. Noverit universitas vestra me caritatis et pietatis intuitu concessisse dedisse et presenti carta mea confirmasse deo et pauperibus hospitalis sancti Petri Ebor' duas bovatas terre de quatuor bovatis meis in territorio de North Dalton, scilicet que iacent propinquiores terre canonicorum de Watton ex parte orientali, cum capitali manso meo et cum duobus toftis et croftis in eadem villa, tenenda scilicet et habenda predictis pauperibus omnia predicta in puram et perpetuam elemosinam liberam quietam et solutam ab omni seculari servicio et exactione sicut aliqua elemosina liberius et melius haberi potest cum omnibus ad predictas terras pertinentibus[121] infra villam et extra. Et ego et heredes mei totam predictam terram cum omnibus suis pertinenciis libertatibus et aisiamentis predictis pauperibus in perpetuam warantizabimus adquietabimus <et> defendemus <in omnibus> contra omnes homines. Hoc tactis sacrosanctis[122] ego cum Roberto primogenito meo et herede meo iuravi[123] et sigillo meo affirmavi. Test(ibus), domino Hamone decano Ebor', magistro Iohanne Rom(ano), Bernardo, Roberto Winton' [et] al(iis)[124] canon(icis) Ebor', Petro succentore, magistro Nicholao ----,[125] Iohanne, Lamb(erto), Radulfo de Fontibus et Alano capellanis[126] ecclesie sancti Petri, Waltero de Vestibulo, Roberto de Tyllol, Radulfo Nuuel, Anketinus de Easingwald, Ingeram de Lesset, Iohanne Iordan, Waltero Iordan et aliis.

The date range is given by the period for Hamo as dean.

# [Ravenser Odd]

For Ravenser Odd, a lost vill near Spurn Point in Holderness, see Poulson, *Holderness*, II, 529–34. There was no section in the Rawlinson volume for Ravenser Odd, which during the second half of the thirteenth century, and the first half of the fourteenth century, was a thriving port. In 1300 there was an inquisition to determine whether it would be to the loss of the king if the master of the hospital, William Langton, were to grant the hospital a plot of his waste land in Ravenser Odd, 220 ft by 120 ft, to hold by charter at a yearly rent of 3s. to the exchequer. Licence was granted the same year (*YI*, III, 137). The vill was abandoned to the sea some sixty years later, half a century before the compilation of the cartulary.

---

[121]   MS: *pertinentiis*.
[122]   MS: *Hoc a tactis factam* for *Hoc tactis sacrosanctis*.
[123]   MS: *curavi*.
[124]   The alternative expansion *Al(ano)* has been rejected as there is no evidence for a canon so named in the appropriate period.
[125]   MS: sic; cf. *CVC*, I, no. 333, where master Nicholas is described as *subcancellarius*.
[126]   MS: *Alanus capellanus*.

# [Stillingfleet]

For Stillingfleet, see R661–R664.

**R811.** Grant at fee-farm by P[aulinus], master, and the brethren of the hospital, to
Henry son of William, for his homage and service, of the 2 bv. land which
they have in Stillingfleet, paying 8s. annually [1194 × c.1202, doubtful]

COPY: BL, MS Addit. 37771 (Selby cartulary), f. 110$^{r-v}$ (old f. 109$^{r-v}$). PRINTED: *Ctl. Selby*,
no. 597, imperfectly.

*Carta Petri*[127] *magistri hospitalis sancti Petri.*
Universis sancte matris ecclesie filiis P[aulinus] magister et conventus fratrum hospitalis sancti Petri Ebor' [f. 110/109$^v$] salutem in domino. Noveritis me dedisse concessisse et hac presenti carta nostra confirmasse Henrico filio Willelmi pro homagio
et servicio suo illas duas bovatas terre quas habemus in Stivelingflet, tenendas et
habendas cum omnibus liberis pertinenciis suis infra villam et extra predicto Henrico
et heredibus suis de nobis in feodo et hereditate, libere quiete integre et honorifice ab
omni servicio et ab omni exactione nobis pertinente, reddendo inde nobis annuatim
tantummodo octo solidos, scilicet iiii$^{or}$ solidos ad Pentecosten et iiii$^{or}$ solidos ad festum
sancti Martini in hyeme. Hiis testibus, Stephano celerario, Anketino, Suano etc.

The unusual form *magister et conventus fratrum hospitalis*, which does not otherwise
appear in grants of this type, and the mixture of singular and plural, are suspicious
features. However, an agreement between the hospital and Byland concerning Skirpenbeck, dating from 1199 × 1201, refers to the *conventum fratrum hospitalis*, and is
attested by members of the York chapter, the three witnesses to the present deed, and
another brother, Gamel (R667). The three witnesses occur as brethren in the time of
Paulinus and later. Stephen became cellarer in 1194 or later. If the deed is a forgery, it
was presumably fabricated in the first half of the thirteenth century, to facilitate one
of the conveyances during that period (HN: Stillingfleet).

# [Skirpenbeck]

For Skirpenbeck, see R665–R667.

**R812.** Letter [of the brethren of the hospital of St Peter] confirming that £20 would
be paid [to the monks of Byland] if they could not warrant the land [granted
to Byland by R667] [probably 27 May 1199 × 4 March 1201]

NOTED: Byland cartulary, f. 115$^r$ (old f. 221$^r$). CALENDAR: *Ctl. Byland*, no. 1155.

Littera [. . .]$^{128}$ eorundem de xx$^{ti}$ libris nobis solvend(is) si dictam terram nobis non
poterunt warantizare.

The limits of date are those of R667.

---

[127] sic.
[128] A word difficult to decipher, apparently of four letters.

**R813.** Grant by Hugh, rector, and the brethren of the hospital, to master John Romeyn subdean of York, of an annual rent of *2m.* which the abbot and convent of Byland were bound to pay the hospital for 1 ct. in Skirpenbeck with tofts and crofts, which the grantors had by gift of Amfrey de Chauncy, with quitclaim in any right in the land [1228 × 1242]

COPY: Easby cartulary, ff. 257<sup>r–v</sup>. NOTED: *EYC*, II, 182; *Ctl. Byland*, no. 1171n.

*Fratres hospitalis quiet' clam' ii.m. redd(itus) I. Rom' q(uod) tanguntur in scripto precedenti.*[129]
*Fratres idem quietam clamat' terram de Skerpn' I. Rom'.*[130]
Omnibus etc. magister Hugo rector et fratres hospitalis sancti Petri Ebor' salutem. Nov(eritis) nos de(disse) conces(sisse) et hac presenti carta nostra confirm(asse) magistro [f. 257<sup>r</sup>] Iohanni Rom' subdecano Ebor' ecclesie pro quadam summa pecunie quam nobis in magna neccesitate nostra premanibus dedit annuum redditum ii.m. quem nobis solvere tenebantur abbas et conventus de Bellaland' ex conventione inter ipsos et nos facta pro una carucata terre cum toftis et croftis et cum omnibus pertinenciis suis in Skerpn' quam habuimus ex dono Amfr(id)i de Chancy, tenend(um) et habend(um) predicto magistro Iohanni et heredibus suis vel assignatis suis predictum redditum libere et solute et quiete in perpetuum. Nos vero predictum redditum prenominato magistro Iohanni et heredibus suis vel assignatis suis warant(izabimus) contra omnes homines in perpetuum. Preterea quiet' clamavimus eidem magistro Iohanni et heredibus suis vel assignatis suis totum ius nostrum quod in predicta terra quocumque modo ad nos pertinere poss(it). In huius autem rei robur et testimonium huic scripto sigillum nostrum appo(suimus).

The date range is the period for John Romeyn as subdean of York.

## [Stockton on the Forest, NR]

For Stockton on the Forest, see R668–R669.

**R814.** Confirmation by Roger de Mowbray of the agreement between the hospital and Thomas Guacelinus concerning 3 ct. in Stockton which Thomas holds of the grantor, for which the hospital pays 20s. annually [1138 × 1148]

ORIGINAL:YAS, MD59/1/77/3, formerly MD59/21/Misc (part), 20 cm. (wide) × 7–11 cm., 14 mm. tongue for seal, of which no trace remains, 7 mm. wrapping tie. Medieval endorsement: *Confirmato R. de Molb'i de carta Thome Guacelin de terra de Stoketun.* PRINTED: *Mowbray Charters*, no. 298, via Lancaster's transcript of the original, where dated 1138 × May 1148. FACSIMILE: Plate VIII.

Roggerus de Molbraio archiepiscopo Eboracensi et capitulo sancti Petri et dapifero suo et omnibus ministris et amicis suis francis et anglis salutem. Sciatis me concessisse et presenti carta et sigillo confirmasse conventionem et pactum quod est inter Thomam Guacelinum hominem meum et fratres hospitalis sancti Petri Eborac' de tribus carucatis terre in Stocatuna quas tenet de me, pro quibus fratres hospitalis

---

[129]  Rubric on f. 257<sup>r</sup>.
[130]  Rubric on f. 257<sup>v</sup>.

reddent supradicto Thome et heredibus suis xx. solidos singulis annis inperpetuum, x. solidos ad festum sancti Martini et decem in Pentecosten, et hoc pro omnibus geldis et consuetudinibus et auxiliis et serviciis, excepta relevatione quam ipsi heredi meo de illa terra facient et danageldo quod per totam Angliam cucurrerit. Ipse autem Thomas Guacelinus et heredes sui facient michi et heredibus meis omne servicium quod super illam terram venerit et ipse Thomas guarantizabit fratribus hospitalis illam terram contra omnes. Teste, Radulfo de Wiuilla et Olyvero de Buci et Gualtero Wincebag et Iohanne capellano et Radulfo de Daiuilla et Rotberto de Buci et Guillelmo de Mamet heremer et Helya de sancto Martino.

Roger de Mowbray came of age in 1138. 3 ct. in Stockton were confirmed to the hospital in 1148 (HN: Stockton). Greenway assigns the witnesses to the 1140s.

## [Wharram le Street]

For Wharram le Street, called Great Wharram in the following deed, and the Fossard interest there, see *EYC*, II, 390–91. The Rawlinson volume did not contain a section for Wharram, and there is no mention of the place in the papal confirmations to the hospital. The hospital interest was limited to two mills, and the sites of, or for, two further mills, which according to the following deed were conveyed to Meaux Abbey in the time of rector Hugh and Abbot Michael, i.e. 1235 × 1245. The deed further states that it was William Fossard who had granted the mills to the hospital (R815). If this can be relied on, the grant to the hospital was made before 1195, when William Fossard II was dead (*EYC*, II, 328). Grants of land in Wharram were made to Meaux by both William Fossard I and his son William II, including the watercourse of Wharram for a mill. William II had large debts, and it is possible that these were a factor in the hospital's acquisition of the mills (*EYC*, II, 390).

In 1234 a fine was made between Hugh, master of the hospital, and Peter de Mauley and Isabel his wife, whom Jordan of Hampton had called to warrant, concerning two mills and the sites of two other mills in Great Wharram (*YF*, 1232–1246, p. 20). Jordan of Hampton's interest is not otherwise attested. He was a clerk,[131] and it is not impossible that this was a fictitious suit in order to improve the title before the assignment of the property to Meaux. The extent of 1287 records 4*m*. rent of the mills of *Wharul* (R903). The reduced rent of £2, as agreed in 1300, was still being paid at the Dissolution (*MA*, V, 396).

**R815.** Agreement between Walter, bishop of Coventry and Lichfield, and master of the hospital, and the brethren, of the one part, and brother Roger, abbot of Meaux, and the convent, of the other part, reciting that Hugh, master, and the brethren of the hospital had granted to Michael, then abbot of Meaux, and the convent, two water mills and the sites of another two mills, in Great Wharram, which the hospital had by grant of William Fossard, for 4*m*. annually. 1*m*. of the rent was to be remised, so Meaux would henceforth pay 40*s*. annually.

---

[131]  For Jordan of Hampton, parson of Kirkburton and of Bentham, see *Reg. Gray*, pp. 28, 36, 192n, 232n; *YD*, IV, no. 505; ibid., V, nos 262, 459n, 465, 467, 469–71. He occurs in 1246 (*Lancs. Fines*, I, 100), and was named as parson of Bentham in an assize roll of 1251–52 (Griffith, 'Yorkshire Clerics', p. 25, citing Assize Roll 1046, m. 72). In 1247, a presentation was made to a mediety of the church of [Kirk]burton (*Reg. Gray*, p. 100). Jordan son of Gilbert of Hampton occurs in 1248 (*YF*, 1246–1272, p. 6). He was presumably dead in 1255, when William of Ouseburn was rector of Bentham (*Ctl. Furness*, II, 327).

Right of distraint in the property, and in the other tenements of the abbey in Great Wharram, if the rent is henceforth in arrears. Friday 25 November 1300.

ORIGINAL: Bodl.,Yorks. Ch. 108, 21 cm. (wide) × 14 cm, bottom turn-up, slit for seal tag, top edge indented, CIROGRAPHUM ABCD cut through; well-preserved seal, good impression, red wax, vessica, 26 mm. × 44 mm., a robed figure standing on a platform, holding a pastoral staff in his right hand and a book in the left; to the dexter a star, moon, and cinquefoil or rose, to the sinister a star, moon, and a [?] bird; +[s]IGILLVM: ABBATIS: DE: MELSA, probably a unique example. Medieval endorsement: *B. De Melsa de molendinis de Wharrum*; no roman numeral or *script'*. FACSIMILES: (including seal), engraved plate of two deeds, entitled 'Antient deeds and seals', 'from the originals in the possession of R. Rawlinson LLD, FRS . . . sumptibus Soc. Antiq. Lond. 1751';[132] Tickell, *Hull*, plate facing p. 178[133] (whence noted Poulson, *Holderness*, II, 314 and whence seal noted *MA*, V, 389–90; seal noted from Poulson at *VCH Yorks*, III, 149). CALENDAR: *Bodleian Charters*, p. 638.

Anno regni regis Edwardi filii regis Henrici vicesimo nono die veneris in festo sancte Katerine virginis apud Ebor' convenit inter dominum Walterum dei <gratia> Coventr' et Lich' episcopum magistrum hospitalis sancti Leonardi Ebor' et fratres eiusdem loci ex una parte et fratrum Rogerum abbatem de Melsa et eiusdem loci conventum ex altera, videlicet quod cum Hugo magister et fratres hospitalis predicti aliquando dimisissent fratri Michaeli tunc abbati de Melsa et eiusdem loci conventui duo molendina aquatica cum stagnis et omnibus aliis pertinentiis suis in Magna Wharrum simul cum omnibus sitibus[134] duorum aliorum molendinorum cum pertinentiis in eadem villa, que omnia habuerunt ex dono Willelmi Fossard', reddendo inde predicto hospitali annuatim quatuor marcas argenti prout in scriptis inde inter eos tunc confectis plenius contineri videtur. Predictus vero Walterus magister predicti hospitalis et fratres eiusdem loci remiserunt ex nunc[135] predictis abbati et conventui de Melsa ----atis[136] [u]nam marcam argenti redditus supradicti, ita videlicet quod singulis annis a tempore confectionis presentium dicti abbas et conventus de Melsa reddant et persolvant hospitali suprascripto quadraginata solidos sterlingos in festis Pentecostes et sancti Martini per equales portiones pro predictis molendinis et eorum pertinentiis ut est premissum. Et si contingat quod predictus redditus quadraginta solidorum de aliquo termino aretro fuerit de cetero bene liceat magistro et fratribus et eorum successoribus qui pro tempore fuerint in predictis tenementis et etiam in omnibus tenementis que idem abbas et conventus habuerunt die confectionis presentium in predicta villa de Magna Wharrum ad quorumcumque manus devenerint distringere et districtionem illam sicut captam quo sibi viderint expedire effugare et eam retinere quousque eisdem magistro et fratribus de predicto redditu annuo quadraginta solidorum plenarie fuerit satisfactum. In cuius rei fidem et memoriam huic scripto

---

[132] An example of the plate is bound in Gough's copy of Burton's *Monasticon Eboracense* (Bodl., Gough Yorks 55). The other deed is an undated grant by John, prior of Drax, to John son of Nicholas de Osgoteby. Two associated deeds, engraved from Rawlinson's collection in other plates, reached the Bodleian Library, but not this one (Bodl.,Yorks. Chs 51, 332).

[133] Annotated 'Hull, published as the Act directs, April 16th, 1790, by T. Browne, R. Millson, G.W. Browne & G. Prince.' Three of those named were amongst the publishers of Tickell's book. Neither the ownership nor the location of the deed is stated.

[134] MS: *situbus*.

[135] Unclear.

[136] MS creased and stained, possibly *memoratis*.

bipartito sigilla partium predictarum alternatim sunt appensa. Dat' apud Ebor' die et anno supradict'.

Meaux's copy of this deed, which was not copied into the Meaux cartulary, was doubtless the main source of the information relating to the acquisition of the mills given in the Meaux chronicle (*Chron. Meaux*, II, 62, 224).

# Extents

The following five documents provide some limited information about the financial affairs of the hospital towards the end of the thirteenth century and a few years prior to its surrender in 1540. The thirteenth-century documents doubtless travelled to Lichfield during the time when Walter Langton was both bishop of Coventry and Lichfield and master of the hospital in the late thirteenth and early fourteenth century.

**R901.** Summary of estimated revenues and expenses of the hospital. 11 October 1280.

ORIGINAL: Lichfield RO, D30/12/113, formerly Qq8. Single membrane, 19–20 cm. (wide) × 60 cm. BRIEF ABSTRACT: Benson, *St Leonards*, pp. 3–4.[1]

Rotulus de terris et redditibus hospitalis sancti Leonardi Ebor' taxat(is) die veneris proxima post festum sancti Dionisii anno domini M°.CC. octogesimo.

[*Marginated*] Grang(ia) de Acum.[2]
Ibidem sunt quatuor caruce[3] cum pratis et pasturis que valent per annum xx. marcas. Summa patet.
[*Marginated*] Docker.
Ibidem sunt due caruce cum pasturis pratis que valent per annum x.li. Summa patet.
[*Marginated*] Heselington'.
Ibidem sunt tres caruce et valent comunibus annis vi.li. xiii.s. iiii.d. Item ibidem sunt iiii.li. redditus de quibusdam terris de dominico tradit(is) ad firmam ad terminum xi. annorum. Summa x.li. xiii.s. iiii.d.
[*Marginated*] Hewrd'.
Ibidem est una caruca et dimidia et valent per annum lxvi.s. viii.d. Summa patet.
[*Marginated*] Benigburg'.
Ibidem sunt quatuor caruce et valent per annum C.s. Item ibidem sunt xviii. acre prati que valent per annum lxxii.s. Item ibidem sunt xii. acre de frisscis que valent per annum xxiiii.s. Summa ix.li. xvi.s.
[*Marginated*] Sutton'.
Ibidem sunt due caruce et valent per annum v. marcas. Summa patet.
[*Entry starts in margin*] Domus de Esingwald' cum clauso valet per annum vi. marcas. Summa patet.
[*Marginated*] Lede.
Ibidem sunt tres caruce et valent per annum x.li. xiii.s. iiii.d. Item ibidem sunt iiii. li. redd(itus) de quibusdam terris de dominico tradit(is) ad firmam ad terminum xviii. annorum. Summa xiiii.li. xiii.s. iiii.d.

---

[1] 'Copy per W.A. Evelyn, translated by R.B. Cook, see Cook MSS, York Museum'.
[2] *Grangia de* is probably intended to apply to all the places named in this section.
[3] sic, not *carucate*, here and elsewhere.

[*Marginated*] Morhamwyk.

Ibidem sunt v. acre terre et quedam magna turbaria que deservit hospitale ad inveniend(um) turbas ad expens(is) hospitalis.

[*Marginated*] Brungflet.

Ibidem sunt quatuor caruce cum prato pastur(a) et aliis pertinenciis que valent per annum lx.li. Summa patet.

[*Marginated*] Bramhop'.

Ibidem est una caruca et valet per annum in omnibus C.s. Summa patet.

[*Marginated*] Eskelby.

Ibidem sunt due caruce que ponuntur ad firmam et valent per annum x.li. Summa patet.

[*Marginated*] Hunton'.

Ibidem sunt tres caruce et valent per annum xii.li. Summa patet.

[*Marginated*] Bowes.

Ibidem sunt tres caruce cum ecclesia eiusdem ville et cum quedam parva collecta que omnia estimantur ad l. marcas que omnia expenduntur in hospitalitate prout a principio fieri consuevit et illa grangiam cum ecclesia et collecta habet quidam frater Willelmus de Eskelbi tota vita sua per scriptum signatum comuni sigillo hospitalis et debet sustinere ibi secum duos fratres hospitalis et recipere magistrum et fratres in eundo et redeundo de partibus Westmerl' et Cumberl'.

[*Marginated*] Garthorn.

Ibidem sunt tres caruce et valent per annum vi. marcas. Non seminatur ibi nisi avena. Summa patet.

Item pasture que pertinent ad hospitale ubique excepta pastura neccesaria ad boves van(ag)iorum xx. marc(as). Summa patet.

Item de placitis perquisitis et portionibus tenent(ium) xx. marc(as).

Summa total(is) C.iiii^xx.vi.li. xvi.s. preter portionem fratris Willelmi de Eskelby que non computatur in ista summa.

## Ecclesie que tenentur in proprios usus eiusdem hospitalis.

Ecclesia de Neuton' valet per annum l. marcas.

Ecclesia de Rufford' valet per annum x.li.

Ecclesia de Saxton' valet per annum l. marcas.

Summa valor(is) ecclesiarum lxxvi.li. xiii.s. iiii.d.

## Collecte eiusdem hospitalis.

Donecast' Upton' Knottinglay Elmete valent per annum C.li.

Coupland' valet per annum iiii.li.

Nona garba de Melton' iiii. marcas.

Loncaster et Wirisdale viii. marcas.

Furneys et Kertmel' lx.s.

Lounesdale et Kendal' viii. marcas.

Parva Wald' Burtun Lokyngton' Brunne et Hugate xxii. marcas.

Insula de Axilholm v.li.

Werueldale cum minutis collectis xx. marcas.

Cravene ix.li.

Burussire xv.li. vi.s. viii.d.

Ridale preter collectam de Malton' xxiiii.li. vi.s. viii.d.

Malton' et Wintringham valent per annum x. marcas.

Harfordlith' xi.li.

Hakenes et Scalleby iiii. marcas
Wytebistrand' ix. marcas.
Cliveland xx.li.
Magna Wald xxxv. marcas.
Richemundschire et collecta de Saureby cum collecta de Karleol' et cum nona
garba de Brigenhal' vii$^{xx}$ marcas.
Spaldigmor xxviii.li. i. marcam.
Holdernesse xx.li.
Inter Huse et Derwent viii.li.
Collecte que pertinent ad grang(ias) dicti hospitalis xx.li.
Collecta de Westmerl' x. marcas.
Collecta que pertinet ad subcelerar(ium) xx. marcas.
Summa CCCC.lxi.li. vi.s. viii.d.[4]

Item de redditu assiso ubique extra civitatem et de firmis molend(inorum) cum
minutis firmis infra civitatem Ebor' ut patet per particulas CC.xiii.li. xi.s. viii.d. ob.
de quibus non possunt levari per annum ix.li. vii.s. ii.d. Et sic remanet de claro
CC.iiii.li. iiii.s. vi.d. ob.
Item de lana et aliis exitis de instauro hospitalis quadammodo placuerit CC. marcas.
Summa CCC.xxxvii.li. xi.s. ii.d. ob.

Summa total(is) extente M.lxii.li. vii.s. ii.d. ob.
Summa total(is) expensarum M.xxxv.li. v.s. iii.d. ob.
Ita remanent ad omnes expens(as) magistri preter panem et ceram qu(ando) est
prope civitatem xxvii.li. xxiii.d.

[*dorse*]
            De diversis rebus que tangunt hospitale sancti Leonardi Ebor'.

    Rotulus de expen(sis) hospitalis sancti Leonardi Ebor' exceptis omnibus expen(sis)
    magistri preter quam in pane et cera per annum dum fuerit iuxta civitatem.

[*Marginated*] De solutione firmarum.
In firmis aliis solvend(is) annuatim xviii.li. xii.s. x.d.
[*Marginated*] De pensionibus solvendis.
In pensionibus aliis per annum debitis per script(os) liiii.li. ix.s. iii.d. ob.
[*Marginated*] De stipendis infra cur(iam).
In stipendis capellorum secularium et famillorum comorant(ium) infra cur(iam)
xxvii.li. ix.s. x.d.
[*Marginated*] De stipendis pastorum.
In stipendis pastorum et custis eorundem ad grangias per annum xliiii.li. vi.s. iiii.d.
Summa C.xliiii.li. xviii.s. iii.d. ob.

[*Marginated*] De duro blado.
In pane ad sustentand(um) expen(sas) consuetas hospitalis in hospitalitate ad portam
et alibi et in aliis expensis necessariis, scilicet in expensis magistri cum fuerit prope
civitatem et in expensis fratrum et sororum capellorum et infirmorum infirmitor(ii)
et familie et liberationum et omnium servientium quorum non est nummarius[5]

---

4   The sum is 6*s.* 8*d.* short.
5   MS: *num'ius.*

videlicet: de frumento qualibet septimana xv. quar(teria), summa per annum DC.lx. quar(teria),[6] prec(ium) quar(terii) v.s., summa C.iiii^xx.xv.li.;

de silig(ine) qualibet septimana xv. quar(teria), summa per annum DC.lx. quar(teria), prec(ium) quar(terii) iiii.s., summa C.lvi.li.;

item de silig(ine) ad festum sancti Leonardi per annum in errogatione pauperibus facienda lx. quar(teria), prec(ium) quar(terii) iiii.s., summa xii.li.

Summa CCC.lxiii.li.

[*Marginated*] De braseo.

In cervisia qualibet septimana ad totam familiam prescriptam preter magistrum videlicet: de braseo avene, qualibet septimana xviii. quar(teria), summa per annum DCC.iiii^xx.xvi. quar(teria), prec(ium) quar(terii) ii.s. vi.d., summa C.xvii.li.;

de braseo ordei qualibet septimana vi. quar(teria), summa per annum CC.lxxii. quar(teria), prec(ium) quar(terii) iii.s. vi.d., summa liiii.li. xii.s.

[*Marginated*] De prebenda.

In prebenda equorum qualibet septimana viii. quar(teria). Summa per annum CCC.lvi. quar(teria), prec(ium) quar(terii) xviii.d., summa xxxi.li. iiii.s.

[*Marginated*] De farina.

In farina ad coquinam de avena de Brungflet per annum vi^xx quar(teria), prec(ium) quar(terii) ii.s., summa xii.li.

Summa CC.xiiii.li. xvi.s.

[*Marginated*] De lardar(ia).

In carnibus grossis qualibet septimana ad totam familiam predictam preter magistrum et hospites scilicet per tres dies cuiuslibet septimane preter sex septimanas Quadrag(esime) xxxvi.s., summa iiii^xx.li. xvi.s.[7]

[*Marginated*] De allece.

In expensis familie predicte annuatim et in errogatione facta pauperibus ad festum sancti Leonardi x. lastes allecis de garnestur(a), prec(ium) cuiuslibet laste l.s., summa xxv.li.

[*Marginated*] De pisce.

In dogedrage[8] empt' ad totam familiam predictam per annum D., prec(ium) cent(enarii) xx.s., summa C.s.

Item in pisce albo empto in Quadrag(esimo) per sex septimanas ad fratres et sorores et capellanos qualibet septimana per tres dies septimane vii.s. vi.d. Summa xlv.s.

[*Marginated*] De caseo empto.

In expensis domus per annum preter caseum de instauro domus DCCC. petr(e), prec(ium) petre vi.d. Summa xxiiii.li.

[*Marginated*] De butiro.

In expensis domus per annum preter instaurum s(cilicet) de butiro empto CC.lx. petr(e), prec(ium) petre ix.d., summa xi.li. v.s.

[*Marginated*] De dupplic(ibus) fest(is) ex antiqua consuetudine.

In expensis fratrum et sororum capellorum et familie per dupplicia festa per annum, scilicet in interferculis vii.li., summa patet.

Summa C.lvii.li. x.s.[9]

---

6    The 'long hundred' (120) is used for *quarteria* and *petre*.

7    recte £82 18s. 0d.

8    A type of fish, possibly cod (*OED*, s.v. dogdrave).

9    The subtotal is 4s. too much. The correct figure is given in the summary account (R902).

[*Marginated*] De hospitibus et forestar(iis).

In expensis iusticiar(iorum) foreste senescalli forestar(iorum) viredar(iorum) rewardator(um) et aliorum ministrorum foreste per communem estimationem per annum xxx.li., summa patet.

Item in expensis aliorum hospitum et supervenientium secundum communem estimationem xx.li. preter panem et cervisiam, summa patet.

Item in expensis eorundem et in exenniis ad supervenientes et alios missis annuatim s(cilicet) de vino tria dolea prec(ium) dolei l.s., summa vii.li. x.s.

Summa lvii.li. x.s.

De variis expensis necessar(iis) domus.

In equis ad fratres et ad carectas per annum xx.li.

In sustentatione officii subcelerar(ii) per annum xx. marc(e).

In reparatione domorum redditual(ium) et domorum infra curiam per annum xx.li.

In expensis fratrum et servientium per annum circa firmas colligend(as) et alios den(arios) de collectis C.s.

In donis datis per annum magnatibus ballivis senescallis cuncur(ialibus) advocatis et aliis. xx.li.

In aquietatione decime domini pape vel domini regis per annum x. marc(e) ad tempus.

In feno per annum preter prata domus singulis annis x.li. ad sustentationem hospitalis et instauri.

In sustentatione et reparatione vasorum et utensilium coquine bracine pistrine et aliarum domuum, nichil per annum, q(uod) de exitibus coquine.

In cera per annum l.s.

In oleo annuatim xxv.s.

Summa iiii$^{xx}$ .xviii.li. xvs.

Summa totalis expens(arum) M.xxxv.li. v.s. iii.d. ob.[10]

This and the following summary were doubtless compiled as a result of the inquiries into the hospital's advowson and indebtedness made in 1280.

**R902.** Summary of the estimated receipts and expenses of the hospital contained in R901, with a narrative account of its indebtedness in 1276–80.

ORIGINAL: Lichfield RO, D30/12/115, formerly Qq10 (part). Single membrane, 18–19 cm. (wide) × 21–22 cm. BRIEF ABSTRACT: Benson, *St Leonards*, p. 3.[11]

Extenta hospitalis.

Memorandum quod die veneris proxima post festum sancti Dionisii anno domini M°.CC. octagesimo [*11 October 1280*] facta fuit extenta hospitalis coram domino Willelmo de Saham et vicomite Ebor' in presencia fratris Thome [de Gaytinton] et R[ogeri] de Malton' quondam custodum, celerar(ii) W. de Eskelby, Laurent(ii), W. de Saham fratrum de omnibus terris redditibus collectis firmis singulis exitibus et omnibus aliis ad hospitali sancti Leonardi pertinentibus hoc modo

---

[10] The sum total of expenses is apparently £1 below the correct figure, which is probably connected with the incorrect figure for pensions and stipends in the summary account (R902).

[11] 'Copy per W.A. Evelyn, translated by R.B. Cook, see Cook MSS, York Museum'.

Summa extente grangiarum C.iiii<sup>xx</sup>.vi.li. xvi.s.
Summa valor(is) ecclesiarum lxxvi.li. xiii.s. iiii.d.
Summa extente collectarum CCCC.lxi.li. vi.s. viii.d.
Summa reddituum assis(orum) et firmarum cum lana et aliis exitibus
CCC.xxxvii.li. xi.s. ii.d. ob.
Summa totius valoris M.lxii.li. vii.s. ii.d. ob.

> Expen(se) dicti hospitalis except(is) omnibus expens(is) magistri preter quam in
> pane et cera per annum dum fuerit iuxta civitate.

In firmis aliis solvend(is) pensionibus et stipend(is) diversorum
C.xliii.li. xviii.s. iii.d. ob.[12]
In DC.lx. quar(teriis) frumenti, prec(ium) quarterii v.s. et DC.lx. quar(teriis) siliginis
per annum, una cum lx. quar(teriis) siliginis ad festum sancti Leonardi, prec(ium)
quarterii iiii.s. — CCC.lxiii.li.
Item [in] DCC.iiii<sup>xx</sup>.xvi. quar(teriis) brasei avene, prec(ium) quarterii ii.s. vi.d.,
et CC.lxxii. quar(teriis) brasei ord(e)i, prec(ium) quarterii iii.s. vi.d., et CCC.lvi.
quar(teriis) avene ad prebendam, prec(ium) quarterii xviii.d., et in vi<sup>xx</sup>. quar(teriis)
avene ad farinam, prec(ium) quarterii ii.s. — CC.xiiii.li. xvi.s.
In lardario allece pisce caseo et butyro C.lvii.li. vi.s.[13]
In expens(is) hospitum et forestariorum per annum lvii.li.
In variis expensis et necessariis domus iiii<sup>xx</sup>.xviii.li. xv.s.

Summa total(is) expens(arum) prout patet in singulis summis per parcellas
M.xxxv.li. v.s. iii.d. ob.

Ita remanent ad omnes expens(as) magistri preter panem et ceram ut superius
dictum est xxvii.li. xxiii.d.

Et compertum fuit coram supradictis circa extentam assisientibus quod collecte
travarum valent plus post adventum dicti Rogeri de ducentis li. quam fecer(un)t
qu(ando) fratres eas collegerunt.
Item compertum fuit eodem die quod omnia bona hospitalis ante tempore dicti
Rogeri per magistres et fratres sepius extenta non sufficiebant ad sustentationem
domus nisi per tres partes anni.

[*dorse*]

Status hospitalis anno septuagesimo sexto.
Memorandum quod die iovis proxima ante nativitatem beati Iohannis baptiste
anno domini M°.CC.lxx. sexto [*20 June 1276*], quo die R[ogerus] de Malton'
fuit institutus ad custodiend(um) hospitale sancti Leonardi Ebor', invenit dictum
hospitale cum quibusdam grangiis obligatum prout patet per parcellas in M.xxviii.
li. xiiii.s.
Quibus satisfecit post adventum suum de D.CCCC.lix.li. xii.s. v.d.
Et preter istam summam solutam apposuit in emptionibus terrarum reddituum

---

[12]  The figure is £1 less than that reported in the main account (R901).
[13]  This figure is reported differently in the main account (R901).

et in finibus pro terris factis et diversis redemptionibus ac construct(i)onibus
domorum novarum per grangias prout patet [per] parcellas CC.lxxv.li. xviii.s. iii.d.
Summa duarum partium M.CC.xxxv.li. x.s. viii.d.

Et memorandum quod in adventu suo invenit dictum hospitale habens defectum
in frumento siligine braseo prebenda farina carnibus pisce allece caseo butiro et
omnibus aliis warnesturis.

Item in secundo anno adventus sui moriebantur per scabiem MMM.CC.v. tam de
bidentibus quam de agnis.

Status hospitalis anno octogesimo.

Memorandum quod in festo sancti Michaelis anno domini M⁰.CC. octogesimo
[29 September 1280] fuit dictum hospitale obligatum prout patet per parcellas tam de
antiquo debito quam de novo in C.lxxvii.li. xix.s. iiii.d. Et remanserunt in octab(e)
nativitatis beate Marie [15 September 1280] in compotum tam in pecunia numerata
quam in arreragiis et aliis debitis prout patet per parcellas CCC.xiiii.li. i.d. ob.
Preterea blada per omnes grangias fuerit dicto die sancti Michaelis integre tam de
decimis quam de dominicis et de collectis que non venduntur.

Item habent de veteri frumento sustentationem sufficientem usque ad natale. Et
de veteri siliginis usque ad festum sancti Martini excepto die sancti Leonardi. Item
empta fuerunt viiˣˣ.xviii. averia ad lardar(ium) tam bobus quam de vaccis. Item
facta est providencia de pisce et allece caseo et butiro pro magna parte.

Memorandum quod dictus R[ogerus] recep(it) ex mutuo de diversis amicis in
primo anno et dimidio octingentas¹⁴ marcas ad providend(um) in supradictis
defectibus et debitis aquietand(is).

**R903.** Extent of the manors and rents belonging to the hospital. August 1287.

ORIGINAL: Lichfield RO, D30/12/106, previously Qq1. A roll of three membranes,
each membrane 20–25 cm. (wide) × 60–70 cm. BRIEF ABSTRACTS: Benson, *St Leonards*,
pp. 6–9;¹⁵ Cullum, 'Hospitals', pp. 111–13.

Rychemund'

[*Marginated*] Eskelby.

Extenta facta ibidem die dominica in festo sancti Laur(entii) anno regni regis
E[dwardi] xv⁰ [10 August 1287] coram H[ugone] de Cressyngham¹⁶ per Walterum
filium Iohannis de Lemyng, Henricum de Lede de eadem, Galfridum le mercer
de eadem, Henricum le pestur de eadem, Alanum Fox de eadem <et> Nicholaum
prepositum de Eskelby iur(atos), qui dicunt super sacramentum suum quod capitale
mes(uagium) cum gardino clauso prato iuxta grangiam et marisco ad capud dicti
mes(uagii) val(et) per annum xxx.s. Summa xxx.s.

Sunt ibi de terra lucrabili viiiˣˣ <vi.> acre, prec(ium) cuiuslibet acre xviii.d.
Summa xii.li. ix.sol.

Sunt ibi de prato falcabili vii. acre, prec(ium) cuiuslibet acre iii.s. iiii.d.
Summa xxiii.s. iiii.d.

---

¹⁴ The first few characters of this word are unclear.
¹⁵ 'Copy per W.A. Evelyn, translated by R.B. Cook, see Cook MSS, York Museum'.
¹⁶ For Hugh of Cressingham and his death at the battle of Stirling in 1297, see *ODNB*.

Est ibi pastura communis in qua possunt sustentari x. vacce i. taurus, et valet pastura illa per annum v.s. Summa v.s.

Item est ibi alia communa pasture in qua possunt sustentari bidentes CC. per estimationem et aliquando plures et aliquando pauciores, qua communa non est incerto. Ideo non extenditur.

Sunt ibi ii. molendina, unum aquaticum et aliud ventricium, et valent per annum xxx.s. Summa xxx.s.

Est ibi de redditu assi(s)o omnium tenentium manerii videlicet de Eskelby, Kirtelington', Rypon', Pykehale et Helagh'[17] vii.li. xviii.s. vii.d. ob. Summa vii.li. xviii.s. vii.d. ob.

Item de firma unius mes(uagii) in Lemyng' quod nunc est in manu magistri hospitalis v.s. iii.d. Summa v.s. iii.d.

Consuetudines liberorum valent per annum xi.s. Summa xi.s.

Placita perquisita valent per annum dimidia marca. Summa dimidia marca.

Item sunt ibi ix. acre terre in manu magistri hospitalis predicti que valent per annum iiii.s. Summa iiii.sol.

Summa totalis extente — xxvi.li. ii.sol. x.d. ob.

[*Marginated*] Hunton'.

Extenta facta ibidem coram H[ugone] de Cressingham die lune in crastino sancti Laur(entii) anno supradicto [*11 August 1287*] per Thomam de Horneb', Henricum filium Gilberti, Ricardum fabrum, Walterum de Burton', Hugonem le bakeler, Robertum filium Rad(ulf)i fabri, Petrum filium Willelmi, Thomam le mare(s)call', Willelmum filium Hugonis, <et> Willelmum filium Rogeri iur(atos) qui dicu(n)t super sacramentum suum quod capitale mes(uagium) cum columbario et herbagio infra clausam valet per annum x.s. Summa x.s.

Sunt ibi de terra lucrabili ix$^{xx}$ acre <et ii. [et][18] dimidia> et valet quelibet acra per annum xviii.d. Summa xiii.li. xiii.s. ix.d.

Sunt ibi de prato falcabili xxv. acre et valet quelibet acre iiii.s. Summa C.s.

Est ibi unum molendinum ventricium quod valet per annum x.s. Summa x.s.

Est ibi communa pasture ad bidentes sine numero sed[19] non extenditur.

Est ibi de redditu assiso omnium tenentium manerii iiii.li. xix.s. viii.d. Item de redd(itu) cotar(iorum) vii.d. Summa C.s. iii.d.

Item sunt <ibi> de pastura separabili iii. acre et valet quelibet acra per annum viii.d. Summa ii.s.

Summa totalis extent(e) xxiiii.li. xvi.sol.

Westmerland'

[*Marginated*] Garthorn'.

Extenta facta ibidem coram H[ugone] de Cressingham hac die martis proxima post festum sancti Laur(entii) anno supradicto [*12 August 1287*] per Adam Attebanke, Iohannem filium Astini, Robertum le wetherhird, Henricum Brune, Walterum filium Gilberti, Henricum le couhirde <et> Robertum de Kendale iur(atos) qui

---

[17]  *Helagh* has not been identified, and may be Healaugh near Reeth, or Healey in Mashamshire, but there is no other evidence for a hospital interest in those places. It is improbable that Healey near Batley, where the hospital did have an interest, is intended.

[18]  Supplied.

[19]  MS: *sz.*

dicunt super sacramentum suum quod capitale mes(uagium) cum curtulagio et herbagio valet per annum v.s. Summa v.s.

Sunt ibi de terra lucrabili CC.xxi. acre et valet quelibet acra per annum viii.d. Summa vii.li. vii.s. iiii.d.

Sunt ibi de prato falcabili iiii<sup>xx</sup> acre et valet quelibet acra ii.s. Summa viii.li.

Sunt ibi pasture separabiles in quibus possunt sustentari per annum lx. vacce cum earum exit(u) <trium> annorum, et M. bidentes, et valet pastura per annum C.x.s. Summa C.x.s.

Est etiam ibi communa pasture in qua possunt sustentari per annum per estimationem MMMM. bidentium et potest valere per annum x.li. Summa x.li.

Est ibi unum molendinum aquaticum quod non molit nisi tantum bladum manerii et non potest sustentare se ipsum et ideo non extenditur.

Est ibi de redditu assiso omnium tenentium manerii xli.s. x.d. ob. Summa xli.s. x.d. ob.

Item est ibi de redditu xxxii. gall(inarum) per annum, prec(ium) cuiuslibet i.d. Summa ii.s. viii.d.

xiiii. bovate terre dant de consuetudine pro respectu habendo <de> secta molendini iii. quart(eria) et di(midio) farme avene, prec(ium) quarter(ii) iii.s. iiii.d. Summa xi.s. viii.d.

Servicia consuetudines liberorum valent per annum xix.s. vi.d. Summa xix.s. vi.d.

Summa totalis extente xxxiiii.li. xvi.s. ix.d. ob.[20]

### Kendale

[*Marginated*] Docker.

Extenta facta ibidem coram H[ugone] de Cressingham die mercurii proxima post festum sancti Laur(entio) anno supradicto [*13 August 1287*] per Nicholaum le Stodhird, Adam filium Nicholai, Adam de Crossedale et Adam de Crosserigge iur(atos), qui dicunt super sacramentum suum quod capitale mes(uagium) valet per annum ii.s. Summa ii.s.

Sunt ibi de terra lucrabili iiii<sup>xx</sup> et x. acre et valet quelibet acra per annum iiii.d. Summa xxx.s.

Sunt ibi de prato falcabili xx. acre et valet quelibet acra xviii.d. Summa xxx.s.

Est ibi pastura separabile in qua possunt sustentari xl. vacce cum exitu trium annorum et valet pastura per annum lx.s.

Est ibi communa pasture in qua possunt sustentari xxiiii. boves et aliquando plures et xl. iumente, scilicet non extenditur communa illa eo quod est incerta etc.

Est ibi quidam boscus in quo nihil potest percipi per annum nisi tantum necessaria in cur(ia), scilicet pannagium inde val(ens) per annum xii.d. Summa xii.d.

Est ibi unum molendinum aquaticum et non potest sustinere se ipsum, ideo non extenditur etc.

Est ibi de redditu assiso quatuor tenentium manerii lii.s. iiii.d. Summa lii.s. iiii.d.

Summa total(is) extente — viii.li. xv.s. iiii.d.

[*Marginated*] Bowes.

Extenta facta ibidem coram H[ugone] de Cressingham die iovis in vigilia assumptionis beate Marie anno supradicto [*14 August 1287*] per Alanum de Eskelby, Uctredum le Stodhird, Willelmum le carpent', Stephanum le tynkeler, Adam filium

---

[20]  1*s.* 3*d.* has been lost from the total.

Roberti, Iohannem le tollere, Willelmum carpent', Iohannem filium Malle et Adam faber iur(atos), qui dicunt super sacramentum suum quod capitale mes(uagium) cum columbario valet per annum vi.s. Summa vi.s.

Sunt ibi de terra lucrabili v^xx.xiiii. acre et valet quelibet acra per annum vi.d. Summa lvii.s.

Sunt ibi de prato falcabili xv. acre quarum quelibet acra valet per annum ii.s. Summa xxx.s.

Sunt ibi ii. molendina, unum aquaticum et aliud ventricium, que non possunt sustinere se ipsa ideo non extenduntur.

Est ibi quedam pastura separabile que valet per annum dimidia marca. Summa dimidia marca.

Ad istud manerium pertinet quedam communa pasture in Staynmore in qua possunt sustentari animalia sine numero et q(ue) est in incerto ideo non extenditur.

[*at the foot of the membrane*] respice intergo.

[m. 1d]

### Adhuc de extenta de Bowes.

Est ibi de redditu assiso omnium tenentium manerii xxiiii.s. vi.d.; item de redditu gallinarum per annum xxii., prec(ium) cuiuslibet i.d.; item de redditu ovorum per annum xi^xx,[21] prec(ium) vi.d. Summa xxvi.s. x.d.[22]

De operibus autumpnalibus per annum xlviii. prec(ium) cuiuslibet i.d. Summa iiii.s. Summa total(is) vi.li. x.s. vi.d. Inde solvuntur per annum Rogero filio Rogeri pro ii. bovatis terre iiii.s. Et sic rem(anet) de claro de total(i) extenta vi.li. vi.s. vi.d.

Ecclesia istius ville pertinet ad hospitale sancti Leonardi et est appropriata eidem hospitale et valet per annum cum decimis hanniletorum[23] ad illas spectantibus per estimationem l. marce. Summa l. marce.

Summa summarum dictorum maneriorum et ecclesie C.xxxiiii.li. iiii.s. ii.d.

### Redd(itus) forinseci pertinentes ad hospitale.

De Ebor' xliii.li. vii.sol. viii.d.

De Heselyngtone per annum ix.li. xiiii.s. x.d.

De Heyworthe et Styuelyngflet xxxiii.s. iiii.d.

De Neutone xxv.li. iiii.s. xi.d.

De Benigburg lxxvi.s. ii.d. extra mol(endinum)

De Flatewathe et Hulveston' lx<x>viii.s. iiii^or.d.

De Huntone lxiii.s. x.d. ob.

De Eregethorn xxxii.s. x.d.

De Neutone et Herneby lxv.s. x.d. ob.

De Eskelby xlviii.s.

De Lemyng' lxx.s. ob.

De Kertlyngtone xlviii.s. viii.d.

---

[21] The number is not entirely certain.
[22] This total includes only 6*d*. sheep rent.
[23] Apparently sic, but meaning unclear.

De Kynigtone ix.li. ii.s. iiii.d.
Howe ix.li. xiiii.sol.
De Heinderby cum vill(a) propinquius liii.sol. vi.d.
De Alvertone et Crakehale iiii.li. xviii.s. vi.d.
De Clyveland xxxv.sol. vi.d.
De redd(itu) ad mens(am) fratrum assignato lv. sol. viii.d.
De firma molend(inorum) de Wharul liii.s. iiii.d.
De Nappay per annum C.xv.s. x.d.
De Holegyle iiii.li. v.sol.
De Bramhope xxx.s. viii.d.
De Middeltone lxx.s. i.d.
De Lethelay et Stochilde xv.li. iiii.d.
De Denecastre vii.li. xvi.s. iiii.d.
De Nottynggelee lxv.sol. v.d.
De Elmete xi.li. ii.s. viii.d.
De Pudesey et Bateley xxvii.s. vii.d.
De Martone lxxii.s. vii.d.
De Ruchford iiii.li. vii.sol. iii.d.
De Coupmannethorn²⁴ cum pertinentiis xxxvi.s. iiii.d. et una libra cere
De Rybbestein xvi.s. ii.d.
De Brungeflet ix.li. xi.s. vi.d.
De Rydale et Waldale xvi.li. xiiii.s. ii.d.
De Hol<der>nesse xiii.s. iiii.d.
De Westmerelaund Cumberlaund Galewey Lonesdale Kendale et Leggardwode
.xiiii.li. ix.s.

Summa totius redd(itus) per annum CC.xliii.li. xi.s. vii.d. ob.

Inde allocatur alibi et oneratur in extent(is) maneriorum diversorum
xxxvi.li. iii.sol. iii.d.
In defen(so)²⁵ redd(itus) in vill(a) Ebor' hoc anno xx.li. xvii.s. vi.d. Summa lvii.
li. ix.d. Et sic rem(anet) ad onerand(um) hic C.iiii^xx.vi.li. x.s. x.d. ob.

Item de travis de collecta blad(i) in comitat(ibus) Ebor' Westmerl' Cumberl' et
Laungcastr' cum nonis garbis quarumdam terrarum et aliis minutis collectis per
annum per estimationem²⁶

[m. 2]

Extenta facta coram H[ugone] de Cressingham et fratre Waltero de Brumpton de
manerio de Beningburg' die lune in crastino sancti Laur(entii) anno regni regis
E[dwardi] xv°. [*11 August 1287*]

Iohannes de Beningburg', Willelmus filius Godewyn', Willelmus de Clifford',
Willelmus filius Henrici de Beningburg', Adam de Benigburg' in Neuton',
Eustachius de eadem, Alanus de Westewod', Iohannes filius S(t)effan(i), Adam filius

---

²⁴ sic, for Copmanthorpe.
²⁵ Unclear.
²⁶ No figure given.

Willelmi filii Godewyn', Iohannes Rotewell', Willelmus filius Wydoni et Henricus filius Rotewell' iurati, dicunt quod capitale messuagium in omnibus exitibus valet per annum dimidia marca. Et sunt ibidem in dominico de terra lucrabili ii<sup>C</sup>.lii. acre terre dimidia acra, quarum quelibet acra valet per annum vi.den. Et est summa vi.li. vi.s. et iii.den.

Sunt etiam in eodem manerio lii. acre terre et dimidia que solebant esse de dominicis, et que Willelmus Paytewyn nunc tenet de feoffamento magistri Galfridi de Haspall' et fratrum hospitalis sancti Leonardi. Et reddunt per annum xxvi.s. viii.den. Summa xxvi.s. viii.d.

Sunt etiam ibi lxi. acre terre que fuerunt de dominico et nunc includuntur [in][27] <novo> parco de Beningburg' ideo non extenduntur hic. Et est summa summarum terre lucrabil(is) in denar(iis) vii.li. xii.s. et xi.den.

Sunt etiam ibi xxxviii. acre prati et iii. rode prati de dominico, et valet quelibet acra per annum iiii.s. Et est summa vii.li. et xv.s.

Sunt etiam ibi lii. plaustrat(e) bosci et marem(ii) <in foresta regis> que capiuntur singulis septim(anis) ad husbot et haybot <et aliquando plus> prout decet quarum quelibet plaustrata valet iiii.den, unde summa per annum xvii.s. iiii.den.

Dicunt etiam quod pastura in foresta regis quam fratres hospitalis habent ibi et habere debent valet per annum ii.s. Et pannag(ium) eorundem ibidem xviii.den. Unde summa utriusque per annum iii.s. vi.den.

Et est ibi quoddam parcum quod continet in se vi<sup>xx</sup> et xvi. acras terre et bosci, et valet in subbosco pannagio et pastura per annum xl.s. Summa xl.s.

Est ibi quoddam molendinum ventricium quod valet per annum x.s. Summa patet. Summa summarum totius extent(e) xix.li. v.s. v.den.

Dicunt etiam xii. iurat(i) quod garba sancti Petri collecta in diversis locis per caruc(as) que adimantur in manerio predicto valent per annum per estimationem xxvi.s. iiii.d. Summa patet.

Summa summarum utriusque xx.li. xi.s. et ix.den.

Predicti xii. iur(ati) dicunt quod in manerio de Neuton' est unum messuagium <cum duabus bovatis terre> quod fuit perquisitum fratrum hospitalis, et preter illud quatuor messuagia et viii. bovate terre unde quelibet bovata continet octo acras que sunt de dominico ecclesie predicte ville. Et que dimittuntur ad firmam per particulas. Et dicunt <quod> predictum mesuagium pro(pin)quiorum <cum predicta terra> valet per annum xli.s. Quatuor mesuagia et viii. bovate reddunt per annum de firma iiii.li. xi.s. iiii.d. Est ibidem aliud mes(uagium) quod pertinet ad ecclesiam et valet per annum v.s. De redditu assiso in predicto manerio xvi.li. xii.s. vii.d. Dicunt etiam quod ecclesie de Neweton' cum alteragio valet per annum xxvi.li. xiii.s. iiii.d.

Item dicunt quod pannagium de bosco valet per annum xii.d. Est etiam ibidem quidam redditus vii.s. qui debet percip(ere) de domino Roberto de Ros de molend(ino) de Linton'. Placita et perquis(ita) ibidem valent per annum dimidia marca.

Summa l.li. xvii.s. xi.d.[28]

---

[27] Supplied.
[28] A large blank space follows, as if allowing the extent of another manor to be inserted.

Extenta facta de manerio de Sutton die martis proxima post festum sancti
Laur(entii) anno supradicto. [*12 August 1287*]

[*Marginated*] Sutton'.
Ricardus Travers de Sutton', Robertus Scharthehalf, Walterus Parvus de Sutton',
Walterus forestarius de Hoby, David' de eadem et Robertus de Ros iurat(i). Dicunt
super sacramentum suum quod capitale mesuagium cum columbar(io) valent i.m.
Et sunt ibi de terra lucrabili iiii^xx et vi. acre et dimidia et valet quelibet acra per
annum vi.den. Summa xliii.s. et iii.den. Sunt etiam ibi vii. acre prati falcabil(is)
et valet quelibet acra per annum xii.den. Summa vii.s. Dicunt etiam quod in
dominicis manerii que includuntur non potest aliquis communicare cum ipsis. Et
valet pastura per annum v.s. Dicunt etiam quod communa pastura infra forestam
ubi communicant et nihil dant <et> cum husbot et haybot in eadem foresta valet
per annum i.m. Dicunt etiam quod pounagium unde sunt quieti in foresta valet
per annum xviii.den.
Summa totius extent(e) iiii.li. iii.s. et v.den.

Dicunt eciam quod garbe sancti Petri collect(e) in diversis locis et adimate in
manerio predicto valent per annum iiii.li. Summa patet.

Summa utriusque viii.li. iii.s. v.d.

Extenta facta de manerio de Esingwald die et anno supradictis.

[*Marginated*] Esingwald.
Predicti iurator(i) dicunt quod capitale messuagium valet per annum v.s. Dicunt
etiam quod sunt ibi ix. acre terre lucrabil(is) et valet quelibet acra per annum
vi.den. Summa iiii.s. vi.den. Dicunt etiam quod sunt ibi xl^a acre de prato falcabi(li)
que per totum annum tenentur in defenso et valent per annum v.m. Dicunt etiam
quod pastura in foresta ubi communicant et nihil dant valet per annum vi.s.
Summa totius extent(e) iiii.li. ii.s. ii.den.

[m. 2d]
Extenta facta apud Hewode die martis prox' post festum sancti Laur(entii) anno
regni regis E[dwardi] xv.[29] [*12 August 1287*]

[*Marginated*] Hewrth.
Duodecim iur(ati) dicunt super sacramentum suum quod capitale messuagium istius
manerii in omnibus exitibus cum columbare valet per annum vii.s. Sunt ibi de
terra lucrabil(i) C.xiiii. acre per minorem centenarium et valet quelibet acra ix.d.
Summa iiii.li. v.s. vi.d. Sunt etiam ibi quatuor acre prati facabil(is) unde due acre
valent per annum viii.s., et due acre alie valent per annum iii.s. Summa utriusque
xi.s. Dicunt etiam quod husbote et heybote que pertinent ad manerium predictum
in foresta regis cum pastura in eadem foresta valent per annum xiii.s. iiii.d. Sunt ibi
duo molendini ventricii que valent per annum preter reprysam xl.s. Et non possunt
extendere ulterius <eo> quod non est ibi secta ad predicta molendina nisi tantum
blada fratrum hospitalis sancti Leonardi que ibidem moluntur.
Summa totalis extente vii.li. xvi.s. x.d.

---

[29] MS: *vx.*

De garbis sancti Petri que coliguntur[30] in diversis villis et adimuntur in manerio
predicto, dicunt quod valent per annum xxvii.s. iiii.d.

Summa utriusque ix.li. iiii.s. ii.d.

Extenta facta in manerio de Lede die mercurii proxima post festum Laurenc(ii)
anno supradicto. [*13 August 1287*]

[*Marginated*] Lede.
Duodecim iur(ati) dicunt super sacramentum suum quod capitale mesuagium cum
columbar(io) et uno molendino aquatico infra situm predicti mesuagii valent per
annum xxxiii.s. iiii.d. Sunt ibi de terra lucrabili CCCC.xxi. acre per minorem
c(entenarium) quarum quelibet acra valet per annum v.d. Et est summa viii.
li. xv.s. v.d. Est ibi quedam terra que spectat ad manerium et vocatur Spitelflate et
continet in se iiii^xx.i. acra et dimidia et dimittitur ad firmam per annum pro iiii.
li. iii.s. vi.d. Sunt ibi de prato separato a pastura xxiii. acre et dimidia, precium
cuiuslibet acre ii.s. Summa xlvii.s.
Item est ibi una acra prati que est de decima ecclesie et valet per annum ii.s.
Summa utriusque xlix.s.
Est ibi quidam boscus qui vocatur le Fal unde habent[31] husbote et haybote et valet
per annum vi.s. Summa xvii.li. vii.s. iii.d.

Dicunt quod garbe sancti Petri collate in diversie villis et adimate in eodem
manerio valent per annum xl.s.
Dicunt etiam quod ecclesia de Saxton' valet per annum xxxiiii.li.

Summa tot(ius) manerii cum ecclesia liii.li. vii.s. iii.d.

Extenta facta in manerio de Bramhop' die mercurii proxima post festum sancti
Laur(entii) anno supradicto. [*13 August 1287*]

[*Marginated*] Bramhop.
Duodecim iur(ati) dicunt super sacramentum suum quod capitale mesuagium ut in
herbag(io) curtilag(io) et gardin(o) valet per annum x.s. Est ibi quedam placea de
herbag(io) inclusa cum duabus acris terre et dimittuntur ad firmam per annum iii.s.
Item sunt ibi duo tofta vasta et dimittuntur ad firmam pro xii.d. et scilicet valet.
Item sunt ibi iiii^xx acre de terra lucrabili, precium cuiuslibet acre vi.d. Summa xl.s.
Item sunt ibi xii. acre prati et valet quelibet acra per annum iii.s. Summa xxxvi.s.
Est ibi quidam boscus in quo percipi potest husbote et haybote et valet per annum
cum herbagio xiiii.s. Item est ibi quedam turbaria et valet per annum xviii.d.
Dicunt etiam quod fratres et familia domus qui sunt in mensa fratrum debent esse
quieti de multura et valet per annum xii.d. Item sunt etiam ibi xviii. precarii qui
debent fieri per unum diem in autumpno et valet xviii.d. preter reprisam cibi.
Sunt ibi duo cottarii qui faciunt vi. precar(ias) in autumpno et valent vi.d. ut supra.
Est ibi pastura ubi debent cum omnibus animalibus suis communicare et valet
per annum xvii.s. vi.d. Placita et perquisita valent dimidia marca. Item sunt xlviii.
<libere> tenentes et faciunt de redd(itibus) per annum xxxi.s. viii.d.

---

30  MS: *que coliguntur* repeated.
31  MS: *habent* repeated.

[*Marginated*] Memorandum de portionibus et redditibus.

Item collecta garbarum sancti Petri per annum que dimittuntur ibidem ad firmam et valent per annum v.s.

Summa totius viii.li. ix.s. iiii.d.

[*Marginated*] Kyrkestall'.
Extenta in predicta villa de Bramhop de manerio de Kirkestall' facta die et anno supradictis. Et quod manerium fratres hospital(is) tenent ad firmam ad terminum xxx. annorum unde unus annus est elapsus et pro <quo> manerio predicti fratres satisfecerunt abbati de Kirkestal de firma pro toto tempore an(te) ingressum eidem manerii.
Predicta iur(atores) dicunt quod capitale mesuagium sicut includitur valet per annum viii.s. Est ibi alia claustur(a) que vocatur la bercar(ia) et continet in se duas acras et valet iiii.s. Sunt ibi de terra lucrabili quinques viginti et quindecim acre, pre(cium) acre v.d. Summa xlvii.s. xi.d. Item sunt ibi xxii. acras i. roda et dimidia pre(cium) acre ii.s. Summa xliiii.s. ix.d. Est ibi communa pastur(a) in qua communicare debent[32] fratres cum omnibus animalibus suis et valet per annum ratione predicti manerii xvii.s. vi.d. Est ibi quodam molendinum aquaticum et valet per annum xl.s. Sunt ibi diversi homines qui tenent ad voluntatem v$^{xx}$ acre terre que sunt de dominicis predicti manerii valent per annum xxxviii.s.
Summa x.li. ii.d.

Extenta de terra Dukett' in villa predicta que fratres tenent ad firmam et pro qua satisfecerunt an(te) ingressum.

Predicti iur(ati) dicunt quod capitale mesuagium valet per annum vi.d. Sunt ibi de terra lucrabili xxxvi. acre et valet quelibet acra per annum v.d. Summa xv.s. Sunt ibi de prato iiii. acre et iii. rode pre(cium) acre xviii.d. Summa vii.s. i.d. ob.
Summa xxii.s. vii.d. ob.

[m. 3]
Extenta facta de manerio de Akum cum appendiciis suis die iovis in vigilia assumptionis beate Marie anno regni regis E[dwardi] xv°. [*14 August 1287*]

[*Marginated*] Acum.
Duodecim iurati dicunt per sacramentum suum quod situs manerii sicut includitur per fossat(um) et hayam valet in omnibus exitibus viii.s. Est ibi aliud mesuagium quod vocatur le Wodehall et valet per annum ii.s. Sunt ibi de terra lucrabili CCC. acre per minorem c(entenarium) precium acre viii.d. Summa x.li. Sunt ibi xxiii. acre prati precium acre xx.d. Summa xxxviii.s. iiii.d. Dicunt etiam quod pastura in dominicis suis tempore aperto valet ii.s. Dicunt etiam quod sunt ibi duo bosci de quibus pastur(is) in eisdem husbote et haybote subboscus et pannag(ium) valent per annum lx.s.
Summa xv.li. x.s. iiii.d.

---

[32] Word unclear.

Collecta bladi sancti Petri facta in diversis locis et adimata in eodem manerio valet per annum v.li. iiii.s. vii.d. ob.

[*Marginated*] Rugford'.[33]

[*Marginated*] Haselinton'.
Duodecim iur(ati) dicunt super sacramentum suum quod capitale mesuagium cum uno clauso adiacente prout includuntur in omnibus exitibus cum uno columbar(io) valent per annum x.s. Item sunt ibidem de terre lucrabili CC. acre per maiorem cent(enarium) et valet quelibet acra per annum x.d. Summa x.li.
Item sunt ibidem xxvi. acre de prato falcabili et valet quelibet acra per annum ii.s. Summa lii.s.
Item est ibidem unum molendinum ventricium quod valet per annum xl.s.
Item sunt ibidem duo homines qui tenent iii. bovatas terre et una mulier que tenet unam cotariam et reddunt per annum de redditu ix.s. iiii.d. Et faciunt predicti diversa opera per annum que valent cum gallinis et ovis que redd(unt) ii.s. iii.d. et non plus q(uod) cibum eis allocatur. Dicunt etiam quod capiunt per annum in manerio pro agistatione averiorum Ebor' v.s. Item sunt ibidem vii. bovate terre que dimittuntur ad firmam et reddet quelibet bovata xi.s. preter una que reddet xiiii.s. Et est summa iiii.li. Est ibidem de redditu assiso liberorum tenetium per annum C.v.s. vi.d. Item placita et perquis(ita) valent annu(atim) iiii.s. Item est quedam turbaria et valet per annum v.s.

Summa totius extent(e) xxv.li. xiii.s. i.d.

Dicunt quod collecta garbarum sancti Petri valet per annum xxiii.s. et adimatur in eodem manerio de Haselington'.

Extenta

[*Marginated*] Morhamwyk'.
Extenta facta ibidem die iovis infra octab(am) assumptionis beate Marie anno regni regis E[dwardi] xv. [*21 August 1287*] coram H[ugone] de Crassngham per Nigellum carpentar', Ricardum filium Roberti, <Rogerum Sparki> Robertum de Ormesby, Rogerum le Ku et Michaelem Snel iur(ati), qui dicunt super sacramentum suum quod capitale mes(uagium) cum omnibus infra circuitum preter eysiamentum domorum valet per annum iii.s. Summa iii.s.
Sunt ibi xiii. acre et dimidia terre lucrabil(is) quarum quelibet acra valet per annum viii.d. Et est summa ix.s. Est ibi pastura seperabil(e) que valet per annum iiii.s. Summa iiii.s.
Est ibi una turbar(ia) que vocatur Inkelmor' que respondet per annum de lxxii. navat(is) turbarum, precium cuiuslibet navat(a) v.s.; et de xl. quar(teriis) sal(is), prec(ium) quar(terii) xviii.d., simul cum dominicis manerii que superius extend(untur), summa xxi.li. Est ibi de redditu assiso trium tenentium cotag(iorum) vii.s. Summa vii.s.

Summa totius extente xxii.li. iii.s.

[*Marginated*] Brungelflet'.
Extenta facta coram H[ugone] de Crassingham die iovis infra octav(am)

---

[33] A blank space is allowed for the extent, which has not been entered.

assumptionis beate Marie [*21 August 1287*] anno supradicto per xii. iuratos, qui dicunt super sacramentum suum quod capitale mes(uagium) cum gard(ino) columbar(io) et toto circuitu valet per annum xv.s.
Sunt ibidem de terra lucrabil(e) CCC.liiii. acre et valet quelibet acra xx.d. Summa xxix.li. x.s.
Sunt ibi de prato frisco lxviii. acre et valet quelibet acra ii.s. vi.d. Sunt ibi de prato salso xxxii. acre et dimidia, valet quelibet acra iii.s. Summa xiii.li. vii.s. vi.d.
Est ibi quedam piscar(ia) que commit(etur) ad firmam pro liii.s. iiii.d. Summa iiii. marce.
Est ibi unum molendinum ventricium quod valet per annum xl.s. Summa xl.s. solvuntur apud <Ebor ideo non non ext(enditur) hic.>
Est ibi quedam communa pastur(a) in qua possunt sustentare MM.v. bidentes et alia averia sin numero. Et q(uod) ignoratur inde valor et est in incertum ideo non adhuc extend(itur).
Est ibi de redd(itu) assis(o) tam liberorum quam nativorum C.xi.s. ii.d. de quo respons(us) in scaccario hospitalis ideo non oneratur hic.
Servicia et consuetudines liberorum et nativorum valent per annum lxxi.s. xi.d.
Placita et perquisita valent per annum i. marca.

Summa totius extente except(is) molend(ino) et redd(itu) assis(o) l.li. xi.s. i.d.

[m. 3d]
Extenta terrarum hospitalis sancti Leonardi Ebor'.[34]

This extent and the following summary were made whilst the hospital was in the king's hands, soon after the death of the master Geoffrey of Aspall in June 1287. Hugh of Cressingham (d. 1297) was a king's clerk and justice. He was the bishop of Ely's steward until 1286, when he became steward of the lands of Queen Eleanor, and a member of her council. Soon afterwards he occurs as a commissioner and a justice of assize (*ODNB*).

**R904.** Summary valuation of the hospital made by Hugh of Cressingham. 18 August 1287.

ORIGINAL: Lichfield RO, D30/12/114, formerly Qq9. Single membrane, 20–22 cm. (wide) × 50 cm. Contemporary endorsement: *Rotulus de valore maneriorum et omnium aliorum spectant(ium) ad hospitale sancti Leonardi Ebor'.*

Rotulus valor(is) maneriorum ecclesiarum et aliorum bonorum spectant(ium) ad hospitale sancti Leonardi Ebor' factus per H[ugonem] de Cressyngham die lune proxima post assumptionis beate Marie anno regni regis E[dwardi] xv^mo.

[*Marginated*] Ebor'

[*Marginated*] Benyngburg.
Manerium eiusdem ville valet per annum except(o) redd(itu) assis(o) xix.li. v.sol. v.d.
[*Marginated*] Neutone.
Manerium eiusdem ville valet per annum xxiiii.li. iii.sol. viii.d.

---

34 Endorsed thus at the head and foot of the membrane.

[*Marginated*] Suttone.
Manerium eiusdem ville valet per annum iiii.li. iii.s. v.d.
[*Marginated*] Esyngwald.
Manerium eiusdem ville valet per annum iiii.li. ii.s. ii.d.
[*Marginated*] Heworthe.
Manerium eiusdem ville valet per annum vii.li. xvi.s. x.d.
[*Marginated*] Lede.
Manerium eiusdem ville valet per annum xvii.li. vii.s. iii.d.
[*Marginated*] Bramhop'.
Manerium eiusdem ville valet per annum vi.li. xii.s. viii.d.
[*Marginated*] Kyrkestal.
Manerium eiusdem ville in quo hospitale habet terminum xxx. ann(orum) valet
per annum x.li. ii.d. Terra Duketti in eadem villa valet per annum xxii.s. vii.d. ob.
Akum. Manerium eiusdem ville valet per annum xv.li. x.s. iiii.d.
[*Marginated*] Heselyngt'.
Manerium eiusdem ville excepto redd(itu) assis(o) valet per annum xx.li. vii.s. vii.d.
Summa vi^xx.li. xii.s. i.d. ob.[35]

## Richemunde

[*Marginated*] Eskelby.
Manerium eiusdem ville excepto redd(itu) valet per annum xviii.li. iiii.s. iii.d.
[*Marginated*] Huntone.
Manerium eiusdem ville valet per annum exc(epto) redd(itu) xix.li. xvi.s. iiii.d.
[*Marginated*] Bowes.
Manerium eiusdem ville valet per annum C.ii.sol.
Summa xliii.li. ii.s. vii.d.

## Westmerland'

[*Marginated*] Garthorn'.
Manerium eiusdem ville excepto redd(itu) valet per annum xxxii.li. xiiii.s. xi.d.
Summa xxxii.li. xiiii.sol. xi.d.

## Kendal'

[*Marginated*] Dolker.
Manerium eiusdem ville excepto redd(itu) valet per annum vi.li. iii.sol.
Summa vi.li. iii.sol.

Ecclesie que tenentur in proprios usus eiusdem hospitalis et valor earundem.

[*Marginated*] Ebor'
Ecclesia de Neutone et valet per annum xl. marcas.
Ecclesia de Rufford et valet per annum x.li.
Ecclesia de Benigburg et valet per annum — non est ibi ecclesia nisi de Neutone.
Ecclesia de Saxstone et valet per annum xxxiiii.li.

---

[35] This sum is written above the entries for Acomb and Heslington, which have been inserted underneath.
Nevertheless the total is intended to include these two manors, but is £10 less than it should be.

[*Marginated*] Rychem'
Ecclesia de Bowes et valet per annum l. marcas.
Summa val(oris) ecclesiarum C.iiii.li.

De thravis et aliis collectis
De travis blad(orum) in comitatibus Ebor' Westmerl' Cumb'laund' et Laungcastr'
cum nonis garb(is) et aliis collectis bladorum per estimationem quia crescunt et
decrescunt iiii$^C$.xl libre. Summa talis.

De redd(itu) assis(o).
De redd(itu) assis(o) infra civitatem et extra ubique in maneriis et aliis villis ubi
redd(itus) debetur CC.xliii.li. xi.s. vii.den. ob. De quibus non possunt levare hoc
anno in civitate q(ui) valet xx.li. xvii.s. vi.d. Et sic remanet de claro hoc anno
CC.xxii.li. xiiii.sol. i.d. ob. Summa CC.xxii.li. xiiii.s. i.d. ob.

De obitibus
Predictum hospitale habere debet de omnibus tenentibus suis medietatem
omnium bonorum suorum cum obierint, si non habuerint uxores et pueros;
quod si habuerint tunc non habebit nisi partem terciam et valet per annum per
estimationem x. marcas. Summa x. marce.

Fines placita et amerciamenta preter ea que extend(itur) in maneriis val(ent) per
annum per estimacionem x. marcas. Summa talis.

De lana et commod(o) instauri.
[*Marginated*] Memorandum de bid(entibus) de Brungesf'.
Lana ii$^M$.vi$^C$.v$^{xx}$ et vi. multon(um) et ovium matric(ium) et vii$^C$.lxxiiii agn(orum)
per maiorem centen(arium) poterit valere per annum per estimatione CC.li. cum
CCC.xvii multon(ibus) v$^C$.<xxxiiii.> ovibus matric(ibus) et iiii.$^C$.xv. agnis de
Brungeflet.
Profectus CC.l. vacc(arum) que nunc sunt in maneriis ut de daer(a) deductis
herbag(iis) et expens(is) et exceptis vicul(is) potest esse per annum per
estimationem xx.li. xvi.s. viii.d., prec(ium) vacce xx.den.
Item xiiii. vacce de Brungeflet et vi. vacce de Morhamwyk' valent per annum
deductis reprisis ii. marcas et dimidiam, prec(ium) vacce ut supra.
Summa lane et daer(e) per annum CC.xxii.li. x.s.

[*Marginated*] Ebor' Morhamwyk.
Item manerium de Morhamwyk valet per annum xxii.li. iii.s.
[*Marginated*] Brunugflet.
Manerium eiusdem ville valet per annum l.li. xi.s. i.d.
Summa lxxii.li. xiiii.sol. i.d.

Summa totalis extente M.CC.lxxvii.li. xvii.s. vi.d.[36]
Summa totalis reprise M.xl.li. xiiii.s. xi.d.
Et sic rem(anet) ad opus magistri CC.xxxvii.li. ii.s. vii.d.

Summa M.CC.lxii.li. v.s. viii.d. ob. Item lx.s. Item x.s.

---

[36]  This is an accurate sum of the totals.

xv.li. xi.s. ix.d. ob. def(iciunt) de prima summa.[37]

**R905.** Summary of income and expenditure of the hospital for the *Valor Ecclesiasticus*
of 1535.

ORIGINAL: PRO, E 344/21/7 (part). PRINTED: *Valor Ecclesiasticus*, V, 17–18.

[m. 27d]
Hospitale sancti Leonardi Ebor'
M(agister) Thomas Magnus incumb(ens) magister ibidem.

Temporal(ibus). Valent in

situ hospitalis predicti, unacum domibus gardinis et edificiis iac(entibus) et scituat(is)
infra civitatem Ebor' predictam ac etiam terr(is) ten(emen)t(is) iac(entibus) in
diversis locis infra dictam civitatem per annum xl.li.

redd(itibus) et firmis divers(is) manoriorum dominiorum terrarum et tenementorum
iacent(ium) in diversis locis infra comitatum predictum, videlicet in redditibus
liberorum tenen(tium) infra ballivatos de Estridding xii.li. xii.s., North Ridding
xx.li. xiii.s. iiii.d., West Ridding xiii.li., graungea de Bennyngburgh xx.li. xii.s., villata
de Newton xxviii.li. xiiii.s. viii.d., villata de Bennyngburgh vi.li. iiii.s. xi.d., villata
de Heslington xxvi.li. xv.d., graungea de Acom xxii.li. xvi.d., villata de Roughfurthe
iiii.li. ii.s. iiii.d., graungea de Heworthe xx.li. xii.s., terr(is) et ten(emen)t(is) in
Nabourne et Fulfurthe xl.s., Flawith x.s., Howe x.li. xiii.s. iiii.d., Ranyngton
ix.li. iiii.s., Exilbye iiii.li. vi.s. viii.d., Kelstwhaitte cvi.s. viii.d., Grenetwhaitt iiii.li.,
grangea de Sutton cxi.s., Lessemyer viii.li., villata de Sutton xxx.s., manerium de
Bromflete xxxvii.li. xv.s., Goyll cvi.s. viii.d., Wheldrake x.li. xiii.s. iiii.d., graungea
de Hunton vi.li., graungea de Lede cum Aberfurth Saxston et Spittell Fall
ix.li. vii.s. iiii.d., mollend(ino) aquat(ico) situat(o) subtus castrum Ebor' xii.li.,
Nappey x.li., dominium de Bramhopp' x.li. vi.s. iii.d., Hovingham xxvi.s. viii.d.,
Skarburgh xlii.s., Kirkeby Fletham xxvi.s. viii.d. In toto in comitatu predicto per
annum CCC.xxxi.li. xvii.s. v.d.

Westm'land'
Adhuc temporal(ibus). Valent in
redditus et firmis divers(is) dominiorum maneriorum terrarum et tenementorum
subscr(iptorum), videlicet in Garethorne viii.li. ii.s., Crosby Banke xxxii.s. viii.d.,
Mebourne xiiii.s., Newby xiiii.s., Asbye v.s. iii.d., Blasterflete xxiiii.s. viii.d.,
Musgrave ii.s., Dokkarr xiii.li. v.s. i. ob. In toto in comitatu predicto per annum
xxvi.li. ix.s. viii.d. ob.[38]

Lincoln'
Temporal(ibus). Valent in
redditis et firmis terrarum et tenementis in Epworthe in comitatu predicto per
annum xxxv.s.

---

[37]  At the foot of the membrane.
[38]  The total for Westmorland is 10s. too much.

[*Sum of temporalities*] CCCC.li. ii.s i.d. ob.

Ebor'

Spiritual(ibus). Valent in
exitibus et proficiis divers(is) rector(iarum) dicti hospital(is) appropriat(arum),
videlicet rector(ie) de Newton super Usam xviii.li. xiiii.s., Saxston xx.li. xx.d. ac
garb(is) dec(imis) et feni rect(orie) de Pikkall xxxii.li., Bowes xvi.li. xiii.s. iiii.d.,
Brignall xx.s., Roughfurth cvi.s. viii.d. In toto in comitatu predicto per annum
iiii<sup>xx</sup>·xiii.li. xv.s. iiii.d.

Casual(ibus). Valent in
vendit(ionibus) bosci tam infra dominium de Benyngburgh quam infra dominium
de Acome communibus annis, vi.li. xiii.s. iiii.d.

Summa totalis valor(is) hospitalis predicti D.li. xi.s. i.d. ob.

[Reprisis]

De quibus

Annual(ibus) resolut(ionibus). Videlicet in
domino regi ad manus forestar(ii) forest(i) de Galtrice pro annuali redditu voc(ato)
lez Methames xlviii.s. vi.d., priori et conventui de Kirkham de annuali penc(ione)
exeunt(i) de Linton c.s., preposito ecclesie sancti Iohannis Beverlaci de redd(itu)
anti(quo) exeunt(i) de albo prato apud Bromflete xxvi.s. viii.d., abbati et conventui
monasterii beate Marie Ebor' pro redditu in Aynderby Whernhowe xv.s., eisdem
pro grangea [m. 28] de Heworth viii.s., priori et conventui monasterii sancte
Trinitatis Ebor' exeunt(i) de Bennyngburgh xvi.s., capitulo ecclesie metropol(itane)
Ebor' exeunt(i) de Neuton super Usam ii.s., abbati et conventui monasterii de
Cristall<sup>39</sup> exeunt(i) de manerio de Bramhop' xl.s., priorisse de Molseby exeunt(i) de
Newton super Usam xii.d., ballivis honoris Pontifract' exeunt(i) de Leede Graunge
ii.s., domino regi castro s' Richmond' pro fin(ibus) et ward(is) ii.s. x.d.; hered(ibus)
domini Fitzhugh et Iohannis Webster exeunt(i) de mollendino apud Lemyng viii.d.;
et vicecomiti Ebor' exeunt(i) de terr(e) in Ranington xii.d.; in toto, ex(tr)a terr(is)
in comitatu Ebor' xiii.li. iii.s. viii.d., div(ersi)s personis exeunt(ibus) de divers(is)
ten(emen)t(is) infra civitatem Ebor' per annum cxix.s. iiii.d. In toto, xix.li. iii.s.

Distribut(ionibus) elemosin(arum). Videlicet in
denar(iis) annuatim solut(is) pro sustentatione sexaginta pauper(um) infra firmarium
dicti hospitalis commorant(ium) iuxta tenorem fundat(ionis) et ordinationes
per progenitores domini regis ibidem, videlicet cuilibet eorundem per annum
xxvii.s. viii.d. In toto, iiii<sup>xx</sup>·iii.li.

Consi(mi)l(is) denar(iis) annuatim distribut(is) in precio pan(is) et allec(iorum)
rub(eorum) in elemosina pauperibus extraneis ad magnas portas eiusdem hospitalis
in die sancti Leonardi confluent(ibus) ex fundatione progenitorum domini regis
predicti per annum xl.s.

---

<sup>39</sup> sic, for Kirkstall.

Cons(imilis) distribut(is) annuatim in die cene domini, videlicet pauperibus in
firmario et pauperibus extraneis ibidem exist(entibus), videlicet in pane vi.s.,
cervisia iiii.s. et in pecuniis x.s., ex antiqua fundatione xx.s.

Distribut(ionibus) in obit(ibus) celebr(andis). Videlicet in
denariis annuatim solutis pro celebratione obit(uum) et funeral(ibus) diebus
divers(arum) personarum videlicet
Rogeri Pipyn v.s.; Rogeri Skelton vi.s. viii.d.; Willelmi Marston x.s.; Rogeri
Swanne; et Katerine consort(is) sue x.s.; Iohannis Arnold, Ricardi Nevell et Petri de
Carnaby xxvi.s. viii.d.; Rogeri Hoode xiii.s.; Isold(e), Willelmi et Roberti Skipwith
xx.s.; Ade Yorke xii.s.; Simonis Hardcorse xiii.s. iiii.d.; Rogeri Barton xxvi.s. viii.d.;
Thome Heslarton xiii.s.; Ricardi Rawinsore xv.s.; Edwardi bone memorie nuper
regis Anglie domine Isabelle matris et Philippe uxoris eiusdem Edwardi ii.s. i.d.;
Willelmi Darrell xi.s. iiii.d.; Iohannis Esyngton xiii.s. iiii.d.; Roberti Skipwith
xiii.s. iiii.d.; Iohannis Yole et uxoris sue x.s.; Thome Lekynfeld vi.s.; Thome Holme
v.s.; Roberti Esyngwold viii.s. xi.d.; Willelmi Brighton vii.s. vi.d.; Thome Peerson
vii.s. vii.d.; Iohannis Toonge et amicorum suorum xi.s. vi.d.; Iohannis Osbaldwike
x.s. vi.d.; Roberti Thixindall viii.s. vi.d.; Iohannis le Scroope vi.s. iiii.d.; Willelmi
Stillington ix.s. iii.d.; Thome Sutton viii.s. xi.d.; Iohannis Twhinge x.s. vi.d. ob.;
Iohannis Usbourne viii.s. ii.d.; Elizabeth' Karr' xxii.s. vii.d.; Iohannis Danyell
vii.s. v.d.; Agnet' Leedes xiii.s. iiii.d.; Willelmi Lee vii.s. x.d. et Thome Esyngwald
xii.s. iii.d.
In toto ex fundat(ionbus) supradict(arum) person(arum) imperpetuum
xix.li. xiii.s. vi.d. ob.

Exhibit(ionibus) choristar(iorum). Videlicet in
denariis annuatim solutis in exhibitione et sustentatione xii$^{cem}$ choristar(iorum) et
clericorum ibidem imperpetuum commoran(tium) ad erudiend(um) tam in cantu
quam in sciencia gramatical(ia) de elemosina dicti hospitalis ex fundatione tam
in esculent(is) et poculent(is) quam in vestitis et aliis quibuscumque necessariis
quiquidem clerici et choristarii quotidie ministr(antes) circa divina officia infra
ecclesiam dicti hospitalis videlicet quilibet eorundem ad l.s. per annum. In toto
xxx.li.

Ordinaria ex fundat(oribus). Videlicet in
cons(imilis) denar(iis) annuatim solut(is) pro oleo pro sustentione ii. lampadum
comburent(ium) cotidie infra firmarium pauperum, ac pro candelis ceriis candelis
cepiis et smigmator(ibus) ac pro pannis lavand(is) et aliis commun(is) expen(sis)
anti(quitus) h(ab)it(is) infra dictum firmarium pauperum, videlicet ii. lampad(ibus)
combur(antibus) noctant(er) per totum annum et quatuor lanternis combur(antibus)
quolibet nocte in ieme a festo annunciationis beate Marie virginis usque
principium iemis e converso ex prima fundatione dicti hospitalis imperpetuum. x.li.

Salar(iis) capellanor(um). Videlicet in
denariis annuatim solutis pro salario sive pencione duorum capellanorum
cantarist(arum) videlicet Willelmi Cowp(er) ad altare beate Marie infra ecclesiam
de Saxston ex fundat(ione) Rad(ulf)i de Wodhowse imperpetuum ad iiii.li per
annum ac in consi(mi)li salario sive pencione annual(i) solut(o) Matheo Smythson
capellano annuatim celebrant(i) infra firmarium pauperum dicti hospitalis et
ministrant(i) dictis pauperibus ex antiqua fundacione ad cvi.s. viii.d. per annum. In
toto, ix.li. vi.s. viii.d.

Sinod(alibus) et procurat(ionibus).Videlicet in
cons(imilis) denar(iis) solut(is) archiepiscopo Ebor' et archidiacono de ibidem pro
senad(alibus) iiii.s. et procurat(ionibus) vii.s. vi.d. pro ecclesia de Saxston; necnon
eidem archiepiscopo et archidiacono de Cleveland pro senad(alibus) iiii.s. et
procurat(ionibus) vii.s. vi.d. pro ecclesia de Newton super Usam per annum. In
toto xxiii.s.

[m. 28d]

Feod(is).Videlicet
feod(o) Georgii Laweson militis auditoris dicti hospitalis xl.s.; Marmaduc(i)
Constable militis capitalis sen(escal)l(i) ibidem xl.s.; Willelmi Maunsell ball(ivi)
libertat(is) dicti hospitalis iiii.li. vi.s. viii.d.; Ricardi Beacham ball(ivi) et collectore
reddit(orum) infra civitatem Ebor' xliii.s. iiii.d.; Roberti Metham armigeri ballivi
d(omi)nii et graungie de Acome iiii.li. iiii.s.; Laurencio Faudington ball(ivo)
dominiorum de Bennyngburgh et Newton super Usam per annum xl.s.; Roberto
Dyneley ballivo dominii de Bramhopp' vi.s. viii.d.; Willelmo Maunsell ballivo
hospitalis in Escr' in com' Ebor' xxvi.s. viii.d.; Willelmo Mennell ballivo de North'r'
Cleveland et Allerton xl.s.; Henrico Burton ballivo ballivat(i) de Westridding xl.s.
In toto per annum xxii.li. vii.s. iiii.d.

Summa repris(arum) C.xxxviii.li.[40]

C.iiii[xx.]xvii xiii.s. vi.d. ob.[41]

Et valet clar(e)

CCC.lxii.li. xi.s. i.d. ob.[42]

CCC.ii.li. xvii.s. vii.d.[43]

Item valet in salario sive pencione solut(a) Matheo Smythson capellano annuatim
celebr(anti) infra firmarium pauperum dicti hospitalis superius deduct(o) unde
dominus rex[44] d(ebet) habere decimam partem et primum fructum suam
attingent(am) per annum ad C.vi.s. viii.d. In toto CCC.lxvii.li. xvii.s. ix.d. ob.

Decima pars inde xxxvi.li. xv.s. ix.d. ob.

Late in 1534, after his break with Rome and the Act of Supremacy, Henry VIII
decided to tax the profits of churches and other religious institutions at 10% annually.
Visitors were appointed in January 1535 to carry out a detailed survey to determine
the amount payable. The resulting reports, known as the *Valor Ecclesiasticus*, were
completed in the following year.[45] The *Valor Ecclesiasticus* may usefully be compared

---

[40]  Revised total of expenses, which excludes *distributionibus in obitibus celebrandis, exhibitionibus choristariorum*,
    and *ordinaria ex fundatoribus*. For the exclusion of these items from the deductions, see *Valor Ecclesiasticus*,
    I, p. v ('General Introduction', often found in vol. VI because printed contemporaneously with it).
[41]  The original total of expenses, which is £1 too high.
[42]  Total of income less revised total expenses.
[43]  Original total of income less expenses.
[44]  MS: *R'*.
[45]  For the *Valor Ecclesiasticus* and its production, see A. Savine, 'The English monasteries on the eve of the

with the five sets of annual accounts of the revenues and expenses from the lands previously owned by the hospital, covering the period from Michaelmas 1541 to Michaelmas 1546 (PRO, SC 6/HenVIII/4601–4605). A summary of the places named in the first of these is printed at *Dissolved Houses*, no. 675.

Dissolution' in *Oxford studies in social and legal history*, I (1909), 1–75 and D. Knowles, *The religious orders in England*, III (Cambridge, 1961), 241–54.

# Appendix I:
## The Masters of the Hospital

### Introduction

Over the four centuries of the hospital's existence, there were changes in what was expected of the master, and in the way he was appointed. For most of the twelfth and thirteenth centuries the appointment was a matter for the dean and chapter, but it is clear that there were tensions regarding the advowson and the master's manner of living. In 1245, after the death of Hugh of Geddington, the dean and chapter laid down conditions as to the dress of the master, if he was a secular man (*secularem personam*), i.e., not a member of a religious order. Hugh, they observed approvingly, had lived simply, and without possessions. Here we see the dean and chapter attempting to reserve the revenues of the hospital for the benefit of its inmates and other deserving poor, rather than for the personal benefit of the master. The twelfth-century masters Robert and Swain, from the little that is known about them, seem likely to have had the charitable objectives of the hospital uppermost in their minds. Paulinus, however, was a king's clerk, a man of affairs, appointed on the wishes of Henry II, and may not have followed the example of his predecessors. As there is little evidence for the lives of the men who held the hospital for the first three quarters of the thirteenth century beyond their work as masters, it is probable that they lived simply, in the manner required by the dean and chapter. Thomas of Geddington, indeed, resigned in 1276 to join the order of Friars Minor. Perhaps Roger of Malton, who had been the archbishop's penitentiary, and was the last master appointed by the dean and chapter, was also a man of that stamp. But the inquiry which marked the end of his mastership found that 'reliefs, perquisites of courts, and altar dues are reserved to him to provide therewith gifts, courtesies, and other matters, as he shall deem expedient' (*CalPat*, 1334–1338, p. 267).

There were periodic attempts to deprive the dean and chapter of their right of presentation. Archbishop Geoffrey installed his own candidate John at the beginning of the thirteenth century, but after a legal battle he was ejected. Henry III also showed an interest, but accepted the findings of inquiries of 1223 and 1246 that the advowson belonged to the dean and chapter (*CRR*, 1223–1224, pp. 142–43; *Ctl. Gisborough*, 1, 52–53n). By the later 1270s the hospital was in debt, and the king appointed first one and then another important layman to supervise its affairs, in conjunction with the master. The hundred inquiry in the city of York in 1274–75 found that the advowson of the hospital had belonged to the king's ancestors, but had been alienated (*YQW*, p. 75), and a commission dated 15 November 1280 for an inquisition into the hospital shows that the king had recently 'recovered' the advowson of the hospital by judgment of his court. The subsequent inquisition found, quite erroneously, that 'the kings used to grant the custody and mastership at will . . . until the time when the dean and chapter possessed themselves of the advowson' (C1029 [*CalPat*, 1334–1338, pp. 266–68]). In October 1280 Archbishop Wickwane had written to the chancellor, Robert Burnell, bishop of Bath and Wells, reminding him that no-one could be instituted as master without the archbishop's approval. Burnell replied immediately saying that he accepted the archbishop's right and did not expect the king, who had recently recovered the advowson, to change the rules (*Reg. Wickwane*, pp. 245, 267). From then onwards the masters were generally important royal clerks, who held the

hospital alongside other valuable benefices. The clerks were accustomed to take the
revenues of prebends for personal use, within certain constraints, and expected to do
the same with the revenues of the hospital. The appointment of Gilbert Stapleton in
1307 was specifically stated to be 'subject to the maintenance of the appointed alms
and other pious works', and doubtless this was always the expectation. But the clear
implication of this reservation was that surplus revenues were the master's property,
and that their use for charitable purposes was not expected. Thus, from 1280, a gift
to the hospital was in effect a gift to the king and his appointee, rather than to a
charitable institution, unless specific conditions were laid down as to the use of the
revenues arising from the gift.

### The Custodes

Apart from the masters, there are occasional references to other men, usually
described as warden (*custos*) of the hospital, who appear to have been entrusted with
the management of the establishment by the non-resident masters.[1] The unnamed
*custos* and his two *garciones* head the list of the hospital's staff made in 1287 (Cullum,
'St Leonard's', p. 21). Sir Robert the *custos* occurs in the 'complaint of the brothers of
the infirmary', made probably at the same time (Benson, *St Leonard's*, p. 11; Cullum,
'St Leonard's', p. 25). William of Yafforth (*Jafford, Yafford*), a chaplain of the archbishop
who had been appointed dean of Christianity in York in January 1289, was probably
warden when the archbishop asked him in December 1293 why the archiepiscopal
presentees to beds at St Leonard's had not been admitted (*Reg. Romeyn*, I, 84, 135).
Yafforth was described as *custos* of the hospital in 1295,[2] when he was said to have
two boys and two horses (Benson, *St Leonard's*, p. 15), and in 1297 (C39 [Cott., f. 6ᵛ]).
A letter, doubtless addressed to Walter Langton, said that Yafforth 'cannot do without
two horses, and two garcons with their robes, and the brothers agree, yet he gives up
his yearly fee of £10 belonging to [the warden's] office' (Benson, *St Leonard's*, p. 11).
Thomas Neville was *custos* in February 1301[/02] (R142); Adam Middelton in 1306
and 1307 (R479n); Robert Pouwer in 1320 (*YD*, VII, no. 161); and Alan Hevede in
1381 (C606 [Cott., f. 118ᵛ]). In 1364 it was stated that there was 'no dwelling-place for
the warden, who fills the place of the master in his absence' (*CalInqMisc*, 1348–1377,
p. 204).

### List of Masters

Lists of masters have been compiled by Baildon (Baildon, *Monastic Notes*, I, 245) and
T.M. Fallow (*VCH Yorks*, III, 343–44).

### Robert of the Hospital (? × 1132 to 1157 × 1164)

Robert of the hospital is first mentioned in the account of the dispute at St Mary's
Abbey contained in Archbishop Thurstan's letter to William de Corbeil, archbishop of
Canterbury. 'Robert, priest (*sacerdos*) of the hospital' was said to be in the archbishop's
party at the meeting in the abbey's chapter house in October 1132 (*Mem. Fountains*, I,
25; Nicholl, *Thurstan*, p. 171).[3] Robert's noble birth and scholarly disposition is attested

---

[1]   It should be noted however, that the masters themselves were also sometimes called *custos*, as were
      the laymen appointed in the 1270s to supervise the administration when the hospital was in debt (see
      below, s.n. Robert of the Hospital, Swain, Thomas of Geddington).

[2]   Called Sir William de Stafford by Benson, whose source was Lichfield RO, D30/12/107, formerly Qq2.

[3]   The authenticity of this letter has been frequently been questioned. If, as seems at least possible, it is a
      forgery or amplification, its date of composition is likely to have been some ten to fifteen years after

by Reginald of Durham, who attributes an elaborate description of the physical appearance of St Oswald to Robert of the hospital, who had found it in old books in English (Simeon of Durham, *Historia regum*, I, 378–79).[4] 'Robert priest (*presbiter*) of the hospital' attested an act of Archbishop Thurstan issued in *c.*1121 × 1138 (*EYC*, VI, no. 9; *EEA*, V, no. 73). He was amongst those who in 1141–43 tried to overturn the election of William FitzHerbert as archbishop of York. 'Robert of the hospital' was addressed with others by a papal letter of 22 April [1142], enjoining them to present their case against William to the pope in person in March [1143], and it seems that Robert undertook the voyage to Rome (Talbot, 'New Documents', p. 10; John of Hexham, *Historia regum*, II, 311, 313).[5] It was probably during the uncertain period of 1140–43 that King Stephen issued a writ to William, earl of York, and the burgesses and men of York, taking Robert, priest of the hospital of St Peter in York, and the men and lands of the hospital, into his protection, and freeing them from claims against their land until the consecration of a new archbishop (C2 [*EYC*, I, no. 172]). In May 1148 'Robert, master of the hospital of St Peter in the city of York', obtained papal confirmation of the hospital's possessions (C178 [*EYC*, I, no. 179]). 'Robert, keeper (*custos*) of the hospital' issued deeds with the assent of the brethren in 1148 × 1156 (R94) and '*c.*1140 × 1156' (C563 [*EYC*, I, no. 215]). Robert attested acta of Archbishop Henry Murdac in favour of Fountains in 1151 × 1153 (*EYC*, I, nos 67, 71; *EEA*, V, nos 113–14). His attestation to Eustace FitzJohn's foundation charter for Malton given in 1151 × 1153 lies between those of Archbishop Henry and Adam, abbot of Meaux (*MA*, VI, 970, no. 1). A probably spurious act of Archbishop William FitzHerbert, ostensibly dating from 1153 × 1154, is witnessed by Robert of the hospital (*EYC*, II, no. 879; *EEA*, V, no. 104). In January 1157 'Robert, master of the hospital of St Peter in the city of York' obtained from Pope Adrian IV a further confirmation of the hospital's possessions, together with a monition to the clergy and laity of the province of York not to withhold the customary payment of thraves, and a letter to the dean and chapter of York urging them to respect and maintain the hospital in York which they had founded (C179, C211 [*EYC*, I, nos 186, 188]; Raine, *Historians*, III, 68–69). He was called 'brother Robert of the hospital' in an act of Archbishop Roger dating from 1154 × 1157 (*EEA*, XX, no. 136). As master of the hospital he witnessed an act of Roger in favour of Furness in 1154 × 1164 (ibid., no. 32). 'Master R[obert] of the hospital and brother Swain, priest, Peter the clerk' are amongst the witnesses to a deed of William Fossard given in 1154 × 1162[6] (*EYC*, II, no. 1095). Swain was perhaps Robert's deputy and the subsequent master of the hospital. Peter the clerk was also almost certainly one of the hospital's brethren.[7] It is likely Robert died or resigned in or before 1164, as Archbishop Roger issued instructions for the procedure for the election of a new master of the hospital in 1154 × 1164 (*EEA*, XX, no. 117).

the events it describes. If the letter were indeed compiled in the 1140s, it would still provide a measure of evidence for Robert's presence in Thurstan's party in 1132. Nevertheless we should not regard it as certain that Robert was master of the hospital in that year. The letter is discussed at Nicholl, *Thurstan*, pp. 251–58; L.G.D. Baker, 'The foundation of Fountains Abbey', *Northern History*, IV (1969), 29–43, at 33–35; Burton, *Monastic Order*, pp. 103–04.

4   Haec Robertus vir ingenuus de hospitali, quod est in Eboraco, se sic in libris veteribus anglicis descripta invenisse retulit, cuius etiam genus dictaminis in modernae linguae modulatione rhythmico pedis metro decurrit.
5   For background, see Norton, *St William*, pp. 76–88.
6   For the date, see FN: Hay.
7   See FN: Peter, clerk of the hospital.

SWAIN OF THE HOSPITAL (1157 × 1164 TO 1178 × 1187)

A mandate of uncertain date, issued by the chapter of York and addressed to the parsons and vicars of Ryedale, stated that the bearer of the mandate, Swain, was the messenger (*nuntius*) of the hospital of St Peter and St Leonard, and the chapter of York (C70 [*EYC*, I, no. 196]). This description of Swain perhaps indicates he was a brother of the hospital and deputy to master Robert, before he himself became master. The attestation to the Fossard deed mentioned above is also suggestive of this possibility.

Master Swain of the hospital witnessed a deed of Juetta of Carlton made in 1167 or before (*EYC*, I, no. 159). A papal confirmation of the possessions of the hospital was addressed to 'Swain, master of the hospital of St Peter in the city of York' in 1173, but when a further confirmation was issued in 1178 or 1179 it was addressed to the nameless proctor (*procuratori*) and brethren of the York hospital (C180, C357 [*EYC*, I, nos 197–98]). A deed issued by the archbishop, dean and chapter made in 1164 × 1177[8] concerning an exchange of property refers to 'brother Swain, called proctor of the hospital', but in Swain's reciprocal deed he describes himself as 'brother Swain, called minister of the poor people (*pauperum*) of the hospital of the Blessed Peter, York' (C881 [*EEA*, XX, no. 126]; *EYC*, I, no. 283). As master of the hospital Swain witnessed five deeds of Roger de Mowbray to Fountains in 1174 × 1175. He attested after the York chapter, the abbots and priors, but before the other witnesses (*Mowbray Charters*, nos 110–12, 119–20). He issued a deed as 'brother Swain, called master of the poor people of the hospital of Blessed Peter, York' (*EYC*, I, no. 300), and another as 'brother Swain, keeper (*custos*) of the hospital of St Peter in York' (R407). A facsimile of an original deed given by 'brother Swain called minister of the poor people of the hospital of the Blessed Peter at York', to which the usual seal of the hospital is attached, is given at *EYC*, XI, no. 147. 'Master Swain of the hospital of the Blessed Peter, York,' with Roger, nephew of the master, witnessed a deed given in the [ruri-decanal] chapter at Kirmington (Lincs.) (Burton transcripts 2, f. 99[r], p. 162, B25 N70). Ellis nephew of master Swain witnessed two gifts to the hospital, both of uncertain date (R660; M: Beningbrough [MS Dods. 120b, f. 49[v]]). Swain's last closely datable attestation was made in 1178 × 1181[9] (*Reg. Gray*, p. 70n).[10] The papal confirmation of 1183 was addressed only to the brethren of the hospital of St Peter, York (C166 [*EYC*, I, no. 199]), and may indicate that Swain had died and that the mastership was vacant.

PAULINUS OF LEEDS (1181 × 1187 TO 1202 × 1203)

For Paulinus, see Carpenter, 'Paulinus'. By 1177 he was vicar of Leeds. He was also a clerk of Henry II, and apparently his confessor. The king offered Paulinus the bishopric of Carlisle in 1186, but he declined it. An inquisition of 1223 found Paulinus had been made master of the hospital whilst there was a vacancy at York, so after the death of Archbishop Roger in 1181. His first datable occurrence as master was in May 1186 or 1187, when he was addressed by a bull of Urban III. He last occurs, as a joint issuer of a deed, on 7 December 1201. He had been dead for some time by 15 May 1203, the date of a papal letter concerning a dispute over the mastership.

---

[8]   Between the legation of Archbishop Roger and the death of master Robert [master of schools].

[9]   As 'master Swain, of the hospital of St Peter, York'. The date range is derived from the death of Archbishop Roger, one of the parties, and the accession of Hamo to the precentorship in or after 1178.

[10]  Some editions give dates later than 1177 for other deeds witnessed by Swain, but the dating does not withstand detailed examination. For example, the gift by Adam son of Peter [of Birkin] to Esholt, which Clay assigned to '*c.*1180 × 1184' (*EYC*, VI, no. 67) may have been issued as early as *c.*1170 (Carpenter, 'Paulinus', p. 29). BL, Harley Ch. 83 C. 38, cited at *VCH Yorks*, III, 343 as evidence for Swain *c.*1184–85, is printed at *Mowbray Charters*, no. 111, where it is assigned to 1174 × 1175.

JOHN (1202 × 1203 TO 1204)

The succession to the mastership after the death of Paulinus was disputed. The brethren unanimously elected John, one of their number, with the support or at the direction of Archbishop Geoffrey. But the dean and chapter, who at that time were involved in several disputes with the archbishop, claimed the right to appoint and attempted to remove John and install their own candidate Ralph of Nottingham. The dean and chapter were eventually successful. The first notice of the dispute is contained in a commission by Pope Innocent III to the dean and subdean of Lincoln and the archdeacon of Bedford, dated 15 May 1203, on complaint by the dean and chapter of York that after the death of P[aulinus], the archbishop had refused to accept their duly elected nominee, who was both respected and learned (*et honestum et literatura perspicuum*), and had intruded another. The judges delegate were to examine the case, and if the facts were as stated they were to remove the intruder and install the elect (*Letters Innoc. III*, no. 475; Raine, *Historians*, III, 111). Their subsequent judgment is undated, but it must have been issued between 1 July 1203 and April 1204,[11] and probably after 23 February 1204, when John was sufficiently secure in his tenure of the mastership to be party to a fine concerning 2 bv. of the hospital's land in Thirsk (*PF John*, p. 84). The judges had examined Archbishop Geoffrey and John, priest of York, as well as original deeds relating to the matter, and they found that the choice of master lay with the dean and chapter, and pronounced their election of master Ralph of Nottingham to be right and canonical. John the priest, who had unlawfully kept the hospital, was entirely removed from it. The judges ordered the chapter's costs of 80*m*. against the archbishop. Afterwards, as the archbishop was unwilling to admit and institute Ralph to the rule of the hospital, the judges themselves instituted Ralph to the rectorship (Raine, *Historians*, III, 110–12). But that was not the end of the matter as John appealed to Rome, saying that he had been a priest of the hospital and had been chosen unanimously by his brethren. He further complained that the matter was under the prior jurisdiction of the bishop of Ely and his co-judges, who had been appointed previously by the pope to investigate.[12] As a result the pope wrote to different judges delegate, the bishop, dean and precentor of Hereford, on 14 May 1204, almost exactly a year after his first letter, repeating the complaints of 'John, master of the York hospital', giving the judges delegate authority to quash any previous actions, and asking them to hear the case and determine it with the agreement of the parties, or to report in writing with a date for the parties to appear before him (*Letters Innoc. III*, no. 559; Migne, *PLCC*, CCXV, 346–47). On 20 May 1204 the pope wrote to the same judges delegate with further information. The brethren and sisters of the hospital of York had intervened in the case, stating they had unanimously elected J[ohn], and did not wish him to be removed and replaced by someone of secular dress appointed by the dean and chapter (*Letters Innoc. III*, no. 560; Migne, *PLCC*, CCXV, 347–48). The second judgment has not survived, but it is likely that the matter had been settled in favour of Ralph by June 1205[13] at the latest, as on 26 July 1205 the pope, acting on complaint of R[alph] rector and the brethren of the hospital, wrote to

[11] Richard, predecessor of the judge delegate Geoffrey as archdeacon of Bedford, last occurs on 1 July 1203; William [de Bramfeld], subdean of Lincoln, another of the judges delegate, was murdered on 25 September 1205. The appeals against the judgment made by master John and the brethren of the hospital must have been made in April 1204 at the latest.

[12] John may have been referring to the commission issued to the bishop of Ely and others on 31 May 1202 to investigate, after many complaints, the competence of the archbishop and his case against the dean and chapter, rather than a separate and otherwise unrecorded commission specific to the hospital (*Letters Innoc. III*, nos 414, 450).

[13] Allowing for the month which was required for a letter to reach Rome from England.

enforce the payment of tithes and other dues owed by Fountains Abbey and certain others to the hospital (C258 [*Letters Innoc. III*, no. 635]). Nevertheless 'master J[ohn] rector of the York hospital' was witness to an act of Archbishop Geoffrey dated 5 July 1205 (*EEA*, XXVII, no. 78). John cannot then have had any control over the hospital, or any chance of recovering the mastership. The archbishop's refusal to acknowledge the fact is entirely in keeping with what we know of his quarrelsome disposition.

The longer version of the inquisition of 1246 states that John was a chaplain of Archbishop Geoffrey (C46 [*Ctl. Gisborough*, I, 53n]) rather than a brother of the hospital, but this information is not contained in the contemporary evidence. There is perhaps a possibility that the archbishop had inserted one of his clerks into the brethren as the future successor to Paulinus. But the absence of contemporary evidence renders it unlikely that it could have been someone as prominent as master John of York, who was amongst the distinguished witnesses to several of Geoffrey's acta, including one of 1191 × 1198 (*EEA*, XXVII, nos 30, 55, 62), and a chapter act of 1191 × 1194 (*YMF*, I, no. 23).

RALPH OF NOTTINGHAM (1204 TO 1214 × 1217)
The dispute over the mastership of the hospital, which led to the ousting of John and the institution of Ralph of Nottingham, apparently between February and April 1204, is detailed above, as is the first dated notice of R[alph] as rector in the papal letter of July 1205.[14] Erneis Balki's quitclaim of land he held in the time of master Paulinus was witnessed by 'Sir S[imon] the dean, H[amo] the treasurer, master Gregory, Ralph, rector of the hospital, successor of master Paulinus and several others of the chapter of St Peter, York' and others named, and was probably issued in 1204 or soon afterwards, before Ralph became well established as master (C644 [*EYC*, I, no. 263]). Ralph's agreement with Haldan son of Baldwin of Leathley was also issued very early in his mastership, as it is witnessed by William of Leathley, who did not live long after Ralph was instituted (R237). On 2 July 1206 Ralph of Woodhouse quitclaimed to master Ralph and the brethren all the debts of master Paulinus, and master John, and the brethren, up to that date (R463).

'Ralph, master of the hospital of St Peter' witnessed a Byland deed in 1207 (*Ctl. Byland*, no. 1157). Master Ralph and the brethren made an agreement with the prioress and nuns of [Nun] Monkton in 1208 (M: Beningbrough [MS Dods. 120b, f. 51ʳ]). In Autumn 1209 master Ralph, rector, and the brethren of the Blessed Peter, York, made an agreement concerning thraves with Geoffrey abbot of St Agatha in Richmond (C284 [Cott., f. 58ʳ]). Ralph made agreements in February 1209[/10] (C247 [Cott., f. 52ᵛ]) and 1212 (M: Sutton [MS Dods. 120b, ff. 45ʳ, 58ᵛ]). He last occurs in 1214, when 'R. master and the brethren of St Peter, York' made an agreement with G[eoffrey] abbot and the convent of Bégard (M: Richmond [Evans, 'Begar', p. 206]). 'Roger, nephew of master Ralph' attested two of the hospital's deeds in 1204 × 1212 (R482, R483).

There were other men associated with the hospital with the name Nottingham. William of Nottingham was a clerk of the hospital in the first quarter of the thirteenth century and frequently attested the hospital's deeds. He, or another of the same name, witnessed two deeds as a secular chaplain (R278, C752 [Cott., f. 149ʳ]). Master

---

[14] Clay's deduction that Paulinus had been succeeded by Ralph in 1201 relies on erroneous assumptions about the succession to the archdeaconries of York and Cleveland (*YMF*, I, no. 31 and n; for discussion see Carpenter, 'Paulinus', n. 66). 'Master Ralph of the hospital', whose successor was in 1207 appointed to a prebend he had resigned in Exeter Cathedral (*RPat*, pp. 75, 81), was a different person, as is clear from his attestation as 'Ralph of the hospital' to a deed of 1184 × 1186 (*EEA*, XI, p. xli n).

Henry of Nottingham seems to have been one of the brethren in *c*.1200 × *c*.1220, but occurs only twice (R109, C236 [Cott., f. 51$^r$]). John of Nottingham was a brother chaplain during the later years of the rectorship of Hugh of Geddington.

HUGH OF GEDDINGTON (1214 × 1217 TO 1244 × 1245),
INTERRUPTED BY WILLIAM (1235 × 1240)
According to an inquisition concerning the hospital made shortly after his death, Hugh of Geddington was admitted as master by the dean and chapter of York, after the death of Ralph of Nottingham, on the petition of Morgan, then provost of Beverley[15] (C46 [*Ctl. Gisborough*, I, 53n]). At an inquiry into the advowson of the hospital held in Michaelmas term 1223 the master, who is not named, said he had custody of the hospital through the dean and chapter of York, whom he called to warrant. The dean and chapter confirmed that the advowson belonged to them (*CRR*, 1223–1224, pp. 142–43). 'H[ugh] rector of the hospital of St Peter, York' made an agreement on 8 September 1217 (R571), and gave another deed in which he was similarly described before March 1218 (R703). He is recorded as master in December 1218 ('Hugh', C123 [*YF*, 1218–1231, p. 8]); February 1219 ('Hugh', C163 [*YF*, 1218–1231, p. 28]); October 1219 ('Hugh', M: Marton [*YF*, 1218–1231, p. 34]); February 1220[/21] ('H.', C317 [Cott., f. 62$^r$]); May 1223 ('brother Hugh de Geitinton', M: Beningbrough [*YF*, 1218–1231, p. 50]; 'H.', C100 [Cott., f. 15$^r$]); April 1226 ('H.', C252 [Cott., f. 53$^v$]); December 1226 ('brother Hugh', M: Pickhill [*YF*, 1218–1231, p. 89]); January 1227 ('Hugh', R4); February 1231 ('Hugh', M: Colburn [MS Dods. 120b, f. 53$^r$]); April 1231 ('Hugh', R385); June 1231 ('Hugh', M: Whitwell [*YF*, 1218–1231, p. 148]); June 1234 ('H.', C103 [Cott., f. 15$^r$]); November and December 1234 ('Hugh', C248 [Cott., f. 52$^v$]; *YF*, 1232–1246, pp. 20, 25]); January 1235 ('Hugh', R595; M: Rainton [*YF*, 1232–1246, p. 35]); and August 1235 ('Hugh', R155, R588). Some time after August 1235, charter evidence shows that Hugh temporarily stood aside from the mastership in favour of one William (see below), who gave a deed as rector in 1239, but is not mentioned in the inquisitions of 1246 or 1280. Hugh occurs again as master in July 1240 ('Hugh', M: Hunton [*YF*, 1232–1246, p. 80]); September 1240 ('Hugh', M: Exelby [MS Dods. 120b, f. 65$^v$]); January 1241 ('Hugh', *YF*, 1232–1246, p. 103); and 1243 ('H.', M: Hemlington [MS Dods. 120b, f. 67$^v$]). On 20 December 1245, after Hugh's death, the dean and chapter made an ordinance as to the dress and manner of living of the master of the hospital, citing Hugh's example, who had since his confirmation worn the dress of the hospital, and lived modestly and without possessions (*continenter et sine proprietate viventum*) (Raine, *Historians*, III, 159). The inquisition of 1246 says that the recently dead master Hugh of Geddington had been successor to Ralph of Nottingham, and so there is no doubt that it was the same Hugh who had returned as master (C46 [*Ctl. Gisborough*, I, 53n]).

There were other men named Geddington associated with the hospital. Thomas of Geddington became master about twenty years after the death of Hugh of Geddington. Ralph of Geddington, chaplain, acted as attorney for master Hugh at Westminster in 1231 (R385), and can doubtless be identified with the 'secular chaplain' who attested many times after *c*.1214 and was instituted to the church of Newton-on-Ouse on 2 October 1238 at the presentation of the hospital (*Reg. Gray*, p. 82). He was still rector of Newton in 1247 (R128). Master John of Geddington, with Ralph his brother, witnessed in *c*.1218 × 1248 (R624). W[illiam] of Geddington

---

[15] Morgan, an illegitimate son of Henry II, was provost by 1212, and had resigned by November 1217 (*Beverley Fasti*, p. 5).

was cellarer, apparently in the second half of Hugh's mastership (M: Crigglestone [MS Dods. 120b, f. 98ᵛ]).

WILLIAM (1245 × 1246 TO 1250 × 1252)
William's interruption to Hugh's mastership is attested by two deeds. 'William rector and the brethren of the hospital of St Peter, York' issued a deed which can be dated with some confidence to 1238 × 1242 (R148). Another grant by 'William rector of the hospital of St Peter' bears the date 7 November 1239 (M: Kirkthwaite [MS Dods. 120b, f. 92ʳ]). The duration of William's interruption to Hugh's tenure of the mastership is unknown, but as far as can be ascertained it fell between August 1235 and July 1240, in which months Hugh was a party to deeds.

It is probable that it was the same William who succeeded to the mastership after Hugh's death but there is no proof of this, and there is no clue to William's identity. He had doubtless been elected on the expectation that he would follow the ordinance of the dean and chapter as to his dress and manner of living. William was master in June 1246, when he made two fines as 'brother William, master of the hospital of St Peter' (R688; YF, 1232–1246, p. 158]), but it was not until 20 October 1246 that the king, as a result of the inquisition, instructed the sheriff not to interfere further with the hospital, the ordination and collation of which belonged to the dean and chapter (Raine, Historians, III, 164–65). It is difficult to determine whether some of William's deeds were issued during his first or second terms as rector (e.g. R687, C734 [Cott., f. 146ʳ]), but his grant to Alan son of Geoffrey of Bugthorpe was undoubtedly issued in 1246 or later (R382). William, master of St Leonard's, was mentioned in a fine of May 1249 (YF, 1246–1272, p. 10), and issued a deed in 1248 × 1250 (M: Easingwold [MS Dods. 120b, f. 54ʳ]). Other grants can be assigned to the second period of his rectorship with varying degrees of confidence (C406, C831 [Cott., ff. 77ᵛ, 165ᵛ]). His last closely datable appearance comes after a case in the king's court of Hilary term 1250, when William, rector of the hospital, handed over Richard, son and heir of Thomas of Stockeld, to Henry de Percy (CRR, 1249–1250, p. 210; Ctl. Percy, no. 460).

ROBERT DE SAHAM (1250 × 1252 TO 1263 × 1265)
Almost nothing is known of Robert de Saham, who occurs as master in April ('Robert', C286 [Cott., f. 58ʳ]), June ('R.', R509) and September 1252 ('Robert', YF, 1246–1272, p. 85), and on 21 March 1262[/63] ('Robert de Saham', CIII [Cott., f. 16ʳ]). A master Robert de Saham witnessed a gift to the hospital of land in Bowes of uncertain date (M: Bowes [MS Dods. 120b, f. 63ʳ]), a gift to the same of land in Hunton in 1240 × 1262 (M: Hunton [MS Dods. 120b, f. 69ᵛ)]); and a gift of land in Beningbrough to St Mary's Abbey in 1219 × 1246[16] (MA, III, 557, no. 34). Whether this was the same man is open to question – if so, all these deeds must belong to the period before he became master of the hospital. It was presumably a different Robert de Saham, clerk, who witnessed benefactions to the hospital made in c.1255 × 1269 (R216), and 1261–62 (M: Hunton [MS Dods. 120b, f. 70ʳ]). A Robert de Saham was presented to the church of Burghwallis in September 1272 (Reg. Giffard, pp. 36–37).

William de Saham was a brother of the hospital in the later thirteenth century. William de Saham, and Robert of the same, witnessed an agreement made by Robert [de Saham], master of the hospital, in 1252 (C286, cf. C649 [Cott., ff. 58ʳ, 127ᵛ]). William de Saham occurs as a brother of the hospital during the mastership of Roger of Malton (R214), and was one of the brethren on the jury of the inquisition of

---

[16]    Whilst Robert of Skegness was steward of the abbey (FN).

*c.* November 1280 (C1029 [*CalPat*, 1334–1338, p. 266]). The extent of October 1280 was made before Sir William de Saham[17] and the sheriff of York, as well as two former masters and W. de Saham, brother of the hospital, and others (R902).

### THOMAS OF GEDDINGTON (1263 × 1265 TO 1275 × 1276)

Thomas occurs as master in November 1265 ('Thomas', R129); October ('Thomas', M: Appleton [St Mary JR, f. 377ʳ (old f. 386ʳ)]) and November 1266 ('Thomas', M: Hunton [MS Dods. 120b, f. 71ʳ]); April 1268 ('Thomas', C257 [Cott., f. 54ᵛ]); February 1268[/69] ('Th.', C937 [Cott., f. 190ᵛ]); July 1269 ('Thomas', YF, 1246–1272, p. 174); April 1272 ('Thomas', M: Thorpe [MS Dods. 120b, f. 101ᵛ]); '1273' ('Thomas', M: Howe [MS Dods. 120b, f. 69ʳ]); May 1274 ('Thomas', C710 [Cott., f. 139ʳ]); and February 1275 ('Thomas', M: Howe [YF, 1272–1300, p. 4]). His surname of *Gaytinton* or *Godington* is known only from a plea of 1270–71 (Baildon, *Monastic Notes*, I, 246), and a 'complaint of the sisters' of the hospital apparently made in 1287 (Cullum, 'St Leonard's', p. 23). He resigned on or before 25 March 1276, when he entered the order of Friars Minor (*Reg. Giffard*, p. 257).[18] As 'brother Thomas, formerly master' he was a witness to the extent of the hospital made on 11 October 1280 (R902).

During Thomas' rule the hospital's indebtedness is first mentioned. On 27 April 1275 Alexander de Kirketon, at that time sheriff of Yorkshire, was appointed by the king, 'during pleasure', to the custody of the hospital of St Leonard 'fallen into debt'. On the same day Kirketon was also appointed to the custody of Newburgh Priory, also in debt. On 20 November 1276 Thomas de Normanville, king's steward, was appointed to the custody of the master and brethren of the hospital, again because of debt (*CalPat*, 1272–1281, pp. 85, 171).

### ROGER OF MALTON (1276 TO 1280)

Sir Roger of Malton, Archbishop Giffard's penitentiary, was elected master by the canons of York on 15 May 1276 (*Reg. Giffard*, pp. 257–59). He occurs as master of the hospital in October 1276 (C914 [Cott., f. 186ᵛ]), January 1276[/67] (Raine, *Historians*, III, 200–03), June 1277 (M: Nappa [MS Dods. 120b, f. 85ʳ]), and Easter term 1278 (Baildon, *Monastic Notes*, I, 246, citing de banco rolls). Malton was said to have been rector for four and a half years at an inquisition into the state of the hospital which was commissioned on 15 November 1280 (C1029 [*CalPat*, 1334–1338, pp. 268]), but had apparently resigned or been ejected from the mastership before that, for he witnessed the extent of 11 October 1280 as 'former master' (R902). In 1286 the executors of master John le Gras were attempting to recover 100*m*. which Gras had loaned Roger of Malton, master of the hospital. It was reported that Roger of Malton had been appointed master by the dean and chapter, in usurpation of the rights of the king's predecessor, but the present king recovered the advowson, Roger was turned out, and all his acts were annulled (Baildon, *Monastic Notes*, I, 246). Roger of Malton, priest, 'formerly master of the hospital of St Leonard', was instituted to the church of Silkstone by Archbishop Wickwane in June 1281, as compensation for the calamity he had suffered (*reparationem ruine quam patitur*). But he was unable to retain possession because of the opposition of the monks of Pontefract, causing the archbishop to complain that after his worthy labours he should be driven to penury in his old age (*post meritorii laboris suis cursum . . . in ultimis iam diebus mendicare miserabiliter cogatur*)

---

[17] For Sir William de Saham (*c.*1225–1292), a justice, who was in Yorkshire in 1280 (*YF*, 1272–1280, p. 46), said to have been a son of Ralph de Saham, of Saham Toney in Norfolk, see *ODNB*.

[18] For the Franciscan Grey Friars of York, probably founded *c.*1230, see *VCH Yorks*, III, 287–91.

(*Reg. Wickwane*, pp. 36, 273–74).[19] At an uncertain date, but probably after the unsuccessful attempt to install him at Silkstone, Roger became master of the hospital of the Blessed Mary Magdalene in Ripon, in which capacity he occurs in 1286 and 1292 (*Reg. Romeyn*, II, 44, 69). He resigned the mastership in May 1294 (ibid., 78). In 1291 Sir Roger of Malton and Sir Hugh of Methley were given licence to go on pilgrimage to the abbey of Pontigny, where Archbishop Wickwane was buried (*Reg. Wickwane*, pp. xx, 333; *Reg. Romeyn*, II, 68). Roger of Malton, priest, gave a rent charge from land in Feasegail, York, held by Nicholas Belle the skinner, to the altar of the Blessed Virgin Mary in the crypt in York Minster and to Peter de St-Nicolas, warden of the altar (*CVC*, I, no. 81).

### GEOFFREY OF ASPALL (1281 TO 1287)

For Geoffrey of Aspall, noted pluralist, administrator and natural philosopher, who took his name from Aspall in Suffolk, see Emden, *Oxford*, pp. 60–61 and *ODNB*. Aspall had apparently begun his ecclesiastical career by 1254, and was called magister in 1262. By 1278 he was keeper of the wardrobe to Queen Eleanor. He served the king in various capacities in the later 1270s and 1280s. He was granted the custody of the hospital of St Leonard for life on 10 June 1281 (*CalPat*, 1272–1281, p. 443) and died (as master) in 'parts beyond the sea' on 11 June 1287 (*CalInqPM*, II, 384–85).

### JAMES DE ISPANIA (1288 × 1290 TO 1293)

For Ispania, see Emden, *Oxford*, pp. 1736–38. He was frequently called nephew, or kinsman, of Edward I's wife Eleanor of Castile, and had a long career as a pluralist and king's clerk. Emden says he was an illegitimate son of Eleanor's brother King Alfonso X of Castile, but the evidence for this statement is unclear. Ispania first occurs in March and July 1281, when, described as the queen's kinsman or nephew, he was allowed oak trees from the forest of Shotover (Oxford) for fuel (*CalCl*, 1279–1288, pp. 79, 96). In August 1282 the king presented him to the church of Crondall (Hants.), in the diocese of Winchester, which was in the king's gift by the voidance of the see (*CalPat*, 1281–1292, p. 32). But the archbishop of Canterbury wanted the church for his chaplain, Peter of Guildford, and wrote to the king and others in May 1283, protesting that Ispania was still a child (*puer, enfant*), and illegitimate to boot (*Reg. Epp. Peckham*, II, 547–49, 554–55, 764). In February and March 1283 the king presented Ispania to the church of Rothbury (Northumberland), in the diocese of Durham (*CalPat*, 1281–1292, pp. 56, 60), and in April 1283 granted him the prebend of Skyrne (*Scren*), in his gift by reason of the voidance of the see of Meath (*CalPat*, 1281–1292, p. 62). In 1284, describing him as king's clerk and nephew of his wife Eleanor, the king granted Ispania a prebend in the church of St Patrick, Dublin, in his gift by reason of the voidance of the see of Dublin (*CalPat*, 1281–1292, p. 137). He was collated to the prebend of Husthwaite, York in September 1287, but the prebend was retained by his predecessor until 1290. Ispania was in possession by January 1293, and resigned the prebend by May 1297. The king presented him to the church of Althorpe (Lincs.) in June 1287 and again in April 1288, the advowson being in the king's hands because of the vacancy of the mastership of St Leonard's Hospital (*CalPat*, 1281–1292, p. 271; C114 [Cott., f. 17ʳ]).[20] There is no record of his institution as master of the hospital, but he was named as master in court proceedings from Easter term 1290

---

[19]   The archbishop came to an agreement with Pontefract Priory in 1284, whereby Silkstone church was appropriated to the priory, saving a vicarage to the archbishop, to which he presented master John of Apperley in August 1284 (*Reg. Wickwane*, pp. 292–94, 317).

[20]   Ispania does not seem to have been instituted to Althorpe. On the presentation of James de Ispania

until Michaelmas term 1292 (Baildon, *Monastic Notes*, I, 246–47, citing de banco rolls). It was during his tenure of the mastership that he became master of arts. Towards the end of May 1291 orders were issued that seventy bucks should be delivered to Oxford for the feast for his inception (*CalCl*, 1288–1296, p. 170). In January 1292 he was described as 'master James de Ispania, king's clerk and member of his household' (*CalPat*, 1281–1292, p. 466). He was described as 'master James de Ispania, clerk, master of the hospital of St Leonard' in March 1293 (*CalChancW*, p. 36), but had resigned the mastership by May 1293, when the king granted it to Walter of Langton (*CalPat*, 1292–1301, p. 15). In that month Ispania acknowledged his debt to Langton of 200*m*., to be levied, in default of payment, of his lands and chattels in co. York (*CalCl*, 1288–1296, p. 317).

Only a brief notice of Ispania's subsequent career can be given. He had papal dispensation to hold a prebend of Wells with other prebends in 1300, a previous dispensation granted by Honorius IV having been lost (*CalPapalL*, 1198–1304, p. 589).[21] In April 1303 he was charged, as a prebendary of St Paul's, with pluralism (*Reg. Winchelsey*, I, 453–54), but in 1304, described as master James de Ispania, nephew of the late Queen Eleanor, canon of London, he had dispensation not to appear or produce to the archbishop of Canterbury, as visitor, the papal dispensation and privileges he had for illegitimacy and plurality of benefices, which were with some of his friends in Rome and Spain (*CalPapalL*, 1198–1304, pp. 612–13). In 1306 a further papal letter was issued, noting his illegitimacy and that he was not ordained, giving a long list of his benefices and confirming his dispensation (*CalPapalL*, 1305–1342, pp. 11–12). As well as York, St Paul's and Wells, at various times he held prebends at Exeter, Lincoln, Lichfield, Salisbury and other places (*FEA*, VI, 82; ibid., VII, 76–77). He was appointed chamberlain of the exchequer in 1317, and had vacated the office by Easter 1323. He served as clerk or receiver of the king's chamber in 1321 (Emden, *Oxford*, p. 1738). In 1331 he was involved in a dispute concerning a prebend in the king's free chapel of Hastings (*CalCl*, 1330–1333, p. 183). He was dead shortly before 22 October 1332, when a successor was collated to his prebend in Lincoln (*Reg. Burghersh*, no. 2769).

## WALTER LANGTON (1293 TO 1307)
For Langton see Thompson, 'Bridgnorth', pp. 67–69; Hughes, 'Langton'; *Reg. Langton*, I, pp. xxxii–xxxix; *ODNB*. He was the son of Simon and Amicia Peverel and took his name from Church Langton in Leicestershire, or one of the nearby settlements also called Langton. Langton is first noted as a wardrobe clerk in the service of Edward I in 1281–82. He was treasurer of the exchequer from 1295, and became bishop of Coventry and Lichfield in 1296. He was granted the mastership of the hospital of St Leonard's no fewer than four times. On 19 May 1293, as king's clerk and one of the household, and keeper of the wardrobe, he was granted the hospital of St Leonard for life after Ispania's resignation (*CalPat*, 1292–1301, p. 15). His fall from grace was rapid after the death of Edward I. Langton was arrested *c.* 7 August 1307, and apparently lost the treasurership on 19 August (Beardwood, *Trial of Langeton*, p. 1). He was probably expelled from the hospital at the same time, as his successor Gilbert Stapleton was appointed on 20 August 1307. Langton was released from prison on 9 November 1308. On the restoration of his temporalities shortly before his release, it seems he was

---

the church was said to be vacant by the death of Adam of Filby. When Roger de Lisle was presented by the Templars in 1290, the same reason for vacancy was given (*Reg. Sutton*, III, 41; ibid., VIII, 20).

21 Not in *Les registres d'Honorius IV*, ed. M. Prou (Paris, 1888). Honorius was pope between 1285 and 1287.

restored to the mastership of the hospital,[22] but resigned it formally on 1 December 1308 (*CalCl*, 1307–1313, p. 132), when it was given to Bishop Reynolds. Langton recovered his position somewhat in subsequent years. He resumed the treasurership in January 1312, and was regranted the mastership of the hospital on 28 January 1314, on Reynolds' resignation. As bishop of Coventry and Lichfield and master of the hospital, Langton was granted protection in October 1314 (*CalPat*, 1313–1317, p. 185). The reason for his subsequent ejection or resignation is unclear, but the hospital was granted to John Hotham on 12 March 1315 (see below). Langton regained the hospital on Hotham's resignation. On 6 August 1316, as bishop of Coventry and Lichfield and master of the hospital, Langton was granted protection for one year. His formal restitution has date 7 August. There it is said that he had held the hospital 'for a long time as well in the time of the late king as afterwards, and from which he was removed by the present king'. Langton occurs as master in May 1317 (*CalPat*, 1313–1317, pp. 525–26, 650), but early the following year resigned the mastership in favour of his nephew Robert Clipston, who was appointed by the king on 30 January 1318 (see below). Langton died in November 1321.

GILBERT STAPLETON (AUGUST 1307 TO AUTUMN 1308)[23]

Gilbert Stapleton appears to have been a younger son of Sir Nicholas Stapleton, and brother to Sir Miles Stapleton, first Lord Stapleton (d. 1314).[24] Gilbert first occurs in September 1288, when as a deacon he was inducted to Normanby church at the presentation of the abbot and convent of St Mary's. In September 1292 he had permission to travel to Rome, or other convenient place, on business connected with his church (*Reg. Romeyn*, I, 167 and n). In February 1304 the archbishop asked his official at York to try the case between Gilbert Stapleton, presented to the church of Terrington by Sir William Latimer senior and Sir Miles Stapleton, knights, and two other clerks who had a claim to the church. Stapleton's claim was unsuccessful (*Reg. Corbridge*, I, 142, 148).

On 20 August 1307, on the fall of Langton, the king granted the custody of the hospital to Gilbert Stapleton, king's clerk, for life, subject to the maintenance of the alms and other pious works of the institution (*CalPat*, 1307–1313, p. 2). Gilbert doubtless owed his preferment to his brother Miles, who was steward to Edward II before and after his succession in July 1307 (*ODNB*, s.n. Stapleton). Gilbert Stapleton, master of the hospital, was ordered to cause the former treasurer of the hospital to appear before those inquiring into Langton's debts on 1 December [1307] (Beardwood, *Trial of Langeton*, p. 134). Stapleton issued a deed as master on 13 January 1308 (M: Pickhill

---

[22] His restoration is mentioned in the writ appointing Reynolds (*CalPat*, 1307–1313, p. 96), but it seems unlikely that the king intended him to take possession.

[23] For the Stapleton family see H.E. Chetwynd-Stapylton, *Chronicles of the Yorkshire family of Stapleton* (1884), reprinted from 'The Stapeltons of Yorkshire', *YAJ*, VIII (1884), 65–116, 223–58, 381–423, 427–74; *Baildon*, I, 319–42; *CP*, XII (1), 259–65. Gilbert Stapleton the clerk has sometimes been confused with Sir Gilbert Stapleton, a younger son of Sir Miles Stapleton (d. 1314). Sir Miles settled his estate of North Moreton in Berkshire, held as 1 k.f. of the earl of Pembroke, on his son Gilbert in 1310. Gilbert Stapleton held North Moreton in 1316. He was apparently living in December 1317, but was dead by 1325, when his heirs were in wardship. His wife was Agnes, one of the daughters and coheirs of Brian Lord FitzAlan. She was said to be aged eight in 1306. If Gilbert's heirs were children by Agnes, they must have died young, for Agnes' heir was her son John by her second husband Thomas Sheffield (*CP*, V, 395–97; *CalInqPM*, V, no. 498; *CalCl*, 1313–1318, pp. 516–17; ibid., 1323–1327, pp. 412, 505; *VCH Berks*, III, 493).

[24] There seems to be no direct proof of this, but the chronology of Miles and Gilbert's careers indicate they were of the same generation. Miles made his settlement on his younger son Gilbert in conjunction with his brother Gilbert Stapleton (*CalInqPM*, V, no. 498).

[MS Dods. 120b, f. 74$^v$]). Some time afterwards the king revoked Stapleton's collation and, at least according to his writ appointing Reynolds, restored the hospital to
Langton. This was apparently on or after 3 October 1308, when Langton's temporalities were restored, although he was not freed until 9 November. Langton did not
take possession. He was said to have surrendered the hospital to the king, and on
10 December 1308 it was Stapleton who was ordered to deliver it to the new master,
W[alter Reynolds], bishop of Worcester. Sir Miles Stapleton had ended his term as
the king's steward in March 1308, and this may be indicative of a reduction in the
family's influence (*CalPat*, 1307–1313, p. 96; *ODNB*). Sir Gilbert Stapleton, rector of
Normanby, was appointed bailiff of Ripon by Archbishop Greenfield in May 1311
(*Reg. Greenfield*, I, 233). In 1312 Sir Gilbert Stapleton was a household clerk of the
archbishop and in 1313 he attested as steward of the archbishop's household. He was
named as a canon of the archbishop's chapel of St Sepulchre in 1315 (*Reg. Greenfield*,
I, 144, 247, 253, 270; ibid., III, 71). He apparently resigned Normanby church in favour
of Richard of Bossall in October 1313, who at the same time resigned the church of
Bossall in favour of William son of Gilbert Stapleton, who was instituted on the presentation of William de Erghum. But it was Sir Gilbert Stapleton who was recorded
as rector of Bossall in March 1316. In July 1317 John de Erghum was presented to
Bossall by Sir William de Erghum, knight (*Reg. Greenfield*, III, 77–78; ibid., v, 258, 262;
*Reg. Melton*, II, 4). Gilbert received a 'commendation' for six months to Womersley
(*Wylmerslay*, *Wylmerleye*) church in December 1313, and was collated and inducted by
lapse by the archbishop in April 1314 (*Reg. Greenfield*, II, 169). He was collated to the
prebend of Monkton in Ripon in May 1314, and was named as a canon of Ripon in
1315 and June 1318 (*Reg. Greenfield*, I, 97n, 285, 296; *Reg. Melton*, I, 1).[25]

But although Stapleton was a member of the archbishop's household, he had not
entirely left the king's service. In March 1312 Gilbert Stapleton, king's clerk, was
appointed to collect the revenues of the Templar's church of Killington, co. York
(*CalFine*, 1307–1319, p. 128). In one of Bishop Kellawe's last acts, Stapleton was collated
to a prebend in the church of Auckland in Durham on 8 October 1316 (*Reg. Kellawe*,
II, 832–33). In September 1317, whilst the see of Salisbury was vacant, the king granted
him the archdeaconry of Berkshire with the prebend of Graham Borealis (*CalPat*,
1317–1321, p. 23), but the grant was ineffective. Gilbert Stapleton, king's clerk, received
the king's pardon in 1319, at the instance of the earl of Pembroke, for acquiring the
manor of Walkingham [Hill] and 1 bv. in *Thorescroft*, held in chief as of the forest of
Knaresborough. He subsequently had licence, dated 3 June 1321,[26] to enfeoff John
Stapleton with the manor (*CalPat*, 1317–1321, pp. 340–41, 594). On 29 January 1320,
as king's clerk, he was made escheator north of Trent (*CalFine*, 1319–1327, p. 15), and
occurs frequently thereafter so described (see e.g. *CalPat*, 1317–1321, pp. 490, 526, 583,
589). He died, according to the date given in a computation of wages due from his
death, on 28 May 1321 (*CalCl*, 1323–1327, p. 416). On 28 June the sheriff of Yorkshire
was ordered to take the lands late of Gilbert Stapleton, tenant in chief, into the king's
hands (*CalFine*, 1319–1327, p. 62).

WALTER LANGTON (AUTUMN 1308)
See above.

---

[25] On 13 December 1323 the pope issued a bull concerning a dispute which had arisen over the prebend
of Monkton after Stapleton's death (*Reg. Melton*, v, no. 171).
[26] The date is apparently a few days after Stapleton's death.

WALTER REYNOLDS (DECEMBER 1308 TO JANUARY 1314)
For Walter Reynolds, a close confidant of Edward II both before and after his accession, see *ODNB*. He was appointed treasurer in succession to Langton on 22 August
1307, and was consecrated bishop of Worcester, the first episcopal vacancy of the reign,
on 13 October 1308. Two months later he was granted the mastership of St Leonard's (see above). Reynolds was translated to Canterbury on 1 October 1313, had his
temporalities on 3 January 1314, and was enthroned on 17 February. He resigned the
mastership of the hospital shortly before 28 January 1314, when it was again granted
to Walter Langton for life (*CalPat*, 1313–1317, p. 80). Reynolds died in 1327.

WALTER LANGTON (JANUARY 1314 TO 1315)
See above.

JOHN HOTHAM (MARCH 1315 to JULY 1316)
For John Hotham, treasurer of England 1317–18, chancellor of the exchequer 1318–20
and bishop of Ely from 1316 until his death in 1337, see *ODNB*. As 'king's clerk' he
was granted the hospital on 12 March 1315 and occurs as master in June of that year
(*CalPat*, 1313–1317, pp. 260, 301). As Langton was regranted the hospital in August
1316, it is likely that Hotham resigned the mastership in July, on the assent of the
archbishop to his election to Ely and his subsequent assumption of the temporalities.
Hotham also resigned his prebend of Stillington in York at that time.

WALTER LANGTON (AUGUST 1316 TO JANUARY 1318)
See above.

ROBERT CLIPSTON (JANUARY TO JUNE × AUGUST 1318)
For Clipston, see Hughes, 'Langton', pp. 73–74. In October 1298 Bishop Walter
Langton had licence to ordain Walter and Robert of Clipston to all the minor orders
(*Reg. Romeyn*, II, 248), and in 1303 had permission to allow his nephews Walter and
Robert, sons of Robert Clipston of the diocese of Lincoln, then aged twelve and ten
years respectively, and only in minor orders, to hold a benefice apiece (*CalPapalL*,
1198–1304, p. 611).[27] Thus Walter and Robert gained prebends in Coventry and Lich-
field at an early age. Walter was collated to the prebend of Tervin in January 1304, and
held it until his death, probably in 1310. Robert was collated to Flixton prebend in
June 1305, but was collated to another prebend, previously held by John Langton, in
September of that year. In September 1312 he was collated to Stotfold prebend, and
in March 1313 to Hansacre, which he held until 1356.
    On 30 January and 24 February 1318 the king granted custody of the hospital of
St Leonard to Robert of Clipston, king's clerk, but on 11 June following he granted
the wardenship to John Walwayn. On 11 August the king revoked Clipston's collation to the hospital, without further explanation, and on 13 August he again granted
the mastership to Walwayn. Clipston's appointment to the mastership had been made
at the request of his uncle Walter Langton, but was revoked because 'the king has
learned that the said Robert is inefficient and unfit to govern the hospital' (*CalPat*,
1317–1321, pp. 75, 105, 196–97). Clipston persistently claimed redress for his expulsion

---

[27] It is probable that the name Clipston derives from the place of that name in Northamptonshire. It lies
about 8 m. south of the Langton villages in Leicestershire, from which Bishop Walter Langton took
his name, and about 6 m. north of Lamport, to which place Robert retired in 1356.

until at least 1333, but was unsuccessful.[28] It is uncertain whether it was the same Robert Clipston, king's clerk, whom the king presented to [East] Leake [Notts.], in York diocese in March 1347. The presentation was revoked in September 1347 (*CalPat*, 1345–1348, pp. 262, 409). In April 1348 the king presented Robert Clipston to the church of Bentham [Yorks.], but in 1349 he presented another to the same church (*CalPat*, 1348–1350, pp. 55, 396). Clipston exchanged his prebend of Hansacre, in Coventry and Lichfield, for Bishopshull prebend in April 1356, and the following June exchanged Bishopshull for the church of Lamport, Northants. He also held the prebend of Buckland Dinham in Bath and Wells, in succession to his brother Walter, from 31 December 1310 until a date before October 1360.

JOHN WALWAYN (AUGUST 1318 TO JUNE × JULY 1326)
For Walwayn, see Emden, *Oxford*, pp. 2224–25; Denholme-Young, 'Vita Edw. II', esp. pp. 202–07, and F.R. Lewis, 'The rectors of Llanbadarn Fawr, Cardiganshire, from 1246 to 1360', *Archaeologia Cambrensis*, XCII (1937), 233–46, at 238–39.[29] At least three royal clerks were referred to as 'master John Walwayn', or 'master John Wawayn' in the reign of Edward II or early in the reign of Edward III. These were: (a) the master of the hospital, who died in June or July 1326, occasionally called 'the elder'; (b) the prebendary of Hereford, Salisbury, St Davids, and Abergwily, and envoy of Queen Isabella, who died in Avignon in 1330, sometimes called 'the younger'; and (c) the constable of Bordeaux and rector of Brancepeth, who died in March 1348, and whose name is usually given as Wawayn rather than Walwayn. Care is needed to distinguish references to the different men, who have frequently been conflated. As Walwayn's namesake and relation master John Walwayn junior appears to have been presented to his first benefice in 1317, and to have been absent for study until at least October 1322, we can be reasonably certain that references to an established master John Walwayn from the first two decades of the century are to the man who was later master of the hospital.[30] From 1302 onwards Walwayn appears amongst the followers of the earl of Hereford. By 1308 he was the earl's 'most trusted clerk, his chief man of affairs' (Denholm-Young, 'Vita Edw. II', pp. 202–03; Davies, *Baronial Opposition*, p. 355n). Master John Walwayn was presented to the church of Old Radnor by Dame Maud de Mortimer in September 1309 (*Reg. Swinfield*, p. 539). The king presented him to the church of Lugwardine in the diocese of Hereford in December 1314, and to the church of Hanslope (Bucks.), in the diocese of Lincoln, in October 1316 (*CalPat*, 1313–1317, pp. 200–01, 550). Master J[ohn] Walwayn, king's clerk, was presented by the king to the prebend of Faringdon in Salisbury cathedral in July 1315 (*CalPat*, 1313–1317, p. 334), but he was unable to retain it.[31] His commission with two others

[28] For details, see Baildon, *Monastic Notes*, I, 248; *Select cases in the court of king's bench under Edward III*, v, ed. G.O. Sayles, Selden Soc., LXXVI (1958), 1.
[29] For his supposed authorship of *Vita Edwardi secundi*, see Denholme-Young, 'Vita Edw. II'; C. Given-Wilson, '*Vita Edwardi secundi*: memoir or journal?', p. 165, and W. Childs, 'Resistance and treason in the *Vita Edwardi secundi*', p. 178n, both in *Thirteenth century England*, VI (1997), at 165–76 and 177–91 respectively; Childs, *Vita Edw. II*, pp. xxiv–xxv.
[30] Emden's accounts of master John Walwayn the elder and master John Walwayn the younger are generally reliable (Emden, *Oxford*, pp. 2224–25). It is unclear whether master John Wawayn, rector of Longnewton and clerk of Queen Philippa, was the same man as master John Wawayn, rector of Brancepeth, proctor of the bishop of Durham, and constable of Bordeaux, who died in March 1348.
[31] Pandulf de Sabellis occurs as prebendary in August 1318 (*FEA 1300–1541*, III, 49). A reference to Sabellis as prebendary of *Farndon* in 1316 (*CalPat*, 1313–1317, p. 400) indicates his tenure of the prebend of Fardon-cum-Balderton in Lincoln cathedral, which he undoubtedly held (*CalPapalL*, 1305–1342, pp. 270, 491; *CalPat*, 1330–1334, p. 243). But it is clear that Sabellis also held the prebend of Faringdon in Salisbury cathedral (*CalPapalL*, 1305–1342, p. 282; *CalPat*, 1327–1330, p. 542).

in April 1316 to treat for peace with Robert Brus shows his standing with the king, as does the earl of Hereford's proposal later in the year that he should be chosen for the vacant bishopric of Durham (*CalPat*, 1313–1317, p. 451; *Hist. Dunelmensis*, p. 98). In 1316 master John Walwayn was recorded as the lord of Stoke Edith, and joint lord of Yarkhill and Weston [Beggard] in the county of Hereford (*Feudal Aids*, II, 389). Master John Walwayn was presented in August 1317 to the church of Llanbadarn Fawr in Cardiganshire by the king, and appears to have held it until his death, as the next recorded rector was presented in November 1326 (*CalPat*, 1317–1321, p. 15; ibid., 1324–1327, p. 333). The king granted the prebend of Weldland in St Paul's, London, to master John Walwayn, king's clerk, on 3 and 8 November 1318 (*CalPat*, 1317–1321, pp. 219, 222). In December 1318, Adam Orleton, bishop of Hereford, found on his visitation the church of Kington held by master John Walwayn, *iuris civilis professor*, as well as Lugwardine and Old Radnor in his diocese, and asked the patron of Kington, Humphrey de Bohun, earl of Hereford, to present another rector (*Reg. Orleton*, p. 88).[32] Walwayn's pluralism in the diocese of Hereford did not prevent the bishop collating him to the prebend of Bullinghope in Hereford cathedral in February 1322 (*Reg. Orleton*, p. 220). Walwayn was later ejected from the prebend as the pope had reserved it for his own collation. The pope's letter of September 1323 confirming it to master Stephen Ledbury DCL was copied to 'John Walwayn, canon of London' (*CalPapalL*, 1305–1342, p. 234).

Walwayn was appointed escheator south of the Trent in February 1315 (*CalFine*, 1307–1319, p. 232), and remained as escheator until he became treasurer on 10 June 1318. He was no longer treasurer on 14 November 1318, having been discharged 'not on account of his demerit but by the importunity of several persons'. On that day the king 'retaining full confidence' in his administrative abilities reappointed him as escheator south of Trent (Tout, *Chapters*, VI, 20; *CalFine*, 1319–1327, p. 78). Walwayn lost the office when the escheatry was divided up in November and December 1323 (*CalFine*, 1319–1327, pp. 251–52, 255).

The king granted the wardenship of St Leonard's Hospital for life to master John Walwayn, king's clerk, on 11 June 1318, and made a further grant 'of the custody' on 13 August, two days after revoking the collation of Robert Clipston (*CalPat*, 1317–1321, pp. 160, 196–97). On 8 November 1318 the king granted Humphrey de Bohun, earl of Hereford and Essex, going beyond seas on the king's service, protection until Easter, with the like to master John Walwayn, Walter bishop of Exeter, master John Walwayn, master of the hospital of St Leonard, York,[33] and Gilbert de Keleshull, clerk, going with the said earl of Hereford and Essex. On 5 December 1318 the king granted Walwayn £100 annually until he could be provided with a suitable benefice (*CalPat*, 1317–1321, pp. 252–53), and on 7 December the king wrote to Robert count of Flanders, requesting him to give credence to the bishop of Exeter, the earl of Hereford and Essex, constable of England, and the king's clerk master John Walwayn, DCL, whom the king was sending to him and also to William count of Hainhault. On 10 April 1319 the king wrote to Hainhault, after the return of his envoys, saying he was sending back master John Walwayn, canon of St Paul's, and asking the count to give him credence as the king's representative (*CalCl*, 1318–1323, pp. 118, 132). On 18 April 1319 master John Walwayn, clerk, had protection going beyond seas on the king's service, and the like was granted to 'the same master John as keeper

---

[32]  Walwayn no longer held Lugwardine in September 1320 when another was presented (*Reg. Orleton*, p. 386).

[33]  As the same master John Walwayn had protection in April 1319 as king's clerk, and separately as keeper of the hospital, this cannot be taken to prove that both John Walwayns were in the party.

of the hospital of St Leonard, York' (*CalPat*, 1317–1321, p. 325). An inquisition held early in 1324 found that many of the allowances to the residents of the hospital had been substantially reduced by master John Walwayn (*CalInqMisc*, 1307–1349, no. 718). Walwayn no longer held the hospital on 15 July 1326, when his successor was appointed. Master John Walwayn was recently dead on 18 July 1326, when John Hampton, escheator in cos Gloucester, Hereford, Worcester, Salop and Stafford, and the march of Wales adjacent, was ordered to take his lands into the king's hands (*CalFine*, 1319–1327, p. 399). Walwayn had exchanged his prebend of Weldland in St Paul's for the rectory of the chapel of Imber, Wiltshire, with Thomas de Burgh, clerk, who had been presented by John le Rous, knight, on 15 May 1326, and instituted on 24 June. Walwayn was presented to Imber by Rous, 'by exchange', on 28 June 1326 and was instituted on 29 June. But he held the chapel for a very short time before resigning it, as Hugh Weymouth was presented on 20 July 1326, and instituted by the bishop 'after the resignation of John Walwayn senior' (*Reg. Martival*, I, 356–58). As Thomas de Burgh occurs on 15 March 1327 as an executor of master John Walwayn (*CalCl*, 1327–1330, p. 104), we can suppose that Walwayn was aware of his own imminent death and arranged the exchange for the benefit of his friend Burgh.[34]

ROBERT BALDOCK (JULY 1326 TO NOVEMBER 1326)
For Robert Baldock, keeper of Edward II's privy seal 1320–23, diplomat, chancellor of the exchequer 1323–26, a protégé of the younger Hugh Despenser, see *ODNB* and Emden, *Oxford*, pp. 96–98. Baldock fell with Edward II. He was captured in November 1326 and died 'miserably abused' in Newgate gaol on 28 May 1327. As master Robert Baldock, king's clerk, archdeacon of Middlesex, he was granted the wardenship of the hospital for life by the king on 15 July 1326 (*CalPat*, 1324–1327, p. 295). The hospital was granted to his successor by the future Edward III, 'guardian of the realm', before 14 December 1326 (ibid., p. 342).

JOHN GIFFARD (DECEMBER 1326 TO 1349)
For a short biography of John Giffard, see *Reg. Hemingby*, p. 200.[35] It is likely that the John Giffard who resigned the church of Cotterstock in 1317 (*VCH Northants*, II, 166)[36] when William Giffard was instituted, and the John Giffard, lord of Cotterstock, who made presentations to Cotterstock in 1320, 1323 and 1333 (*Reg. Burghersh*, nos 1192, 1246, 1464), can both be identified with the master of St Leonard's. In May 1312, as a clerk of Queen Isabella, John Giffard was given dispensation at the queen's request to accept two benefices to the value of 200*m.*, and he was doubtless one of her eight clerks given licence to enjoy the fruits of their benefices as non-residents for three years (*CalPapalL*, 1305–1342, p. 97). Giffard was granted protection on 3 May 1313 as he was going beyond seas with the queen (*CalPat*, 1307–1313, p. 580). Described as king's clerk, in November 1316 he was granted land from the wastes of the forest of Rockingham in Northamptonshire (*CalFine*, 1307–1319, pp. 311–12). His collation by Lewis, bishop elect of Durham, to the church of Haughton[-le-Skerne]

---

34  In 1291 the prebend of Weldland was assessed at £2 annually, and the church of Imber £10 (*Taxatio Ecclesiastica*, pp. 19b, 180b, 185b), but these figures presumably do not represent the true value of the benefices to the incumbents. Weldland was assessed at £7 17s. 4d. in 1535 (*Valor Ecclesiasticus*, I, 363).
35  His contemporaries included John Giffard, rector of Lanivet, Cornwall, and canon of Exeter, and John Giffard, rector of Inwardleigh, Devon, later vicar of Okehampton, Devon, for both of whom see Emden, *Oxford*, p. 762.
36  No reference given, but presumably from Lincoln Record Office, Episcopal Register 2 (Bishop Dalderby's register), f. 133[v].

in that diocese, which must have been made in 1317–18, was confirmed by the king in January 1328 (*CalPat*, 1327–1330, p. 201). In June 1318, at the queen's request, Giffard was provided with a canonry at Wells, with reservation of a prebend, notwithstanding that he was rector of Haughton in the diocese of Durham, and a canon of York with expectation of a prebend (*CalPapalL*, 1305–1342, p. 177). Giffard was described as Queen Isabella's 'notary' or 'clerk for the queen's letters' and acted as her steward north of Trent (Tout, *Chapters*, III, 34n; ibid., v, 276, 285). On 14 December 1326 the grant for life of the wardenship of the hospital made to John Giffard, king's clerk, by letters patent 'under testimony of Edward, the king's firstborn son, when guardian of the realm' was ratified (*CalPat*, 1324–1327, p. 342). The grant 'by the late king' was confirmed by Edward III on 1 February 1327 (*CalPat*, 1327–1330, p. 9). Giffard's estate as the keeper of the hospital for life was again ratified in March 1335, together with his estates in the church of Haughton, and his prebends in York and Wells 'in consideration of his service to the king and Queen Isabella' (*CalPat*, 1334–1338, pp. 86–87). Giffard acquired the prebend of Givendale in York in 1322; a prebend in Wells in 1322 × 1335; and a prebend in Salisbury in 1339. As John Giffard, son of Osbert [Giffard], of Cotterstock, clerk, he received a pardon in September 1340 in consideration of his good service to Queen Isabella and the king. He was going to Rome on the king's business and feared his enemies might cause him trouble (*CalPat*, 1340–1343, p. 36). For Giffard's foundation in 1339 of the chantry college of Cotterstock, comprising a provost and twelve chaplains, see *VCH Northants*, II, 166–67 and *Reg. Burghersh*, no. 1621. A clerk was instituted to a vicarage at Giffard's presentation on 20 June 1349 (*Reg. Shrewsbury*, p. 611), and it is likely that he was then still living; but he was dead on 20 August 1349, when the mastership of St Leonard's was granted to Brembre. Thus Giffard died at the height of the Black Death in the north, in possession of the hospital and his prebends in York, Salisbury, and Wells. Giffard's heir was his kinsman John son of Roger Giffard (*CalCl*, 1354–1360, p. 537).

## THOMAS BREMBRE (AUGUST 1349 TO 1361)

Thomas Brembre first occurs in August 1337, when, described as king's clerk, he was granted the chapel of the tower of Botehaut,[37] which was in the king's possession with the lands of the count of Eu (*CalPat*, 1334–1338, p. 498). In March 1343, the king granted him the prebend of Stratton in Salisbury cathedral, and in July of the same year the prebend of Milton Manor in Lincoln cathedral (*CalPat*, 1343–1345, pp. 12, 104, 258). In July 1345, again described as king's clerk, he was granted the 'office of the chirography' in the common bench, which he was allowed to perform by deputy (*CalPat*, 1343–1345, p. 534). Brembre received the prebend of Sutton in Lincoln cathedral by the king's gift in February 1347 (*CalPat*, 1345–1348, p. 256), and doubtless resigned Milton Manor at that time. In November 1348 he occurs as receiver of the king's chamber (*CalPat*, 1348–1350, p. 212; cf. *CalCh*, 1341–1417, p. 99); in 1345, 1348 and 1349 he was referred to as the king's secretary (otherwise the receiver of the king's chamber),[38] and in 1349 clerk of the king's secret seal (*CalPapalP*, 1342–1419, pp. 101, 135, 142, 157; Tout, *Chapters*, v, 180). On 20 August 1349 he was granted the wardenship of the hospital of St Leonard for life (*CalPat*, 1348–1350, p. 368). As Sir Thomas Brembre he was mentioned in the Norwich bailiff's accounts of 1350–51 (*Norwich Records*, II, 39). Brembre was named as master of the hospital in 1355, 1358 and 1359 (*CalPat*, 1354–1358, p. 231; C214, C686 [Cott., ff. 48ʳ⁻ᵛ, 133ʳ⁻ᵛ]). He was

---

37  Otherwise Buttehaut, in Wighton in Norfolk.
38  On this point, see Tout, *Chapters*, IV, 261–62.

granted the deanery of Wimborne Minster in August 1350, and held the dignity until his death. There he founded a chantry of four chaplains in 1354 (*CalPat, 1348–1350*, p. 555; *VCH Dorset*, II, 110–11). In 1354 he was collated to the prebend of Sneating in St Paul's. He became keeper of the privy seal in the same year (Tout, *Chapters*, IV, 259), and so occurs in 1355–56. In 1357 he was indited by Thomas, bishop of Ely, by papal authority, causing the king to complain to the pope on Brembre's behalf, calling him his secretary. But the pope rejected the king's complaints, and instructed him to take care of the behaviour of his servants (Tout, *Chapters*, III, 219; ibid., V, 34; *CalPapalL*, 1342–1362, pp. 625, 627). Brembre occurs as master in February 1361, when he had a grant to the hospital from the king, and was living in May 1361, when he had licence to return to a prebend he had exchanged. He was dead on 24 October of that year (*CalCh, 1341–1417*, p. 169; *CalPat, 1361–1364*, pp. 30, 96, 99).

RICHARD RAVENSER (APRIL 1363 TO MAY 1386)
For Richard Ravenser, see *ODNB*; Foss, *Judges*, IV, 78–79. He was attorney to Queen Philippa in 1343, and in 1353 was described as a chancery clerk. Ravenser became keeper of the hanaper in the chancery in 1357. He was granted the archdeaconry of Norfolk in 1359, and the archdeaconry of Lincoln in c.1368. Ravenser acquired the provostship of Beverley by exchange in 1360, and resigned it before 20 January 1368. He held the prebend of Knaresborough in York Minster from 1371 until 1381. On 8 February 1363 the unnamed master and the brethren of the hospital were granted a licence for alienation in mortmain (*CalPat, 1361–1364*, p. 313), but it is probable that the mastership was then vacant. As king's clerk, Ravenser was granted the mastership for life on 26 April 1363 (*CalPat, 1361–1364*, p. 331). He occurs as master in June 1365, July 1367 (*CalPat, 1364–1367*, pp. 128, 422), June 1369 (*CalPat, 1367–1370*, p. 275), July 1373 (*CalPat, 1370–1374*, p. 389), October 1376 (*CalPat, 1374–1377*, p. 356), February 1380 (*CalPat, 1377–1381*, p. 465), July 1382, July and November 1383, January 1384 (*CalPat, 1381–1385*, pp. 157, 305, 366), and apparently held the mastership until his death in May 1386. He was buried in Lincoln cathedral. Ravenser had an interest in hospitals and charitable provision which extended beyond St Leonard's. With his brother Robert Selby, he set up the hospital or hostel for twelve poor men in Hull, sometimes known as Selby's Hospital, in or before 1375 (*MA*, VI, 275; *Ctl. Gisborough*, nos 1087a, 1089a; *VCH Yorks*, III, 313; *CalPat, 1377–1381*, pp. 561–62).

NICHOLAS SLAKE (JUNE 1386 TO C.1389)
For Slake, see Thompson, 'Bridgnorth', pp. 38–39, 77–79. Nicholas Slake was said to be the favourite chaplain of Richard II (Tout, *Chapters*, III, 405), and his career advanced accordingly until the accession of Henry IV in 1399. In February 1379, the king collated him to the first prebend to become free in the collegiate church of Howden (*CalPat, 1377–1381*, p. 330). In May 1382 he was appointed for life to the mastership of the hospital of St Mary, Rounceval, in Westminster,[39] and in the same month was granted a prebend in the king's free chapel of St George, in Windsor castle. In July 1384, as king's clerk, he was granted a prebend in the king's free chapel of Hastings (*CalPat, 1381–1385*, pp. 117, 123, 195, 443; *CalInqMisc, 1377–1388*, no. 170). In October 1385 he became archdeacon of Chester during the voidance of the see of Coventry and Lichfield (*CalPat, 1385–1389*, p. 23). He was granted the hospital of St Leonard by the king on 5 June 1386 (*CalPat, 1385–1389*, p. 158). Slake was one

---

[39] For this hospital, originally a dependency of the Augustinian priory of Roncevalles in Navarre, see *VCH London*, I, 584–85; G. Rosser, *Medieval Westminster 1200–1540* (Oxford, 1989), pp. 310–20.

of those imprisoned by the 'Merciless Parliament' of 1388 (Tout, *Chapters*, III, 429, 435), and may have lost the mastership as a result, although his successor was not appointed until January 1390. In November 1391 Slake was granted the archdeaconry of Wells (*CalPat*, 1388–1392, p. 492). He was twice granted the deanery of the college of St Mary, Bridgnorth, firstly in 1387, resigning it in 1391, and secondly in 1401, but there is no evidence the second grant was effective (Thompson, 'Bridgnorth', pp. 51, 79). In May 1392 he was granted the wardenship of the hospital of St John, Bridgnorth;[40] in August 1395 a prebend in the king's chapel of Tamworth; and in September 1395 the wardenship of the hospital of Sherborne [Dorset][41] (*CalPat*, 1391–1396, pp. 52, 621). He was made dean of the king's free chapel of St Stephen in the palace of Westminster in April 1396, and so occurs in 1398, 1401, 1407 and 1411. The deanery was held by another by 1425 (*CalPat*, 1391–1396, pp. 684–85; *CalCl*, 1399–1402, p. 418; *VCH London*, I, 570–71; *CalInqMisc*, 1422–1485, no. 16). Slake held the deanery of Wells from 1398, but was said to be 'late dean of Wells cathedral' on 1 November 1400 (*CalInqMisc*, 1399–1422, no. 160). His arrest and imprisonment in the tower was ordered on 4 January 1400, apparently because he was suspected of involvement in the Epiphany rising.[42] In 1403, Slake, described as 'late dean of Wells', was being pursued by a canon of Wells for a debt (*CalCl*, 1399–1402, p. 34; ibid., 1402–1405, p. 276; *CalPat*, 1399–1401, p. 214). There were more actions against him for debt in 1404, 1406, and 1409, but in that year he seems to have recovered his position somewhat, when five bonds, by five separate individuals, each in the sum of £2000, were made out to him (*CalCl*, 1402–1405, pp. 360, 376; ibid., 1405–1409, pp. 145, 497, 527–28). In 1414 Nicholas Slake, now described as rector of Croston in Lancs., released all actions against those who had issued bonds to him in 1409 (*CalCl*, 1413–1419, p. 192). He had been presented to Croston by the king in 1409, and was presumably dead in 1418, when another was presented to the rectory (*VCH Lancs*, VI, 87).

## ROBERT BAYS (JANUARY 1390 TO 1391)

Robert Bays first comes to notice in 1372 as a clerk of the diocese of Wells in his twenty-first year, when he was granted a papal dispensation, in addition to a previous dispensation for illegitimacy, to hold a benefice with cure of souls, as long he took orders as soon as he was of age, and appointed a vicar in the interim. As vicar of Yeovil and 'priest and scholar of civil law' he received further dispensations in 1375, allowing him to hold any number of benefices as long as they were mutually compatible, and to be non-resident for seven years, so that he could further his studies in civil law at a university (*CalPapalL*, 1362–1404, pp. 181, 212, 216). In 1376 the king

[40] For the hospital of Holy Trinity and St John the Baptist in Bridgnorth, see *VCH Salop*, II, 98–99. Slake's appointment to the mastership was ineffective.

[41] For the hospital of St Thomas, Sherborne, see *VCH Dorset*, II, 105. Slake's appointment to the wardenship names his predecessor as John Wendelyngburgh, deceased. Wendelyngburg's estate in 'the chapel of St Thomas on the Green, Shirburn, co. Dorset' had been confirmed the previous June (*CalPat*, 1391–1396, p. 576). M.E. Cornford has erred in claiming Slake and his predecessor as masters of the hospital of SS Lazarus, Martha and Mary, Sherburn, co. Durham (*VCH Durham*, II, 116). The advowson of the Sherburn hospital belonged to the see of Durham, which was not vacant in 1395.

[42] Richard Maudelyn, whose arrest was ordered at the same time, was certainly part of the plot. His name appears on a list of dead, which includes Thomas earl of Kent, John earl of Huntingdon, and William earl of Wiltshire, whose goods were to be delivered to Westminster (*CalCl*, 1399–1402, p. 225). Maudelyn was apparently executed with William Feriby in London about the end of January 1400. His body was said by some to have been passed off as that of Richard II (Given-Wilson, *Chronicles*, pp. 50, 228, 244).

ratified his estate as vicar of the church of Yeovil, in the diocese of Bath and Wells (*CalPat*, 1374–1377, p. 241). He occurs as a canon of Bath and Wells in 1379, holding the prebend of Combe Tertia. In July 1383, as vicar of Yeovil, he was granted protection for a year as he was going to Ireland; and in both January and May 1386 he had a year's protection as he was going to Ireland in the king's service (*CalPat*, 1381–1385, p. 290; ibid., 1385–1389, pp. 95, 126). He was confirmed in his estate as canon of Wells and prebendary of Combe in August 1386 (*CalPat*, 1385–1389, p. 185).

Bays was granted the hospital of St Leonard by the king on 15 January 1390 (*CalPat*, 1388–1392, p. 172).[43] He had resigned his mastership of the hospital, or been ejected, by 8 June 1391, when his successor was appointed (*CalPat*, 1388–1392, p. 428). At about the same time he lost his prebend and vicarage: in October 1391 the king ratified Thomas Redman as vicar of Yeovil (*CalPat*, 1388–1392, p. 490); and in June 1392 William Excestre was appointed to Combe Tertia. The losses may have been connected with outlawry: in April 1391, Robert Bays, vicar of Yeovil and canon of Wells, received a pardon for outlawry for non-appearance to answer for debts (*CalPat*, 1388–1392, p. 396). He appears to have continued to dispute the possession of his Wells prebend, acting as 'Robert Bays, canon of the cathedral church of Wells' in July 1395 (*CalCl*, 1392–1396, p. 472). In view of his connections with Yeovil it is likely he was the Robert Bays, clerk, of Somerset, who occurs in 1395 and 1397 (*CalCl*, 1392–1396, p. 486; ibid., 1396–1399, p. 225). The king presented Robert Bays to the church of Hemyock (co. Devon) in the diocese of Exeter in December 1396 (*CalPat*, 1396–1399, p. 60). In March 1399 Bays was said to be a clerk of the duke of Exeter (*CalCl*, 1396–1399, pp. 374–75). This was John Holland, Richard II's half-brother. Holland's part in the Epiphany rising, for which he was executed on 9 or 10 January 1400, doubtless ended Bay's career. He can perhaps be identified with Robert Bays, clerk, who was impleaded in Trinity term 1401 for non-payment of a bond dated 1 August 1399 in the sum of 20*m*., to be repaid at Braunton in Devon (PRO, CP 40/562, rot. 213d), and with Robert Bays, clerk, who made a recognisance for 100*s*. in January 1404, to be levied in default of payment of his lands and chattels in Yorkshire, and of his church goods (*CalCl*, 1402–1405, p. 296).

WILLIAM BOTHEBY (JUNE 1391 TO JANUARY 1399)

Not much is known of Botheby beyond his tenure of the hospital. The king granted William Botheby, chaplain, the prebend of Strensall in York Minster on 26 February 1388, and his estate as prebendary was ratified on 28 July the same year (*CalPat*, 1385–1389, pp. 413, 497). But Francis Carboni, archdeacon of York, had a prior claim, and Botheby resigned his right in the prebend before 15 July 1389 (*CalCl*, 1389–1392, p. 47).[44] On 23 October 1389 Botheby and Nicholas Catton, clerks, 'the king's lieges', had licence to pass to the Roman court to obtain benefices from the pope, but this expedition, if it took place, left no trace in the papal registers. Botheby obtained a prebend in the church of St Martin le Grand in London from the king in February 1390 (*CalPat*, 1388–1392, pp. 154, 194). William Botheby, chaplain, occurs with others

---

43 It is possible that Bays owed the mastership to his predecessor Slake, as the two must have been acquainted. Slake had acquired the rectory of Yeovil between 1385 and 1387, some years after Bays had become vicar, and appears to have lost the rectory before October 1391, when John Bell was presented [to the vicarage] (Lyte, 'Somerset Incumbents', p. 82; *CalPat*, 1388–1392, p. 486). Slake was said to be 'late parson of Yeovil' in September 1394, when he was granted protection, and in April 1396 was 'late parson of Yeovil and patron of the vicarage', the church being in the king's hands because of Slake's outlawry (*CalPat*, 1391–1396, pp. 483, 703). Slake's outlawry probably came about as a result of non-appearance to answer for a debt (see e.g. *CalPat*, 1396–1399, p. 396).

44 *FEA 1300–1541*, VI, 81, citing YML, Torre MS, p. 1027, has Botheby vacating the prebend by death.

in October 1393 as a trustee of land in Thirsk for John Kilvington and his wife Isabel (*CalPat*, 1391–1396, p. 326).

William Botheby, king's clerk, was granted the wardenship of the hospital for life by the king on 8 June 1391 (*CalPat*, 1388–1392, p. 428). In February 1398, Botheby was ordered to allow John Danyell, a brother of the hospital,[45] to have his chamber in the hospital, with access to the chapel adjoining, with his meat, raiment and other things. There had been arguments between Botheby and Danyell and others over the governance of the hospital, and Danyell had 'long been suing with the king and council for the better ruling thereof' (*CalCl*, 1396–1399, p. 250). Matters were not resolved, and on 11 December 1398 master Ralph Selby, William Feriby, archdeacon of the East Riding, Robert Ragenhill and John Harwod were commissioned to inquire into the state of the hospital on information of 'diverse defects' arising from the negligence of the masters, and the strife between Botheby the master and various members of the hospital, with power to suspend the master from the administration of the hospital's goods if there was reasonable cause (*CalPat*, 1396–1399, p. 507; *CalCl*, 1396–1399, p. 363). The inquiry forced Botheby's resignation on 16 January 1399 (*VCH Yorks*, III, 344, citing Chan. Misc. bdle. 20, file 3, no. 1), and on 21 January his successor was appointed. In Easter, Trinity and Michaelmas terms, 1400, the then master, William Waltham, was suing William Botheby, clerk, to give up a book, worth 100s., and chattels, worth £40 (Baildon, *Monastic Notes*, II, 82). Nothing is known of Botheby after this date.

## WILLIAM FERIBY (JANUARY 1399 TO AUGUST × SEPTEMBER 1399)

For Feriby, see Emden, *Oxford*, pp. 678–79.[46] Several men called William Feriby were active towards the end of the fourteenth century.[47] There seems no reason to doubt Emden's assertion that the William Feriby who was appointed master of the hospital in 1409 was the man of that name who had held the mastership in 1399. William Feriby had gained his MA by 1364, when he was a fellow of Balliol college. He was junior proctor of Oxford university in 1368–69, and senior proctor in 1369–70. His early benefices included Foxholes (Yorks.), Littlebury (Essex), and Whiston (Yorks.). He was granted a canonry in Lincoln, with expectation of a prebend, by papal provision in 1389, notwithstanding his rectory of Whiston. The king granted him the archdeaconry of the East Riding in 1393, but the dignity was disputed. It was again granted to Feriby in February 1397. In November 1397 the king granted his clerk master William Feriby, chaplain, because he had been appointed his chief notary, 40*m.* annually, until he could be provided with benefices to the value of 100*m.* (*CalPat*, 1396–1399, pp. 62, 262). In April 1399 Feriby was granted the archdeaconry of Lincoln, but the grant was ineffectual. Described as archdeacon of the East Riding, Feriby was a member of the commission appointed to investigate the state of St Leonard's Hospital in December 1398. The then master resigned, and on 21 January 1399 William Feriby, king's clerk, had a grant of the wardenship. On 30 April 1399 Feriby

---

45  Sir John Daniel, brother of the hospital of St Leonard, was bequeathed 20s. in the will of William Waltham, a later master, made in 1416 (*Test. Ebor.*, III, 57).

46  For Feriby's supposed authorship of an antecedent to 'Giles' Chronicle' see M.V. Clarke and V.H. Galbraith, 'The deposition of Richard II', in *Bulletin of the John Rylands Library Manchester*, XIV (1930), 125–81, at 150–53.

47  William Feriby of Ferriby, who with seven others was commissioned to inquire into the detention of thraves in April 1399, during Feriby's mastership, was probably a layman (*CalPat*, 1396–1399, p. 584), and can possibly be identified with the knight who was captured with Richard II at Flint castle. For master William Feriby, rector of Blakeney, Norfolk, who may possibly be identical with the rector of Blofield mentioned in the following note, see Emden, *Oxford*, p. 679.

had special protection for the hospital and its men, on his petition alleging much dilapidation by former masters, particularly Botheby (*CalPat*, 1396–1399, pp. 468, 542, 565). Feriby's first term as master lasted less than eight months, and his successor was granted the hospital on 15 September 1399. Richard II had been imprisoned in the tower of London on 2 September, and the future Henry IV was issuing letters under Richard's great seal. Feriby probably lost the mastership because his loyalty to the new regime was doubted. Sir William Feriby, a layman, and doubtless a kinsman of the master of the hospital, was with Richard II when he was captured at Flint castle in August 1399 (Given-Wilson, *Chronicles*, pp. 140, 150). A different master William Feriby was executed for his part in the Epiphany rising of January 1400.[48] But Henry IV took pains not to upset the established order and administration any more than was necessary (Tout, *Chapters*, IV, 63–65, 148), and Feriby's career as king's clerk continued. He undertook an embassy to Cologne in 1400, and was chancellor to Henry, prince of Wales, later Henry V. In June 1400 the king presented him to Horncastle church (Lincs.) and in March 1402 he issued William Feriby, chaplain, master in arts and bachelor in canon law, a pardon for obtaining a bull concerning dignities and prebends in York, Lincoln, and Beverley (*CalPat*, 1401–1405, p. 54). On 13 July 1409, master William Feriby was again granted the wardenship of the hospital (*CalPat*, 1408–1413, p. 88), apparently by exchange with the previous master William Waltham, who gained Feriby's East Riding archdeaconry. Feriby occurs as master in November 1413 and February 1414, when he had royal confirmation of certain hospital deeds. He was dead before 15 March 1415, when his successor was appointed (*CalPat*, 1413–1416, pp. 119, 159, 283).

## WILLIAM WALTHAM (SEPTEMBER 1399 TO 1409)

For Waltham, see Emden, *Cambridge*, p. 614; *FEA 1300–1541*, passim; *Test. Ebor.*, III, 55–59. According to unpublished notes of A. Hamilton Thompson, he was brother to John Waltham, bishop of Salisbury (Tout, *Chapters*, III, 215–16n). He was admitted to King's Hall, Cambridge, in 1377, and was ordained in 1378. He became archdeacon of the East Riding in 1386, but was displaced in 1389. In 1393 he was readmitted to the York chapter, when he was collated as canon of York and prebendary of Dunnington, and in 1399 exchanged the prebend for that of South Cave, which he held until his death. In 1396 he held prebends in York, Wilton Abbey, St Paul's and Salisbury. Master William Waltham was appointed keeper of the hanaper of the chancery in October 1393, on the death of John Ravenser, clerk, and held the office until the fall of Richard II (*CalCl*, 1392–1396, p. 216 and passim; Tout, *Chapters*, IV, 63n). But Waltham did not fall with the king, for on 15 September 1399, after power had passed to Bolingbroke, William Waltham, king's clerk, was granted the wardenship of St Leonard's Hospital (*CalPat*, 1396–1399, p. 595). In July 1400 Waltham had protection for a ship which he had freighted in London with 'divers victuals for the expenses of his household at the hospital' (*CalPat*, 1399–1401, p. 266). Waltham was admitted to the hospital's rectory of Althorpe in April 1407 (C1046 [Cott., f. 216ᵛ]). He occurs as master of the hospital in July 1407 (*CalPat*, 1405–1408, pp. 339, 345; C1035 [Cott., f. 212ᵛ]). In July 1409 he appears to have given up the mastership and the rectory of Althorpe to William Feriby in exchange for the archdeaconry of the East Riding. Waltham held the archdeaconry until his death. His will, which included

---

[48]  Master William Feriby, clerk, rector of Blofield, Norfolk, the son of Christine Feriby, who was executed on 28 January 1400, has frequently been confused with Richard II's favoured clerk (*CalPat*, 1399–1401, pp. 225, 236; *CalCl*, 1399–1402, p. 225; *CalInqMisc*, 1399–1422, no. 245; *CalPapalL*, 1396–1404, p. 396).

a codicil dated 5 October 1416, was proved on 9 October 1416, and included a request for burial in Lincoln Cathedral next to the tomb of his uncle Sir John Ravenser.

## WILLIAM FERIBY (1409 TO 1415)
See above.

## ROBERT FITZHUGH (MARCH 1415 TO 1431)
For Robert FitzHugh, diplomat, chancellor of the university of Cambridge and bishop of London, see Emden, *Oxford*, pp. 689–90; and *ODNB*. His first known benefice was Mottram, Cheshire, which he held in October 1398, when he was granted licence to study at Oxford for two years. As Robert FitzHugh, son of the king's knight Henry FitzHugh [of Ravensworth], the king's chamberlain (d. 1425), he was granted the wardenship of the hospital of St Leonard, vacant by the death of William Feriby, on 15 March 1415 (*CalPat*, 1413–1416, p. 283). FitzHugh occurs as master in July 1428, 1429, and 3 September 1430 (*CalPat*, 1422–1429, p. 494; *CalCl*, 1429–1435, pp. 23, 165). He presumably resigned the mastership some time after his provision to the bishopric of London on 30 April 1431. FitzHugh was consecrated on 16 September 1431, and died as bishop in January 1436.

## WILLIAM SCROPE (1431 TO 1456)
For Scrope, see Emden, *Oxford*, pp. 1660–61, and the further biographical references given there. He was a son of Stephen, second Lord Scrope of Masham. In May 1410 he had papal dispensation to hold a benefice, even though he was only sixteen years old. In 1411 he gained a canonry in Ripon, and was admitted to the rectory of Catton in the same year. In 1428 he had licence to hold an incompatible benefice in addition to his canonries and prebends of Ripon and Beverley and the rectory of Catton. The king 'by advice of the council' granted the wardenship of St Leonard's to William Scrope, king's clerk, bachelor of both laws, on 28 November 1431 (*CalPat*, 1429–1436, p. 183). He resigned the mastership in 1456 in favour of George Neville[49] (C1047 [*CalPat*, 1452–1461, p. 277]). In *c*.1443 Scrope obtained the archdeaconry of Stow, which he held until 1448, when he became archdeacon of Durham. He was master of Greatham Hospital, Durham, from 1451 until his death on 12 May 1463. He was buried in St Stephen's chapel in York Minster.

## GEORGE NEVILLE (1456 TO 1458)
For Neville, see Emden, *Oxford*, pp. 1347–49 and *ODNB*. George Neville was born in 1432, the fourth and youngest son of Richard earl of Salisbury, and so was brother to 'the Kingmaker', Richard Neville, earl of Warwick and Salisbury. He held the archdeaconry of Durham by 1452, and was elected chancellor of Oxford university in 1453. Master George Neville, clerk, was granted the wardenship of the hospital on 24 January 1456 'in lieu of a grant thereof to the king's clerk, William Scrop, bachelor of either law, by letters patent, surrendered' (C1047 [*CalPat*, 1452–1461, p. 277]). Neville was elected bishop of Exeter in February 1456, but his consecration was postponed until he reached his twenty-seventh year and took place on 25 November 1458. This was probably the occasion of his resignation from the mastership of St Leonard's, as Hals was appointed early in December. Neville later regained the mastership, and appears as George, bishop of Exeter, master of the hospital, on 30 October 1462.

---

[49] Emden says he exchanged the mastership in 1448, but the authority cited (*YD*, IV, 82) makes no reference to Scrope or the hospital.

Neville was translated to the archbishopric of York in 1465, and occurs as George, archbishop of York, master of the hospital, on 19 November 1465 (*CalPat*, 1461–1467, pp. 247, 477). He was implicated in the brief restoration of Henry VI in 1470–71, and as a result was arrested on Edward IV's entry to London in April 1471. Though he was pardoned a few days later, he does not appear to have been allowed to return to York. He was rearrested on a charge of treason in April 1472, his temporalities were seized, and he was imprisoned in Calais. In November 1474 he was again pardoned and released, returning to England in December. He died at Blyth, Notts., on 8 June 1476.

### JOHN HALS (1458 TO 1458 × 1462)

For Hals, see Emden, *Oxford*, pp. 856–57 and *ODNB*. He was born *c.*1407, the second son of John Hals, a justice of the king's bench, of Keynedon, near Kingsbridge, Devon. Hals was a trusted servant of Edmund Lacy, bishop of Exeter, and in 1438 he gained a prebend in Exeter cathedral. Hals occurs as a chaplain of Queen Margaret in 1446 and 1457. In 1455 Hals was provided to the bishopric of Exeter by the pope, at the king's request, but Richard, duke of York, protector of the realm during the king's insanity of that year, was successful in installing his own candidate George Neville. Hals had a papal dispensation to hold a benefice incompatible with his archdeaconry of Norfolk in 1457, and on 3 December 1458 was granted the wardenship of St Leonard's for life (*CalPat*, 1452–1461, p. 470). He was consecrated bishop of Coventry and Lichfield in November 1459, and this may have been the occasion for his resignation of the mastership. He was keeper of the privy seal during the brief restoration of Henry VI in 1470–71 and was pardoned by Edward IV in July 1471. Hals died about 30 September 1490.

### GEORGE NEVILLE (1458 × 1462 TO 1472 × 1474)

See above.

### WILLIAM EURE (1474 TO 1477)

For William Eure or Evre, see Emden, *Cambridge*, p. 217. He was a son of William Eure of Witton-le-Wear in Durham and his wife Maud, daughter of Henry FitzHugh, baron of Ravensworth.[50] Eure was ordained subdeacon in 1445, and held the rectory of Brompton in Pickering in 1449. From 1453 until 1483 he was warden of St Mary's Hospital in Bootham in York. He obtained the archdeaconry of Salisbury in 1471 and held it until his death. On 14 February 1474 king's chaplain William Eure, archdeacon of Salisbury, was granted the custody of St Leonard's Hospital (*CalPat*, 1467–1477, p. 421). Eure surrendered the hospital before 3 September 1477, when George FitzHugh, a son of Eure's cousin Henry FitzHugh, and a nephew of Eure's predecessor George Neville, was appointed. This suggests that Eure's short tenure of the mastership was organised by Neville's allies in England in order to reserve it for FitzHugh. Eure was dead by December 1483.

### GEORGE FITZHUGH (1477 TO 1488)

For George FitzHugh, see *Test. Ebor.*, IV, 245 and Emden, *Cambridge*, p. 231. He was born *c.*1461, a son of Henry Lord FitzHugh of Ravensworth (d. 1472) and Alice, a daughter of Richard Neville, earl of Salisbury. He owed his early preferment to his uncle George Neville, archbishop of York from 1465 until 1476. FitzHugh held

---

[50] For the Eure family see *Test. Ebor.*, II, 284–87; *Hist. Northumberland*, XII, 494–97; *CP*, V, 179–80; Hedley, *Northumberland Families*, I, 184–91.

the prebend of Weighton in York Minster from 1475 until his death, and acquired a Lincoln prebend at about the same time. 'George FitzHugh, clerk' can have been no more than seventeen years old when on 3 September 1477 the king granted him the custody of the hospital of St Leonard 'in lieu of a like grant of the same to the king's chaplain William Eure, by letters patent, surrendered' (*CalPat, 1476–1485*, p. 54). FitzHugh resigned the mastership of the hospital early in 1488. In 1483 he was installed as dean of Lincoln. He was master of Pembroke Hall, Cambridge, from 1488 until his death, and also served as chancellor of the university. FitzHugh is recorded as chaplain to Henry VII in 1500. He died on 20 November 1505 and was buried in Lincoln cathedral. His protégé John Constable was an executor of his will, proved on 11 May 1506.

## JOHN CONSTABLE (MARCH 1488 TO JULY 1528)

For John Constable, see Emden, *Cambridge*, p. 155. He was brother and executor to Sir Marmaduke Constable of Flamborough (d. 1518), and so a son of Sir Robert Constable (d. 1488) (*Gentleman's Magazine*, February 1835, p. 154; *ODNB*, s.n. Constable family and Sir Marmaduke Constable). It is likely that Constable gained the prebend of Dunham in Lincoln cathedral in 1494 through the patronage of George FitzHugh, who as noted above was dean of Lincoln from 1483 until his death in 1505. Constable was later successively treasurer of Lincoln (1508), archdeacon of Huntingdon (1512), and dean of Lincoln (1514). On 7 March 1488 the king granted the wardenship of St Leonard's to John Constable, clerk, for life. The hospital had been surrendered by George FitzHugh in his favour (*CalPat, 1485–1494*, p. 269; *Mat. Henry VII*, II, 423).[51] Constable occurs as master of the hospital in 1510 and 1515 (*LPFD*, I, 179; ibid., II, 302). He died on 14 July 1528, holding the deanery of Lincoln and also the mastership, despite having agreed to surrender it in March 1528 in exchange for prebends to the same value of £43 clear (*LPFD*, IV, 1776, 1973). He was buried in the nave of Lincoln cathedral, near the tomb of George FitzHugh.

## THOMAS WYNTER (JULY 1528 TO LATE 1529)

For Thomas Wynter, said to have been an illegitimate son of Cardinal Wolsey, see *ODNB* and the biographical references there cited. Wynter was born *c.*1510, and through Wolsey's influence was dean of Wells, provost of Beverley, and held the archdeaconries of York, Richmond, and Suffolk by the end of 1526. To these trophies Wynter added the wardenship of the hospital on 17 July 1528 (*LPFD*, IV, 1975, 1977, 2717). But by then Wolsey's influence was waning and with it Wynter's prospects. Wynter soon came under pressure over his multiple benefices and in late 1529 returned to England from Paris, where he was studying, to relinquish most of them including the mastership. Nevertheless he remained archdeacon of York, provost of Beverley, and canon of Southwell. He became a royal chaplain, and in 1537 acquired the archdeaconry of Cornwall through the influence of Thomas Cromwell. In May 1543 he resigned the Cornwall archdeaconry, and at about the same time the provostship of Beverley, and appears no further in the records.

---

[51]   No doubt the beneficial resignation was facilitated by Marmaduke Constable's access to the king. Sir Marmaduke Constable had been a knight of the body under Richard III, but was also prominent under Henry VII, occurring again as knight of the body in 1486, and becoming sheriff of Yorkshire in November 1488. In 1492 he accompanied the king to France (*ODNB*).

THOMAS MAGNUS (DECEMBER 1529 TO DECEMBER 1539)
For Thomas Magnus, 'a notable example of the civil service pluralist who was instru-
mental, through assiduous royal service, in consolidating the Henrican Reformation',
see *ODNB*; *Clifford letters of the sixteenth century*, ed. A.G. Dickens, Surtees Society,
CLXXII (1962), 42–44; Thompson, 'Bridgnorth', p. 87; *York clergy wills 1520–1600*, I
(Minster clergy), ed. C. Cross, Borthwick Texts and Calendars, x (York, 1984), 86–87.
He was apparently born in 1462 or 1463[52] but nothing is known of his early years.
Thompson gives his first benefices as Sessay (instituted 2 October 1497) and South
Collingham, near Newark (instituted 16 November 1498), but it was as rector of
*Northborow* (Northborough, Northants.), diocese of Lincoln, that he gained papal
dispensation to hold an additional benefice, or on resignation of Northborough to
hold any two other benefices (*CalPapalL*, 1492–1498, no. 820). He became archdeacon of the East Riding in June 1504 and held several other benefices, including
the sacristy of the archbishop's chapel of Holy Sepulchre. Magnus was a member of
the privy council, and was constantly employed on matters of state during the reign
of Henry VIII, particularly on diplomatic missions to Scotland. Thomas Magnus,
clerk, was granted custody of the hospital of St Leonard, in place of Thomas Wynter,
clerk, on 11 December 1529 (*LPFD*, IV, 2717, 2719). He held the mastership for
almost exactly ten years, before surrendering it to the Crown on 1 December 1539
(*LPFD*, 1539, XIV (2), no. 623). In lieu of the mastership Magnus received an annuity,
a dwelling house, the grange of Beningbrough in Yorkshire, and other grants in satisfaction of his pension of £100 (*VCH Yorks*, III, 343). He died in August 1550 and was
buried at Sessay.

---

[52] The date is deduced from a chantry certificate, apparently drawn up in 1549, which states his age to
be 86 (*Yorks. Chantry Certs*, II, 428).

# Appendix II:
## The Early Stewards of Pontefract

*The Lords of the Honour*

The lands which later formed the honour of Pontefract were held in 1086 by Ilbert de Lacy.[1] Ilbert was succeeded by Robert, his son, in the reign of William II (*EYC*, III, nos 1416–17). At a date between 1109 and 1115[2] Robert de Lacy suffered forfeiture and exile for an unrecorded misdemeanour. The honour of Pontefract then passed to Hugh de Laval (*EYC*, III, 148). Laval was dead in 1130, when William Maltravers owed 1000*m.* for his land, and £100 for his wife (*EYC*, III, 183, citing *PR*, 31 Hen. I, p. 34). Maltravers was killed in 1136 by Pain, a knight of the honour of Pontefract, and Stephen regranted the honours of Pontefract and Clitheroe (also known as the honour of Blackburnshire) to Ilbert de Lacy II, son of the banished Robert (*EYC*, III, 183, 185). Ilbert de Lacy died between February 1141 and June 1143, when his widow Alice was remarried to Roger de Mowbray (*EYC*, III, 185; *Mowbray Charters*, pp. xxviii n, 138). Ilbert was succeeded by his brother Henry de Lacy, who confirmed to Selby the gift made by Ilbert his grandfather, Robert his father, and Ilbert his brother (*EYC*, III, no. 1506). Henry de Lacy left England on crusade in about May 1177 and is said to have died in the Holy Land on 25 September of that year. His heir was his son Robert. Robert de Lacy died on 21 August 1193 and was buried in Kirkstall Abbey. Robert's heir was Aubrey de Lisours, his cousin, who on 21 April 1194 settled the whole estate 'which had been Robert de Lacy's' on her grandson Roger the Constable [of Chester], who assumed the name of Lacy. In that year Roger accounted for scutage of his honour of Pontefract, and in 1195 fined for the king's confirmation, and had livery of Robert de Lacy's possessions, excluding the castle of Pontefract. Roger de Lacy died on 1 October 1211, but his son and heir John de Lacy did not obtain seisin of his lands until the end of July 1213 when he agreed the fine for his inheritance. In 1232 John was created earl of Lincoln, by right of his wife. He died on 22 July 1240. John de Lacy's son and heir Edmund was underage, and was still underage on 26 May 1249, though he appears to have had seisin of his lands in about May 1248, probably as a result of his marriage. Edmund died on 2 June 1258, when his son Henry was seven years old. Edmund's widow Alice purchased her son's wardship for £3,755. Henry was contracted to marry Margaret, coheir of Sir William Lungespee, and on 1 June 1268, still underage, Henry did homage with her and had livery of her inheritance. From 1272 Henry was active in the king's service. He lived until 5 February 1311, his heir being his daughter Alice, who died without issue on 2 October 1348 (*VCH Lancs*, I, 300–11, 318–19; *CP*, VII, 676–88).

---

[1]  For the Lacy family, see *VCH Lancs*, I, 282, 300–19; *EYC*, III, 148, 185, 199; *CP*, VII, 676–88; Sanders, *English Baronies*, p. 138.

[2]  He had been dispossessed by the time of the Lindsey survey, which has now been dated to 1115 (T. Foulds, 'The Lindsey Survey and an unknown precept of Henry I', *Bulletin of the Institute of Historical Research*, LIX (1986), 212–15).

## The Lacy Stewards

Several deeds referred to in the Family Notes have been dated by the attestation of one of the stewards of the Lacy honour of Pontefract. Richard Holmes included a list of stewards and their dates in his edition of the Pontefract cartulary (*Ctl. Pontefract*, I, 316).[3] Though it has long been known that Holmes' list is unreliable,[4] a revised list has not hitherto been attempted. The evidence for twelfth- and thirteenth-century Lacy stewards is limited, and so it is difficult to establish their roles and chronology. Further research into the chronology of families holding of Lacy will doubtless enable the present list to be improved. The analysis depends on the assumption that the stewards held office continuously for a period of years, and were not chosen afresh each year.[5]

There is no twelfth-century evidence to show that there were then separate stewards for the honours of Blackburnshire and Pontefract. Waleys occurs as steward in both Blackburnshire and Pontefract during the tenure of Roger de Lacy, and may have been steward in both places concurrently. A deed of Roger de Lacy granting the church of Rochdale to Stanlow Abbey, witnessed by *Roberto Wallensi tunc senescallo, Willelmo de Lungvillers tunc senescallo hospitii mei* (*Ctl. Whalley*, p. 137), shows there was also a household steward. During the time of Roger de Lacy we find Adam of Dutton and Hugh of Dutton attesting Blackburnshire but not Pontefract deeds as steward (*Ctl. Whalley*, p. 22; *Ctl. Kirkstall*, p. 194n), suggesting that each honour had its own steward. Waleys' attestation as 'steward of Pontefract' in 1205 × 1209 is possibly a further indication. His successor as steward of Pontefract, Robert of Kent, may have been steward in Blackburnshire as well. Gilbert of Notton attested both Pontefract and Blackburnshire deeds as steward, as did Henry Waleys. But Waleys appears to have held the stewardship of Pontefract before that of Blackburnshire, and it is possible that Notton too held the stewardships at separate times. Both Hugh of Dutton and Geoffrey of Dutton attested Blackburnshire deeds as steward in 1213 × 1232 (*Ctl. Whalley*, pp. 73, 138, 279, 806, 1075); G[eoffrey] of Dutton was addressed as steward by John de Lacy, constable of Chester, in a deed concerning [Lower] Acreland [in Sawley, in the honour of Blackburnshire] given at Pontefract in November 1223 (*Ctl. Sallay*, no. 207), and we know that Robert of Kent was steward of Pontefract at Michaelmas of that year. Further evidence for the separate stewardships in *c.*1230 is provided by a Pontefract deed witnessed by *domino I[ohanne] de Lasci constabulario Cestrie, dominis Hugone Butel' et Gaufrido de Dutton senescallis ipsius domini I.* (*Ctl. Pontefract*, no. 282). The Dutton stewards do not otherwise occur in Pontefract deeds, and Butler does not attest Blackburnshire deeds. Later in the century Nicholas de Burton occurs as steward of Blackburnshire, and on another occasion as steward of Pontefract. Peter de Santon does likewise. The chronology is not sufficiently clear for us to say whether either of them held both stewardships concurrently.[6]

---

3   A list of stewards and constables of Pontefract 'extracted from the coucher book of the abbey [sic] of Pontefract' was printed in 1827 (Fox, *Pontefract*, pp. 64–69).

4   On Holmes' belief that there were two stewards named Hugh Butler, Baildon states 'Holmes gives no reason for the distinction . . . and I doubt its accuracy'; and later says '[some of] these alleged dates . . . seem very arbitrary' (Baildon, 'Saville and Butler', pp. 70–71). Clay commented that 'these dates and the order of these holders of the stewardship must, however, be regarded as subject to modification' (Clay, 'Wridlesford', p. 243).

5   This was certainly the case in the fifteenth century, when grants of the stewardship were frequently made for life (Somerville, *Lancaster*, I, 513–23).

6   A list of the Blackburnshire stewards is at Whitaker, *Whalley*, I, 268–69, but is not of great value for the period before 1274.

*List of Stewards*

There are notes on the stewards of Blackburnshire and the officers of the honour of Pontefract from the late thirteenth century onwards in Somerville, *Lancaster*, I, 347, 350–51, 355, 362–63, 372–73, 378, 500, 513–523. J.R. Maddicott, *Thomas of Lancaster 1307–1322: a study in the reign of Edward II* (Oxford, 1970), p. 340, adds a few stewards and constables of Pontefract to Somerville's lists.

## HERBERT (STEWARD TO HUGH DE LAVAL)

Hugh de Laval's grant of churches to Nostell Priory, dated 1119 × 1129 by Farrer, is witnessed by Thurstan archbishop, Herbert *dapifero meo*, Richard Guiz and another. Farrer postulated that the steward was Herbert de Morville, noting that Morville and Richard de Guiz are named in the pipe roll of 1130 immediately after the entry by which Laval's lands were assigned to Maltravers after Laval's death (*EYC*, III, no. 1488; *PR*, 31 Hen. I, p. 34).

## RALPH SON OF NICHOLAS (STEWARD TO HENRY DE LACY)

Adam son of Swain's notification of his gift of the church of Lund (later Monk Bretton Priory) to Pontefract Priory, dating from 1154 × c.1156,[7] is witnessed by Osbert the archdeacon, Ralph *dapifer* and others (*Ctl. Pontefract*, no. 380; *EYC*, III, no. 1669). A deed of Henry de Lacy, dated to 1155 by Farrer without explanation, was attested by Ralph son of Nicholas, *dapifero suo* (*EYC*, III, no. 1769). Ralph son of Nicholas held 1 k.f. of Lacy in 1166 (*EYC*, III, no. 1508). Not described as steward, he followed Osbert the archdeacon in the witness list to a deed of Robert de Lacy made in 1177 or later (*EYC*, III, no. 1509). He gave land in Bradley (Huddersfield) to Fountains and was succeeded by his son Adam of Cridling during the last quarter of the twelfth century (*EYC*, III, no. 1762 and n).

## OSBERT OF BAYEUX THE ARCHDEACON (STEWARD TO HENRY AND ROBERT DE LACY)

Apart from the dubious act of Archbishop Thurstan to Durham Priory, apparently dating from c.1121 × 1128 (*EYC*, II, no. 936; *EEA*, v, no. 43), Osbert the archdeacon first attests in 1135 × 1139 (*EYC*, I, no. 62; *EEA*, v, no. 44). In 1139 × 1140 Archbishop Thurstan surrendered the mill belonging to the prebend of St Peter [York], which prebend Osbert the archdeacon, his *nepos*, was holding (*EYC*, I, no. 154; *EEA*, v, no. 81). After the death of Archbishop William in June 1154, Osbert was accused of causing his death by poison. Osbert denied the accusations, but he was eventually ousted from his archdeaconry. His expulsion is normally assigned to c.1157. This date is suggested by a letter from Archbishop Theobald to Pope Adrian IV, believed to have been written towards the end of 1156, stating that Osbert would appear before him on the octave of Epiphany following; and by the first attestations of Bartholomew archdeacon, said to be Osbert's successor, which apparently date from c.1157 × c.1158 (Clay, 'Archdeacons', pp. 278, 409–10; *EEA*, v, 127; John of Salisbury, *Letters*, I, 26–28, 42–43, 258–62; *FEA*, vi, 47; Norton, *St William*, pp. 144–46). But the evidence for the succession of prelates to the five archdeaconries of York in the mid-twelfth century is rather tenuous, so the date cannot be regarded as entirely secure. The archdeaconry continued in dispute for several more years. Osbert appeared in person before Adrian IV's successor, Alexander III, claiming that he had obtained a letter from Adrian stating that he had

---

[7]  Archbishop Roger's confirmation of the gift, made at Adam son of Swain's request, has similar witnesses, including Osbert the archdeacon, suggesting the same occasion (*EYC*, III, no. 1670; *EEA*, xx, no. 72). Adam son of Swain was dead in 1159 (*EYC*, III, 319).

performed his purgation, and granting him immunity from trial by the archbishop or anyone else, except in the presence of the pope or his legate. Nevertheless Archbishop Roger had deprived him of the archdeaconry and confiscated the letter. Further, the archbishop promised Osbert's unnamed son an annuity of 30*m.* until he could be provided with a prebend of the same value, but had stopped paying the money and done nothing about the prebend. The archbishop's messengers countered that Osbert had resigned his archdeaconry voluntarily. The pope's letter asked the abbots of Ford, Evesham and St Albans to investigate the matter, and if Osbert's allegations were true, to admonish the archbishop and see to it that the archdeacon recovered his letter and the archdeaconry (Caenegem, *English Lawsuits*, pp. 574–76). The date of the pope's letter cannot be earlier than 1164, for Archbishop Roger is described as legate, and the latest date is 1181, when both Roger and Alexander were dead. Morey suggests a date of *c.*1175 × *c.*1180, noting that the pope uses the uncommon phrase *apud nos vel apud successorem nostrum*, indicating a date late in his career (Morey, 'Canonist Evidence', p. 352). The final judgment is unknown.

Whatever the formal situation may have been, it is clear that Osbert did not remain an active member of the York chapter for long after the consecration of Archbishop Roger on 10 October 1154. His only appearance in chapter in the time of Archbishop Roger is as witness to a confirmation by the dean and chapter to Fountains of lands specified *in carta domini nostri Rogeri Eborac' archiepiscopi*. This is also the only appearance of Ralph, bishop of Orkney, after the death of Archbishop William, so an early date is likely (*Ctl. Fountains*, p. 708; *EEA*, xx, no. 20; Carpenter, 'Paulinus', p. 12 and n). Osbert the archdeacon is first witness to Archbishop Roger's confirmation to Whitby, addressed to the dean and chapter, taking precedence over a York canon and the archbishop's steward (*EYC*, ii, no. 880; *EEA*, xx, no. 105). Walter of Huggate's gift to Watton is witnessed by Roger, archbishop of York, John treasurer, Osbert the archdeacon, Simon canon of Beverley and others named (*EYC*, i, no. 158).

Osbert the archdeacon is frequently found as a witness to deeds belonging to the Lacy fee during the archiepiscopate of Roger. In some of the earliest, like the archbishop's confirmation of Adam son of Swain's gift of Lund to Pontefract, he maintains some archidiaconal gravitas (*EYC*, iii, no. 1670; *EEA*, xx, no. 72); but in later years, though still described as archdeacon, he witnesses without senior ecclesiastical companions, in less important transactions, and it seems his archidiaconal power has ebbed away (e.g. *EYC*, iii, nos 1500, 1623). By 1166 Osbert the archdeacon had been enfeoffed with ½ k.f. by Henry de Lacy (*EYC*, iii, no. 1508). The land lay in Middle Haddlesey, and probably in Bradley (Huddersfield).[8] After a period Osbert was no longer usually described as archdeacon, and in his own deeds he calls himself Osbert of Bayeux.

Osbert is named but once as steward to Henry de Lacy, and that appearance has previously been misinterpreted. The witnesses to Jordan Foliot's grant to Pontefract, given in 1166 × 1177,[9] include Henry de Lacy, and *Ottone de Tilli, Osberto archidiac' tunc dapifero Hug' de Tilli*. The cartulist has omitted his usual point between witnesses, so Holmes expanded Hugh in the genitive (Pontefract cartulary, f. 33/26ʳ; *Ctl. Pontefract*, no. 89; *EYC*, iii, no. 1527). But Hugh de Tilly, possibly the younger brother of Otes de Tilly, and the rector of Rotherham (FN), was not a man of such substance as to

---

[8]  See below. I have not seen 'Farrer, MS. Notebook 21', apparently Wightman's source for his assertion that the Lacy lands of Osbert the archdeacon lay 'in Manningham, Idle, Frizinghall and Haworth' (Wightman, *Lacy Family*, p. 102), nor any other supporting evidence for this statement.

[9]  Also attested by Roger Peitevin, so definitely after 1166 and possibly after 1173, when his father Robert apparently still held the fee (FN), and before the death of Henry de Lacy.

require a steward of the status of Osbert the archdeacon, who elsewhere precedes Hugh de Tilly, and sometimes Otes de Tilly, in attestations (*EYC*, III, nos 1529, 1624). Osbert was steward to Henry de Lacy, not Hugh de Tilly.

Osbert also served as steward during the tenure of Robert de Lacy, apparently after an interval during which Adam de Reineville held the stewardship. Osbert, steward of Robert de Lacy, witnessed a deed of Robert son of Alan de Torp in 1178 × 1189[10] (*EYC*, III, no. 1744). *Hosb[ertus] tunc dapifer* witnessed a quitclaim by Roger of Roall to Robert de Lacy and the monks of Pontefract (*EYC*, III, no. 1624). Osbert the archdeacon appears as first witness to a deed of Robert de Lacy to Kirkstall. Osbert of Bayeux was the first witness to an agreement made in the county court in York in summer 1184. Important tenants of the Lacy fee followed in the witness lists to both these deeds, and it is possible that Osbert owed his precedence to the steward-ship, though he is not so described (*Ctl. Pontefract*, no. 311; *EYC*, III, nos 1509, 1779). Before 1188,[11] as Osbert of Bayeux, he gave 1 bv. in Middle Haddlesey to Pontefract, whilst Adam de Reineville was steward (*EYC*, III, no. 1718). The gift by Osbert of Bayeux of ½ ct. in Bradley and common pasture for sixty cows and sixty horses was confirmed to Gisborough Priory by Henry II in 1175 × 1189[12] (*EYC*, II, no. 673). This was identified by Brown, followed by Clay, as Bradley near Grimsby, apparently because Hugh of Bayeux gave Gisborough the church of Kelstern, some 10 m. to the south (*Ctl. Gisborough*, I, 17, 247n; *EYC*, index to I–III). But the tenure of land in Bradley, Huddersfield, by Ralph son of Nicholas, Osbert's predecessor as steward, suggests this was the place, as does Prior Roald of Gisborough's attestation to Adam son of Ralph son of Nicholas's deeds concerning Bradley (Huddersfield) in 1194 × 1198[13] (*Ctl. Fountains*, pp. 122, 127).[14]

As well as his Lacy holdings, in 1166 Osbert the archdeacon held 11 ct., where 14 ct. made a fee, of the honour of Skipton (*EYC*, VII, no. 47). Clay established that the land lay in Airton and Calton, par. Kirkby Malham, and Elslack, par. Broughton, and later passed to the family of Staveley and thence to FitzHugh of Ravensworth (*EYC*, VII, 216–17). Osbert the archdeacon witnessed several deeds of Alice de Rumilly and her husband William son of Duncan, lords of the honour of Skipton, given in some cases shortly before, and in others shortly after, the accession of Archbishop Roger (*EYC*, VII, nos 13, 14, 17, 18). In the 1170s and 1180s he witnessed, as Osbert of Bayeux, deeds of Alice de Rumilly and her tenant Walter Fleming (*EYC*, VII, nos 28, 29, 87).

Osbert also held of Paynel. In or before 1188,[15] Osbert of Bayeux confirmed to Drax Priory 1 ct. in Bingley, which William Paynel, his *antecessor*, had given to the canons (*CalCh*, 1300–1326, pp. 175–76; *EYC*, VI, no. 68). Land in Bingley, given by Osbert the archdeacon, was confirmed to the hospital of St Peter, York, by Pope Lucius III in 1183 (C166 [*EYC*, I, no. 199]). As this gift is not mentioned in previous papal confirmations, it was probably made in or after 1178. The extent of the lands of the Templars of 1185 includes an assart given by Osbert the archdeacon, then held by Alice of Bingley for 2s. annually (*EYC*, VI, no. 68n; *MA*, VI, 831a). Osbert of Bayeux gave a toft in Bingley to the Hospitallers (*EYC*, VI, no. 69). He was almost certainly dead in 1191, when William of Bayeux, son of Osbert the archdeacon, owed £15 in

---

[10]  Whilst Hamo was precentor of York and Rainer [of Waxham] was undersheriff of Yorkshire.

[11]  The witness Mauger de Stiveton was dead in that year (FN: Stiveton of Steeton in South Milford).

[12]  Between the consecration of John, bishop of Norwich and the king's death.

[13]  Witnessed by Roger Bavent as sheriff of Yorkshire.

[14]  There is no other mention of Bradley in *Ctl. Gisborough*, nor in the sixteenth-century accounts for Gisborough at *Valor Ecclesiasticus*, v, 80–81 and *Dissolved Houses*, no. 681.

[15]  Witnessed by Mauger de Stiveton.

a schedule of debts due to Aaron the Jew, by pledge of Gerard, canon of York (*EYC*, VI, 159; *PR*, 3&4 Ric. I, p. 23). At Michaelmas 1194 the debt remained unpaid and the pledges were said to be Gerard, canon of York, Osbert, clerk of Sherburn, and Robert, chaplain of *Burc* (*PR*, 6 Ric. I, p. 157).[16] The debt disappears from the roll the following year.

### WILLIAM VAVASOUR (STEWARD TO HENRY DE LACY)
A deed of Henry de Lacy confirming the church of Blackburn to Henry clerk of Blackburn is witnessed by William Vavasour, *dapifero nostro* (*Ctl. Whalley*, pp. 75–76). William Vavasour held a third of a fee of Lacy in 1166 (*EYC*, III, no. 1508).

### ADAM DE REINEVILLE (STEWARD TO HENRY AND ROBERT DE LACY)
Adam de Reineville, steward, witnessed a deed of Henry de Lacy, when Henry was departing for Jerusalem, at Easter, probably in 1177 (*EYC*, III, no. 1629). Thus it seems Adam succeeded Osbert as steward to Henry de Lacy. A deed of Gilbert de Lacy to Pontefract is witnessed by Robert de Lacy, Adam de Reineville then steward, and others, indicating Reineville was also steward after the succession of Robert de Lacy (*EYC*, III, no. 1786; *Ctl. Pontefract*, no. 5). Adam de Reineville, *dapifer*, witnessed Osbert of Bayeux's gift to Pontefract made in or before 1188[17] (*EYC*, III, no. 1718).

### IVO OR EUDO DE LONGVILLERS (STEWARD TO ROBERT DE LACY)
Ivo, steward of Sir Robert de Lacy, attested a deed of Thomas Campion (*EYC*, III, no. 1640; *Ctl. Pontefract*, no. 297). Eudo de Longvillers, steward, attested an undated deed given before the wapentake court at Clitheroe (*Ctl. Pontefract*, no. 240). He attested similarly a deed of Hugh, prior of Pontefract, witnessed by Adam son of Peter [of Birkin], who died in 1190 × 1194, and John his son (*Ctl. Pontefract*, no. 486; FN: Birkin). It is not at the moment possible to assign accurate dates to any of these appearances. Some details of Eudo's career are given at Clay, 'Longvillers', pp. 43–44.

### SAMSON OF WOODLESFORD (STEWARD TO ROBERT DE LACY)
Samson of Woodlesford (*Wridlesford*) attested two deeds of Robert de Lacy as steward, neither of which can be precisely dated (*EYC*, III, nos 1521, 1818; *Ctl. Pontefract*, no. 9). He was the leading witness to two other deeds of Robert de Lacy, without description, but probably owed his precedence to the stewardship (*Ctl. Fountains*, p. 138; *Ctl. Kirkstall*, p. 197). He attested early in 1199, not as steward (*EYC*, III, no. 1755), and was witness to a fine of September 1201, when Robert Waleys was steward (*EYC*, III, no. 1526). Before 1202 he made a grant of 13 a. in Fixby (*YD*, IV, no. 187). He was mentioned as holder of an abutment in Morley in 1202 (*PF John*, p. 33). Further references to him were collected by Clay, but these are not extensive, and do not identify his parentage or heir (Clay, 'Wridlesford', pp. 251–52). As he does not appear

---

16 The pledges may also have been sons of Osbert the archdeacon. Gerard canon [of York], son of Osbert, witnessed a deed dated 1155 × 1165 by Farrer but possibly earlier (*EYC*, III, no. 1776; for the date, see Carpenter, 'Paulinus', p. 14 and n). Another son witnessed a Baldersby deed in 'c.1160 × c.1180' as Thurstan of Bayeux, son of Osbert the archdeacon (*EYC*, XI, no. 280). In 1194, the sheriff accounted for 42s. 8d. for half a year's rent for Bingley 'of Osbert of Bayeux' (*PR*, 6 Ric. I, pp. 12–13). This was presumably after the death of Robert son of Robert son of Harding in the year to Michaelmas 1194, and the resulting escheat of the Paynel estates during the wardship of Maurice de Gant, his son, who was still under age in 1200, but was holding Bingley in 1212. The rent does not appear in subsequent rolls as the wardship was sold to William de Ste-Mère-Église (*EYC*, VI, 34–35, 156). The high level of the rent indicates that Osbert's lands had also escheated, presumably on the death of his son William.
17 See n. 11 above.

in the time of Henry de Lacy, and occurs during Robert de Lacy's tenure only as
steward, or as leading witness, it is likely he held the stewardship towards the end of
Robert de Lacy's tenure.

### ROBERT WALEYS (STEWARD TO ROGER DE LACY)

Robert Waleys[18] served Roger de Lacy as under-sheriff whilst Roger was sheriff of
Yorkshire in 1204–1209. He also served as steward, possibly for the entire period of
Roger's tenure which ran from 1193 to 1211. He witnessed frequently as steward
(*Ctl. Pontefract*, nos 174, 176, 212, 458), and also as [under-]sheriff, though doubt-
less acting in his capacity as steward (*Ctl. Pontefract*, nos 177, 181, 194, 211, 316, 431).
Final concords were made before Robert Waleys, steward, and others, in the court of
Roger de Lacy at Pontefract, in September 1201 and May 1206 (*EYC*, III, no. 1526;
R468). He was steward of the same court in March 1209 (*EYC*, III, no. 1695n; *Ctl.
Fountains*, pp. 357–58). He attested a gift to Byland by Roger de Lacy, constable of
Chester, as his steward (*EYC*, III, no. 1525). On one occasion he attested as 'Robert
Waleys [under-]sheriff of Yorkshire and steward of Pontefract' (*Ctl. Pontefract*, no. 175).
Robert Waleys was named as *dapifer* in a final concord made in the Lacy court of
Clitheroe in 1195–96 (*EYC*, III, no. 1524), and attested Roger de Lacy's grant of the
church of Rochdale to Stanlow Abbey as steward (*Ctl. Whalley*, p. 137).[19] This suggests
that he also held the stewardship of Blackburnshire, possibly concurrently with that
of Pontefract.[20] After Roger de Lacy's death Waleys proffered 1000*m.* not to have to
render account for the period when he was Roger's steward (*PR*, 13 John, p. 33).

### ROBERT OF KENT (1213 ? TO 1223 × 1225)

Robert of Kent attested many deeds in the Pontefract cartulary as steward, often with
John of Birkin. As steward, he attested a deed of John de Lacy, constable of Chester,
given at Damietta (Egypt), during the fifth crusade (*Ctl. Pontefract*, no. 21). Holmes
dated the deed to 1218, in which year the city was besieged, but it may have been
issued in 1219 or early 1220 (*ODNB*, s.n. John de Lacy and Ranulf [III], sixth earl of
Chester). There is no evidence that Robert of Kent was steward to Roger de Lacy,
John de Lacy's father, or that he had a predecessor as steward to John de Lacy. He
attested as steward of Pontefract at Michaelmas 1223 (*Ctl. Pontefract*, no. 250). It is
tolerably certain that he was steward before Gilbert of Notton.[21] *Roberto de Chenet,
tunc senescallo Iohannis de Laci*, who attested a deed with John and Roger of Birkin,
was doubtless the same man (*EYC*, III, no. 1636). Kent may also have served as steward
of Blackburnshire, for he witnessed as steward a deed of John de Lacy, constable of
Chester, granting to Salley ½*m.* annually to be paid at Clitheroe (*Ctl. Sallay*, no. 210).

### GILBERT OF NOTTON (1223 × 1225 TO 1223 × 1227)

Gilbert of Notton, 'steward of John de Lacy', attested a deed of Adam the chaplain,

---

18  For the Waleys family, which provided two other stewards during the thirteenth century, see FN:
    Ste-Marie.
19  The deed is also witnessed by *Willelmo de Lunguillers tunc senescallo hospitii mei.*
20  Waleys was not the only steward of Blackburnshire during Roger de Lacy's tenure, for Hugh of Dutton,
    steward, attested a confirmation by Roger to Stanlow (*Ctl. Whalley*, p. 22).
21  See below. We are here discounting the somewhat remote possibility that Adam the chaplain's deed,
    attested by Gilbert of Notton as steward, was issued in 1219, and immediately preceeded a change of
    steward to Robert of Kent, who then dashed off to Damietta before the withdrawal of English forces in
    1220. Gilbert of Notton, not described as steward, was the leading witness to a Bradley (Huddersfield)
    deed at Whitsuntide 1219 (*Ctl. Fountains*, p. 128), and may perhaps as served as steward of Pontefract
    in the absence of Lacy and Kent on crusade.

son of Richard son of Lesing of Ledston, with John of Birkin, Hugh of Toulston, John of Heck, Adam son of Thomas de Reineville and others (*Ctl. Pontefract*, no. 190). Hugh of Toulston was probably dead in October 1226, and John of Birkin was certainly dead in October 1227. John of Heck succeeded his father Ilard between Easter 1219 and October 1226 (FNs). Adam son of Thomas de Reineville succeeded his grandfather Adam de Reineville after December 1218 (*EYF*, p. 74; *YF*, 1218–1231, pp. 9–10). Thus it is reasonably safe to assign this deed to 1219 × 1226. Gilbert of Notton, steward, attested two other deeds with Birkin, Toulston, and Heck (MS Dods. 133, ff. 124$^v$, 126$^r$). It follows that Gilbert of Notton was steward after Robert of Kent and before Henry Waleys. As steward, Gilbert of Notton attested a deed of Simon Butler, and also attested with him (*Ctl. Pontefract*, nos 98, 130, 476). If, as is likely, this was the Simon Butler whose widow Mathania quitclaimed any right in dower in lands Simon had given to William of Campsall and Pontefract Priory in 1224[/25] (*Ctl. Pontefract*, no. 115), then Notton had become steward before Lady Day 1225. Notton also served as steward of Blackburnshire. He witnessed several deeds in the Whalley cartulary as steward, including two of John de Lacy, constable of Chester (*Ctl. Whalley*, pp. 32, 420 and passim).

## Henry Waleys (1223 × 1227 to 1226 × 1230)

Henry Waleys, as steward, witnessed a deed of Gilbert son of Hugh son of Ailburn of Pontefract, by which Gilbert surrendered all right in an assart in Preston to Pontefract. In return the monks gave him a grazing place nearby, and 3*m*. The deed by which Prior S[tephen] and the convent confirmed the grazing place follows in the cartulary. The attestation is truncated after three witnesses with the word 'etc.'. These witnesses are the three leading witnesses to Gilbert's surrender, except that Henry Waleys is not described as steward. As Holmes pointed out, it is very likely that the cartularist has omitted the witnesses because they were the same as those to the preceeding deed (*Ctl. Pontefract*, nos 160–61). It is therefore safe to assign the two deeds to the same date. It follows that Henry Waleys was steward at some point during the rule of Prior Stephen, i.e. between November 1226 and February 1238.[22] Henry Waleys attested as steward of Pontefract with John of Birkin (*Ctl. Pontefract*, no. 252), who was dead in 1227 (FN). Thus Waleys was steward after Gilbert of Notton, and before Hugh Butler, who was steward in 1230 as is shown below. It appears that Waleys was subsequently steward of Blackburnshire, as he witnessed as steward the deed of John de Lacy, earl of Lincoln and constable of Chester, confirming to Stanlow the church of Eccles, which must have been issued in 1232 × 1234[23] (*Ctl. Whalley*, pp. 36, 64).

## Hugh Butler (1226 × 1230 to 1232 × 1238)[24]

Unlike his predecessors, Hugh Butler (*Pincerna*)[25] does not occur as steward with John of Birkin, who died in 1227 or shortly before (FN), but so attested with Eudo de Longvillers, who died in 1229–30 (*Ctl. Pontefract*, no. 165; Clay, 'Longvillers',

---

22  Stephen's predecessor Hugh was party to a fine in November 1226; Stephen was named as prior in January and December 1235; his successor Peter occurs on 13 February 1238 (Clay, 'Priors of Pontefract', pp. 462–63).

23  After Lacy became earl of Lincoln, and before the confirmation by Alexander, bishop of Coventry and Lichfield (*Ctl. Whalley*, pp. 37–38).

24  Holmes' supposition that Hugh Butler also served early in the tenure of John de Lacy appears to be based on a deed of Adam son of Roger of Crosland made to Pontefract, 'for the health of my soul and of my lords Henry, Robert, and Roger de Lacy', witnessed by Hugh Butler, steward of Sir John, constable of Chester, which he dated 'circa 1212' (*Ctl. Pontefract*, no. 456).

25  For Hugh Butler and his family see Baildon, 'Saville and Butler', esp. pp. 68–75.

pp. 44–45). He may have served as steward to the dowager Maud de Lacy, widow of Roger de Lacy, before becoming steward to her son John de Lacy.[26] Butler attested as steward [of Pontefract] after Michaelmas 1226, during the widowhood of Alice Haget, formerly wife of Jordan de Ste-Marie (*Ctl. Pontefract*, no. 306; FN: Ste-Marie). Hugh Butler, and Geoffrey of Dutton,[27] stewards, attested together with John de Lacy, constable of Chester, i.e. in or before 1232 (*Ctl. Pontefract* no. 282). Butler attested as 'steward of the earl of Lincoln' (Burton transcripts 1, f. 113ʳ, p. 173, B20 N41); and attested a deed of John de Lacy, earl of Lincoln and constable of Chester, as steward (MS Dods. 133, f. 129ʳ, cited 'Dodsworth's Yorkshire Notes', *YAJ*, VI, 449), so was also steward in 1232 or later. There can be little doubt that Hugh of Armthorpe, steward of Pontefract, who witnessed Henry of Shelley's gift of land in Cudworth to Roche made before August 1242[28] (*YD*, I, no. 156), was the same man, as the Butler family held in Armthorpe in the reign of John (*SY*, I, 87).

## ALAN THE CLERK (1232 ? × 1238 TO 1232 × 1238)

Alan the clerk, then steward, and Peter the receiver witnessed a deed of sale by William son of Robert Mey of Marsden to Pontefract Priory of 1 bv. in Marsden (Lancs.), which he and his father held of William de Vescy, for 2*m*. 3*s*. (*Ctl. Pontefract*, no. 283). The monks paid ½*m*. for a quitclaim by Maud, widow of Robert Mey, in her dower in the same land. Her deed is attested by Alan the clerk, steward, and five other witnesses, all of whom also attest William son of Robert Mey's deed (*Ctl. Pontefract*, no. 283c). It is clear that the two deeds were given on the same occasion, after the death of Robert Mey. Robert Mey himself issued no fewer than four surrenders or quitclaims to the priory concerning the bovate. Three of these have similar witnesses, including Sir J[ohn] de Lacy, constable of Chester (indicating 1232 or before), Hugh Butler (indicating 1226 or later) and Geoffrey of Dutton, stewards of Sir J[ohn], and Walter the receiver (*Ctl. Pontefract*, nos 281–82, 283a, 283b). William de Vescy issued a quitclaim to the priory, with similar witnesses, including Sir John constable of Chester, Hugh Butler, Geoffrey of Dutton, and Peter the receiver (*Ctl. Pontefract*, no. 230). We can therefore be confident that Alan the clerk was steward after Hugh Butler.[29] Alan's appearance with Peter the receiver makes it reasonably clear that he

---

[26] A deed of Roger of Thornton giving land in Allerton, near Bradford, to Robert son of Robert Smith was attested by 'Hugh, steward of the lady of Bradford' as last witness. By a later deed, issued in 1238 or not long before, with first witness 'Hugh Butler then steward', Roger quitclaimed the same land to Pontefract Priory (*Ctl. Pontefract*, nos 303–04; for the date, see FN: Scot of Calverley). Holmes postulated that the 'lady of Bradford' was the mother of the lord of Pontefract, holding the manor of Bradford as part of her dower. However, Holmes has misdated Thornton's second deed, and so identified the 'lady of Bradford' as Margaret, widow of John de Lacy, earl of Lincoln, rather than Maud, widow of Roger de Lacy. The latter occurs in 1212, 1219, and 1226 × 1228 and held several manors in Lincolnshire in dower 'besides the demesne of the barony of her son' (*VCH Lancs*, I, 304; *Bk of Fees*, pp. 163, 249, 285, 360, 362). There is evidence that Bradford, a demesne manor of the honour of Pontefract, was held in dower by a Lacy widow in 1316 (*WYAS*, p. 331; *Ctl. Pontefract*, no. 304n).

[27] See above. Dutton was steward of Blackburnshire.

[28] Also witnessed by Henry, rector of Rothwell. Henry the clerk of Nottingham, son of Henry physician (*medici*) of Nottingham, was instituted to Rothwell in 1191 × 1202, and occurs as rector in 1208 × 1237 ('Ctl. Nostell', nos 519–20, 1021 [ex pp. 166, 336]). William Blundell was instituted to Rothwell in August 1242 (*Reg. Gray*, p. 92).

[29] There are also two grants by William de Vescy to William son of Robert May of the 1 bv. in Marsden which his father held beforehand, at 3*s*. annually, for which grant William son of Robert had given Vescy 1*m. in gersuma*. The witnesses to these include Sir Henry Waleys, steward of the constable of Chester (*Ctl. Pontefract*, nos 283d, 283e). As it has been established that Henry Waleys was steward before Hugh Butler, it seems that Robert May surrendered the land in Marsden to Vescy, who regranted it to William, Robert's son. But Robert then surrendered it to the priory, ignoring the previous transactions.

was steward before Adam de Nairford.[30] Sir Alan the clerk, steward, attested several deeds in the Whalley cartulary, including examples before and after John de Lacy became earl of Lincoln in 1232, showing he held the stewardship of Blackburnshire, apparently before he became steward of Pontefract (*Ctl. Whalley*, pp. 288, 394, 398, 578, 750, 837–38, 870; *Ctl. Sallay*, no. 254).

## ADAM DE NAIRFORD (1232 × 1238 TO 1240 × 1246)

Adam de Nairford attested as steward of the earl of Lincoln in March 1237[/38] (*Ctl. Pontefract*, no. 126a) and June 1238 (ibid., no. 26), and as steward in May 1240 (ibid., no. 475). There is no evidence that he continued as steward after the death of John de Lacy. He also served as steward to the countess of Warenne at some time during the period 1240 to 1248[31] (*EYC*, VIII, 247), and was sheriff of York in 1246.

## WALTER OF LOWDHAM (1240 × 1246 TO 1247 × 1250)

Sir Walter of Lowdham (*Ludham*) attested as steward of Pontefract in May 1246, apparently before Edmund de Lacy had obtained seisin of his lands (*Ctl. Pontefract*, no. 200). He attested as steward with Sir Henry Waleys, who was dead in October 1251 (*Ctl. Pontefract*, no. 153; FN: Ste-Marie); and whilst Dalmatius was prior of Pontefract and Sir Robert de Eu was constable of Pontefract (*Ctl. Pontefract*, nos 135, 551). As steward, he attested a deed of Richard Waleys, which must have been made after the partition of the lands of Richard's grandmother Alice Haget, following the inquisition after her death, and so after February 1247 (*Ctl. Pontefract*, no. 291; FN: Ste-Marie). Ralph of Horbury, steward of John de Warenne, and Walter of Lowdham, steward of Edmund de Lacy, together witnessed a Fixby deed (Clay, 'Wridlesford', p. 251).

## JOHN OF HODROYD (1247 × 1250 TO 1258 × 1260)

John of Hodroyd (*Hoderode*) attested as steward, or steward of Pontefract, in November 1250 (*Ctl. Pontefract*, no. 480[B]), December 1250 (*YD*, III, no. 85), summer 1251 (*Ctl. Pontefract*, no. 553), September 1251 (*Ctl. Pontefract*, no. 554), 1252[/53] (MS Dods. 139, f. 57ᵛ), November 1253 (*Ctl. Pontefract*, no. 169), 1257[/58] ('Ctl. Nostell', no. 126 [ex f. 20ᵛ]), Easter 1258 (*MA*, v, 503, no. 7) and May 1258 (*Ctl. Pontefract*, no. 29). Clay gives some notes on his family at *YD*, IV, 164–65.

## HENRY WALEYS (1258 × 1260 TO 1264 × 1276)

Henry Waleys,[32] steward of Pontefract, witnessed a quitclaim made apparently in 1260 (A2A: DD/SR/A11/1).[33] An inquisition was held before Sir Henry Waleys, steward

Matters were only rectified some time after Robert's death, by the priory's payments to his widow and son.

30  Walter the receiver occurs with stewards Robert of Kent (*Ctl. Pontefract*, nos 125, 257, 258), Henry Waleys (ibid., no. 22), and Hugh Butler (ibid., nos 23, 118, 123, 225, 227, 282, 285, 452, 456). He witnessed with Roger de Stapelton, sheriff of York, implying 1236 × 1239 (*Ctl. Fountains*, p. 144). He attested a deed dated 1235 (ibid., no. 154), and was dead in January 1241, when the king granted to master Peter de Alpibus, the queen's doctor, the prebend in the chapel of St Clement in Pontefract castle, which had belonged to Walter, sometime receiver of J[ohn] earl of Lincoln (*CalPat*, 1232–1247, p. 243). Peter the receiver, who is not to be identified with Peter de Alpibus, seems to have overlapped with Walter, as he witnessed the deed of William de Vescy with Sir John, constable of Chester, made apparently in 1226 × 1232 (*Ctl. Pontefract*, no. 230). Robert the receiver occurs when Adam de Nairford was steward and John de Lacy was earl of Lincoln (ibid., nos 25, 202), and during the stewardship of Walter of Lowdham in the time of Prior Dalamatius (ibid., no. 551).

31  During her widowhood.

32  He was a younger son of Henry Waleys, steward of the 1220s (FN: Ste-Marie).

33  NottsA, Savile of Rufford papers.

of Pontefract, on 9 September 1264 (*YI*, I, 97). He was therefore steward when Alice de Lacy was holding the honour of Pontefract as guardian of her son. Robert de Ripairis, steward to Alice de Lacy, was given safe conduct in November 1265 (*CalPat*, 1258–1266, p. 503), but no evidence has been discovered to show he was steward of Pontefract.

NICHOLAS DE BURTON (DATES UNKNOWN, BETWEEN C.1250 AND 1280)
William of Ryther, John Vavasour, Ralph of Normanville, William Vavasour, then constable of Pontefract, knights, and Nicholas de Burton, steward of the same, witnessed a deed of Ralph of Ryther son of John *de Toftona*[34] giving land in Oglethorpe to Nostell Priory. The gift was included in the general confirmation of Edward I made in 1280 ('Ctl. Nostell', no. 622). The Vavasour witnesses make a date before *c.*1250 unlikely,[35] but it is not currently possible to determine where Burton should be placed. Nicholas de Burton also attests two deeds as steward of Blackburnshire, but these deeds too are difficult to date (*Ctl. Whalley*, pp. 956, 960).

PETER DE SANTON (? TO 1275 × 1276)
Peter de Santon was steward of Pontefract in 1275 (*CR Wakefield*, p. 104). He was also steward of Clitheroe, and so attested deeds, one of which was issued March 1274[36] (*Ctl. Whalley*, pp. 1077, 1112).

SIMON OF THORPE (1275 × 1276 TO 1278 × ?)
Simon of Thorpe, steward of Pontefract, attested a bond for 10*m*. to be paid at Easter 1276 (*Cat. Anc. Deeds*, III, A.5779). He witnessed as steward on 1 May and 29 June, 1278 (Fox, *Pontefract*, pp. 19–20; MS Dods. 155, f. 83ᵛ).[37]

*Other Stewards Connected with Pontefract*

Thomas was *dapifer* of the monks of Pontefract. He attested in 1154 × 1159 (*EYC*, III, nos 1321, 1669, 1670). He witnessed with his brother William in '1175 × 1185' (*EYC*, III, nos 1550, 1555), and with his son Michael (*EYC*, III, no. 1866). William *dapifer*, who witnesses Henry de Lacy's confirmation to St Peter's hospital (R121), does not otherwise occur in connection with the honour of Pontefract. He was perhaps associated with the archbishop.[38]

---

[34]  i.e. Towton ?
[35]  See pedigree at *EYC*, VII, 167.
[36]  Peter de Santon, steward, witnessed a grant of Adam son of Hugh to his brother Robert. Robert's subsequent grant of the land was witnessed by Gilbert de Clifton, steward. Clifton was steward in March 1274 (*Ctl. Whalley*, pp. 649, 1111–13; Somerville, *Lancaster*, I, 347).
[37]  He also attested *YD*, VI, no. 193, which shares several witnesses with MS Dods. 155 and was probably given on the same occasion.
[38]  William the steward is a witness to acta of Archbishops Thurstan, William, and Roger (*EYC*, I, nos 62, 105, 154, 161, 280; ibid., III, no. 1565).

# Index of Manuscripts

BROUGHTON HALL
MS Tempest                                    R809

JOHN RYLANDS UNIVERSITY LIBRARY, MANCHESTER
MS Latin 219 (Meaux chronicle)                R725

LEEDS DISTRICT ARCHIVES
MS Ingilby                                    R102, R702–R705

LICHFIELD RECORD OFFICE
Records of Lichfield Dean and Chapter         R901–R904

NORTHAMPTONSHIRE RECORD OFFICE
Fitzwilliam (Milton) Charters                 R600

YORKSHIRE ARCHAEOLOGICAL SOCIETY, LEEDS
MD59 (Middelton deeds)                        R357, R417–R423, R426, R668–
                                              R669, R742–R750, R752–R756,
                                              R800, R803–R804, R806–R808,
                                              R814
DD57 (Woolley Hall deeds)                     R728

YORK MINSTER LIBRARY
Reg. Mag. Alb.                                R769
MS Add. 271 (Walbran transcripts)             R785

# Index of Headnotes

Editorial notes have been included at the beginning of each topographical section of the cartulary. These give an overview of the tenure of the place and the hospital's interest there. They are referred to in the text by the abbreviation 'HN'. This index serves primarily to indicate where these notes may be found, but also includes references to each topographical section in 'Supplementary Documents'. Thus, in similar manner to the seventeenth-century Contents List (pp. 1–3), it provides a finding aid for deeds belonging to a particular location.

# Index of Family Notes

This index is designed to facilitate access to the main entry for a family or individual, which may be no more than a reference to another work. These entries are referred to in the text by the abbreviation 'FN'. Bold indicates that the family appears in a chart pedigree.

# Index of Persons and Places

Italic type is used for references when the name appears in a document text: the name may appear additionally in the editorial notes on the page indicated. Roman type is used if the name appears only in editorial notes. Italics are used to indicate references in the Lacy deed printed on p. 307 n. 10 and the Octon deeds printed on pp. 710–11 as well as the St Leonard's documents. No attempt has been made to indicate multiple occurrences of a name on the same page. 'Richard son of John' is normally indexed under 'Richard' and not 'John', although a few well known figures are indexed under e.g. FitzJohn, FitzStephen. The hospital is referred to as 'St Leonard's' to avoid confusion with York Minster, dedicated to St Peter. Field names are not usually indexed.

In many cases an attempt has been made to distinguish between different individuals of the same name, but these distinctions are rarely absolutely certain. The identification of different members of the hospital fraternity is an area of particular difficulty. There are several men who appear as 'William the chaplain', for example. It is likely that some of them appear elsewhere with a topographical description, e.g. 'William of Garendon'; or perhaps as 'William the clerk', 'William the deacon', 'Master William', 'brother William', 'brother-chaplain William'. The reader should therefore bear in mind that different men may appear under a single index entry, and that the same man may appear in several different entries. Those who wish to explore the challenges encountered in indexing charters accompanied by extensive editorial notes should read Charles Clay's introduction to his index to Farrer's volumes of *Early Yorkshire Charters* (*EYC*, index to I–III, Introduction).

Nicholas of, 721
Robert of, 721–2, *727*
Roger of, *268*
Ackton (nr Featherstone), Aiketona, Oketon,
    306–7, 309, 311–12, *464*
  family, 311
  John son of William, 312
  Peter of, *see* Toulston
  Reiner of, 308, 311–12, 335, *464*
  —, heirs of, 312
  William of, 312
  —, his son, 312
Aclum, *see* Acklam
Acomb, Acom(e), Acum(b), Akum, *1*, *4–8*, 73,
    *448*, *458*, *825*, *919*, *922*, *925*
  Acomb Gates in, Acum gatas, *452*
  Acomb Grange in, 4, *905*, *924*, *927*
  —, bailiff of, *see* Metham
  Acomb hag in, Akumhag, *445*, *447*, *820*
  Woodhall in, Wodehall, *919*
  Alan of, *173*, *353*, *456*
  Gilbert (son of Alan of), *447–9*, *457*
  Oliver of, *451*, *825*
  Ralph of, *264*
  Ralph of, chaplain of St Leonard's,
    *453*
  Thomas le franktenant of, *see* Franklin
  Thomas son of Richard of, *353*
  William of (of St Leonard's), *488*
Acre (Palestine), 110
Acreland, *see* Sallay
Acton, Actun, *see* Aughton
Acum, Acumb, *see* Acomb
Ad Fontem, *see* Atwell
Ad Gotam, *see* German
Ad Pontem, *see* Attebrigg
Adala, *see* Adel
Adam, *229*, *321*, *815*, *893*
  abbot of Kirkstall, 201, 469
  abbot of Meaux, 711–12, 719, 742, 744,
    752, 931
  abbot of Welbeck, 77
  archdeacon of York, *see* Thorner
  brother of St Leonard's, *460*, *797*
  chaplain, *255*
  chaplain, *see* Greasbrough
  chaplain, *see* Ledston
  chaplain of Otley, *34*, 370
  chaplain of St Leonard's, *7*, *75*, *225*, *230*,
    *233*, *365*, *559*, *644–5*, *676*, *741*, *815*
  clerk (mid 12th cent.), *862*
  clerk of Burnby, *575–6*
  clerk of Calverley, 393
  —, Mary his wife, 393
  clerk of Cleveland, *723*
  clerk of Poppleton, *264*

clerk of Rufforth, *343–4*, *448*, *823*, *and see*
    Rufforth (Adam)
clerk of St Leonard's, *136*, *704*
deacon, *186*, *814*
dean, 154
—, his dau., wife of Henry de Redman,
    154
forester of Leathley, *295*
forester of Otley, *289*, *294*, *297–301*, *543*
forester of Rufforth, *451*
goldsmith, *204*, *206*
hermit, *687*
parson of Burton, *354*
parson of Calverley (son of Jordan ?), *392*,
    393, *395–6*
—, his brothers, *see* Hugh, William
parson of Hemsworth, *811*
parson of Hooton, *see* Hooton·Roberts
parson of Knapton, 74
parson of Thwing, 713
priest (of Greasbrough ?), *218*, *see also*
    Greasbrough
prior of Hooton, *in error for* parson, 805
prior of Monk Bretton and Pontefract,
    *193*, *see also* Northampton
rector of Arncliffe, *see* Adam (rural dean)
reeve of Upton, *532–3*
rural dean of Brodsworth (*i.e.* Doncaster),
    8, 159, *see also* Brodsworth
—, Vincent his son, 159
rural dean of Craven, rector of Arncliffe,
    251, 503, *872–3*
smith, *914*
brother of Alan son of Peter, *see* Noizeby
brother of Hamelin, 253
brother of Peter dean of Wakefield, 247
brother of Thomas parson of Kellington,
    180, 192
son of Austin, 388
son of Burnel, *see* Elmsall
son of Copsi, 414, 580
son of Ellis son of Baldwin, 255
son of Eudo, *9*
son of Guy (of Rufforth), *450–51*
son of Hugh, *966*
—, Robert his brother, *966*
son of Ketel, *354*
son of Laurence, *605*
son of Nicholas, *913*
son of Norman, 10, 23, 129, 272–3, 277,
    357, 524, 525
—, fee, 276
—, his dau., wife of Hugh of Leathley,
    *see* Christiana
son of Orm, *354*
son of Peter, *see* Birkin

Akenberg, *see* Lockington
Aketon (nr Spofforth), Aicatuna, Aycton,
    Ayketon, Eyketon, 357, 410, 415
    John of, *199*
    Jolain of (12th cent.), *428*
    Jolain, Jodlan of (13th cent.), *67, 198–9,*
        *366, 420, 425*
Akum, Akumhag, *see* Acomb
Alan
    abbot of Roche, *808*
    brother of St Leonard's, *676*
    brother-knight of St Leonard's, *233*
    butler, *see* Butler
    canon of York, 181, *478, 871*
    —, his chaplain, *see* Nicholas
    chamberlain (of Henry de Lacy), *168*, 169
    chaplain of York Minster, *899*
    clerk, steward of Pontefract and
        Blackburnshire, 964–5
    clerk of Acomb, *7, and see* Alan (parson of
        Knapton)
    clerk of Langton, *320*
    clerk (of St Leonard's ?), *198*
    clerk of Sinderby, *766*
    clerk, nephew of Maltalent, *549*
    cook (of St Leonard's ?), *577*
    I, count of Brittany, 380, 596, 758, 765
    III, earl of Richmond and count of
        Brittany, 108, 163, 603
    forester, *547, 553*
    lecher (*lecator*), *192*
    parson of Knapton, 7, *452*
    priest (12th cent.), *809*
    prior of Drax, 322
    provost of Beverley, 584
    rector of Adel, 68
    reeve (of Bramhope ?), *26, 29*
    serjeant of St Leonard's, *669*
    steward of Pontefract and Blackburnshire,
        *see* Alan (clerk)
    subprior of Pontefract, 180
    villein of Peter de Fauconberg, *454*
    son of Alan son of Maltalent, *548–9*
    son of Alexander, *see* Sancton
    son of Arnald, 60
    son of Augustin, *398–9*
    son of Brian, *see* FitzBrian
    son of Elinant, *see* Barton
    son of Ellis, *822, and see* Catterton,
        Hammerton
    son of Forn, *see* Bramhope
    son of Geoffrey (of Weston), *543*
    son of Henry, *254*
    son of Hereward, *see* Bramhope
    son of Osbert, *814*
    son of Peter, *see* Noizeby

    son of Romund, *227*
    son of Serlo, *280*
    son of Theobald son of Vuiet, 147
    son of Thomas, *see* Butler
    son of Torfin, *see* Allerston
Alan
    Peter, *391–2, 395, 397*
    Roger, *392, 395, 818*
    Swain, 388
    William (son of Swain), 388
Albeneio, Alben', *see* Aubigny
Albin, master, 109
Albourne, 655
Albus, *see* White
Alby, Simon, *189*
Alda, Henry de, 16
Aldborough, 93–4, 147–9, 373, 534, *see also*
    Burgh
    church of St Andrew, 147
Aldeford, Stephen de, *881*
Alderges (in Sancton), Haldeherges, 774, 865
Alderthwaite, Allerwaith
    John son of Henry of, 84
    Thomas of, 491
Aldewaldelaye, *see* Alwoodley
Aldewerc
    Norman de, *431*
    Osbert de, *400*
    Reiner de, *230*
    *cf.* Aldwark, Aldwarke
Aldiges, Henry de, *432*
Aldort, Robert, *253*
Aldred, Alred, *551, 562*
    priest (of Heslington), *602–3*
    nephew of Robert Brun, *549, 563*
    son of Besing, 13, 406, 413, 439, 442
Aldwaldeslay, *see* Alwoodley
Aldwark (nr Alne, NR), 130, *cf.* Aldewerc
Aldwarke, 842–4, *cf.* Aldewerc
    Robert of, 842–3, 845
    —, Joan his wife, *see* Clarel
Aldwoldelay, *see* Alwoodley
Aldwulf, pre-Conquest tenant, 433
Alebaster, *see* Arbalaster
Alemare (*lost*, in Wheldrake), 685
Alerdale, *see* Allerdale
Alestanbothuna, *see* Elsingbottom
Alewaldelay, *see* Alwoodley
Alexander I, king of Scotland, 837
Alexander
    abbot of Kirkstall, 169, 473
    abbot of Meaux, 212–13, 440, 719, 771,
        816
    bishop of Coventry and Lichfield, *see*
        Stavensby
    bishop of Lincoln, 5, 742

Bath and Wells, *see also* Wells
  bishop of, *see* Burnell
  prebend of, *see* Buckland Dinham
Batheleia, *see* Batley
Bathonia, Bada, Henry de, sheriff of York,
    362
Batley, Batelay, Batheleia, 249, 386, *915*
  Gamel son of Liulf of, *249*
  John of, *250*
  William son of Richard of, *249–50*
Baumees, *see* Beaumes
Bavent, Batevent, Batvent
  Lettice dau. of Nicholas son of Maud
    de, 130
  Roger de, sheriff of York, 12, 200, 273,
    276, 374, 427, 438, 467, *510–11*, 593, *788*,
    *810*, 876–7, 960
  Roger de (*another ?*), *337*
Bavill, Eudo de, *890*
Baxby, 884
Bayeux, Baius
  Alan de, *364*
  Hugh de, 742, 960
  Osbert de, archdeacon, steward of
    Pontefract, 103, 105, 112, 183, *479*, 875,
    958–61
  Ranulf de, 742
  Thurstan de (son of Osbert), 961
  William de, 960–61
Bayldun, *see* Baildon
Baynton, *see* Bainton
Bays, Robert, king's clerk, master of St
    Leonard's, 948–9
Beacham, Richard, bailiff and collector of
    rents for St Leonard's, *927*
Beal, 183
Bealeys (nr Lockington), Belaugh, Belhagh,
    312, 854
Beamsley, Bethmeslay, 269–70, 502
  Reginald of, *271*
Béarn, Constance de, wife of Henry of
    Almain, 806
Beasley, Reginald or Reynold (16th cent.),
    registrar of jurisdiction of Durham, xliii
Beatrishil, *see* Betteros Hill
Beatrix, tenant of manor of Rotherham, 114,
    *and see* Wickersley
Beauchamp (*Bello Campo*), Richard de, *9*
Beaufitz
  Alice, wife of William Plumpton, 404,
    406, 412, 414, 416–17
  Henry, 404, 406, 414, 416
  —, Cecily his wife, *see* Plumpton
    (Huckeman's descendants)
Beaufort, Henry, bishop of Winchester, king's
    chancellor, 619

Beaumes, Baumees, Beaumys, Beumys, *see
    also* Beum
  William de, steward of St Leonard's, 35,
    *142, 336, 339, 485, 514, 612, 625, 628, 674,
    727, 776, 833–4, 891*
Beaumont, Beaumunt (*Bello Monte*)
  Lewis de, bishop of Durham, 945
  William de, *262, 562*
Beauvais (dép. Oise), Belvaco
  abbey, 659
  Vincent de, xlix
  Walter de, *140*
Beauver
  John de, 854
  Ralph de, 519
  Robert de, 519
Bec, William de, *254*
Beckard
  John, 93
  —, Margery or Mary his wife, 93
  Peter, 93, *779*
Becket, Thomas, archbishop of Canterbury,
    king's chancellor, 148, 159, 474, 606
Beckingham (Notts.), 209
Bect', Ivo de, *225*
Bedale (NR), 130, 866, *see also* FitzAlan,
    FitzBrian
Bedford, archdeacon of, *933, and see* Geoffrey,
    Laurence, Richard
Beeford (Holderness), 438
  rector of, *see* Calverley (William)
  Robert of, 438
  —, Alice his wife, *see* Bretton
Beellum, Philip de, 688
Beeston, Beston, Bestun, 41, 119
  Adam of, 276, *393*
  Ralph of, *390*
Bégard (dép. Côtes-d'Armor)
  abbey, 934
  —, abbot, *see* Geoffrey
Beighton (Derbs.), 106, 116–18, 120
Beines, William de, *228*
Bek
  Alice, wife of William of Willoughby, 520
  Anthony, bishop of Durham, 264, 519–20
  Margaret, wife of Richard de Harcourt,
    520
  Nigel de, 416
Bekwith
  Adam, 739
  —, Elizabeth his wife, 739
  John, 635–6
Belaugh, *see* Bealeys
Belby, Beleby, Ellis of, *894*
Beler
  Hamo, *604*

Beningwurd, Beningwurdhe, *see* Benniworth

Bennesson, Robert, *615*

Bennetland, Hugh of, *538–9*

Benniworth, Beningwurd(he), Benigburg, 346

    Geoffrey of, 346

    Gilbert of, 346, *348–9*

    —, Sarah his wife, *see* Warwick

    Lucy of, wife of Philip de Chauncy, 346, 444

    Maud of, wife of — Mortimer, 346, 444

    William of, 346, *348*

Bennyngburgh, *see* Beningbrough

Benson, Roger de, 608

Benstede, John, rector of Spofforth, 514

Bentelay, *see* Bentley

Bentham, church, 943

    rector or parson of (*named*), 943, *and see* Hampton, Ouseburn

Bentley (in Chapel Allerton), 476

Bentley (nr Doncaster), Bentelay, Benetleia, lxi, *1*, 83, 85–6, *100*, 158, *163–4*, 489, 803, 848

Benton, Bentun, Walter of, steward, *872*

Benyngburt, *see* Beningbrough

Beolton, *see also* Bolton

    Hugh son of William de, 234

    William de, 234

    —, Alice his wife, 234

Berard, Thomas, master of Temple in England, 274

Berb', Roger de, clerk of St Leonard's, *385*

Bercarius, *see* Shepherd

Berclai, Henry de, *190*

Bergh, *see* Burgh

Berghthorp, *see* Belthorpe

Berkeston, *see* Barkston

Berkeworth, John son of John, champion, *637*

Berkin, *see* Birkin

Berkshire, archdeaconry of, 941

Berlay, Berley, *see also* Barlow

    Henry de, 15

    Henry de (of Heslington), *633*

    Robert de, knt, 84, 284

    Stephen de, rector of Bolton-upon-Dearne, 84

    William, 86

Bernaburg (*unident.*), clerk of, *see* Thomas

Bernake, Richard de, 47

Bernard

    bishop of Carlisle, 374

    brother-chaplain of St Leonard's, *30*, 65–6, *135–6, 139, 141–3, 172, 197, 225, 231, 332, 334–6, 350, 381, 460–61, 494–5, 540, 557, 585, 591, 594, 692, 759, 815, 824, 829, 856*

    canon of York, *445, 821, 899*

    chaplain of Sherburn, 292, *494*

    clerk, *609*

    I clerk (of Ripley), 382, *383*

    II clerk (of Ripley, son of Norman), 382–3

    parson of Normanton, 466

    prior of Newburgh, 212

    prior of York Holy Trinity, *348*

    serjeant of St Leonard's, *753, 887*

    son of Gamel, *see* Ripon

    son of Orm, *354*

    son of William, *see* Araines

Bernard

    Ellis, parson of Tickhill, 529

    Richard, 868

    Thomas, *634–6*

Bernerthorpe, Gilbert de, *741*

Bernestona, *see* Barmston

Bernevale, Bernevall, Bernewele, Gilbert de, *285–6, 339, 826*

    —, Aubrey his dau., 339

    —, Cecily his dau., 339

Bernulf, priest of Sitleswrdia, *166*

Bernville, Richard son of Peter de, 746

Berton, *see* Burton

Bertram

    prior of Durham, *781*

    prior of Pontefract, 193

    son of Fulk, *see* Hammerton

Bertram, Roger, justice, *674*

Bertrand, master, steward of Tickhill, 844

Bertrard, serjeant of St Leonard's, *228*

Berweby, *see* Barrowby

Berwick-in-Craven, 508

Besacra, *see* Bessacarr

Besing, Basing (of Woolthwaite), 527, 529, *846*

Besingbi, *see* Bessingby

Bessacarr, Besacra, 122–3, 360, 804

    Peter of, *9*

Bessingby, Besingbi

    Mauger of, *862*

    William of, *862*

Beston, Bestun, *see* Beeston

Beswick, 439, 854, 879–80

Bete, Richard, 209

Bethmeslay, *see* Beamsley

Béthune, Baldwin de, earl of Aumale, 664, 744, 746

    —, his wife, *see* Hawise

Betteros Hill (Hillam), Beatrishil, Betricehill, 60

Beugrant, Bheugrant

    John (son of William), 414, 417–18, *427*, 429

    Peter (son of John), 405, 417, *420, 422–4*, 426

Bolton (in Craven), Bouelton, lxi, 273, *674*
  Lobwood in, *q.v.*
  priory, 251–2, 278, 361, 369, 377, 502, 659,
    728, *and see* Embsay
  —, cartulary, 68
  —, prior, *674*, 848, *and see* John, Robert,
    Thomas
Bolton by Bowland, 127, 275, 277–8, 410
  church, 278
  Richard of, 278
Bolton upon Dearne, Bouilton, 83–8, 124–5,
  861
  church, 83–4, 88, 124–5
  rectors or parsons of, *see* Bellewe
    (William), Berlay, Haringby, Richard
    (rector), Went Hill, William (parson)
Bolton Percy, 242, 372, 555, 863
Bolumer, *see* Bulmer
Bona Villa, *see* Boneville
Bonde, Bund
  Alan, *62–3*
  Roger, *61*
Bondholm (Ledston), 496
Boneville, Bonevile, Bonneville (*Bona Villa*)
  Alice de, wife of Richard de Arnhale,
    455
  William de, *28, 218–19, 222–3, 232*, 455
  —, Thomas brother of (*in error for* son
    of ?), *223*
  —, Thomas son of, *219, 222, 232*
  William de, master, clerk of St Leonard's,
    7
Boniface
  Alan, 876, 879
  Thomas, 438, 878
Bonneville, *see* Boneville
Bootham, *see under* York
Bordeaux (dép. Gironde), constable, *see*
  Wawayn
Boroughbridge (*Pons Burgi, Pons Bergi*),
  147–9, *150*, 373, 376
  clerk, *see* Jeremy, Stephen
  rural dean, *see* Herbert, Staveley
  smith, *see* Walter
  Jeremy of, *see* Jeremy (clerk)
  Richard of, rector of Askham, 436
Borton, Bortone, *see* Burton
Boscer, Boscher, Robert, 596, *609*, 610
Bosco, *see* Bois
Boseville, Bosevill, Bosevilla
  Peter de, 803
  Thomas de, brother of Ralph Nowell,
    124, *164*, *513*
  Thomas de (*another*), 803
  —, Elizabeth his wife, 803
  William de, *164*, 806

Bossall, Bozhale
  rectors (*named*), 941
  Maud of (dau. of Richard), 591
  Richard I of, 591, 752
  —, Mabel his wife, *see* Stuteville
  —, Maud his wife, *see* Ganton
  Richard II of, *591*
Bosse, Agnes, 311
Botehaut, Buttehaut (Norf.), tower, 946
Botelrie, William, *787*
Botheby, William, master of St Leonard's,
  king's clerk, canon of London St
  Martin le Grand, 949–51
Botheme, Bothum, *see* York (Bootham)
Botilder, John, 319
  Olive his wife, 319
Botiller, *see* Butler
Bouelton, *see* Bolton
Bouer, Beuur, Buuer
  Daniel, *219–23, 231–2*, 555
  —, James his brother, *219, 221–3, 231–2*
  —, Laurence his brother, *219, 221–3, 231–2*
  Robert, *293*
  William, *697, 699–700*
Bouhcton, *see* Bucton
Bouilton, *see* Bolton
Bouis, *see* Bowes
Boulogne, Bolonia, Bulonia
  Nicholas de, *219, 222, 232–3*, 491
  Roger de, *365*
Bourton, *see* Burton
Bouuington, *see* Boynton
Boville, Sewal de, chancellor of archbishop
  Gray, canon, dean and archbishop of
  York, 241, 521, *532*, 610–11
Bovington, *see* Boynton
Bowelton, *see* Bolton
Bowes, Boghes, Bohes, Bouis, *906, 913–14*,
  *922*, 936
  capital messuage, *914*
  church, *906, 914, 923, 925*
  grange, *906*
  watermill, *914*
  windmill, *914*
  Percival (16th cent.), 571
  Robert of, chaplain of St Leonard's, 136,
    *141, 258, 336, 350, 523*, 591
  William of, clerk, deacon, chaplain of St
    Leonard's, rector of York St Margaret
    Walmgate, *99, 135, 332, 494, 696, 705*
Bowtheronfeilde, *see* Boldron Hill
Boxgrove (Sussex), priory, 679–80
  —, prior, 684
Boynton, Bovington, Bouuington, 592
  Adam of, *650*

Joan of, wife of Ralph de Vermelles, 122, 124
Branton (Northumb.), 608
  John of, 608
Brattleby (Lincs.), 813
Bratton (Wilts.), 640
Braunch
  Ellis, *282, 293–4*
  Jordan son of Ellis, *282*
Braunton (Devon), 949
Brawby, Braweby, John, chaplain, 657–8, 738, 851
Bray, Turgis de, 743–4
  —, Maud his wife, *see* Scures
Braydeford, *see* Bradford
Braytheywelle, Braythwell, *see* Braithwell
Brayton, Braitona, lxx, *1*, 76, 78, *89–90*, 183, 341, 518
  church, 179
  Haldan of (son of Robert), lxx, 76, *89–90*
  John of (son of Haldan), lxxi, 76, *89–90*
Brayzwele, *see* Bracewell
Brearey, *see* Breary
Brearton (nr Scotton), Brereton, 101
  Richard of, *96–7, 176*
  Robert of, *97*
  William of, *402*
Breary (nr Bramhope), Brearey, Brerehage, Brerehagh, Brerehale, Brerehaw, Brerehaye, Brerhage, Brerhale, 17, *26*
  family, 17–18
  Adam of, *23*
  Alan of (son of Robert), 17–18, *25, 38*
  John of, *32, 45*
  Robert of (12th cent.), 15, 17–18, *25–8,* 252
  —, Agnes his wife, *see* Frank
  Robert of (son of Robert, late 13th cent.), 18
  Robert of (son of William, 13th cent.), *18, 21*
  Robert of (son of William, 14th cent.), 18
  Samuel, succentor of York (d. 1735), 18
  William of (late 12th cent.), *24, 27*
  William of (13th cent.), *19*
  —, Margaret his wife, 18
Breauté, Faukes de, 278
  —, his wife, *see* Margaret 'countess'
Brebazun, *see* Brabazon
Breddale, *see* Burdale
Breddesword, *see* Brodsworth
Bredewell, *see* Braithwell
Bredon
  John, *537*
  Richard, *537*

Brembre, Thomas, king's clerk, master of St Leonard's, canon of St Paul's, dean of Wimborne, 738, 946–7
Brenna, *in error for* Braham, 357
Brentingham, *see* Brantingham
Brerehage, Brerehagh, Brerehale, Brerehaw, Brerehaye, Brerhage, Brerhale, *see* Breary
Brereton, *see* Brearton
Bressenay, Agnes de, 871
Bret, Bret'
  John, 80
  Richard, *592*
  Walter, *620, 730*
  William de, *490*
Bretel
  Richard, elder, 215
  —, Ragenild his wife, *see* Ste-Marie
  Richard, younger, 215
Bretewelle, *see* Braithwell
Bretgate, *see under* York
Breton, *see* Bretton
Bretteby, Robert de, *42–3*
Brettegate, *see* York (Bretgate)
Bretteville, Richard de, *766*
Brettgate, *see* York (Bretgate)
Bretton, Breton, Bretun, Brito(n), Britonil, Brytonus
  Adam, 342
  Alan, *897, see also* Rufforth
  Alice, wife of Robert of Beeford, 438
  Avice, wife of Peter de Setona, 438
  Emelina, wife of Roger of Grainsby, 438
  Geoffrey (12th cent.), *see* Bugthorpe
  Geoffrey (d. *c.*1247), *see* Rufforth
  Jordan, *see* Bugthorpe
  Maud, wife of Richard de Setona, 438
  Peter, *see* Bugthorpe
  Ralph, 111
  Robert, *see* Bugthorpe
  Robert son of William, *see* Pool
  Roger, *342, and see* Bugthorpe
  William, *400, and see* Pool
Bretton, Brettun, Broctone, *see also* Burton (Salmon)
  family (of Burton Salmon), 60–61
  Adam de (son of Roger), *61–2, 64*
  Gervaise de, 60, *193*
  John son of Robert de, *61–2*
  John de (*in error for* le ?), 373
  Osbert de, 60
  Peter de, 60
  Pigot de, 60–61
  —, Agnes his dau., 61
  Robert de (brother of Osbert), 60
  Robert de (son of Serlo), 61

Bruncet, *see* Brunet
Bruneby, *see* Burnby
Brunehou, *see* Brown Howe
Brunesford, *see* Brinsworth
Brunet, Bruncet, John, *161*
Brungelflete, Brungareflet, Brungelflete,
    Brunge(r)flet, Brungesf', Brungflet,
    Brunkerfleth, *see* Broomfleet
Brunne, *see also* Kirkburn
    Adam de, *613, 627–8, 632*
    John de, *see* Westbrunne
    Robert, *616–17*
Brunnebi, Brunneby, *see* Burnby
Brunnehum, Brunnun, *see* Nunburnholme
Brunolvesheved, Gilbert de, 151
Brunugflet, *see* Broomfleet
Brursel, Geoffrey, *195*
Brus, *see also* Bruce
    fee, 82, 120, 133, 138, 155, 234, 236, 266,
        272, 343, 433, 442, 444–5, 534, 593,
        599–600, 721
    Adam I de, 568
    Adam II de, 133, 266–7, 313, 433, 568
    —, Juetta his wife, *see* Arches
    Agnes de, wife of Walter de Fauconberg,
        266
    Laderina de, wife of John de Bellewe, 78,
        81–2, 433, 437
    Lucy de, wife of Marmaduke of Thwing,
        600, 715–16, 727
    Margaret de, wife of Robert de Ros,
        442, 721
    Peter I de, 134, 266–7, 459, 568, 599
    —, his steward, *see* Henry son of Conan
    Peter I or II de, 268
    Peter III de, 78, 81, 151, *154*, 155, 266, 433,
        437, 442, 444, 721
    —, his coheirs, 81
    —, his steward, *see* Pickering
    Robert, king of Scotland, *see* Robert
    Robert I de, 47, 272, 534, 784
    Robert II de, 266
Brytonus, *see* Bretton
Bubwith, 383
    Nicholas, clerk, *634*
Bucard, Burchard, treasurer of York, *see*
    Puiset
Bucchtton, Buchton, Buchtton, *see* Bucton,
    Buhtton
Buci, Bucei
    Oliver de, *902*
    Robert, *321*
    Robert de, *775–6, 902*
Buckingham, marquess of, *see* Grenville
Buckland, Bukland, Richard, *637*

Buckland Dinham, prebend (Bath and Wells),
    943
Buckrose wapentake, bailiff of, *see* Drewton
Buckton (nr Bempton), 652
    Arnald, Arnulf, Ernald of, *652–3*
    Geoffrey son of Arnald of, 652
    Walter son of Arnald of, 652–3
    William son of Arnald of, *652, 653*
Bucton, Bouhcton, Buchton, *see also* Buhtton
    Fulk de (of St Leonard's, son of
        Geoffrey), 225, 386, *389*, 547, *558, 560*
    Nigel de, knt, *198*
Buet, Thomas, 374
Bugthorpe (*unident.*), Bugatorp
    Gamel of, *781, 814*
    Hugh brother of Nicholas of, *722*
    Nicholas of, 8, *164*, *722*
    —, Alice his wife, *8*
    —, Alice his dau., wife of William
        Fairfax, *7–8*
Bugthorpe (ER), Bugethorp, Buggethorp,
    Buketorp, *1*, 436–7, 439, 455, *577*
    prebend (York), 765
    Alan of, *see* Rufforth
    Geoffrey I of, *alias* Geoffrey Bretton,
        steward of Amfrey de Chauncy, 434,
        437–8, *577*
    —, Dera his wife, 434, 438
    Geoffrey II of (d. *c*.1247), *see* Rufforth
    Geoffrey of, *alias* Geoffrey Bretton (son
        of Geoffrey), 434, 438
    Jordan I of, *alias* Jordan Bretton, king's
        officer, 434, 436, 438–9, 646, 712, 774,
        853
    —, Mabel his wife, *see* Octon
    Jordan II of (son of Geoffrey of
        Rufforth), 434, 437, 443, *451, 882*
    Peter of, *alias* Peter Bretton, 434, 438–9
    Robert of, *alias* Robert Bretton, 434,
        438–9, *882*
    Roger of, *alias* Roger Bretton (son of
        Jordan), 434, 438
    William de (*c*.1230), *447, 454–5, 457*
    William (14th cent.), 437
    —, Alice his wife, 437
Bugthorpe (WR, nr Maltby), 57
    Geoffrey of, 57
    Hamelin of, 54–7, *529*
    —, Eleanor his dau., wife of Reginald, 57
    —, Margaret *or* Margery his wife, *see*
        Oldcotes
    —, Maud his dau., wife of Robert
        Drincof, 57
Buhtton, Buhton, Bucchtton, Buchtton', *see
    also* Bucton
    Ralph de, clerk of St Leonard's, *19–20*,

Ralph of (son of German), knt, *19*, 20, *41*,
    131, *and see* Mansel
Burn (in Brayton), 76, 78, 81, 83–4, 86–8
Burnby (nr Pocklington), Brumeby, Bruneby,
    Brunnebi, Brunneby, *1*, *574–5*, 647
    church, 574
    clerk of, *see* Adam
Burnel, *see* Aumenil, *and cf.* Burel
Burnel
    Adam, *see* Elmsall
    Robert, bishop of Bath and Wells, king's
        chancellor, 929
    Thomas, 248
    William, canon of York (Ampleforth
        prebend), 597
Burnus (Kirkburn ?), Burnu', Ralph de, *195*,
    *see also* Ralph (priest)
Burri, Thomas, 720
Burrough Green (Cambs.), 82
Burs, *see* Biria
Bursea, 714, 853, 855, 875
    Michael son of Thurstan of, 853
Bursel, Alan, *70*
Burshill, 744
Burstall, Burstal, William de, *9*
    —, Hugh his brother, *9*
    —, Robert his son, *9*
Bursyre, *see* Burghshire
Burton, *see also* Brandesburton, Hundburton,
    Kirkburton
Burton (*unident.*), Berton, Borton, Bourton,
    Burtone, Burtun, *906*
    parson of, *see* Adam
    Ellis de, *811*
    Henry de, *723*
    Henry, bailiff of St Leonard's, *927*
    Henry de, clerk, *390*
    Hugh, 738
    John, *44*
    John, bailiff of Hedon, *673*
    John (antiquary), xliv–xlv, lxvii, lxxiii, 773
    Michael de, *alias* Michael of the hospital,
        chaplain of St Leonard's, *324–5*, 326,
        *730–32*
    Nicholas de, steward of Pontefract and
        Blackburnshire, 957, 966
    Richard de, *634*
    Thomas de, *369*
    Thomas, abbot of Meaux, 744, 752
    Walter de, *912*
    William de, *124*
    —, Nicholas his son, *see* Lumby
Burton Agnes, 655–6, 720, *and see*
    Annaisburton
Burton Constable, xliv
Burton Fields, *see* Hundburton

Burton Fleming, 652
Burton Hall (nr Brayton), 76, 84, 180, 183
Burton-in-Kendal (Westm.), 155
    Roger de, knt, *155*
Burton Leonard, Borton, Bortone, *1*, *93–4*,
    *95–9*
    church, 99
    Westschowe in, 97
    Adam son of Morand of, 97
    Durand of, *95–6*, *99*
    Henry of, *98–9*
    Henry Atwell of, 97
    Henry son of William of, *96*
    Nicholas of, *96*, *98–9*
    Robert of (son of Muriel), *96–9*
    William son of Aldred of, *95–6*, *99*
Burton Salmon, Bretton, *1*, 60, *61–4*, *see also*
    Bretton
Burun, Erneis de, *174–5*, *257*, *404*, *538*, *758*
Burussire, *see* Burghshire
Bury St Edmunds, 786
Busli, Builly, Bulli, *see also* Bully
    Gilbert de, *163*
    Hugh de, 804
    Idonea de, wife of Robert de Vipont,
        528–30, 805, 825
    John de (son of Richard), *530*, 804–5, 841
    Richard de, 489, 527, 799, 801, 804
    Robert de, *219*, *233*
    Roger de, Domesday tenant, 51, 115, 209,
        247, 489, 491, 527, 791, 799, 840, 848
    William de, 804
Bustard, Buistard, Bustarde
    Henry, 75, *140*, *173*, 220, *707*, *822*
    Robert, 73–4, *173*, *446–7*, *449*, *457*, *707*
Bustardthorpe (*lost*, nr York), Bustardethorp,
    Bustardthorppe, Thorp Bustard, *1*,
    73–4, *75*, *172*, *822*
Butare, Walter son of Richard de, *731*
Buteler, Butelier, *see* Butler
Butevilain, Robert, archdeacon of York, dean
    of York, *347*, *430*, *478*, 490, *550–52*, *761*,
    *859*, *862*
    —, his chaplain, *see* Robert
    —, his clerk, *see* Richard
    —, his son, *see* Hugh (canon)
Butler, Botiller, Buteler, Butelier, Butiller,
    Buttiller (*Pincerna*)
    Adam, *427*
    Agnes, wife of Hugh Pingel, *419*
    Agnes, wife of William of Middleton, 419
    Alan, 419
    Alan son of Thomas, 133, *417–18*, *504*
    Geoffrey, 652
    Henry, *619*, *707*
    Hugh, *alias* Hugh of Armthorpe (*q.v.*),

Coleby, Colebi, William de, *327–9, 331, 334–5, 469, 545, 547, 557–8, 560*
Coleton, Colet'
    Roscelin, Recelin de, *549, 562*
    Simon de, *562*
Coletorp, Walter de, *428*
Colevill, *see* Colvill
Coley (nr Halifax), *278*
Colingham, *see* Collingham
Coll', John, *569*
Colling, son of, *see* Girard
Collingham, Colingham, Colyngham, *23*
    Robert of, brother-chaplain of St
        Leonard's, *135, 139, 301, 349, 370, 577, 594, 696, 756, and cf.* Robert (brother-chaplain)
Collingham, South (nr Newark), rector of,
    *see* Magnus
Collum, *see* Cowlam
Cologne, *951*
Colton, *441–2*
    Adam son of Thomas, *43–4*
    Geoffrey son of Thomas de, *875*
    Henry of, *450*
    Henry of, clerk, *143*
    Robert son of Thomas de, *875*
    Thomas de, *875*
    William of, *450–51*
    William son of Thomas, *43–5*
    —, Alice his wife, *45*
Colvill, Colevill
    John de, *342*
    Philip, *873*
    Robert de (son of William), *342*
    Thomas, knt, *634*
    William de, *342, 873*
Colyngham, *see* Collingham
Combe Tertia prebend (Wells), *949*
Compton (nr Collingham), *23, and cf.*
    Cumpton
Conan
    earl of Richmond, *408, 599, 605*
    son of Henry, *alias* Conan of Kelfield
        (dead 1251), *598–600*
    son of Henry (dead *c.*1285), *598, 600–1*
    —, Petronilla his wife, *see* Conyers
    son of Henry (14th cent.), *601*
    son of Torfin, *alias* Conan of Manfield,
        *alias* Conan of Kelfield, *478, 596, 598–9, 605, 606*
    —, Juetta his wife, *605*
Condeio, *see* Cundy
Coney Street, *see under* York
Conisbrough, Kunigheburgh, *209*
    court, *108*
    clerk of, *see* Ellis

constable of, *see* Hersy
earl of, *see* Warenne
Coniston, Cold, *131*
Constable (of Flamborough)
    John, master of St Leonard's, archdeacon
        of Huntingdon, treasurer, dean and
        canon of Lincoln, *584, 954*
    Lettice, wife of Thomas Houton, *657*
    Marmaduke, knt, *658*
    Marmaduke, knt (d. 1518), sheriff of York,
        *954*
    Marmaduke, knt (mid 16th cent.),
        steward of St Leonard's, *927*
    Richard, *713*
    Robert I, *10, 519*
    Robert II, *713*
    Robert III, *10, 272, 407, 521, 657, 789*
    Robert IV, knt, *657, 711, 886*
    —, Joan his wife, *see* Hook
    Robert (d. 1488), *954*
    William I, *10, 521, 735, 774, 789, 854*
    William II, knt (d. 1319), *657, 711*
Constable (of Burton Constable), William
    (18th cent.), xliv
Conyers, Coigners, Coiners
    family, *601*
    Geoffrey de, *772*
    Helen de, wife of Bernard de Araines, *772*
    Petronilla de, *alias* Petronilla of Kelfield,
        wife of Conan son of Henry, *598, 600–1*
    Roger de, *145, 146*
    Roger son of Roger de, *145*
Conyngeston, *see* Conistone
Cook
    Alexander, *125*
    William, master, *614*
    *and see* Alan, Gilbert, Holdebert, Kippax,
        Norman, Ralph, Richard, Roger,
        Simon (master), Walter, Weston
        (Roger)
Cookridge, *15, 251, 474*
Copeland (Westm.), Coupland, *906*
    Richard of, knt, *154*
    William of, *881*
Copgrove, Coppegrave
    Osgot of, *97*
    Walter of, *96–7, 99*
Copmanthorpe, Copmantorp,
    Coupemanthorp, Coupmanthorp,
    Coupmannethorn, *1, 8, 138–43, 793–4, 915*
    Henry granger of, *142*
    —, Alice his wife, *142*
    Henry son of Peter of, *139*
    Hugh son of Osbert of, *142*

Robert of, constable of Knaresborough,
  bailiff of Spofforth, sheriff of York,
  149, 362
Robert of (*another* ?), 444
Cresaker, Cresacre
  John, 84
  William de, 652
Creskeld, Cressekelled, Cressekelde, Kreskeld,
  16, 27, 33
  Hugh of, 25–29
  Roger son of Peter of (*alias* Roger of
    Arthington ?, *q.v.*), 14
Cressingham, Crassingham, Cressyngham,
  Hugh of, steward of Eleanor of
  Castile and bishop of Ely, 779, 911–13,
  915, 920–21
Cresswell, 76, 79, 85–6
Cressy
  family (of Hodsock), 58
  Hugh de, justice, constable of Rouen,
    58, 109
  Hugh de, son of Roger and Eustacia, 58
  —, Margaret his wife, *see* Chesney
  John, 58
  Roger de, 58, 59, 113
  —, Cecilia wife of, *see* Clifton
  William de, 58, 846
Cressyngham, *see* Cressingham
Creswolde (*in error for* Creskeld ?), 27
Creyk, *see* Crayke
Crich (Derbs.)
  church, chantry in, 87
  Robert of, 80
  Roger of, 79
Cridling Stubbs, Credelyng, Crideling,
  Cridlinc, 795
  Adam of, 215–16, 795, 958, 960
  —, Alice wife of, *see* Dor
  Alexander son of Thomas of, 170
  Ralph son of Nicholas of, steward of
    Pontefract, 795, 958, 960
Crigglestone, Criggeliston, Crigleston
  Adam of, 210, 216
  —, Sybil his wife, *see* Ste-Marie
  Alan of, 210, 214, 216
  Hugh of, 189, 215
  John of, 884–5, 886–8, 892
  —, his wife, *see* Hook
  Margaret of, wife of Roger of Hook, 884
  Robert son of Adam of, 213, 810
  Thomas of (son of Adam), 210, 213, 216, 810
  —, Christiana his wife, 213, 216
  William of, 887, 888–9
Crimple, Cremple, beck, 420–21, 503
Cristall, *see* Kirkstall
Crocheslei, William de, 604

Croft, William of, 232
Crompton (Lancs.), 316
Cromwell, Thomas, 954, *and cf.* Crumbwell
Crondall (Hants.), rector of, *see* Ispania
Crookes, Crookesmoor (Eccleshall,
  Sheffield), 87
Crosby Bank (nr Crosby Ravensworth,
  Westm.), 924
Crose, Robert atte, *see* Atcross
Crosland, Adam son of Roger of, 963
Cross, Robert atte, *see* Atcross
Crossby, Crosseby, Nicholas de, steward of St
  Leonard's, 167, 282, 285, 336, 339, 485,
  587, 674, 727, 756, 776
Crossdale, Crossedale, Adam of, 913
Crosseman, William, 756
Crosserigge, Adam de, 913
Crossum (*unident.*), 681
Crosthwaite, Crostwaite, 410
Croston (Lancs.), rector of, 948
Crouchback, *see* Edmund
Croxton (Cambs.), 716
Croxton (Lincs.), 76
  family, *alias* Kersall, 76
  Hugh of, 108
  Richard of, 76, 108
  Robert son of Richard of, *see* Robert,
    Kersall
Crumbwell, John, 489, *and cf.* Cromwell
Cryol, Geoffrey, 805, *and cf.* Clarel
Cuckney (Notts.), 701
Cudworth, 367, 753, 964
Cuerdley (Lancs.), 86
Cuinterel, *see* Quintrell
Cumberland, 373, 906, 915, 923
  earl of, *see* Clifford
Cumin, John, archbishop of Dublin, 430, *and
  cf.* Cunin
Cumpton, *cf.* Compton
  Geoffrey de, 293
  Ive (son of Geoffrey de), 293
  John de, 139
  Robert son of John de, clerk, 22, 23, 24
  —, Alice his mother, 24
  Walter de, 736
Cundall, Cundal, Robert de, 562
  —, Odo his brother, 562
Cundy, Cundi, Condeio
  Gilbert de, 339
  Roger de, 604, 609, 778
Cunegeston, *see* Conistone
Cunesgast', *see* York (Coney Street)
Cunigdes Doding, Swain de, 431
Cuniggeston, *see* Conistone
Cunin, Kunin, William, 433, 459–60, 823, *and
  cf.* Cumin

Easington, Esyngton, John, *926*
Easingwold, Esingwalde, Esyngwald,
    Esyngwold, Hesigwald, 293, 714, 716,
    *905, 917, 922*
    Alan of, master, *263*
    Anketin of, *760, 899*
    John of, master, *176, 391, 484, 586*
    —, Emma his mother, *391*
    Robert, *926*
    Thomas, *926*
East Riding, archdeaconry of, sequestrator
    in, *see* Darreyns
    archdeacon, 446, *and see* Feriby, Magnus,
    Skirlaugh, Waltham, Wisbech
East Riding
    rebellion, xlii
    queen's feodary of, *see* Smetheley
Eastburn, 81
Eastby (in Embsay), Estby, *728*
Eastfield, Estefeld, William, 806
Easthorpe (*lost*, in Heslington), Estorp, 596,
    *613, 633*
Easthorpe (nr Londesborough), 714, 716–17,
    772, 854–5
Eastrington, 770
Ebberford, Eberford, *see* Aberford
Eboracum, Ebor', *see* York
Eborard, *see* Everard
Eburfordia, *see* Aberford
Ecclefelde, *see* Ecclesfield
Eccles, church, 963
Ecclesall (Sheffield), 87
Ecclescliffe, *see* Egglescliffe
Ecclesfield, Ecclefelde, 79–81, 84–6
    Robert of, *849*
Eccleshill, Robert de, *818*
Eccup, 17–18, 252
Écuires (dép. Pas-de-Calais), 742
Eda, Ede, son of, *see* Richard
Edburford, *see* Aberford
Edderthorpe, Edrictorp, Roger of, *189*
Edelingtona, *see* Edlington
Edenthorpe, *see* Streetthorpe
Edingley (Notts.), 87
Edington, *see* Arthington
Edith dau. of Forne, wife of Robert d'Oilly,
    638–40, *641, 643,* 644, *645*
    Alice her dau., supposed dau. of Henry I,
    wife of Ernulf de Mandeville, 638,
    640, *643*
    Robert her son, *see* FitzRoy
Edlington, Edelingtona, Edlincton,
    Eldinctun, 77
    clerk of, *see* Robert
    Denise of, sister of John son of Ellis, wife
    of Peter of Wadworth, *160, 162*

    Ellis of, *321*
    John son of Ellis of, 162
    Peter of, *see* Wadworth
Edmund
    king of East Anglia, saint, 138
    earl of Cornwall, lord of Knaresborough,
    *alias* Edmund of Almain, xlviii, 147,
    149, *150,* 714
    —, his household, 150
    —, his steward, *see* Pierrepont, Russell
    earl of Lancaster, Leicester and Derby, *alias*
    Edmund Crouchback 113, 714, 716
    —, his steward, *see* Octon (John III)
    *cf.* Admund
Edneshal
    Peter de, *184*
    Richard de, *184*
    William de, *184*
Edric, Edryck, William, *167*
Edrictorp, *see* Edderthorpe
Edward, *644*
    I, king of England, lxvii, 10, 81, 514,
    807–8, 844, 883, 939, 966; before
    accession, 113, 471
    —, Eleanor his wife, *see* Castile
    II, king of England, 802, 940, 942, 944–6;
    as prince of Wales, 317
    —, Isabella his wife, *see* France
    III, king of England, 739, 843, *926,* 945–6
    —, Philippa his wife, *see* Hainhault
    IV, king of England, xlii, 953
    dispenser, *837*
Edward, son of, *see* William
Efward, *91*
Eggborough, Egborough, Egburc, Egburgh,
    Egdburg, Egeburg, *1, 168, 169,* 178–83,
    *184–7*
    windmill, *187*
    Adam of, 179, *814*
    Adam son of Henry of, *187*
    Adam son of Margaret of, *187*
    Birlet, widow of, *184*
    Simon of, *186*
    Thomas miller of, *187*
Egglescliffe, Ecclescliffe, Stephen of, *818*
Eggleston (co. Durham), abbey
    —, abbot of, *155*
Egle, John del, *191–2*
Egmanton (Notts.), 768
Egypt, *see* Damietta
Eldeberge (*lost*, in Brampton Bierlow), 848
Eldmire (NR), Elvetemere, 126
Eldstanbodhum, *see* Elsingbottom
Eleanor
    queen, wife of Edward I, *see* Castile
    queen, wife of Henry III, *see* Provence

Foulford, *see* Fulford
Fountains, *see also* Fontanis, Fontibus
   abbey, xxxix, 13, 22, 94, 101, 116, 120,
      133–4, 145–8, 165, 212–14, 216, 275,
      277–80, 309–10, 319, 323, 343, 347,
      360–61, 370, 373–4, 376, 382–3, 408,
      410, 412–13, 415–16, 435–6, 440, 444,
      454–5, 468, 470, 473, 492, 524–5, 579,
      738–9, *740*, 768, 871, 931–2, 934, 958–9
   —, cartulary, xlvii, lviii, lxiii, lxvii, 101,
      120, 134, 216, 278, 378, 738, 768
   —, president's book, 735
   —, abbot, 13, 133, 276, 346, 416, 442, 685,
      770, *and see* Allerton, Eston, Haget,
      John, Murdac (Henry), Reginald,
      Richard
   —, cellarer, *see* Eston
Fox, Alan, *911*
Foxholes, 721–2
   church, 571
   rector of, *see* Feriby
   Roger of (son of Adam), 463, *480–82, 487*
   —, Margaret his wife, 463, *487*
France, 54, 844, 954
   Isabella of, queen of England, wife of
      Edward II, 739, *926*, 943, 945–6
Franceys, Francigena, Frankys, Fraunceis,
      Fraunceys
   Adam, *285–6*
   John, burgher and mayor of Hedon, *673*
   Nigel, *880*
   Peter, 197, *495, 523, 618, 755–6*
   Richard, lxxi, *47–9, 288–9, 291, 294*
   William, *190,* 591, *592,* 685
   —, Maud wife of, *see* Ganton
Franchomo, *see* Freeman
Francigena, *see* Franceys
Francis, serjeant of Gilbert de Gant, *652*
Franctenant, *see* Franklin
Franfer, Franser, Fraunfer
   Richard, 167
   Thomas, *167*
Frank
   Agnes dau. of Richard, wife of Robert
      of Breary, 17
   Thomas son of Robert, 363
Frankland, William (16th cent.), 649
Franklin, Frankelaine, Frankelein, Frankeleyn,
      Franctenant, Fraunkeleyn
   Adam, *584*
   Godfrey, 789
   Robert, *139, 451, 789, 825*
   Thomas, *173, 447–51, 456–7*
   William, 72
Frankys, *see* Franceys
Franley, *see* Farnley

Franser, *see* Franfer
Fraunceis, Fraunceys, *see* Franceys
Fraunfer, *see* Franfer
Fraunkeleyn, *see* Franklin
Freeman, Franchomo
   William (of Lotherton), *338*
   William (of North Duffield), *703*
Frettenham (Norf.), 716
Freville
   Baldwin de, 314
   —, Isabel his wife, *see* Scalers
   Roger de, 314
   —, Margaret his wife, *see* Kellythorpe
Freybergh, *see* Thrybergh
Fribi, Ralph de, *797*
Fribois, Robert de, *781*
Frickley, 214
   John, 803
Fridaythorpe, 309–10
Friseby, *see* Firsby
Frisemarays, Frisemaris(e), *see* Frismarsh
Friseton, *see* Friston
Frismarsh (*lost*, nr Patrington), Frisemarays,
      Frisemaris(e), Frismareis, Frismariss,
      1, *589*
   Osbert of (son of Walter), *589*
   Robert of, *674*
   Stephen of, *674*
   Walter of, 589
Fristona, Fristone, *see* Fryston
Frith (*unident.*), river, 816
Frithebi, *see* Firby
Frizinghall, 959
Fryston, Friseton, Fristonia
   church, 214
   fee, 215
   rector of, *see* Feugers, Waleys (Robert)
   serjeant of, *see* William (son of Fulk)
   John of, 129, 212–13
   Robert, rector of Heaulagh, 738
   William of, 210, 212–13, *307*
   —, Alice Haget dau. of, wife of Jordan
      de Ste-Marie, *see* Haget
   William of, parson of Healaugh, 216
Fryston, Ferry, *see* Ferry
Fryston, Monk, 246
Fryston, Water, Fristone, 213 14
Fublet, William de, 761
Fugerol, William de, 234
Fulford, Gate and Water, Foulford, Fuleford,
      Fulefort, Fulfurthe, 12, *637*, 706, 707,
      758, *924*
   John of, *589*, 707
   Richard of, *708–9*
   Thomas of, clerk, *707–9*

Grawelleflat(h), see Crawelflat
Gray, Grey
  Hawise de, 73, 531
  Isolda de, 79
  John, 172
  John de, bishop of Norwich, 412, 417
  Richard, 462
  —, Isabel his wife, 462
  Robert de (archbishop's brother), 79, 521, 531
  Robert de (later 13th cent.), 73, 172
  Robert de, rector of Campsall, 163, 164
  Walter de, archbishop of York, 73, 79, 130, 149, 201, 213, 263, 276, 284, 391, 393, 446, 455, 462, 521, 531–2, 841, 844
  —, chancellor of, see Boville
  —, clerk of, see Bocland
  —, steward of, see Boyville, Rivere, Widdington
  Walter de (archbishop's nephew), 437, 521, 531
Graynesby, see Grainsby
Grayrigg (Westm.), Grarig, Crarig, 151, 152
  William son of Swain of, 32–3
  —, Ascelot or Ascilia his wife, 32–3, cf. Bramhope (Ascelot)
Grayve, see Grave
Greasbrough, Gresbroc, Gresbroke, Gresebroch, Gresebrock, Greseby, Gressebroc, 1, 88, 106, 112, 209, 217–24, 226–33
  Barbot Hall in, q.v.
  millpond, 217–18
  'old vill', 230
  Adam of, chaplain, 217, 219, 222–3, 226, 228, 232–3, see also Adam (priest)
  Ailsi of, 231–2
  Erneis of, 223
  Geoffrey son of Swain of, 228
  Godric of, 228
  Henry of, 229
  Hermer, Heremer of, 231–2
  Hugh son of Goding of, 219, 225
  Hugh son of Helewise of, 225
  Mabel of, 230–31
  Ohkil, Othkil of, 219, 222, 233
  Peter of, 227
  Richard smith of, 232
  Robert son of Peter of, 217
  Roger of, 223
  Roger son of Moses of, 233
  Swain smith of, 219, 225, 230–31, 233
  Walter of, 227
Greatham (Durham), hospital, master of, see Scrope
Green, Grene (in South Kirkby ?), 1, 241

Green (de Viridi)
  Jordan de la, 390–91
  Simon de la, 388
Greenfield, William, master, canon of York, dean of Chichester, archbishop of York, 84, 601, 941
  —, his register, 85
Greenford, John de, bishop of Chichester, 438, 679
Greenogue (co. Meath), 54
Greenthwaite (nr Sutton on the Forest), Grenetwhaitt, 924
Greenway, Greneway, Robert, 493
Greenwood, see Grenewode
Greetwell (Lincs.), 106–7, 112–13
  church, 107
Greg, William, 860
Gregory
  clerk (of St Leonard's ?), 897
  master, canon of York, 427, 777, 934
  prior of Bridlington, 752
  son of Arnald, 646
Gregory, Thomas son of Nicholas, 637
Greindorge, Grein de Ekge, see Graindeorge
Grendal', Walter de, 594, see also Kirby (Grindalythe)
Grene, see Green
Grene in Balne, see Balne
Grenetwhaitt, see Greenthwaite
Greneway, see Greenway
Grenewode, John, bailiff and coroner of the liberty of St Leonard, 569
Grent, Geoffrey, 894
Grenville, George Nugent-Temple-, marquess of Buckingham, lxviii
Gresbroc, Gresbroke, Gresebroch, Gresebrock, Greseby, Gressebroc, see Greasbrough
Gressenay, Agnes de, 871
Gresshop, Greshop, Robert de, squire of master of St Leonard's, 615, 628
Greta dau. of Hagen, 580
Grewelthorpe, alias Thorpe (Malzeard), alias Thorp in Kirkebysiria, 416–17, 768
Grey, see Gray
Greynesby, Greygnesby, see Grainsby
Greystoke
  fee, 638, 640, 644
  Ranulf son of Walter of, 638
  Thomas of, 588
  Thomas son of William of, 638
  William of, 588
Gribthorpe, 54
Grimbald
  knight, 153
  Joseph, 665–6, 668

Loscoe, 311

Lotherton, Lotrington, Luter(incton),
    Luterington, Luteryngton,
    Lutringthona, Lutrington,
    Lutterington, 239, *338*, *552–3*
  mill, *190–92*
  priest of, *see* Gerard
  Henry of, *190*
  Hugh of, *190*
  Ivo of, *549*
  Jordan of, *190*
  Richard of, *254, 272, 285–6, 451, 547, 549,*
    *552, 558, 560, 825*
  Robert of, *190, 555–6*
  Thomas of, *549*
  William son of John of, *795*
  William son of Jordan of, *796*
  William son of Walter of, *552*
  —, William his brother, *552*

Lounesdale, *see* Lonsdale

Louth, Luda
  Gilbert of, *717*
  Jeremy of, *625*
  Nicholas, *717*
  Robert of, *458–60*

Louth Park (Lincs.), Parcum de Luue, Luwe,
  abbey, 212, 884, *886, 888–9, 892*
  —, abbot, *see* John

Louthorp, *see* Lowthorpe

Louvain, Loven, Luvayn
  Henry de, *579–80*
  Jocelin de, *579—81, 733, 735, 873*
  —, Agnes his wife, *see* Percy
  —, his steward, *see* Percy (Geoffrey)
  John, *64*

Louweder, Lowther, Richard de, *161*

Lovel, Luuel, Luvel
  family, 531
  Adam, *775–6, 874*
  Peter, *176, 351*
  Robert, *348, 741*
  Roger, master, king's clerk, 506

Loven, *see* Louvain

Loversall, 8, 360, 803, 878–9
  chapel, 160

Lovetot, *see* Luvetot

Lowcock, Lucok, Luuecoc, Luuekoc
  John (of Fairburn), *61–4*
  John (of Haddlesey), *185*
  Richard, *811–12*

Lowdham (Notts.), Ludeham
  Eustace of, undersheriff of Yorks, 347, *865*
  Walter of, steward of Pontefract, 965

Lowther, *see* Louweder

Lowthorpe, Louthorp, 655, *656*
  church, 655

mill, 655
  rector of, *see* Heslerton (Robert)
  Cecily of, wife of Robert Heslerton,
    654–5
  Margery of, wife of John Heslerton,
    654–5
  Thomas of, 654–5
  Walter of, *653*

Loxley (in Plumpton), Loxlay, Loxleia, 358,
  *421, 429*

Lu, William le, *163*

Lucius III, pope, 151, 960

Lucok, *see* Lowcock

Lucy
  Geoffrey de, 110–11
  Reginald de, 373
  —, Amabel his wife, *see* Rumilly
  Thomas, 665

Luda, *see* Louth

Ludeham, *see* Lowdham

Luel, Peter, *321*

Lugwardine, rector of, 943–4

Luke, Lucas, *452*
  son of Richard son of Siward, *see* Hedon

Lumby, 124, 522
  Nicholas of (son of William), 124
  Robert of, *167*

Lumley (co. Durham), 710, 879
  family, 718, 752
  John, baron Lumley (16th cent.), 710, 879

Lund
  Adam de, de la, *64, 262, 815*
  Geoffrey de, 768
  Richard de la (son of William), *185–7*
  Robert de, prior of Warter, 854
  Simon de, *184*
  William de la, *186*

Lund (in Gateforth ?), 2, 178, *341*

Lund (in Hemingbrough), 341

Lund 'subtus Brek' (nr Catton ?), 784

Lund church, *later* Monk Bretton priory,
  958–9

Lund-on-Wold (nr Lockington), *711*, 716–17,
  739
  rector of, *see* Arnhale

Lundres, *see* London

Lune, river, Lon, *152–3, 354*

Lune or Luve, Robert de, *605*

Lung, Thomas le, *627*

Lungboys, Lungthois, William, *253–4*

Lungespee, *see* Longespee

Lungvillers, *see* Longvillers

Lupset, 809

Lupus, Robert, constable of Knaresborough,
  149

clerk of Peter dean of Wakefield, *247*
cook (of Kippax), *184*
cook (of Ribston), 417
deacon (12th cent., of St Leonard's ?), *205*
deacon (13th cent.), *495*
Domesday tenant, 258
earl of Westmorland, *see* Neville
falconer, *see* Falconer
forester of Bramhope, *39, 792*
'of the hospital' (*de hospitali*), *see* Hospital
marshall, 79
master of St Leonard's, *see* Nottingham
parson of Helmsley, *208, 422–3, 425–6,*
  *522–3, 669,* 731
parson of Kirkleatham (*Lium*), 268
physician, *89–90*
priest of Bir', *184*
priest or chaplain of Burnus
  (Kirkburn ?), *321, 478, 580, 588*
priest of Duckmanton, 77
priest of Ravenfield, *399*
priest (12th cent., of St Leonard's ?),
  *551, 581, 701, 722, 752, 765, 786, and see*
  Ralph (chaplain)
prior of Blyth, 59
prior of Nostell, 117
rector of Newton-on-Ouse, *see*
  Geddington
rural dean of Craven, 872
sheriff of Hedon, 664
smith (of Leathley), *281, 290*
steward, *see* Cridling
brother of Baldwin, *see* Bramhope
brother of Robert priest (mid 12th
  cent.), *602–3*
great-grandfather of Richard Malebisse,
  655
son of Aldelin, 145
son of Baldwin, *see* Bramhope
son of Geoffrey, *515*
son of Gunnild, *221–2*
son of Hugh (of Doncaster), 161
son of Hugh (of Ribston), 417–18, 504
son of Hugh (of Sutton), 132
son of Juetta, carpenter of Brampton, 49
son of Lews, *224*
son of Mauger, *893*
son of Nicholas, *see* Cridling
son of Pain (clerk of Doncaster ?),
  159–60, *847*
son of Ralph (of Grimthorpe ?), *269,*
  *360, 724*
son of Reginald, serjeant of Scoter, *819*
son of Robert son of Pain, *see* Wilsic
son of Roger, 382
son of Syre, *see* Everthorpe

son of Thurstan, 894
son of Toke, *193*
son of Walter, *25–7*
son of Warin, 626
son of William, *572*
son of Wimund, *304,* 308, *312–14, 320–22,*
  *729, 859*
—, his fee, *314*
—, his brothers, *see* Peter, Robert
—, his sons, *see* Kellythorpe (Thomas),
  Leon
Rambold, *227*
Ramkil, *see* Ranchil
Ramkille, John, *732*
Rampan, Hugh de, *858*
Ramsden, William (16th cent.), 373, 463
Ramsey abbey (Hunts.), *729*
Ramsholme (Pollington), 182
Ranchil, Ramkil, Ranchel, *alias* Ranchil of
  Coney Street, *431, 551, 563*
Ranchil, son of, *see* Thomas
Ranchil, *see also* Ramkille
Rand, William, *287*
Randulf, Randolf
  son of Ingram, sheriff of Nottingham,
    119
  son of Randulf, 116
Randulf
  Geoffrey, *658*
  Richard (13th cent.), *573*
  Richard (14th cent.), *658*
Ranes (*unident.*), 418
Ranington, *see* Rainton
Ranson, John (17th cent.), keeper of records
  in St Mary's tower, xlv, lii, lviii
Ranulf
  (of North Cave), *690–92*
  brother-chaplain or brother-priest of St
    Leonard's, *553, 872, 898*
  chaplain of Saxton, *553, and see* Saxton
    (Ranulf)
  clerk, *664*
  clerk of Brignall, *736*
  clerk (of Swaythorpe), *753, 756*
  deacon, *553*
  earl of Chester, 106–8, *609*
  priest, *549, and see* Elsingbottom
  priest, son of, *see* Hugh
  reeve (of Heslington), *617–19, and see*
    Heslington
  sheriff of Holderness, 664
  son of Henry, 897
  son of Robert, 12
  son of Simon, *777*
  son of Walter, *see* Greystoke

Richmond, honour of, 380, 408, 492,
    596–600, 603, 708, 765, 896
  extent of, 747
  sheriffs of, *see* Valognes, Wigan
Richmond, 721
  abbey of St Agatha, *see* Easby
  castle, *925*
  castle guard, 599
  earl of, 599, 601, *and see* Alan, Britannia,
    Conan, Geoffrey
  — of, *198*
  Osbert of, *247*
Richmondshire, xliv, *907, 911, 922–3*
Ricstorp (*lost berewick of* Hunmanby), 649
Rictun, *see* Reighton
Rida, Rid'
  Arnulf de, *186*
  Gilbert de, *186*
  William kinsman of Adam de, *588*
Ridale, *see* Ryedale
Ridel
  Geoffrey, 846
  Geoffrey, bishop of Ely, 128
Riding, William del, *170*
Ridrefeld, Nicholas de, *399*
Ridware, Redewale, Ridwale, Ridewal
  family (of Hamstall Ridware, Staffs.), 212
  Adam of, 210–12
  Nicholas of, 211
  —, — his supposed wife, dau. of Isolda
    de Ste-Marie, 211
  Thomas, 84, 212
Rie, *see* Ryther
Rievaulx, abbey, xxxix, 107–8, 126, 128–9,
    159, 312, 645, 718
Rievill, *see* Riville
Rigsby, Gilbert of, knt, 89
Rigton, 10, 277–9, 416, 524
  mill, 278–9
Rigura, Peter, *385*
Rigwood, Rigwde, *see* Ringwood
Rilleston, *see* Rylstone
Rillington, 593, 877
  John of, 438
Rimington, 10, 129, 132, 255–6, 277–9, 524
  Ellis of (son of Walter), *256*
  Philip of, 279
  Walter son of Philip of, 279
Ringwood (Greasbrough), Rigwde, Rigwood,
    Ringwde, *217, 227, 231–2, 233*
  Gilbert of, *217, 227*
Riparia, Ripairis, Ripariis, *see* Rivere
Ripley, Rippel(eia), 149, 283, 363, 376, 382–3,
    412–13, 454
  church, 133, 382–3
  mill, 382

clerk of, *see* Bernard
Avice dau. of Bernard of, 383
Bernard of, *see* Bernard (clerk)
Richard of (son of Norman), 358, 382–3
Robert of (son of Bernard), 382–3
Robert son of Huckeman of, *see* Robert
William of, *184*
William I of (son of Richard), 383
William II of (son of William I), 383
Riplingham, William of, *687*
Ripon, 77, 145–6, *912*
  collegiate church, prebend in, *see*
    Monkton
  —, canon of, 941, 952
  hospital of Blessed Mary Magdalene,
    master of, *see* Malton
  liberty, 477
  bailiff, *see* Bellewe (Stephen), Daiville
    (Peter), Stapleton, Tocotes, Warin
  Bernard son of Gamel of, *145*
  Osbert of, chaplain or vicar of St Wilfred,
    Ripon, *145*
  Peter of, *329*
  Robert of, *604*
  Roger son of Osbert or Osbern of, *145*
Rippel(eia), *see* Ripley
Riston (Long), Ristun, Ryston, 2, 742–7, *748,*
    772
  church, 744
  windmill, 747
Rithe, Rither, *see* Ryther
Rivallis, Peter de, keeper of Knaresborough,
    149
Rivel, William, 280
Rivere, Ripairis, Riparia, Ripariis
  Henry de la, 430
  John de la, 886
  —, Isabel his wife, *see* Hook
  Nicholas de la, 431
  Richard I de la, knt, 430–31
  Richard II de la, 431
  Richard III de la, 431
  Robert de la, steward of archbishop and
    Alice de Lacy, 8, 532, 966
  Thomas de la, 867, 869, 886
  —, Joan his wife, *see* Ughtred
  Walter de la, *430, 567*
Riville (dép. Seine-Maritime), Rievill,
    Ryvile, Ryvill, Ryvyle, 546
  family, 546
  Alexander de (12th cent.), *549, 551, 582*
  Alexander de (13th cent.), *191–2*, 305, *325,*
    *328–9, 332, 337, 484, 541, 558, 560*
  Goda de, wife of Ralph of Woodhouse,
    545–6, *560*
  Henry son of Richard de, *236–7*

127, *136*, *162*, 181, 544, *550*, *552–3*, 567,
569, *602–3*, *662*, *781*, 929–31
master of St Leonard's (13th cent.), *see*
Saham
master of schools at York Minster, *see*
Magnus
master of Swine priory, 709
miller of Lead, 305, *328*
parson of Adel, 68
parson of Leathley, *34*, *see also* Leathley
(Robert)
priest (12th cent.), 252, *641*
priest (mid 12th cent.), brother of Ralph,
*602–3*
priest of Catterick, *603*
priest of Doncaster, 159–60
priest 'of the hospital', *see* Robert (master
of St Leonard's)
prior of Bolton, 735
prior of Carlisle, 55
prior of Malton, 853
prior of Nostell, 117
prior of Warter, *see* Lund
prior of Worksop, 122
receiver of Pontefract, 965
rector of Campsall, attorney of Adam de
Neufmarché, 164
rector of Long Preston, *see* Robert (rural
dean)
rector of Manfield and rural dean of
Richmond, *51*, 52
rector of Hemingford, 845
rural dean of Craven, rector of Long
Preston, 503
rural dean of Richmond, *see* Robert
(rector of Manfield)
serjeant of St Leonard's, *220*, *326*, *760*
serjeant of Skyrack, *226*
shoemaker, *788*
smith (of Ganton), 591–2
vicar of Calverley, 393
vicar of Campsall, *163*
vicar of Thomas de Reineville, *52*
warden of St Leonard's, 930
wetherherd, *912*
brother of Adam son of Hugh, 966
son of Amary, *176*
son of Amfrey, *895*
son of Angor, *see* Angers
son of Arnold (mid 12th cent.), *641*
—, Gamel his brother, *641*
son of Arnold (early 13th cent.), 638, *646*
—, Christiana his dau., wife of John of
Millington, 638, *646*
—, Helewise his wife, 638, *646*
son of Astin, *193*

son of Bernard, *780*, *and see* Ripley
son of Copsi, 596–8, *602–5*, 634
—, his son, *see* Torfin
—, his wife, *see* Eva
son of Cristin, *259*
son of David, *857*
son of Edwin, 415
son of Elinant, *766*
son of Ernis son of Ace the moneyer, *899*
son of Eudo or Ivo, *641*
son of Fulk, 127, 132–3, *675*, *723–4*, 733,
735
son of Gamel, *641*, *822*, *824*, *862*
son of Geoffrey, *364*, *646*, *895*
son of Gerbod (of Braithwell), 159, *804*
son of Gilbert, *493*, *and see* Stockeld
son of Golle, *602*
son of Huckeman, forester, of Ripley,
412–13
—, his sister, *see* Avice
—, his sisters Sigerith and Agnes, 413
—, his nephews Hugh and Thomas, 413
son of Huckeman, *see* Plumpton
son of Hugh, 79, *207*, *282*, *299*, *303*, 785
—, Robert son of, *299*, *303*
son of Hugh son of Ypolitus, *see*
Middleton (in Wharfedale)
son of Ingram, *814*
son of John, *283*
son of John (of Woolthwaite), *536*
son of Jollan or Joldan, *392*, *395–6*
son of Jordan, *see* Bugthorpe
son of Ketel, *145*
son of Langus, *701*
son of Mauger, *895*
son of Meudre, 608
son of Muriel, *see* Burton
son of Oren, *785*
son of Osbert (of Ripon ?), *145*
son of Pain, 159, 161, *398–9*, 527, 800,
*802–5*, 841, *847*
—, Godit wife of, *see* Wilsic
son of Paulinus, *see* Pool
son of Peter, *384*, *810*
son of Ralph, *89–90*, *and see* Middleham
son of Ralph the smith, *912*
son of Randulf, 182
son of Raynald (of Ribston), 404
son of Richard, *231*, *427*, *510–11*
son of Richard (of Croxton), 76
son of Robert (mid 12th cent.), *603*
son of Robert (of Ribston), 432
son of Robert son of Fulk, steward of
William de Percy, 127–8, 309, 407
—, Alice his mother, *see* St-Quintin
son of Robert son of Harding, 474, *961*

4, 433, 435–7, 445–61, 819–24, 915, 920,
924
church of All Saints, 433, 435–6, 820, 821,
822, 823, 825, 906, 922, 925; altar of St
Katherine, 433
grange, 343
clerk of, see Adam, Rufforth (Ellis)
rector of, see Rufforth (Ellis)
family, 234
Adam of, 452–4, 456, 460, 825, and see
Adam (clerk)
Alan of, master, alias Alan Bretton (q.v.),
alias Alan of Bugthorpe (son of
Geoffrey I), 433–4, 436–7, 455–6, 936
Ellen or Eleanor or Helen of, wife of
Geoffrey of Rufforth and Simon de
Halton, 343, 433–7, 445–51, 454, 456–8,
461, 819–20, 822, 824; her seal, 824
Ellis of, rector of Rufforth, clerk, 434–6,
452, 823
Fulk of, 75, 130, 234, 413, 433–6, 441, 443,
445, 447, 452, 458–61, 785, 819–25
Geoffrey I of, knt, alias Geoffrey Bretton,
alias Geoffrey II of Bugthorpe,
129–30, 172–3, 343–4, 352, 366, 376,
422–3, 426, 433–7, 439, 443, 445–54,
456–60, 513, 577, 704, 819, 822, 824–5,
865, 882
—, Ellen his wife, see Rufforth (Ellen)
—, Jordan his son, see Bugthorpe
Geoffrey II of (son of Geoffrey I), 434,
437, 451
John of (unident.), 452
John of (brother of Fulk), 434–6, 452–3,
461, 825
John son of Adam of, 449
John of (son of Fulk), 434, 436, 447
John of (son of William brother of Fulk),
434, 436
Jordan son of Geoffrey of, see Bugthorpe
Ralph of, 435
Robert of (son of Fulk), 434, 436
W. of (son of Geoffrey I ?), 434, 436
William of (12th cent.), steward of Roger
de Flamville, 434–5, 549
William of (brother of Fulk), 434, 436,
823
William of (son of Fulk), 75, 434, 436
Rufus, Ruffus
Baldwin, 748
Geoffrey, bishop of Durham, 606
Henry son of Walter, 415
Peter, 70
Ralph, 9
Reginald, 701
Simon, 698, and see Follifoot

Swain, 195
William, 897–8
William, brother of St Leonard's, 585
Rugford, Rugheford, Rughford, see Rufforth
Rugherthorn, see Rowthorne
Rughmares, Ruhemares, see Rawmarsh
Rugley (nr Alnwick), 317
Rugthorp, Ruhthorp, see Thorpe le Street
Ruhal(a), see Roall
Ruhcford, Ruhford, see Rufforth
Rumilly
Alice de, wife of William son of Duncan,
837, 960
Alice de (d. c.1215), 664
Amabel de, wife of Reginald de Lucy, 664
Amice or Avice de, wife of William de
Curcy II, 251
Cecily de, wife of William earl of
Aumale, 664, 674
Cecily de, wife of William Meschin, 251,
837
Robert de, 251
Runcie, Runcin, Runsi, Jordan son of
Robert of, 10, 21, 45
Rupe, see Roche
Rupella, see Rochelle
Ruppehale, Ruppe Halenay, Tupehale, Joel,
28–9
Russell, Rossel, Rushill
family, 58
Alan, in error for Alexander, 64
Alexander, 63–4
Geoffrey, steward of Edmund earl of
Cornwall, knt, 150
John (of Naburn), 616–17, cf. Naburn
(John)
Robert, 58
Roger son of William, 697, 699–700
Walter, 703
William, 698
William (of Azerley), 101
William (de Feria), 260
—, Alice his wife, 260
William (of Normanton), 466, 468
—, Emma his wife, see Peitevin
Ruston, 720
Ruston Parva, Rouston, 720
Ruswick, 380
Rutepel (unident.), 841
Ruthorp, see Thorpe le Street
Rutland, 716
Rutter, Ruttur, Robert, 64
Rybbestaine, Rybbesteine, Rybstayne, see
Ribston
Rye, see Ryther
Ryedale, Ridale, Rydale, 906, 915, 932

Gundreda de, 720
Herbert de, 720–22
—, Agnes his wife, 722
Idonea de, 120, 211
Robert de, 119–20, 210–11
—, Aubrey his wife, see Chevercourt
William de, 720–22
William son of Anthony de (15th cent.),
    722
St-Samson (de Sancto Sampsone), Nicholas de,
    priest, 203
St-Sauveur (de Sancto Salvatore)
Robert de, chaplain, 323
Thomas de, chaplain of St Leonard's, 824
Ste-Barbe (de Sancta Barbara)
W. de, chaplain, 323
William de, dean of York, bishop of
    Durham, 661–2, 859
Ste-Colombe (de Sancta Columba), Ralph de,
    canon of York, 661–2
Ste-Marie (de Sancta Maria)
family, 209
Adam de, 81, 119, 210–12, 215–16, 219,
    229–30, 233, 491, 841
—, Alice his wife, 210–11
—, Aubrey his wife, see Chevercourt
Agatha de, 210, 215
Bartholemew de, 210–11
Elizabeth de, supposed sister of Jordan,
    216
Elizabeth de, wife of Henry Waleys, 210,
    212
Isolda de, wife of Adam of Ridware,
    210–12
—, — her dau., supposed wife of
    Nicholas of Ridware, 211
Jordan de, 115, 180, 210–16, 219, 230, 233,
    274, 441, 469, 561, 841
—, Alice his wife, see Haget
Katherine de, wife of — Braithwell, 210,
    215
Lucy de, wife of Reginald of Annesley,
    210–12
Nicholas de, 210, 212, 215, 219, 222, 225–6,
    229–30, 232, 491, 798, 841
—, Ragenild, Rahenild, his wife, 219, 233
Nicola de, wife of Robert of Cockfield,
    210, 212, 214–16
Pain de, 209–13, 215–16
Ragenild de, wife of Richard Bretel, 210,
    215
Richard de, 210, 213–14, 216
Sybil de, wife of Adam of Crigglestone,
    210, 212–13, 215–16
Sybil de, wife of Jordan de Reineville, 78,
    80–81, 210–12, 491

William de, rector of Healaugh, 216
Ste-Mère-Église, William, rector of
    Harewood, bishop of London, 68, 961,
    and cf. William (parson of Harewood)
Saintelai, see St-Éloi
Sakespye, Henry, 216
Salceto, see Saucey
Sale Wyyeton, Henry de la, 369
Salicosa Mara, Salcusemare, see Saucusemare
Salisbury
bishopric of, 941
bishop of, see Waltham
Salisbury, archdeacon of, see Eure
Salisbury
cathedral, prebends in, 939, 946, 951,
    and see Faringdon, Graham Borealis,
    Stratton
—, canons of, see Ispania, Walwayn
—, dean of, see Oxford
earls of, see Longespee, Neville, Salisbury
    (Patrick)
Patrick of, earl of Salisbury, 639
Sallay, Sawley
abbey, xxxix, 132, 255, 273, 275–6, 278,
    357, 407, 501–3, 581, 871, 962
—, cartulary, 503
—, abbots, see Brewer, Eston, Geoffrey,
    Richard, Walter
Acreland in, 957
Salmonby, Salmandreby, Salmundby,
    Salmundeby, William of, 347, 450–51,
    454
—, Margery his wife, see Tuschet
Salsemare, see Saucusemare
Salso Marisco, Salsomarisco, see Saltmarsh
Salter, Alan, 674
Saltmarsh (de Salso Marisco), Elvard de,
    891
Saluzzo, Boniface de, rector of Tickhill
    chapel, 844–5
Salvage, Ralph, 323, cf. Savage
Salvain, Salvayn, Salvein, Salvey, Selveyn
Anketin, knt, 868
—, Isolda his wife, 868
Geoffrey, 789
Gerard, 634, 788, 789, 879–80
John son of Gerard, 656
—, Emma his wife, 656
Osbert, 701
Ralph, 399, 530, 810
William, 675, 741, 874
Sambec, see Sandbeck
Sampson, Samson
saddler, see Saddler
son of Josce, 505
son of Toke, 701

Eneas of (son of Hugh), *alias* Eneas of
 Middleton, *271*, 356–7, 360–62, *366*,
 *370–71*
—, his wife, *see* Avice
—, Robert his brother, *see* Middleton
Stubham, *in error for* Stubhus, *289*
Stubhus
 Geoffrey de, *253*
 Henry de, 16, *253–4, 289–90, 295*
Stubhus(um), *see* Stubham
Stubley, Richard de, *367*
Studley, 101
 William son of Richard of, *101*
Studley Roger, 145
Stultus, *see* Swain
Sturdi, Hugh, *367*
Sturton-le-Steeple (Notts.), 54
Stute, Osbert, *195*
Stuteville, Estutevill, Stuttavilla
 fee, 313, 470, 578, 591
 Agnes de, *720*
 Alice de, 718
 Anselm de, 718
 Geoffrey de, *874*
 Mabel dau. of Robert de, wife of
  Richard of Bossall, *591*
 Nicholas de, 148, *696*
 Robert de, sheriff of York, 109, 148
 Robert de (d. *c.*1205, son of William),
  148, 412
 Robert de (mid 13th cent.), *363*, 866
 Roger de, knt, *720*
 William de, justice, 69, 93–5, 133–4, 148,
  234, 267, 373, 408, 412–13, *510–11*
Stutton, 275, 279, 462, 607
 William of, *337*
Styketon, John de, 419
Styrrup (Notts.), Stirapa, 53–7, 106–7
 windmill, 53
 Alice of (dau. of Ranulf), *alias* Alice of
  Oldcotes'), 53–7
—, Ingram her son, *see* Styrrup (Ingram)
—, John her son, *see* Clowne
—, Maud her dau., wife of Bartholomew
  de Overton, 55
—, Philip her son, 55
—, Robert her son, *see* Blyth
 Gerard of (son of Ranulf), *alias* Gerard of
  Oldcotes, 53–5, 57, 59, 527, 804
—, his wife, *see* Maud (dau. of Ingram)
 Ingram of (son of Alice), 53, 55–6
—, Denise his wife, 56
—, Richard his son, *see* Mattersey
 John son of Ingram of, 56
 John of (son of Robert), 53
 Norman of (son of Alfred of Barnby), 54

Ranulf or Randulf of, 53
Richard (son of William), 56
Robert of (son of Ranulf, brother of
 Gerard), 53, *59*
Simon son of Ingram of, 56
William of (son of Richard of
 Mattersey), 56
Styvelyngflet, *see* Stillingfleet
Styvethon, *see* Stiveton
Suala, *see* Swale
Sualedala, *see* Swaledale
Suart, Robert, *725*
Suatorp, Suauethorp, *see* Swaythorpe
Suell, *see* Southwell
Suffolk, 123
 archdeacon of, *see* Wynter
Suhtdigton, -dightona, *see* Deighton
Suinish, *see* Swineshead
Suintona, *see* Swinton
Sully, Henry de, nephew of King Stephen, 5
Sumenur
 Roger le, *881*, 882
 Thomas le, *881–2*
Sumerville, Somervile, Summervilla
 Roger, 655
 William de, *162, 307*, 877
Summerscales (Beamsley), 269
Sunderland, Richard (17th cent.), 278
Sunderlandwick, 714
 Adam son of Arnald of, 774
Suply, Henry, *see* Copsi
Surdeval
 Richard de, 47
 William de, *see* William
Surrais, Godwin, *218*
Surrey, earl of, *see* Warenne
Sussex, sheriff of, *see* Hay (Roger)
Suthcava, *see* Cave (South)
Suthkirkeby, Sutkirkebi, *see* Kirkby (South)
Sutor (shoemaker)
 Henry (of Leathley), *281, 287, 290*
 Jordan (of Leathley), *296*
 *see also* Robert
Sutors Road, *see* Hedon
Sutthull, *see* Stockeld
Sutton (*unident.*)
 John of, *628*
 Margery, *843*
 Oliver of, parson of Harewood, bishop of
  Lincoln, 68
 Roger of, *241*
 Thomas, *241, 637, 926*
 William of, heir of Gilbert of Saxton, 305
Sutton (nr Byram), 132
 Adam of, *61–2*
 John of, *61–2*

Tadcaster, *3*, 408, 501, 505–6, 581, 686, *840*
    church, 275–6
    rectors or priests of, *see* Arnald, Leathley
        (Robert), Nicholas, Paulinus
    vicar of, *see* Saxton (Roger)
    Jordan of, marshall, *549*
Tagun, *see* Tacun
Tailor, Taillur, Tailur, *see* Taylor
Takel, Ralph, 398, *400*
    Simon son of Ralph, 398
Talemunt, Thalemunt
    Benedict de, *763*
    *cf.* Thalamo
Talliator, *see* Taylor
Talun, Talon
    John, *668*
    Robert, 718, 752
    Stephen, *695*, *857*
    Walter, 679, *701*
    William, *691–2*, *698*
    William son of Godfrey, 774
Tamworth (Staffs.), chapel, prebend in, 948
Tanay, Tanet, — de, wife of — de Cressy,
        58, 109
    Avice de, wife of William de Clairfait, 58,
        106–8, 220, 247
    Luke de, steward of Knaresborough,
        149
    William de, 58, 106–7
Tanfield, 599
    Avice of, wife of Robert Marmion,
        598–600
    Hugh II of (d. *c.*1203, son of Jernegan II),
        382, 598–9
    —, his wife, *see* Maud (dau. of Torfin)
    Jernegan II of (d. 1182, son of Hugh I),
        382
    Jernegan III of (d. *c.*1214, son of
        Hugh II), 598–9
    Roger of (son of Jernegan II), 382
Tang(a), Tange, Tanghe, *see* Tong
Tankersley, 319
    church, 317
    manor, 318
    Alice, dau. of Richard, knt, wife of
        Richard Tyas, 317–19
    Henry of, knt, 477
    —, Agnes, his wife, *see* Peitevin
    Joan, dau. of Richard, knt, wife of Sir
        Hugh Elland, 319
    Richard of, 477
Tanner, Ellis son of Richard, 386, *397*
Tattersall, Robert of, 380, 649
Taunton, William of, 514
Tautona, *see* Towton
Taverner, Ellis, *167*

Taylor, Cissore, Scissore, Talliator, Taillur,
        Tailor, Tailur
    Adam, 443
    —, Isolda his wife, 443
    Hugh, *371*
    John, *150*, *343–4*, *448*, *456*, *823*
    Reginald (of Doncaster), *161*, *165*
    Reginald, bailiff of York, 130
    Simon, *173*
    *see also* Arnald, Godfrey
Tempest, Roger, *728*
Templar, William, *329*
Templars, lxviii, 105, 138, 169, 178–82, 184,
        274, 276, 278, *307*, 355, 362, 367, 388,
        404, 431, 569, 580, 598, 603, 616, 706,
        747, 754, 769, 773, 776, 939, 941
    deeds of, 307
    extent of lands, 104, 169, 431, 960
    brother of, *see* Hastings
    master in England, 569, *and see* Berard,
        St-Maur, Saunford
    master in Yorkshire, *see* Halton (Robert)
Tenneslowe, *see* Tinsley
Tenterer, Teynterer, Nicholas, *371*
Terrington, 720, 868
    church, 940
Testard, William, archdeacon of Nottingham,
        323
Teutonicus, *see* Tyas
Textor, *see* Weaver
Teynterer, *see* Tenterer
Thalamo, Robert de, *381*, *cf.* Talemunt
Thalemunt, *see* Talemunt
Thanest', Thomas de, *575–6*
Thanghe, *see* Tong
Tharlesthorpe, Margaret dau. of Richard,
        wife of Henry du Bois, 94
Thehamtuna, *see* Trehampton
Theobald
    archbishop of Canterbury, xlii, 132, 234,
        307, 517, 542, 569, 596, 604, 687, 701,
        710, 767, 958
    brother of St Leonard's, *22*, *898*
    chaplain, *603*
    clerk, *644*
    —, Murdac his brother, *644*
    lorimer, *see* Lorimer
    prior of Blyth, 56
    son of Pain, 583
Theweng, *see* Thwing
Thicket, 681, 683, 686
    priory of St Mary, xl, 680–81, 683–6
    —, prioress, *see* Eva, Joan
Thickley, East (co. Durham), *formerly*
        Thickley Punchardon, 606
Thilem', *see* Tillmire

St Mary Magdalene, friary, 82
York, St Peter's or St Leonard's hospital of
advowson of, 929
altars, St Edmund, 138, *141*, *794*
—, St Katherine, 433, 821
—, St Leonard, *9*, *459*
archive, xliii–xlvii
cartulary, xlv–lxiii
chapel (of St Margaret), *173*
church of St Leonard in, xlii, 138, *141*,
234, *389*; consecration of, *542*, 687, 847
court, *846*, *896*
exchequer of, *612*
hall, *143*
history, xl–xlii; *Historia fundationis*, xl–xli,
lvii, 6; 'destroyed by fire', xli
infirmary, 138, *143*, *658*, *926*
liberty of, coroner of, *see* Grenewode
(John)
—, coroner's roll, xlvii
thraves, xxxix, xli–xlii, xlviii, lvi, 91, 258,
343, 345, 659–60, 663, 749, *750*, *910*,
*915*, *923*, 931, 934, 950
York, St Peter's or St Leonard's hospital of,
personnel
auditor, *see* Lawson (George)
bailiffs, *see* Beacham (Robert), Burton
(Henry), Dyneley (Robert),
Grenewode (John), Mansel (William),
Mesnil (William), Standeven
(Thomas)
brothers, *see* Adam, Alan, Alexander,
Alfred, Ambrose, Astin, Balke
(William), Brompton (Walter), Daniel
(John), Dolfin, Exelby (William),
Gamel, Geoffrey, Heck (William),
Henry, Hervey, Humphrey, Hunton
(John), Knaptoft (Alan), Laurence,
Leomar, Nicholas, Nottingham
(Henry), Osmund, Pain, Palmer
(Walter), Ralph, Reginald, Robert,
Roger, Rufus (William), Saham
(William), Sandal (Ellis), Simon,
Siwath, Stephen, Stephen (of the
cellar), Stockton (Walter), Theobald,
Thomas, Trent (William), Udard,
Wakefield (Richard), Wigan,
William (cellarer), William (smith),
Wintringham (Walter), Yol
(Thomas)
brother-chaplains, *see* Bernard,
Collingham (Robert), Garendon
(William), Henry, John, Laurence,
Nottingham (John), Ranulf, Robert,
Roger, Stowe (Laurence), Thomas,
William

brother-knights, *see* Alan, Robert
brother-priests, *see* Pain, Ranulf, Robert
cellarers, *573*, *and see* Exelby (William),
Geddington (William), Godfrey
(lay-brother), Herbert (lay-brother),
John (lay-brother), Robert
(brother), Roger (brother), Stephen
(lay-brother), Thomas, Udard, Walter
(lay-brother), William
chaplains, *see* Acomb (Ralph), Adam,
Alexander, Aquila (William), Bowes
(Robert, William), Burton (Michael),
Ellis, Fontanis (Philip, Ralph),
Fontibus (Ralph), Fulk, Geddington
(Ralph), Geoffrey, German, Henry,
Hugh, Ingram, Lambert, Laurence,
Matthew, Michael, Nicholas, Peter,
Philip, Ralph, Richard, Robert,
Roger, St-Sauveur (Thomas), Thomas,
Walter, William
chapter, *645*, *836*, 934
clerks, *see* Adam, Alan, Berb' (Roger),
Boneville (William), Bowes (William),
Buhtton (Ralph), Cave (Henry),
Derby (Roger), Eustace, Fossard
(Richard), Garton (Richard),
Geoffrey, Gilbert, Gregory, Harpham
(John), Henry, Hugh, John, Lada
(John), Langwath (Thomas), London
(Nicholas), Myton (Hugh), Nicholas,
Nottingham (William), Paulinus,
Peter, Philip, Ralph, Reiner, Richard,
Roger, Simon, Stow (Robert),
Thomas, Walter, William
cook, *see* Alan
deacons, *see* Agmund, Bowes (William),
Cave (Henry), Fossard (Richard),
Fulk, Henry, Ralph, Robert, William
keeper, *see* warden
lay-brothers, *see* Anketin, Girard, Godfrey,
Herbert, Hugh, John, Peter, Richard,
Stephen, Swain, Tuschet (Thomas),
Walter, William, William (brother of
Godfrey)
marshall, *see* Mauger
master, *645*, 929–55, *and see* Aspall,
Baldock, Bays, Botheby, Brembre,
Clipston, Constable, Eure, Feriby,
FitzHugh, Geddington, Giffard, Hals,
Hotham, Ispania, John, Langton,
Leeds, Magnus, Malton, Neville,
Nottingham, Ravenser, Robert,
Saham, Scrope, Slake, Stapleton,
Swain, Waltham, Walwayn, William,
Wynter
—, champion of, *see* Berkeworth

Yreby, *see* Ireby
Ysaacman, *see* Isaacman

Yun, deacon of South Kirkby, *241*
Yverthorpe, *see* Everthorpe